Mental Health and Wellness in Healthcare Workers:

Identifying Risks, Prevention, and Treatment

Clint A. Bowers
University of Central Florida, USA

Deborah C. Beidel
University of Central Florida, USA

Madeline R. Marks
University of Maryland, USA

Kristin Horan
University of Central Florida, USA

Janis Cannon-Bowers
Cannon-Bowers Consulting, USA

A volume in the Advances in Psychology, Mental Health, and Behavioral Studies (APMHBS) Book Series

IGI Global
PUBLISHER of TIMELY KNOWLEDGE

Published in the United States of America by
IGI Global
Medical Information Science Reference (an imprint of IGI Global)
701 E. Chocolate Avenue
Hershey PA, USA 17033
Tel: 717-533-8845
Fax: 717-533-8661
E-mail: cust@igi-global.com
Web site: http://www.igi-global.com

Library of Congress Cataloging-in-Publication Data

Names: Bowers, Clint A., editor. | Beidel, Deborah C., editor. | Marks, Madeline R., 1990- editor. | Horan, Kristin, 1989- editor. | Cannon-Bowers, Janis A., editor.
Title: Mental health and wellness in healthcare workers : identifying risks, prevention, and treatment / Clint Bowers, Deborah Beidel, Madeline Marks, Kristin Horan, and Janis Cannon-Bowers, editors.
Description: Hershey, PA : Medical Information Science Reference, [2022] | Includes bibliographical references and index. | Summary: "This book draws attention to the emerging issue of stress-related illness in healthcare and reviews the state-of-the-art of multiple individual topics within this domain and outline the additional research that needs to be conducted to best serve this population"-- Provided by publisher.
Identifiers: LCCN 2021045856 (print) | LCCN 2021045857 (ebook) | ISBN 9781799888130 (hardcover) | ISBN 9781799888147 (ebook)
Subjects: MESH: Occupational Stress--psychology | Occupational Stress--prevention & control | Health Personnel--psychology | Health Promotion | COVID-19--psychology
Classification: LCC RC963.48 (print) | LCC RC963.48 (ebook) | NLM WA 495 | DDC 158.7/2--dc23
LC record available at https://lccn.loc.gov/2021045856
LC ebook record available at https://lccn.loc.gov/2021045857

This book is published in the IGI Global book series Advances in Psychology, Mental Health, and Behavioral Studies (APMHBS) (ISSN: 2475-6660; eISSN: 2475-6679)

British Cataloguing in Publication Data
A Cataloguing in Publication record for this book is available from the British Library.

For electronic access to this publication, please contact: eresources@igi-global.com.

Advances in Psychology, Mental Health, and Behavioral Studies (APMHBS) Book Series

Bryan Christiansen
Global Research Society, LLC, USA
Harish C. Chandan
Argosy University, USA

ISSN:2475-6660
EISSN:2475-6679

Mission

The complexity of the human mind has puzzled researchers and physicians for centuries. While widely studied, the brain still remains largely misunderstood.

The **Advances in Psychology, Mental Health, and Behavioral Studies (APMHBS)** book series presents comprehensive research publications focusing on topics relating to the human psyche, cognition, psychiatric care, mental and developmental disorders, as well as human behavior and interaction. Featuring diverse and innovative research, publications within APMHBS are ideally designed for use by mental health professionals, academicians, researchers, and upper-level students.

Coverage

- Developmental Disorders
- Counseling & Therapy
- Socialization
- Human Interaction
- Mental Health & Disorders
- Treatment & Care
- Eating Disorders
- Neurological Disorders
- Psychiatry
- Human Behavior

IGI Global is currently accepting manuscripts for publication within this series. To submit a proposal for a volume in this series, please contact our Acquisition Editors at Acquisitions@igi-global.com or visit: http://www.igi-global.com/publish/.

The Advances in Psychology, Mental Health, and Behavioral Studies (APMHBS) Book Series (ISSN 2475-6660) is published by IGI Global, 701 E. Chocolate Avenue, Hershey, PA 17033-1240, USA, www.igi-global.com. This series is composed of titles available for purchase individually; each title is edited to be contextually exclusive from any other title within the series. For pricing and ordering information please visit http://www.igi-global.com/book-series/advances-psychology-mental-health-behavioral/110200. Postmaster: Send all address changes to above address.

Titles in this Series

For a list of additional titles in this series, please visit: www.igi-global.com/book-series/advances-psychology-mental-health-behavioral/110200

Handbook of Research on Neurocognitive Development of Executive Functions and Implications for Intervention
Francisco Alcantud-Marín (University of Valencia, Spain) María Fernanda López-Ramón (University of Valencia, Spain) Esperanza Navarro-Pardo (University of Valencia, Spain) Veronica Moreno-Campos (University of Valencia, Spain) and Yurena Alonso-Esteban (University of Valencia, pain)
Medical Information Science Reference • © 2022 • 400pp • H/C (ISBN: 9781799890751) • US $345.00

Provision of Psychosocial Support and Education of Vulnerable Children
Simon George Taukeni (University of Namibia, Namibia) Joyce Mathwasa (University of Fort Hare, South Africa) and Zoleka Ntshuntshe (University of Fort Hare, South Africa)
Information Science Reference • © 2022 • 335pp • H/C (ISBN: 9781799888963) • US $195.00

Digital Therapies in Psychosocial Rehabilitation and Mental Health
António Marques (School of Health, Polytechnic Institute of Porto, Portugal) and Ricardo Queirós (Polytechnic Institute of Porto, Portugal)
Medical Information Science Reference • © 2022 • 414pp • H/C (ISBN: 9781799886341) • US $345.00

Digital Innovations for Mental Health Support
Julie Prescott (University of Bolton, UK)
Medical Information Science Reference • © 2022 • 409pp • H/C (ISBN: 9781799879916) • US $345.00

Strategies and Methods for Implementing Trauma-Informed Pedagogy
Carianne Bernadowski (Robert Morris University, USA)
Information Science Reference • © 2022 • 335pp • H/C (ISBN: 9781799874737) • US $195.00

Handbook of Research on Clinical Applications of Meditation and Mindfulness-Based Interventions in Mental Health
Sanjeev Kumar Gupta (All India Institute of Speech and Hearing, India)
Medical Information Science Reference • © 2022 • 439pp • H/C (ISBN: 9781799886822) • US $425.00

Handbook of Research on Applied Social Psychology in Multiculturalism
Bryan Christiansen (Global Research Society, LLC, USA) and Harish C. Chandan (Independent Researcher, USA)
Information Science Reference • © 2021 • 358pp • H/C (ISBN: 9781799869603) • US $235.00

IGI Global
PUBLISHER of TIMELY KNOWLEDGE

701 East Chocolate Avenue, Hershey, PA 17033, USA
Tel: 717-533-8845 x100 • Fax: 717-533-8661
E-Mail: cust@igi-global.com • www.igi-global.com

Table of Contents

Section 3
Prevention and Treatment Issues

Detailed Table of Contents

The COVID-19 pandemic has placed tremendous strain and presented unprecedented challenges for health systems and healthcare workers (HCW) across the world. Research shows that HCW on the frontline are at higher risk of burnout, anxiety, depression, and symptoms of post-traumatic stress disorder, just to name a few. Traditionally, research on mental health and HCW has predominantly focused on the generalized healthcare professional workforce. Largely missing from this conversation are immigrant HCW. This is surprising given that immigrant workers are crucially important in treating Americans fighting COVID-19 and over-represented in various healthcare occupations and States. Through an intersectionality lens, the authors identify unique factors during the COVID-19 pandemic that can impact the mental health of immigrant HCW. The authors discuss the negative attitudes towards immigrant HCW and mental health outcomes and the unique intersecting factors of race, immigrant status, and class. Recommendations for future interventions, research, and practical implications are provided.

Healthcare providers are at risk for stress-related illness (e.g., burnout, compassion fatigue, and secondary traumatic stress) due to the nature of their jobs. Healthcare providers who work in pediatrics face unique challenges compared to those who work in adult healthcare. This chapter reviews three common challenges pediatric healthcare providers face, including working with children who may die or may be facing death, managing difficult family dynamics, and responding to cases of suspected child abuse and neglect. In addition, pediatric providers face additional challenges during public health crises (e.g., natural disasters and the COVID-19 pandemic), including specific challenges related to telehealth, navigating a lack of services and mental health programs and managing adverse childhood events. Several recommendations are made throughout this chapter to assist pediatric providers with these challenges.

Interventions addressing healthcare workers' mental health should build upon an exhaustive understanding of the major causes of both work-related stress conditions (i.e., job demands) and positive mental health (i.e., job resources) in the workplace at all the levels they might unfold, namely the individual, the group, the leader, and the organization. The chapter draws upon a multilevel workplace mental health needs assessment exercise performed within three different departments of a large healthcare institution and involving both managers and employees. It aims to illustrate the job demands and resources at multiple levels in the targeted organization, differentiate among healthcare workers' mental models of their working conditions, and discuss the research and practical implications of such findings. Also, it offers practical recommendations on how to effectively conduct such activities by, on the one hand, considering both healthcare workers' mental health risk and protective factors and, on the other hand, encompassing multiple workplace levels of analysis.

The purpose of this chapter is to explore a model of health-oriented leadership in which healthcare leaders' attitudes and cognitions precipitate their health-oriented leadership behaviors and ultimately impact frontline healthcare workers' health and well-being. To better understand these relationships, this chapter will explore this model at different levels of specificity of leadership including general (e.g., transformational), specific (e.g., health-oriented), and targeted (e.g., sleep). The authors separately examine the ways in which healthcare leaders' health-oriented attitudes, cognitions, and behaviors can impact followers' health and well-being. In doing so, they highlight that internal antecedents (e.g., attitudes and cognitions) are necessary precursors for effective health-oriented leadership behaviors. Then they provide recommendations for research and practice based on the model and the current state of the literature in order to better their understanding of health-oriented leadership while simultaneously improving the health and wellness of frontline healthcare workers.

This conceptual chapter offers a critical review of contemporary theory and research in relation to 'burnout' and 'moral injury' to consider how understandings of burnout and moral injury can be usefully applied to healthcare workers during the COVID-19 pandemic. The authors find that whilst there are significant overlaps in the conceptualisation of 'burnout' and 'moral injury', there is also significant potential in drawing on systemic understandings of moral injury originating in military literature to understand and support healthcare workers. A focus on the systemic and organisational support needed to work with moral injury in healthcare staff would reduce staff burnout, time-off, and turnover improving patient outcomes and offering economic advantages to healthcare organisations. Whilst much research has been undertaken in relation to healthcare staff burnout, this chapter offers an original contribution to knowledge by offering a conceptual account of the usefulness of systemic understandings of moral injury in healthcare settings during the COVID-19 pandemic.

Chapter 11
How the Prevalence of Work Stress Influences the Quality of Life and Performance of Hospital Employees 213
Navneesh Tyagi, Noida Institute of Engineering and Technology, India
Preeti Tyagi, ICRI, India

Recently the COVID-19 pandemic has very clearly revealed the enormous challenges and risks our healthcare workers are facing globally while working in difficult situations. They are more prone to make mistakes which can lead to harmful effects on them and their patients leading to work stress which has become a part of their daily lives. A dearth of studies has examined this concept in an organizational context as it affects an individual's life and work. This study is examining the influence of work stress on employee performance and quality of life of healthcare workers. Data collected from employees of selected hospitals with the help of a structured questionnaire were analyzed using SPSS version 23. Findings of correlation and regression analysis revealed a significant positive influence of the work stress on employee performance and quality of life.

Section 3
Prevention and Treatment Issues

Chapter 12
A Creative Intervention for Supporting the Mental Wellness of Nurses: The Ameliorative Promise of Graphic Testimonials 227
J. Blake Scott, University Central Florida, USA
Christa L Cook, University of Central Florida, USA
Nathan Holic, University of Central Florida, USA
University of Central Florida, University of Central Florida, USA
Aislinn Woody, University of Central Florida, USA

Mental health challenges are prevalent among nurses who have been on the front lines of the COVID-19 pandemic, with dangerous and demoralizing working conditions, mental health stigma, and limited mental health support contributing to such challenges. A wide range of interventions have been developed to support nurses' mental wellness therapeutically, through organizational and broader advocacy, and by educating communities and publics about nurses' experiences. Nurses have produced various forms of artistic expressions, including comics or "graphic testimonials," to document, process, and share their experiences. Yet such forms, as examples of "graphic medicine," remain a relatively untapped and unique

Preface

Mental health amongst healthcare professionals has long been recognized as a matter of importance within society. In the pre-coronavirus disease 2019 (COVID-19) pandemic world, working in healthcare brought with it the reputation as a profession known for its difficult and taxing nature. However, media coverage of the plight of healthcare professionals during the COVID-19 pandemic heightened awareness amongst researchers, practitioners, and the general public on the imperative to protect the mental health and wellness of healthcare professionals. For example, nurses reflecting on their status as "angels or heroes" of the pandemic, pointed out the World Health Organization had already slated 2020 as the 'year of nursing.' This amplification placed nurses on the frontlines and raised public awareness of the value of nurses in healthcare (Mendes et al., 2021).

The same can be said of our work for this book. Our journey in organizing this textbook began before the COVID-19 outbreak. The burden of work-related stressors was already apparent within the healthcare workforce, with examples of long-standing issues including higher injury rates, exposure to workplace violence, higher levels of burnout, and more physical and mental health challenges than the general population (National Occupational Research Agenda Healthcare and Social Assistance Council [NORA HCSA Council], 2019). The onset and duration of the pandemic reinforced the importance of the broad topic of mental health and shaped several chapters of the book. With the continuation of the pandemic into 2022, the book ostensibly took on new meaning and purpose throughout the pandemic's evolution.

It is important to note that despite increases in public awareness of the importance of frontline healthcare workers, this recognition alone was not enough to protect the mental health and wellness of healthcare professionals during the pandemic. The early stages of the COVID-19 pandemic prompted a precipitous drop in healthcare utilization for non-urgent procedures, coupled with new challenges for healthcare systems regarding urgent or emergent care. The burden placed on the healthcare system was compounded with the care of COVID-19 patients without adequate levels of personal protective equipment, therapeutics, and vaccines (Grimm, 2020). Several professionals found themselves laid off, furloughed, or redeployed to new work locations; others found themselves part of skeleton crews coping with extraordinary demands. These demands included burdensome routines, donning and doffing of available personal protective equipment, worries regarding bringing the virus home to their families, and high levels of burnout and moral distress over caring for dying patients in isolating conditions (Grimm, 2020). These conditions created an enormous and lasting burden, as evidenced by high levels of burnout, anxiety, depression, and posttraumatic stress disorder and unprecedented levels of turnover within the profession. Specifically, a meta-analysis revealed that globally, 21% of health care workers reported depression, 22% reported anxiety, and 21.5% reported posttraumatic stress disorder (PTSD) as a result of dealing with COVID-19 patients (Li et al., 2021). According to an integrative review, COVID-19 increased the mean turnover intentions of nurses and introduced a novel set of predictors of turnover, such as disease-related worry (Falatah, 2021).

Together, the historical and current challenges associated with work in the healthcare profession require action on the part of researchers, practitioners, healthcare systems, and the general public. If the moniker of "healthcare hero" is to carry any weight, then we owe it to those in these essential occupations to quickly and comprehensively address mental health and wellness.

The editors of this book represent expertise in Clinical Psychology and Industrial-Organizational Psychology. They have advocated for healthy workplaces, particularly for those in industries or occupations that are at high risk for stress, injury, or illness. Their work addresses occupational stressors ranging from routine to traumatic. This book follows our previous focus on first responders, as our goal is to reveal the mental health burden associated with stressful occupations. The editors' passion for the subject matter only deepened throughout the course of the COVID-19 pandemic. The clinicians offered no-cost therapeutic consultations for healthcare workers and the researchers among the group launched projects identifying the needs of healthcare professionals. As society moves forward into a post-pandemic reality, we must capitalize on lessons learned to address the pressing need for mental health and wellness support among healthcare professionals.

The editors are thankful to those who contributed to this book, as their work addresses topics of importance for healthcare professionals. The editors' hope is for readers to internalize the content and apply the knowledge to make meaningful changes in healthcare environments and open avenues for future research.

ORGANIZATION OF THE BOOK

The goal for the book is to create resources for therapists, managers, and researchers. Each of the three sections within this book highlight important themes facing healthcare professionals. The themes address threats to mental health and wellness, the role of healthcare organizations, and action to promote mental health and wellness. We will provide a brief description of each chapter within these sections, explaining their relevance to the purpose of this book.

Section 1: Stress in Healthcare

While employees of any industry or occupation face stressors in the workplace (American Psychological Association [APA], 2008), researchers, practitioners, and undoubtedly healthcare professionals themselves recognize that the frequency and severity of certain stressors are increased within the healthcare industry (NORA HCSA, 2019). This section covers contemporary research related to stressors at the job, organization, or even societal level that influence healthcare professionals' mental health and well-being.

The first chapters in this section highlight how the COVID-19 pandemic either introduced new stressors or exacerbated existing stressors in healthcare environments. Chapter 1, "Lived Experiences of Healthcare Professionals During COVID-19 Public Health Emergency: A Qualitative Exploration," uses an interpretive phenomenological analysis to understand the experiences of healthcare professionals during the COVID-19 pandemic. The theme of their interviews reflected both the burden of healthcare work during the COVID-19 pandemic and the process of finding meaning in this work. Chapter 2, "Perceived Stress Levels of Medical and Non-Medical Staff in the Face of COVID-19," provides the results of a descriptive study examining the perceived stress levels of medical and non-medical staff, also differentiating stress levels by employment contract type, gender, and whether or not the individual takes medication. The results are important for preventing, monitoring, and treating stress in healthcare environments. Chapter 3, "The Impact of COVID-19 on Mental Health and Well-Being of Immigrant Healthcare Workers: Intersectionality Matters," highlights the mental health risks that exist at the intersection of race, class, and immigration status for immigrant healthcare workers. In addition to describing interventions and future research possibilities focused on immigrant healthcare workers, the authors make a case for increased attention to intersectionality in healthcare research.

The remaining chapters in this section focus on the benefits of accounting for contextual details, such as the specialty area of the healthcare professional or barriers and facilitators to wellness that exist within their environment. Chapter 4, "Pediatric Healthcare Providers: Unique Challenges and Strategies to Improve Wellness," focuses on stressors faced within the pediatric specialty area, including the mentally healthy management of unique challenges such as working with terminally ill children, suspected child abuse, or difficult family dynamics. Finally, Chapter 5, "Barriers to Healthy Nutrition and Exercise Behaviors Among Healthcare Workers," discusses the workplace challenges, or barriers, that can make it more difficult to develop and implement healthy behaviors that promote wellness. The chapter concludes with a discussion of facilitators and initiatives that can help promote wellness in healthcare environments.

Section 2: Organizational Issues

For far too long, the burden of promoting physical and mental health has been assigned solely to the employee. That is, traditional intervention paradigms offer programming geared toward individual action, which ignores powerful interpersonal and environmental determinants of mental health (Martin et al., 2016). The chapters in this section illustrate the importance of an organization-focused approach to improving mental health and wellness in healthcare environments.

Chapter 6, "Prioritizing Well-Being for Healthcare Professionals," examines a trend within the healthcare industry; despite being imperative to protecting and promoting patients' health, healthcare professionals often neglect their well-being. She addresses systemic factors at the organization and societal level that contribute to this phenomenon and proposes integrative solutions. Chapter 7, "Conceptual Understanding of Providers' Responses to the Complexity of Healthcare Delivery," discusses complexity science as an important tool in healthcare environments. Complexity science recognizes the complex nature of healthcare systems and argues that stakeholders must account for the interconnected nature of each part of that system. The chapter then discusses complexity science in relation to the affective experiences of healthcare professionals and their well-being. Chapter 8, "Mentally Healthy Healthcare: Main Findings and Lessons Learned from a Needs Assessment Exercise at Multiple Workplace Levels," describes possibilities for intervention to promote mental health at the individual, team, leader, or organization level. The authors argue for interventions that address risks and protective factors across multiple levels within a healthcare environment.

Chapter 9, "Health-Oriented Leadership in Healthcare: The Role of Supervisor Attitudes, Cognitions, Behaviors," examines the role of supervisors in promoting health and well-being in healthcare employees. Their model asserts that leader cognitions, attitudes, and behaviors are important in promoting healthy outcomes among frontline workers. Chapter 10, "COVID-19 and Healthcare Staff Well-Being: Is Burnout Really a Systemic Issue of Morality?" argues for the increased use of systemic, organization-level supports that allow employees to cope with moral injury in healthy ways. Finally, Chapter 11, "How the Prevalence of Work Stress Influences the Quality of Life and Performance of Hospital Employees," describes a study examining occupational stressors, quality of life, and performance of hospital staff. The results underscore the importance of minimizing occupational stress in healthcare professionals' work lives to promote both qualities of life and performance.

Section 3: Prevention and Treatment Issues

Those interested in promoting health and safety in the workplace can adopt several approaches. Those adopting primary prevention methods provide interventions to employees who are not exhibiting any signs of poor mental health or wellness. In contrast, those adopting secondary and tertiary approaches provide intervention to employees exhibiting risk factors for illness or those diagnosed with occupational illness or injury, respectively (Quick, 1999). The chapters in this section illustrate the value of a comprehensive approach in healthcare environments, with solutions geared toward both prevention and treatment.

Chapter 12, "A Creative Intervention for Supporting the Mental Wellness of Nurses: The Ameliorative Promise of Graphic Testimonials," examines the use of graphic medicine as a novel intervention to address mental health challenges in the healthcare profession. The authors describe graphic testimonials as an intervention and outline an agenda for future research using this technique. Chapter 13, "Mindfulness-Based Approaches to Reduce Injuries Among Nurses and Nursing Aides," describes the usefulness of mindfulness-based approaches to address physical and psychological injuries in healthcare professions. The authors explore methods to improve mindfulness-based interventions by preserving the fidelity to the Eastern philosophies that gave birth to the mindfulness-based approaches and promoting more meaningful integration of East-West concepts and techniques.

Chapter 14, "Working With Medical Personnel in the Aftermath of a Mass Shooting: Lessons Learned From Nickel Mines," discusses often-overlooked occupational stressors, traumatic events, and occupational violence. This chapter focuses on steps that hospitals can take before or after a mass casualty event to best preserve the mental health of hospital staff. Finally, Chapter 15, "Team Resilience in Healthcare," summarizes the topic of team resilience in the healthcare industry. Team resilience is relevant to healthcare professionals' mental health and well-being. Work tends to be highly interdependent, and the quality of social interactions in the workplace influences well-being. Furthermore, team resilience is a collective protective factor against the stressors present in a healthcare environment.

CONCLUSION

Healthcare employees are essential to the health and wellbeing of society. Yet, systemic stressors and organizational issues promote poor quality of work-life and jeopardize these essential employees' mental health and wellness. By recognizing the stressors faced by healthcare employees, by leveraging the role (and responsibility) of organizations in promoting positive quality of work-life, and by developing comprehensive prevention and treatment solutions, stakeholders can promote the mental health and wellness of healthcare professionals and better ensure a healthy experience for employees and patients.

Kristin A. Horan
Madeline R. Marks

REFERENCES

American Psychological Association (APA). (2008). *Stress in America*. Accessed on March 12, 2022 from https://www.apa.org/news/press/releases/2008/10/stress-in-america.pdf

Falatah, R. (2021). The Impact of the Coronavirus Disease (COVID-19) Pandemic on Nurses' Turnover Intention: An Integrative Review. *Nursing Reports*, *11*(4), 787–810. doi:10.3390/nursrep11040075 PMID:34968269

Grimm, C. A. (2020). *Hospital experiences responding to the COVID-19 pandemic: Results of a national pulse survey March 23-27, 2020*. U.S. Department of Health and Human Services Office of Inspector general. Retrieved on March 12, 2022 from https://oig.hhs.gov/oei/reports/oei-06-20-00300.pdf

Li, Y., Scherer, N., Felix, L., & Kuper, H. (2021). Prevalence of depression, anxiety and post-traumatic stress disorder in health care workers during the COVID-19 pandemic: A systematic review and meta-analysis. *PLoS One*, *16*(3), e0246454. doi:10.1371/journal.pone.0246454 PMID:33690641

Martin, A., Karanika-Murray, M., Biron, C., & Sanderson, K. (2016). The psychosocial work environment, employee mental health and organizational interventions: Improving research and practice by taking a multilevel approach. *Stress and Health*, *32*(3), 201–215. doi:10.1002mi.2593 PMID:25044861

Mendes, M., Bordignon, J. S., Menegat, R. P., Schneider, D. G., Vargas, M. A. D. O., Santos, E. K. A. D., & Cunha, P. R. D. (2021). Neither angels nor heroes: Nurse speeches during the COVID-19 pandemic from a Foucauldian perspective. *Revista Brasileira de Enfermagem*, 75. PMID:34614072

National Occupational Research Agenda Healthcare and Social Assistance Council (NORA HCSA Council). (2019). *National Occupational Research Agenda for Healthcare and Social Assistance*. Retrieved on March 11, 2022 from https://www.cdc.gov/nora/councils/hcsa/pdfs/National_Occpational_Agenda_for_HCSA_February_2019-508.pdf

Quick, J. C. (1999). Occupational health psychology: The convergence of health and clinical psychology with public health and preventive medicine in an organizational context. *Professional Psychology, Research and Practice*, *30*(2), 123–128. doi:10.1037/0735-7028.30.2.123

World Health Organization. (2022). *Weekly epidemiological update on COVID-19 - 8 March 2022*. Retrieved on March 11, 2022 from https://www.who.int/publications/m/item/weekly-epidemiological-update-on-covid-19---8-march-2022

Section 1
Stress in Healthcare

Chapter 1
Lived Experiences of Healthcare Professionals During the COVID-19 Public Health Emergency:
A Qualitative Exploration

Rajbala Singh
LNM Institute of Information Technology, Jaipur, India

Anu Malik
LNM Institute of Information Technology, Jaipur, India

ABSTRACT

Against the backdrop of the COVID-19 pandemic, this study used an interpretative phenomenological analysis to explore the lived experiences of healthcare professionals (HCPs). Twenty in-depth interviews were conducted with nine physicians and 11 paramedical staff. The analysis is summarized into five superordinate themes: initial reaction, perceived challenges, existential distress, the building of support mechanisms, and growth in adversity. While the first three themes broadly reflect the difficulties encountered by HCPs while serving COVID-19 patients, the last two themes demonstrate the scope of finding meaning in work and personal growth during this unprecedented public health emergency. This study also highlights the heavy toll of the physical and psychological burdens on HCPs due to the COVID-19 health crisis. The insights gained from this study can be utilized in designing an effective intervention program to promote resilience and well-being among HCPs.

INTRODUCTION

The World Health Organization (WHO) announced the COVID-19 outbreak as a pandemic on March 11, 2020, and made an emphatic call to all the countries to take necessary actions to combat and control

DOI: 10.4018/978-1-7998-8813-0.ch001

the pandemic outbreak. India accounts for a significantly larger population density of about 1.3 billion people than other countries globally. The demographic complexity of India already has the issues of clean drinking water, poor sanitation, densely populated living conditions, access to healthcare, etc. These issues have posed a significant threat to India's mission to control Coronavirus transmission and offer effective treatment (Pal & Yadav, 2020).

The crisis of COVID-19 has reaffirmed the significance of an efficient healthcare system to bridge the gap between demand and supply. India has a mixed healthcare model consisting of government and private healthcare systems (Chokshi *et al.,* 2016). According to a report published in the *Economic Times* (Goel, 2019), WHO recommended a 1:1000 doctor-population ratio to manage health necessities effectively in any country. However, India had a 1:1445 doctor population ratio in 2019. According to Kumar and Pal (2018), India would achieve the WHO's prescribed doctor-population ratio by 2024-25 only with the intervention of government policies. In the light of these facts, it can be argued that healthcare professionals (HCPs) are facing an enormous amount of workload to manage the uncertainties resulting from the pandemic of COVID-19. The burden of the pandemic has also led to a variety of psychological issues on HCPs (Hummel *et al.,* 2021). The health and well-being of HCPs are essential as they provide sustainable health care services to the patient population.

The study investigates the lived experiences of HCPs involved in treating COVID-19 patients using an interpretive phenomenological approach (IPA). There is a dearth of in-depth studies in the Indian context examining the lived experiences of HCPs and understanding their psychological and occupational challenges in mitigating the demand. The study may contribute to the extant literature by identifying critical factors that are imperative for the mental health and efficiency of HCPs. The study also discusses significant recommendations to promote resilience and well-being.

BACKGROUND

HCPs are essential for any healthcare system. During the times of health emergencies, apart from treating the patients, it is also expected that HCPs will be involved in public health education, epidemiological surveillance, quarantine management, fever clinics, staging facility operation, and more' (Seale et al., 2009, p. 2). However, they are also the people who remain on the frontline, making themselves vulnerable to get infected (Ives et al., 2009).

The Coronavirus outbreak in the world has left the healthcare system overwhelmed. The unexpected surge of heightened workload for HCPs has posed many questions ranging from managing occupational workload to maintaining mental health amid the crisis. According to Pollock et al. (2020), HCPs are at a greater risk for developing mental health and well-being related issues that include:

...concern about exposure to the virus; personal and family needs and responsibilities; managing a different workload; lack of access to necessary tools and equipment (including personal protection equipment, PPE); feelings of guilt relating to the lack of contribution; uncertainty about the future of the workplace or employment; learning new technical skills; and adapting to a different workplace or schedule (p.8).

HCPs play a key role in managing the hardships and challenges associated with COVID-19 despite a significant mismatch between the doctor-patient ratio in India (Ghosh, 2021). Studies have reported that HCPs are at a higher risk of mental health problems during the current pandemic (Gupta et al.,

2021; Mohindra et al., 2020). Mental health issues like anxiety, depression, and occupational stress are common among Indian HCPs (Parthasarathy et al., 2021, Suryavanshi et al., 2020; Wilson *et al.,* 2020). Increased exposure, long working hours, resultant stress, and fatigue also increase the risk of infection among healthcare workers (Banerjee et al., 2020). HCPs have also witnessed several other challenges. The editorial of the Lancet (2020) mentioned that along with testing and treatment, healthcare workers also have to handle different levels of violence due to misinformation, fear, and stigma among people regarding the pandemic. Several reports of not letting HCPs stay in rented houses (Joy, 2020) and incidences of violence have also surfaced in the media (Iyengar, Jain & Vaishya, 2020; WHO, 2020).

The sudden outbreak of the Coronavirus has given very little time to prepare for this pandemic. The world is still attempting to strategize the ways of dealing with COVID-19. The health and well-being of people are essential, and besides, the well-being of those providing healthcare services is also equally important. According to Ghebreyesus (September 17, 2020), the Director-General of WHO, 'no country, hospital or clinic can keep its patients safe unless it keeps its health workers safe.' Teoh, Hassard and Cox (2020) suggest the need for organizational support for doctors regarding autonomy in decision-making, a sense of belongingness to feel valued and supported, competence to deal with challenging situations, and healthcare workers prioritizing themselves to rest and recover. Mental health problems of healthcare workers should be a priority for psychiatric interventions. Thus, in this context, the present study explores the lived experiences of HCPs during the COVID-19 crisis using a phenomenological approach.

Framework

Qualitative research is inspired by the influence of culture and appreciates the knowledge gathered from stakeholders' experiences. The phenomenological approach in qualitative research understands the meaning in experiences pertaining to the context in which these experiences are rooted. The phenomenological approach is an integrated approach of description and interpretation. The philosophy of the phenomenological approach focuses on descriptions of events, emphasizing that the interpretation is rooted in the lived experiences of individuals in those specific events.

According to Smith and Osborn, (2015), the phenomenological approach enables the researchers to examine the participant's living world experiences in detail. It aims to gauge "an individual's personal perception or account of an object or event, as opposed to an attempt to produce an objective statement of the object or event itself" (p. 53). In other words, it allows the researcher to access the "insider's perspective" in terms of personal lived accounts rather than guided by any theoretical framework (Conrad, 1987; Smith & Osborn, 2015). Since the phenomenological approach stresses understanding how individuals "perceive and make sense of things," it recommends flexible data collection techniques such as personal accounts, personal diaries in general, and semi-structured interviews. The study will employ a semi-structured interview technique for data collection.

METHOD

Participants

The sample consists of nine physicians (four females and five males) and 11 paramedical staff (seven female nursing staff, three male nursing staff, and one ward boy), who served in COVID-19 designated

Table 1. Characteristics of participants

Participant's Code	Gender	Age	Designation	Marital Status	Total Work Experience
1	Female	27	Doctor (MBBS)	Married	2 years
2	Female	29	Doctor (MBBS, perusing P.G.)	Unmarried	3 years
3	Female	36	Doctor (BAMS)	Married	4 years
4	Female	42	Doctor (BAMS)	Divorced	7 years
5	Female	56	Nurse	Married	7 years
6	Female	46	Nurse	Married	7 years
7	Female	38	Nurse	Married	10 years
8	Female	28	Nurse	Unmarried	2 years
9	Female	25	Nurse	Unmarried	2 years
10	Female	23	Nurse	Unmarried	3 years
11	Female	28	Nurse	Married	7 years
12	Male	30	Doctor (MBBS)	Unmarried	4 years
13	Male	32	Doctor (MBBS)	Separated	4 years
14	Male	31	Doctor (MBBS)	Unmarried	2 years
15	Male	32	Doctor (MBBS, pursing P.G.)	Unmarried	3 years
16	Male	31	Doctor (MBBS)	Married	4 years
17	Male	41	Pharmacist	Married	8 years
18	Male	39	Pharmacist	Married	10 years
19	Male	35	Wardboy	Unmarried	8 years
20	Male	34	Nurse	Married	4 years

wards/hospitals in the northern part of India. The average age of participants is 34 years, and the average work experience is of 4.3 years. In this sample, 11 participants are married and live with their families, whereas eight participants are unmarried and stayed in shared accommodation with their friends or colleagues. In addition, two participants are divorced/ separated and live with their extended family. Table 1 represents a detailed description of the sample characteristics:

IPA is idiographic (Smith & Osborn, 2015); therefore, there is a consensus for using a smaller sample size (Reid, Flowers & Larkin, 2005) as the analysis of larger data sets can impede in maintaining "subtle inflections of meaning" (p. 626, Collins & Nicolson, 2002).

Data Collection

The study employs a semi-structured interview method for data collection. It is one of the best-suited methods of data collection for IPA as it allows a deeper glance into the social and psychological spheres of the life of the participant. In addition, the semi-structured interviews enable a researcher to explore novel areas, in-depth details and generate rich data (Smith & Osborn, 2008).

Participants were duly informed about the aim and scope of the study. Participants' confidentiality was ensured. The interviews were scheduled as per the convenience of the participants. The data was collected between March 2021 and mid of April 2021. Interviews were conducted either face-to-face or through telephone at mutually convenient times. Purposive sampling is used for data collection guided by the maximum variation strategy (Patton, 2002). The authors conducted the interviews, who possess Ph.D. degrees and have prior experience conducting interviews. As guided by the qualitative research norms (Given, 2016), researchers have decided that data would be collected till the point of data saturation. According to Faulkner and Trotter (2017), in qualitative research, data saturation refers to a point when additional data fail to lead to new information or emergent themes. In this study, both authors conducted the interviews independently. However, after each interview, they listened to recorded interviews together on the same day and discussed their observations and reflections. The authors unanimously decided that repetitive content in the last three interviews would indicate data saturation.

During the in-person interviews, adequate safety measures and COVID-19 protocol were adhered. The in-person interviews were conducted in a quiet atmosphere without interruptions. The telephonic interviews were pre-scheduled as per the availability of the participants. Both in-person and telephonic interviews were recorded and saved in MP3 files. To maintain the anonymity, each participant was given a specific code. The interview continued from 35-55 minutes for each participant. The interviews were conducted in Hindi, as this was the primary spoken language of the participants. However, occasional use of the English language was also evident during the interview. Field notes and important observations were maintained in English. The recorded interviews were transcribed and translated into English.

Interview Outline

The semi-structured interview outline is created after consulting with the relevant literature in the concerned field and informal interaction with two HCPs. Both the authors duly discussed their observations and prepared an initial draft. The interview outline was open to modification to encompass new spheres which emerged during the interviews. It consisted of open-ended questions, beginning from broad areas of exploration then moving to sensitive topics (Smith & Osborn, 2003). It helped in good rapport building with the participants and encouraged them to share their experiences without apprehension. The following questions were broadly asked to the participants:

1. How do you feel about the current situation?
2. What is the difference between providing healthcare services before and during the COVID-19 pandemic?
3. What are your unique experiences and challenges of taking care of COVID-19 patients?
4. What support did you get to manage the current public health crisis?
5. Do you feel emotionally and physically exhausted?
6. Have you ever hesitated to work during COVID-19 and felt susceptible to COVID-19 infection?
7. What are your personal insights about the current situation?

The interviewer has engaged in subtle prompting wherever required to generate rich data. Necessary probes such as "tell me something more about it," "how did you feel about it," etc., were used to understand the depth of a concept.

Ethical Consideration and Rigor

The present study has been approved by the Institute Ethics Committee of LNM Institute of Information Technology, Jaipur. Participants' due consent was sought before data collection.

To maintain the rigor in qualitative research, bracketing is used to ensure the validity of data collection and analysis process. According to Chan, Fung and Chien (2013), bracketing advocates that researchers should lay aside their preconceived notions about phenomena understudy to understand, interpret, and analyze the participants' lived experiences in a reasonably unbiased manner. The authors remained neutral while conducting the interviews and built a good rapport with the participants. The interviewers opted for active listening and seeking clarification wherever required to maintain the collected data's authenticity and avoid researchers' biases. The authors rigorously discussed emergent themes, superordinate categories of themes, and related subthemes during the data analysis phase to arrive at a consensus.

ANALYSIS

The authors have used the IPA framework (Smith & Osborn, 2003) to analyze the data. Recorded interviews are transcribed and translated manually into the English language. The first step in the IPA analysis suggests reading the transcripts several times. Researchers independently read the transcripts carefully and repeatedly to obtain a first-hand impression of the data content. It has also allowed researchers to immerse into the data that further facilitated the search for common words, sentences, and phrases across the transcript and identified common themes at the initial level. In other words, the search for common words, sentences, and phrases has helped the researchers to condense the data.

Moreover, re-reading the transcripts and re-listening the original interviews (whenever required) allowed researchers to obtain clarity. The second step of analysis involves identifying and naming themes through the process of abstraction. Significant interaction with the data has helped in naming themes that vividly depict the participant's incidences, actions, and interactions within appropriate contexts. Authors adopted the following two ways to label themes at this stage:

- By adopting the words/ phrases reflected in the data, or
- By employing a higher level of abstraction where researchers used concise phrases reflecting a deeper psychological conceptualization of themes.

Next, the authors prepared independent lists of emergent themes. To ensure the trustworthiness of the data (Lincoln & Guba, 1985), both authors critically discussed their lists of emergent themes and prepared a comprehensive list of common themes.

The third step of analysis is known as theme clustering. The purpose of theme clustering is to put similar experiences under a meaningful category. The authors collectively and critically analyzed the connections across themes and prepared a coherent table of themes (Callary, Rathwell & Young, 2015). It is important to note here that the analysis process was not strictly sequential but cyclical. Finally, in consultation with each other, the authors prepared a table of superordinate themes by considering commonality among sub-themes and relevant short extracts reflecting participants' lived experiences to substantiate each sub-themes.

RESULTS

Five major superordinate themes emerged from the data analysis: initial reaction, existential distress, perceived challenges, the building of support mechanisms, and personal growth in adversity. The following section provides a detailed description of the results:

Theme 1: Initial Reaction

Denial and Uncertainty

Initially, when participants encountered the news of COVID-19 from different sources, they were in a state of denial that something like this could happen in India. However, when the first few cases were reported in India, they were not ready to accept that the Coronavirus could spread rapidly in India:

Participant 1: *Even the people in top administration cannot think that it would come to India. Our CMO (Chief Medical Officer) said that there is significantly less likelihood of this virus spreading in India.*
Participant 4: *When the cases started coming, we were perplexed, and everyone in the department and Government was in a panic mode.*

Participants shared that several of their personal and professional plans became uncertain due to the public health emergency of Covid-19. They had to withhold their plans, such as getting married on scheduled dates, attending family functions, deciding whether to go for higher studies, etc. They were also unsure about the timeline of executing and fulfilling their personal and professional plans in the near future due to the uncertainty caused by the COVID-19. The uncertain nature of the disease led to mental shock and panic among the HCPs. They were perplexed, and it was difficult for them to accept that now they had to deal with this crisis.

Undefined Nature of Disease and Challenges

The state of denial could not withstand long. Regulatory bodies had to accept the presence of disease after having reported COVID-19 cases across India. Regulatory bodies prepared policies, and subsequently, various measures came in force to curb the spread of the disease, including testing, tracking, and symptom-based treatment. The undefined nature of the disease has created much confusion that also led to frequent changes in the guidelines regarding testing and treatment protocols. It has further made testing and treatment of COVID-19 patients quite difficult and precarious for HCPs:

Participant 16: *It is a new illness, and there are no well-defined treatment and preventive guidelines, which makes it difficult.*
Participant 20: *Due to lack of proper information and research, we have to draw inferences from earlier pandemics.*

Initially, fever clinics were set up in the hospitals to segregate the probable COVID-19 patients based on certain symptoms or travel history in the past fortnight. It created an additional workload on HCPs.

At this stage, it was not easy for HCPs to filter out possible COVID-19 cases as individuals were pretentious about providing honest details:

Participant 14: *If a doctor is on screening duty, he/ she has to decide whether the person is Covid positive or not...patients tend to trick and bypass the screening process.*

Since it was a new disease, there was no well-defined treatment action plan, making the situation difficult for HCPs. Along with uncertainty and confusion regarding the disease, they also shared many psychological issues related to their existential statuses, such as social and emotional distancing from their friends and family, fear of getting infected, and fear of death.

Theme 2: Existential Distress

While working in the Corona ward, the majority of HCPs have reported that they feel an existential crisis for themselves and the family due to the following reasons:

Social-Emotional Distancing and Well-being Concerns

Due to the infectious nature of the disease, HCPs distanced themselves from their family members that further has led to social-emotional seclusion, feeling of helplessness, and depression at times. Participants' felt that it was even more difficult for female HCPs as many of them send their children either to grandparents or to distant relatives:

Participant 20: *I could not meet family for months...This was depressing. I have a one-and-a-half-year-old son... My wife is also worried about me as several HCPs have lost their lives.*
Participant 19: *I got separated from the family at the onset of the pandemic.*
Respondent 7: *My children are emotionally attached to me. It was difficult for us whenever I went for COVID-19 duties.*

The concern for the well-being is reciprocal as both HCPs, and their family members are facing existential crises. It was observed that the concern about well-being was two-fold: if HCPs get infected, the family cannot actively support them; and if any family member gets infected, they would not be in a condition to provide active support, unlike any other disease before the pandemic:

Participant 5: *I could not meet my daughter; she had got a liver infection during this duration, she wanted to meet me, but I could not as I was in the COVID-19 duties.*

Participants also expressed that they were tense and were going through the fear of getting infected.

Fear of infection

Participants expressed immense fear of getting infected with the unpredictable disease of COVID-19. They fear that if they got tested positive, they also had to stay in similar situations like other patients.

Participant 13: *Fear of getting infected from the patients is so high that the staff is frightened to take vital parameters of the patients.*

HCPs shared that they were also apprehensive about getting tested for COVId-19. With the passage of time, there was also a rise in the number of infected patients and HCPs, leading to the fear of death among participants.

Fear of Death

Feeling of loneliness, burnout, and the unpredictable nature of disease have instilled a fear of death among HCPs, especially when they witness the death of their colleagues. Along with this, they also witnessed news of HCPs dying while serving COVID-19 patients from various other sources such as social media, newspapers etc., leading to an existential crisis about themselves and their family members:

Participant 6: *If we are going for the COVID duty, we do not know whether we would return home safely or not...The fear of death is always there as the colleagues get infected and succumb to death.*
Participant 3: *I experienced the COVID symptoms once, and the only thought that I had was if I died, what would happen to my children.*

Participants shared that they lived in constant fear of death amid certain personal and professional challenges caused by the disease of COVID-19.

Theme 3: Perceived Challenges

The undefined nature of the disease posed many challenges to HCPs both at the personal and professional levels.

Personal Challenges

The following sub-themes emerged in this category:

Isolation and Feeling of Loneliness

As per the treatment protocol, after fortnight duty in the COVID-19 ward/hospital, HCPs have to quarantine themselves for a certain number of days as per the guidelines. Participants have reported heightened levels of loneliness as they could not go home or visit their family members and friends. Even if they were staying at home, it was total segregation from the entire family. Virtual mediums were the only option to combat extreme loneliness/isolation:

Participant 16: *Staying in isolation for 14 days is strenuous. There is no escape from this situation. One has to deal with this alone, which is the most challenging part.*

Fear of Being Contagious

Participants shared that since they are actively involved in treating COVID-19 patients, they also fear that their family members could get infected through them. Participants feared that they could be a possible threat to their elderly parents, especially those with comorbidities.

Participant 15: *The fear of being a contagion is very high... I felt that I could be asymptomatic and a carrier of disease because the efficacy of the test* (COVID-19 diagnostic test) *was also not 100 percent. I separated myself from my parents as they had comorbidities.*

They also reported that many patients did not follow COVID-19 safety protocols despite many suggestions and awareness campaigns from the Government and hospital management. It led to dissatisfaction among HCPs as they felt that whom they are treating with great concern are indifferent about HCPs' health status.

Participant 10: *When the OPD started, we told them to cover their faces with masks, but they did not do that. No one wants to believe in Covid and follow the rules.*

Due to fear of being contagious to family members, most participants separated themselves from their families. As a result, they had to face the challenge of managing household chores alone.

Management of Household Chores

Apart from the hectic schedule at the hospital, managing the household chores such as cooking food and cleaning the house, etc., were the primary concerns. Due to the severely contagious nature of the disease and recommended hygiene protocols, it became compulsory to cook healthy food by oneself or by any family member if available. Reporting the Corona positive cases through delivery persons in the media has also created a compulsion to be self-reliant on nutritional requirements. The lockdown has also restricted services of house help that added burden along with tedious jobs at the hospital. It is especially true in the case of females and unmarried HCPs. Although, in many cases, hospital management arranged meals for the HCPs in the hospital canteen during duty hours, most of them were reluctant to have it:

Participant 18: *After so much workload, we have no support for food and other household activities, which is the most challenging. We have not eaten properly, and we are not getting help from anywhere.*
Participant 19: *We have to cook for ourselves as we could not eat in the canteen. It has increased our work.*

These shreds of observation show that participants were constantly battling their mental and physical sphere. For example, they were dealing with psychological fears and managing household chores simultaneously. Moreover, they also had to face direct or indirect forms of social discrimination occasionally.

Social Discrimination

Participants reported that occasionally they had to face social discrimination from their neighborhood people and the local community. People in the neighborhood tended to avoid interacting with them as they perceived fear of getting infected. In some cases, discrimination was also extended to family members, such as restricting children during playtime by the neighbors, sharing the pooled transport system, and not renting their houses to HCPs. In other words, this attitude has made them become silent sufferers of social seclusion:

Participant 7: *The discrimination was always there as people would not let their children play with our children...I usually travel by pooled auto-rickshaw, and when the fellow passengers learned that I served in the COVID-19 ward, a few of them showed non-verbal cues and feared that they could also get infected.*

Participant 14: *Some friends and colleagues were asked to vacate their houses....In a building adjacent to ours, the staff was asked to leave.*

Professional Challenges

Apart from personal challenges, participants also have reported several professional challenges while serving in the Corona ward:

Working in Personal Protective Equipment (PPE)

The participants have revealed that performing medical procedures with a PPE kit was one of the most significant challenges during the pandemic. Generally, the PPE kit is ill-fitted, and due to this, carrying out critical care responsibility is even more challenging. Face shields cause decreased visibility, and as a result, reading the vital parameters of a patient is relatively tough. In addition, doffing a PPE kit is somewhat more complicated than donning as there are chances of contracting the virus from the surface:

Participant 12: *Due to ill-fitting and big sizes of PPE kit, walking in the ward is difficult... Every minute counts and even a minute's delay can result in loss of lives.*

Participant 7: *Moreover, fogging on the face shield blocks visibility. I was not able to read the pulse-oximeter and other vital parameters of the patient.*

Participant 11: *Doffing of PPE kit is complex, and one has to be very careful because the kit might have already infected from outside.*

Moreover, having layers of mask on face, communicating, and breathing properly is a real challenge. Since the possibility of the virus being airborne, the use of air conditioners in the hospitals are also restricted:

Participant 9: *Wearing a PPE kit during summer is a real challenge due to a long hectic schedule and working in a non-air-conditioned environment. It has led to dehydration and dizziness at times.*

Responding to natural needs such as hunger, thirst, and excretion, they said it is difficult to mitigate. Moreover, female HCPs experience greater discomfort during their menstruation cycle while working in a PPE kit. Since a few of the female HCPs are nursing mothers, it is tough for them to decide whether to breastfeed the baby or not:

Participant 17: *We have to take care of daily necessities such as water and urine, as after wearing PPE, we cannot do that. We cannot take food for eight hours.*

Participant 1: *Covid duties are challenging during menstruation because of fatigue and pain. Doffing and donning of the PPE is not easily possible whenever one require to use the utilities.*

Negligence of Other Diseases and Delay in Treatment

Participants have expressed that the pandemic altered the routine preventive and curative process. The pandemic has brought severe consequences for those who wanted to get treated for other illnesses, both acute and chronic in nature. The regular outpatient departments (OPDs) are closed due to the pandemic, an obstacle to running routine healthcare. Due to this, several patients have to postpone their diagnosis, necessary surgeries, and follow-ups:

Participant 15: *Patients suffer during this pandemic. The asthma patients cannot be nebulized; this hinders the treatment. The required surgeries are postponed and it has affected the health of the patients.*

Role of Touch in Clinical Practice

Participants have revealed that COVID-19 protocols impacted the traditional diagnosis procedure. In standard diagnosis procedure, there is a significant role of physical touch, that is, physical examination to determine if there is an early sign of any illness, which has wholly restricted during this time of pandemic:

Participant 2: *Examination of a patient before Covid was better; we would auscultate the patient. The physical touch, which is most important in a physician's diagnosis, is missed now...Only urgent procedures are allowed. The diagnosis is completely based on lab test results.*

Feeling of Burnout and Negative Transference

The long working hours, lack of sleep, isolation, psychological fears, managing personal work at home, limited contact with the family members, etc. have resulted in physical and emotional exhaustion leading to the feeling of burnout among HCPs. Along with these factors, one of the critical reasons for burnout among HCPs was the negative transference of patients' rough emotions on HCPs. HCPs occasionally became the victims of patients' wrath and rude behavior. Getting diagnosed with COVID-19 makes patients both physically and mentally stressed, and occasionally they let it out on HCPs. It at times makes HCPs demoralized for the amount of effort they use to put towards making the condition of the patients better:

Participant 16: *We are frustrated and disturbed. My patience is getting tested. I think at several points that I cannot take this anymore. It is physically and mentally exhausting, and I want to go home and sleep.*

Participant 1: *Handling the patients and their agitation was challenging. Those asymptomatic think they have no illness; they do not want to stay in quarantine facilities. It was not that difficult to handle disease and symptoms than patients' rude behavior.*

Along with several challenges at the personal and professional level, HCPs reported systemic support and self-management to cope with the situation.

Theme 4: Systemic Support and Self-Management

Social support has been imperative to coping while working in a crisis. Participants acknowledged the external support from colleagues and the hospital administration and developed their internal support mechanisms. The presence of both internal and external support mechanisms has emerged from the verbatim reports of the participants. HCPs have shared that they receive ample support from their colleagues and hospital administration. The adverse period of COVID-19 and related challenges facilitate new levels of cohesiveness and social support system among the colleagues:

Participant 5: *The staff is very cooperative...and the cohesiveness among the colleagues has been increased in this period.*

Participant 8: *The support from the administration is there; we do not have to face many issues in this context.*

HCPs developed specific self-management strategies such as self-reliance for personal needs, thinking about their role models in their profession or observing their colleagues stay active and positive, trusting the efficacy of the Corona vaccine to effectively deal with the adverse situation created by COVID-19:

Participant 11: *One has to rely on self-management. I am mentally prepared by myself... If you trust the vaccine, it gives mental strength, and there is nothing more one can do.*

Participant 4: *When everyone around is doing the duties...we get stronger when we look at our colleagues and friends working.*

The majority of the participants also shared that this situation has strengthened their belief in the almighty God. Furthermore, they believed this belief enables them to be active in the current status of crisis.

Participant 3: *God will help us in dealing with this problem. This belief gives us the power to go on in life.*

Systemic support and self-management enabled them to identify a scope of personal growth amid the crisis of COVID-19 and motivated them to work.

Theme 5: Personal Growth in Adversity

Despite the challenging situation and fight against COVID19, personal growth under pressure is also evident. Participants have reported that their professional responsibility has prompted them to take charge of the current crisis. The participants were able to view their profession's value and find self-satisfaction and meaning in their work.

Finding Meaning in Work and Self-Satisfaction: Participants shared that they could find meaning in their work while dealing with the overwhelming demands of a sudden public health emergency. It helped them to derive a sense of purpose and new learning experiences. In some cases, they also got encouragement from family and friends to perform their duties diligently:

Participant 12: *I can find meaning in work. We have done so many medical procedures to save lives, and that all seems fruitful.*

Participant 6: *I never say no to duties as it is always a good learning experience.*

Finding meaning in an adverse situation like COVID-19 also helped them derive self-satisfaction from their work. Therefore, the HCPs have expressed that they have joined this profession as it gives them an internal satisfaction in providing medical care and support to the people, and this remains true during the present pandemic:

Participant 12: *You are a doctor, so you have to do it. You have studied for this, so the sense of responsibility is there. We joined the profession because we like doing this, and we do it on humanitarian grounds.*

Participant 10: *Working during Covid provides self-satisfaction. We can serve the people when it is required.*

HCPs as a Counselor and Facilitator: The attendants of the patients are not allowed to visit in the Corona ward, HCPs have to adopt an extra role behavior such as a counselor or a facilitator. They use to soothe the patients emotionally, counsel them appropriately so that patients would not get panic. At times, they also serve as a communication medium between patients and their family members:

Participant 13: *The patient cannot meet the family and you are the only one with whom they can communicate. You have to counsel the patient and sometimes enable them to speak to their family through personal phone or tab in distress, which increases the workload. In this process, I have developed empathy towards patients.*

An Identity of Corona Warrior: In the time of the current pandemic, HCPs have been risking their lives to save people from the health complexities caused by COVID-19. The Indian Government has recognized their unconditional dedication and called them Corona warriors. HCPs shared that it feels good to know that they are being recognized as Corona warriors:

Participant 18: *My friends felt proud of me when they realized that I am working in the COVID wards. They expressed their happiness. I even helped a few people who got tested and suggested the treatment.*

DISCUSSION

The impact of COVID-19 has been quite overwhelming for the HCPs due to the unavailability of preventive and curative treatment. This public health emergency has imposed unprecedented challenges to the physical and psychological health of people. This study has adopted a qualitative approach to inquire about the lived experience of healthcare providers who served in the medical care of COVID-19 patients using IPA.

At the beginning of the 21st century, a part of the world had witnessed different forms of SARS-associated Coronavirus disease (WHO, 2003). However, India did not face any such health emergencies at a broader level. Thus, initially, even in the presence of COVID-19 related news coming from different parts of the world, denial and uncertainty plagued the mind of HCPs. HCPs used denial to cope with the stress and uncertainty caused by the impact of COVID-19 in the other part of the world. Denial has also been reported as one of the defense mechanisms under extreme stress situations in the literature (Ritchie, 2014).

After the initial stage of denial and uncertainty, HCPs had to acknowledge the presence of disease. However, the indeterminate nature of the disease and rapidly changing guidelines posed a significant challenge to the testing, tracking, and treating of COVID-19. According to Gupta and Sahoo (2020), "lack of proper communication from the higher authorities to the frontline HCWs and rapidly changing guidelines regarding infection control measures could lead to uncertainty, apprehension, lack of knowledge and a sense of uncontrollability over the situation" (p. 6).

The disease of COVID-19 has also challenged the existential status of the HCPs. They have been facing episodes of social exclusion due to social-emotional distancing from their near dear ones. It is especially true for the female HCPs, who raise a younger child or are nurturing mothers. Sahin *et al.* (2020) has reported similar findings. Moreover, working in an unpredictable environment and witnessing critical cases of COVID-19 might have promoted a feeling of emotional exhaustion among HCPs. Pessin *et al.* (2015) reported that the fear of death, experience of negative emotions, death, and anxiety are the typical characteristics of existential distress. Gama, Barbosa, and Vieira (2014) reported that emotional exhaustion promoted fear of death among nursing staff. Similarly, Browall et al. (2014) found that witnessing discomforting situations like death and dying deeply affects HCPs as they feel powerless to control uncertainty.

HCPs also have experienced the fear of getting infected as they are engaged with the caring duties of COVID-19 patients. Similar findings have also been reported in other studies. Sun et al. (2020) have reported that the feeling of fear, a kind of negative emotion, is evident among HCPs serving their duties in the Corona ward. Ness et al. (2021) has found that management of stress due to the fear of the unknown has been prevalent among HCPs involved in treating COVID-19.

HCPs have reported several challenges, both personal and professional in nature. Among the personal challenges, loneliness, household chores management, the fear of being contagious and social discrimination are major factors. Loneliness observed in the study could be attributed to either mandatory COVID-19 protocol or forced separation from family due to the fear of contracting and unfurling COVID-19 to family members. Ness et al. (2020) also have observed that HCPs deliberately have isolated themselves from their close family members due to the fear of being contagious.

HCPs have to go through an additional burden of taking care of household chores along with hectic schedules at the hospitals. Crimi and Carlucci (2021) also found that HCPs, especially female HCPs, have to adjust to their household chores. Occasional episodes of social discrimination are also evident among HCPs. The neighbors, local community, and even family members sometimes unintentionally make them the victims of social discrimination leading to temporary social exclusion episodes. Mohindra et al. (2021) have found that neighbors and landlords are the primary sources of social stigma against the HCPs. One of the main reasons for this social discrimination could be attributed to the perceived health stigma that promotes a person's perception in the form of an object that could threaten society. Since HCPs are serving in the ward of COVID-19, an infectious disease, local community and neighbors might have unconsciously motivated to discriminate against them even in the absence of any valid ethical concerns. Such discrimination and stigma have been evident throughout the history of infectious diseases like HIV, SARS-COV, MERS, and Ebola (Sevimli, 2020).

Among the professional challenges, handling the PPE kit while working in the Corona care unit was one of the most significant challenges faced by HCPs. Doffing the PPE kit was relatively more challenging than donning and other issues such as walking in the PPE kit, visibility issues due to face protective equipment, etc. Moreover, female HCPs found it even more challenging to work in PPE kits, especially during their menstruation days. Several studies have reported that female HCPs face relatively more discomfort than their male counterparts in using PPE kits. Scholars pointed out that human factor engineering should be considered to control the design deficiency of the PPE kit, including the gender requirement (Parush et al. 2020). Fan et al. (2020) have reported that failure to comply with precautions for handling PPE kits could lead to the transmission of pathogens.

The pandemic also has altered the routine preventive and curative processes of other diseases. According to Rosenbaum (2020), the pandemic has shifted the medical attention on COVID-19 patients, ignoring the criticality of other diseases. This shift has suddenly affected the quality of medical care adversely due to drastic changes in medical practice in recent times compared to the pre-pandemic period. It has also raised serious concerns regarding the campaigns to eradicate communicable diseases such as tuberculosis, polio, etc., from the world (Roberts, 2021).

Moreover, COVID-19 protocols have also altered the role of physical examination, that is, touch in the overall diagnosis process. According to Horton (2019), touch plays a significant role in clinical examination. It helps build an empathetic understanding of a health professional to her/his patient. Horton further suggests that "touch builds trust, reassurance, and a sense of communion. Touch is about fostering a social bond of sympathy, compassion, and tenderness between two strangers. Touch can even convey the idea of survival" (p. 1310). However, the current pandemic curtailing the physical examination in clinical practice is the need of the hour for the well-being of HCPs (Hyman, 2020).

The long hectic work schedule and other psychological factors such as loneliness, the fear of death, social and emotional distancing paved the way for burnout among HCPs. Azoulay et al. (2020) reported that fear, frustration, physical and emotional exhaustion are the significant determinants of psychological burden among HCPs. Benfante *et al.* (2020) reported COVID-19 related psychological trauma such as anxiety, depression, and insomnia among HCPs. HCPs also experienced vicarious trauma as they witnessed the pain and suffering of patients. Negative transference (anger, frustration, etc.) of patients on HCPs even fosters the feeling of burnout. Sahoo et al. (2020) report that due to treatment protocol, COVID-19 patients have to live in isolation away from the emotional warmth of the family that instills fear of death, stigma, and mental distress in them. In such uncontrollable situations, patients might have used the defense mechanism of displacement and directed it on already physically and emotionally fatigued HCPs. The study recommends that the government device a strategic policy to recruit a significant number of HCP's to share the workload. It would also improve the doctor-patient ratio as recommended by WHO.

Apart from subtle challenges, HCPs also report several mechanisms that help them cope with the overwhelming situation of COVID-19. Participants have expressed that they receive ample unconditional support from hospital administration and their colleagues. Kovner et al. (2021) have found that institutional and peer support protect against negative feelings of fear, anxiety, and depression. George et al. (2020) have reported that cohesiveness and trust are two major factors that created a conducive environment to combat the challenges that occurred during the Ebola outbreak. Peer support mechanisms have paved the way for a sense of togetherness and encouragement in the tough times of the pandemic of COVID-19. Apart from institutional and peer support, participants also have developed their internal support mechanisms. To maintain the motivation to work, HCPs rely on observational learning regarding how their role models keep them motivated to work efficiently. Frontline workers in India have received both doses of the COVID-19 vaccine; HCPs reflected their faith in the efficacy of the vaccination for

COVID-19. Singhania, Kathiravan and Pannu (2021) have found in their study that 80% HCPs support vaccination for COVID-19.

Finally, participants also have reflected their faith in the supreme power of God and transcendental beliefs to cope with the adversity caused by the pandemic. Kowalczyk et al. (2020) suggest that transcendental beliefs positively correlate with keeping a positive attitude in difficult times. Roman, Mthembu, and Hoosen (2020) have proposed that transcendental or spiritual beliefs may help people cope with perceived sufferings, fear of death, and adversity of illness.

The study findings reveal that most HCPs have reported personal growth even under adverse circumstances. HCPs have found value and meaning in their work and have felt a sense of responsibility and satisfaction to serve COVID-19 patients. Similar findings are also reported by Sun et al. (2020) among female nurses who are involved in the COVID-19 treatment process. Besides this, HCPs are also instrumental in providing emotional calmness to distressed patients. They are receptive to patients' fear and emotional distress and give patients hope to overcome the disease. Such activities of health workers could be instrumental in promoting well-being among patients.

Despite having many in-depth reflections, this study has a few limitations. First, most participants (70%) were interviewed telephonically due to lockdown protocols, the participants' non-verbal cues, and other significant field notes could not be kept. Second, the sample composition only consisted of HCPs; however, the future study can incorporate experiences of hospital management staff (both support and administrative staff) to understand the complexity of care given during the pandemic of COVID-19. There is a dearth of a validated questionnaire explicitly designed for HCP's to assess the severity of mental health issues. The themes identified in the study can be employed to construct a questionnaire that could aim to assess the severity of challenges and mental health issues for HCPs. The findings also highlighted gender-specific issues concerning female HCPs. Future research can examine the challenges and mental health issues of female HCPs.

The study recommends strengthening systemic support to improve the efficiency of HCPs and healthcare delivery. The study's findings provide insights to identify critical factors imperative for designing interventions to promote resilience and well-being among HCPs. The study highlights that Indian HCPs face tremendous mental health issues such as loneliness, burnout, existential distress, including fear of death and contagion. The study recommends periodic screening of mental health issues and providing appropriate psychological interventions to resolve these issues among HCPs. Gupta and Sahoo (2020) also urged mental health support system for HCPs. D'Rozario (Sepetember7, 2021) suggested that recommendations of the Center for Disease Control and Prevention, U.S. can be incorporated such as 'counseling, dedicated "quiet spaces," and training seminars for healthcare professionals.' In addition, findings revealed problems related to the PPE kit. The study recommends acknowledging human factor engineering and gender-specific requirements in designing the PPE kits.

HCPs witnessed negative transference from patients and social discrimination from the neighborhood. Such an attitude of citizens demoralizes HCPs. The Indian Government has declared 'violence against healthcare workers a non-bailable offense through the Epidemic Diseases (Amendment) Ordinance, 2020, much more can be done' (D'Rozario, September 7, 2021). The study suggests that different forms of media reporting may initiate a campaign targeting the attitudinal change of citizens towards HCPs. It may help change the attitude of citizens towards the HCPs and strengthen the HCP-patient relationship. The stable doctor-patient relationship could lead to patients' access and satisfaction with the health care system

HCPs also faced challenges in mitigating household chores. Proper care of young children was also a vital issue among female HCPs with a lack of active social support. Females are directly responsible for daily chores, child development, and extended family as per the prevailing gender norms in India. According to Chauhan (2020), working women bear three significant responsibilities: unpaid household chores, reproductive work, and professional employment compared to their male counterparts. The study proposes robust systemic support for HCPs taking care of their essential needs and a safe crutch facility for female HCPs. Finally, findings also indicated the scope of finding meaning in work, self-satisfaction and building a social support mechanism among HCPs. The study recommends that teaching self-regulation strategies as a part of psychological interventions would be effective for HCPs to manage their thoughts, emotions, and behaviors. It would enable them to find meaning, hope, and satisfaction with work even under dreadful situations.

The findings of the study also have important implications for building a resilient healthcare system in India. A resilient healthcare system is a prerequisite for the effective management of present and future health threats (Nuzzo et al., 2018). According to Kruk et al. (2015), a resilient healthcare system can be defined as "the capacity of health actors, institutions, and populations to prepare for and effectively respond to crises; maintain core functions when a crisis hits; and, informed by lessons learned during the crisis, reorganize if conditions require it" (p. 1990). Narwal and Jain (2021) have suggested that HCPs or health workforce are integral to any resilient healthcare system. Therefore, this study recommends working out of a comprehensive intervention program to protect the holistic well-being of HCPs. It would enable them to bear the physical and psychological burden caused by the present and future health crises.

CONCLUSION

This study presents an in-depth understanding of the lived experiences of HCPs involved in the treatment of COVID-19 using IPA. This study highlights how HCPs have comprehended the disease, how their personal and professional challenges are encountered in this process, how they have faced existential and social issues, and how they own an extra role behavior of a counselor or a facilitator with a scope of personal growth. The insights gained from the study can be utilized to design a comprehensive intervention program to strengthen resilience and promote the well-being of HCPs.

ACKNOWLEDGMENT

We thank Dr. Tilak Singh (Medical Officer, Dist. Shamli, Uttar Pradesh, India), who helped us in the data collection. We are also grateful to our participants for taking time from their hectic schedules and sharing their experiences with us.

FUNDING

This research received no specific grant from any funding agency in the public, commercial, or not-for-profit sectors.

REFERENCES

Azoulay, E., Cariou, A., Bruneel, F., Demoule, A., Kouatchet, A., Reuter, D., Souppart, V., Combes, A., Klouche, K., Argaud, L., Barbier, F., Jourdain, M., Reignier, J., Papazian, L., Guidet, B., Géri, G., Resche-Rigon, M., Guisset, O., Labbé, V., ... Kentish-Barnes, N. (2020). Symptoms of anxiety, depression, and peritraumatic dissociation in critical care clinicians managing patients with COVID-19. A cross-sectional study. *American Journal of Respiratory and Critical Care Medicine*, *202*(10), 1388–1398. doi:10.1164/rccm.202006-2568OC PMID:32866409

Banerjee, A., Mukherjee, K., Bhattacharjee, D., Garai, D., & Chakraborty, R. (2020). Status of Healthcare Workers in Relation to COVID-19 Infection: A Retrospective Study in a Level 4 COVID Hospital in Eastern India. *The Journal of the Association of Physicians of India*, *68*(12), 55–57. PMID:33247643

Benfante, A., Di Tella, M., Romeo, A., & Castelli, L. (2020). Traumatic stress in healthcare workers during COVID-19 pandemic: A review of the immediate impact. *Frontiers in Psychology*, *11*, 2816. doi:10.3389/fpsyg.2020.569935 PMID:33192854

Browall, M., Henoch, I., Melin-Johansson, C., Strang, S., & Danielson, E. (2014). Existential encounters: Nurses' descriptions of critical incidents in end-of-life cancer care. *European Journal of Oncology Nursing*, *18*(6), 636–644. doi:10.1016/j.ejon.2014.06.001 PMID:24996512

Callary, B., Rathwell, S., & Young, B. W. (2015). Insights on the Process of Using Interpretive Phenomenological Analysis in a Sport Coaching Research Project. *Qualitative Report*, *20*(2), 63–75. doi:10.46743/2160-3715/2015.2096

Chan, Z. C., Fung, Y., & Chien, W. (2013). Bracketing in Phenomenology: Only Undertaken in the Data Collection and Analysis Process. *Qualitative Report*, *18*(30), 1–9. doi:10.46743/2160-3715/2013.1486

Chauhan, P. (2020). Gendering COVID-19: Impact of the Pandemic on Women's Burden of Unpaid Work in India. *Gender Issues*. Advance online publication. doi:10.100712147-020-09269-w PMID:33132690

Chokshi, M., Patil, B., Khanna, R., Neogi, S. B., Sharma, J., Paul, V. K., & Zodpey, S. (2016). Health systems in India. *Journal of Perinatology*, *36*(3), S9–S12. doi:10.1038/jp.2016.184 PMID:27924110

Collins, K., & Nicolson, P. (2002). The meaning of 'satisfaction for people with dermatological problems: Reassessing approaches to qualitative health psychology research. *Journal of Health Psychology*, *7*(5), 615–629. doi:10.1177/1359105302007005681 PMID:22113145

Conrad, P. (1987). The experience of illness: recent and new directions. Research in the sociology of health care. Vol. 6: the experience and management of chronic illness, 1-31.

Crimi, C., & Carlucci, A. (2021). Challenges for the female healthcare workers during the COVID-19 pandemic: The need for protection beyond the mask. *Pulmonology*, *27*(1), 1–3. doi:10.1016/j.pulmoe.2020.09.004 PMID:33087308

D'Rozario, A. (2021, September 7). *Supporting India's Healthcare Workers. New Asia Perspective.* Retrieved from https://www.csis.org/blogs/new-perspectives-asia/supporting-indias-healthcare-workers

Fan, J., Jiang, Y., Hu, K., Chen, X., Xu, Q., Qi, Y., Yin, H., Gou, X., & Liang, S. (2020). Barriers to using personal protective equipment by healthcare staff during the COVID-19 outbreak in China. *Medicine, 99*(48), e23310. doi:10.1097/MD.0000000000023310 PMID:33235088

Faulkner, S. L., & Trotter, S. P. (2017). *Theoretical saturation. In The International Encyclopedia of Communication Research Methods*. John Wiley & Sons.

Gama, G., Barbosa, F., & Vieira, M. (2014). Personal determinants of nurses' burnout in end of life care. *European Journal of Oncology Nursing, 18*(5), 527–533. doi:10.1016/j.ejon.2014.04.005 PMID:24888265

George, C. E., Inbaraj, L. R., Rajukutty, S., & de Witte, L. P. (2020). Challenges, experience and coping of health professionals in delivering healthcare in an urban slum in India during the first 40 days of COVID-19 crisis: A mixed method study. *BMJ Open, 10*(11), e042171. doi:10.1136/bmjopen-2020-042171 PMID:33208338

Ghosh, S., Moledina, N., Hasan, M. M., Jain, S., & Ghosh, A. (2021). Colossal Challenges to the healthcare workers combating the second wave of COVID-19 in India. *Infection Control and Hospital Epidemiology, 1-5*. Advance online publication. doi:10.1017/ice.2021.257 PMID:34075871

Given, L. M. (2015). *100 Questions (and Answers) about Qualitative Research*. SAGE publications.

Goel, S. (2020, January 31). The doctor-population ratio in India is 1:1456 against WHO recommendation. *Deccan Herald*. Retrieved from https://www.deccanherald.com/business/budget-2020/the-doctor-population-ratio-in-india-is-11456-against-who-recommendation-800034.html

Gupta, S., & Sahoo, S. (2020). Pandemic and mental health of the frontline healthcare workers: A review and implications in the Indian context amidst COVID-19. *General Psychiatry, 33*(5), 1–10. doi:10.1136/gpsych-2020-100284 PMID:34192235

Horton, R. (2019). Offline: Touch—the first language. *Lancet, 394*(10206), 1310. doi:10.1016/S0140-6736(19)32280-9 PMID:31609215

Hummel, S., Oetjen, N., Du, J., Posenato, E., de Almeida, R. M. R., Losada, R., ... Schultz, J. H. (2021). Mental health among medical professionals during the COVID-19 pandemic in eight european countries: Cross-sectional survey study. *Journal of Medical Internet Research, 23*(1), e24983. doi:10.2196/24983 PMID:33411670

Hyman, P. (2020). The disappearance of the primary care physical examination—Losing touch. *JAMA Internal Medicine, 180*(11), 1417–1418. doi:10.1001/jamainternmed.2020.3546 PMID:32832987

Ives, J., Greenfield, S., Parry, J. M., Draper, H., Gratus, C., Petts, J. I., Sorell, T., & Wilson, S. (2009). Healthcare workers' attitudes to working during pandemic influenza: A qualitative study. *BMC Public Health, 9*(1), 1–13. doi:10.1186/1471-2458-9-56 PMID:19216738

Iyengar, K. P., Jain, V. K., & Vaishya, R. (2020). Current situation with doctors and healthcare workers during COVID-19 pandemic in India. *Postgraduate Medical Journal, 0*, 1–2. doi:10.1136/postgradmedj-2020-138496 PMID:32817496

Joy, S. (2020, March 25). Amidst COVID-19 outbreak, landlords ask doctors, nurses to vacate houses; govt warns owners. *Deccan Herald.* Retrieved from https://www.deccanherald.com/national/amidst-covid-19-outbreak-landlords-ask-doctors-nurses-to-vacate-houses-govt-warns-owners-817435.html

Kovner, C., Raveis, V. H., Van Devanter, N., Yu, G., Glassman, K., & Ridge, L. J. (2021). The psychosocial impact on frontline nurses of caring for patients with COVID-19 during the first wave of the pandemic in New York City. I-II, 1-11. *Nursing Outlook, 69*(5), 744–754. Advance online publication. doi:10.1016/j.outlook.2021.03.019 PMID:33894986

Kowalczyk, O., Roszkowski, K., Montane, X., Pawliszak, W., Tylkowski, B., & Bajek, A. (2020). Religion and Faith Perception in a Pandemic of COVID-19. *Journal of Religion and Health, 59*(6), 2671–2677. doi:10.100710943-020-01088-3 PMID:33044598

Kruk, M. E., Myers, M., Varpilah, S. T., & Dahn, B. T. (2015). What is a resilient health system? Lessons from Ebola. *Lancet, 385*(9980), 1910–1912. doi:10.1016/S0140-6736(15)60755-3 PMID:25987159

Kumar, R., & Pal, R. (2018). India achieves WHO recommended doctor population ratio: A call for paradigm shift in public health discourse! *Journal of Family Medicine and Primary Care, 7*(5), 841–844. doi:10.4103/jfmpc.jfmpc_218_18 PMID:30598921

Lancet. (2020). India under COVID-19 lockdown. *Lancet, 395*(10233), 1315. doi:10.1016/S0140-6736(20)30938-7 PMID:32334687

Lincoln, S. Y., & Guba, E. G. (1985). *Naturalistic inquiry.* Sage. doi:10.1016/0147-1767(85)90062-8

Mohindra, R., Ravaki, R., Suri, V., Bhalla, A., & Singh, S. M. (2020). Issues relevant to mental health promotion in frontline health care providers managing quarantined/isolated COVID19 patients. *Asian Journal of Psychiatry, 51*(3), 102084. doi:10.1016/j.ajp.2020.102084 PMID:32289728

Mohindra, R., Soni, R. K., Suri, V., Bhalla, A., & Singh, S. M. (2021). The experience of social and emotional distancing among health care providers in the context of COVID-19: A study from North India. *Journal of Human Behavior in the Social Environment, 31*(1-4), 173–183. doi:10.1080/10911359.2020.1792385

Narwal, S., & Jain, S. (2021). Building Resilient Health Systems: Patient Safety during COVID-19 and Lessons for the Future. *Journal of Health Management, 23*(1), 166–181. doi:10.1177/0972063421994935

Ness, M. M., Saylor, J., Di Fusco, L. A., & Evans, K. (2021). Healthcare providers' challenges during the coronavirus disease (COVID-19) pandemic: A qualitative approach. *Nursing & Health Sciences, 23*(2), 1–9. doi:10.1111/nhs.12820 PMID:33580590

Nuzzo, J. B., Meyer, D., Snyder, M., Ravi, S. J., Lapascu, A., Souleles, J., Andrada, C. I., & Bishai, D. (2019). What makes health systems resilient against infectious disease outbreaks and natural hazards? Results from a scoping review. *BMC Public Health, 19*(1), 1–9. doi:10.118612889-019-7707-z PMID:31623594

Pal, R., & Yadav, U. (2020). COVID-19 pandemic in india: Present scenario and a steep climb ahead. *Journal of Primary Care & Community Health, 11*, 1–4. doi:10.1177/2150132720939402 PMID:32644871

Parthasarathy, R., Jaisoorya, T. S., Thennarasu, K., & Murthy, P. (2021). Mental health issues among health care workers during the COVID-19 pandemic–a study from India. *Asian Journal of Psychiatry, 58*, 102626. doi:10.1016/j.ajp.2021.102626

Parush, A., Wacht, O., Gomes, R., & Frenkel, A. (2020). Human factor considerations in using personal protective equipment in the COVID-19 pandemic context: Binational survey study. *Journal of Medical Internet Research, 22*(6), e19947. https://preprints.jmir.org/preprint/19947

Patton, M. Q. (2002). *Qualitative research and evaluation methods.* Sage Publications.

Pessin, H., Fenn, N., Hendriksen, E., DeRosa, A. P., & Applebaum, A. (2015). Existential distress among caregivers or professionals taking care of dying patients. *Current Opinion in Supportive and Palliative Care, 9*(1), 77–86. doi:10.1097/SPC.0000000000000116

Pollock, A., Campbell, P., Cheyne, J., Cowie, J., Davis, B., McCallum, J., McGill, K., Elders, A., Hagen, S., McClurg, D., Torrens, C., & Maxwell, M. (2020). Interventions to support the resilience and mental health of frontline health and social care professionals during and after a disease outbreak, epidemic or pandemic: A mixed methods systematic review. *Cochrane Database of Systematic Reviews, 2020*(11). Advance online publication. doi:10.1002/14651858.CD013779 PMID:33150970

Reid, K., Flowers, P., & Larkin, M. (2005). Exploring lived experience.. *The Psychologist, 18*(1), 20–23.

Ritchie, T. D. (2014). Denial. In T. R. Levine (Ed.), *Encyclopedia of Lying and Deception.* Sage Publications. doi:10.4135/9781483306902.n107

Roberts, L. (2021). How COVID hurt the fight against other dangerous diseases. *Nature, 592*(7855), 502–504. doi:10.1038/d41586-021-01022-x PMID:33883727

Roman, N. V., Mthembu, T. G., & Hoosen, M. (2020). Spiritual care–'A deeper immunity'–A response to Covid-19 pandemic. *African Journal of Primary Health Care & Family Medicine, 12*(1). Advance online publication. doi:10.4102/phcfm.v12i1.2456 PMID:32634003

Rosenbaum, L. (2020). The untold toll—The pandemic's effects on patients without Covid-19. *The New England Journal of Medicine, 382*(24), 2368–2371. doi:10.1056/NEJMms2009984 PMID:32302076

Sahin, T., Aslaner, H., Eker, O. O., Gokcek, M. B., & Dogan, M. (2020). Effect of COVID-19 pandemic on anxiety and burnout levels in emergency healthcare workers: a questionnaire study. doi:10.21203/rs.3.rs-32073/v1

Sahoo, S., Mehra, A., Suri, V., Malhotra, P., Yaddanapudi, L. N., Puri, G. D., & Grover, S. (2020). Lived experiences of the corona survivors (patients admitted in COVID wards): A narrative real-life documented summaries of internalized guilt, shame, stigma, anger. *Asian Journal of Psychiatry, 53*, 102187. doi:10.1016/j.ajp.2020.102187 PMID:32512532

Seale, H., Leask, J., Po, K., & MacIntyre, C. R. (2009). "Will they just pack up and leave?"–attitudes and intended behaviour of hospital health care workers during an influenza pandemic. *BMC Health Services Research, 9*(1), 1–8. doi:10.1186/1472-6963-9-30 PMID:19216792

Sevimli, S. (2020). Healthcare professionals acting ethically under the risk of stigmatization and violence during COVID-19 from media reports in Turkey. [doi:https://philpapers.org/rec/SEVHPA]. *Eubios Journal of Asian and International Bioethics; EJAIB, 30*(5), 207–211.

Singhania, N., Kathiravan, S., & Pannu, A. K. (2021). Acceptance of Covid-19 vaccine among healthcare personnel in India: A cross-sectional survey during the initial phase of vaccination. *Clinical Microbiology and Infection*. doi:10.1016/j.cmi.2021.03.008

Smith, J. A., & Osborn, M. (2003). Interpretative phenomenological analysis. In J. A. Smith (Ed.), *Qualitative psychology: A practical guide to research methods* (pp. 51–80). Sage Publications, Inc.

Smith, J. A., & Osborn, M. (2008). Interpretative phenomenological analysis. In V. Eatough & J. A. Smith (Eds.), *The Sage Handbook of Qualitative Research in Psychology* (pp. 179–194). Sage Publications.

Smith, J. A., & Osborn, M. (2015). Interpretative phenomenological analysis as a useful methodology for research on the lived experience of pain. *British Journal of Pain, 9*(1), 41–42. doi:10.1177/2049463714541642 PMID:26516556

Sun, N., Wei, L., Shi, S., Jiao, D., Song, R., Ma, L., Wang, H., Wang, C., Wang, Z., You, Y., Liu, S., & Wang, H. (2020). A qualitative study on the psychological experience of caregivers of COVID-19 patients. *American Journal of Infection Control, 48*(6), 592–598. doi:10.1016/j.ajic.2020.03.018 PMID:32334904

Suryavanshi, N., Kadam, A., Dhumal, G., Nimkar, S., Mave, V., Gupta, A., Cox, S. R., & Gupte, N. (2020). Mental health and quality of life among healthcare professionals during the COVID-19 pandemic in India. *Brain and Behavior, 10*(11), e01837. doi:10.1002/brb3.1837 PMID:32918403

Teoh, K. R., Hassard, J., & Cox, T. (2020). Individual and organizational psychosocial predictors of hospital doctors' work-related well-being: A multilevel and moderation perspective. *Health Care Management Review, 45*(2), 162–172. doi:10.1097/HMR.0000000000000207 PMID:29957704

Wilson, W., Raj, J. P., Rao, S., Ghiya, M., Nedungalaparambil, N. M., Mundra, H., & Mathew, R. (2020). Prevalence and predictors of stress, anxiety, and depression among healthcare workers managing COVID-19 pandemic in India: A nationwide observational study. *Indian Journal of Psychological Medicine, 42*(4), 353–358. doi:10.1177/0253717620933992 PMID:33398224

World Health Organization. (2003). *Consensus document on the epidemiology of severe acute respiratory syndrome (SARS) WHO/CDS/CSR/GAR/2003*. Retrieved from https://www.who.int/csr/sars/en/WHOconsensus.pdf

World Health Organization. (2020a). *Attacks on health care in the context of COVID-19*. Retrieved from https://www.who.int/news-room/feature-stories/detail/attacks-on-health-care-in-the-context-of-covid-19

World Health Organization. (2020b). *Keep health workers safe to keep patients safe*. Retrieved from https://www.who.int/news/item/17-09-2020-keep-health-workers-safe-to-keep-patients-safe-who

Chapter 2
Perceived Stress Levels of Medical and Non-Medical Staff in the Face of COVID-19

Sajedeh Rabipour
Islamic Azad University, Dubai, UAE

ABSTRACT

The sudden outbreak of COVID-19 as a deadly disease worldwide has caused widespread psychological problems as well as physical problems. Due to the importance of prevention and control of psychological problems in exposed individuals, the present study was conducted to investigate the perceived stress of medical and non-medical staff in the face of the epidemic of COVID-19 disease. 90.2% of the subjects had moderate job stress and 4.2% had severe stress. The level of stress in students was higher than formal and contract employees. Also, women had more stress than men, and people with medication, people without medication, and people with medical occupations more than non-medical occupations. Vulnerable groups in society, such as women, students, and healthcare workers, need more prevention and care in the COVID-19 crisis, which should be strengthened over time as effective coping strategies and disease epidemic management, access to medical resources, and mental health systems also plan national strategies and first aid in crises through telemedicine and online services.

INTRODUCTION

In December 2019, pneumonia erupted following the release of Covid 19 in Wuhan City, Hubei Province, China, and subsequently attracted worldwide attention (Chan et al., 2020). From the beginning of the outbreak to mid-April 2020, the Global Assessment Website has identified 204,952 patients with Covid 19 in Iran, of which 9,623 have died from the virus. According to statistics, Iran ranks ninth in the world in terms of the number of deaths due to Covid 19 to mid-April (Parker, 2021). Covid-19 has been repeatedly described as a deadly virus (Sheahan et al., 2020). "Covid infections are mild in humans, but epidemics of the two beta-coronavirus (SARS Covid 19) cause severe respiratory syndrome, so much so that in the Middle East, Covid 19 acute respiratory syndrome occurs," said Chalvin Huang, Quoting

DOI: 10.4018/978-1-7998-8813-0.ch002

the World Health Organization. "There have been thousands of deaths in the last two decades." Rapid transmission is a feature of such diseases and occurs as a result of close contact, pandemic or epidemic (Wang et al., 2020). The rapid rate of transmission and spread of the disease increases the vulnerability of people due to the fear of contracting the disease. Also, the ambiguous nature of the disease and its unfamiliarity, as well as the implementation of quarantine measures that have been strictly applied in some countries, such as China, caused a large number of people to be isolated and, consequently, many aspects of life were affected and caused Further increase in disease burden and widespread psychological problems such as panic disorder, anxiety and depression have been accompanied by physical problems (Wong et al., 2005). Stress and anxiety caused by the fear of being in the community cause people not to enter shopping centers, students not to enter educational centers and workers and tourists do not enter work and leisure institutions and as a result feel reduced independence and stress and worries about income and job security and Other cases have led to psychological problems, with governments in China, Singapore, and Australia expressing concern about the psychological side effects of Covid 19 and seeing the long-term effects of this isolation and fear in society as a serious threat to mental health (Wong et al., 2005).

Stress has long been considered as an important concept (Xiao et al., 2020). In fact, stress refers to the process of adaptation of a person when faced with internal and external challenges. It promotes psychological (anxiety, depression, memory loss, burnout) and pain disorders and is also associated with various physical health outcomes and diseases such as cancer, diabetes, cardiovascular disease and asthma and rheumatoid arthritis (Qiu et al., 2020). Perceived stress is considered as a result of the interaction between the person and his environment (Rosmond, 2005). Of course, the biggest debate in measuring stress is whether we should limit ourselves to measuring visible external stressors (shocking and big life events or the sum of small events) or whether we should focus on personal stress reactions (Suryadevara et al., 2020).

Research on previous epidemics in recent years has reported a wide range of psychosocial effects on individuals at the individual, social, and international levels during the outbreak of infectious infections (Parker, 2021); During the H1N1 flu epidemic, about 10% to 30% of the general public feared infection with the virus and disease (Mina et al., 2016; Hellhammer & Hellhammer, 2008), and in a study on the Ebola outbreak, people feared getting sick or dying. They experienced weakness, disability and social stigma (Liu et al., 2020). Also, health care professionals, especially those who work with patients with confirmed or suspected Covidus 19, are most at risk for both infection and mental health problems, and experience the fear of transmitting the virus to family, friends, or colleagues. they do. For example, a study in China during the SARS epidemic showed that nurses working in a high-risk clinical ward such as the SARS unit in a Beijing quarantine hospital were more likely to develop symptoms of acute post-traumatic stress (Suryadevara et al., 2020). Another study of hospital physicians and nurses in Wuhan, China, reported that 55% of health care workers experienced high levels of depressive symptoms, 44% experienced anxiety, and 34% experienced insomnia (Sheahan et al., 2020). "In the fight against the Covid epidemic, 19 health care workers are under a lot of pressure, including the risk of infection, insufficient pollution protection, overwork, frustration, discrimination, isolation, patients with negative emotions, Contact and contact with families and severe burnout; This condition caused psychological problems such as stress, anxiety, depressive symptoms, insomnia, denial, anger and fear. These mental health problems not only affect the attention and perception and decision-making ability of staff, but may also slow down the ability to fight Covid 19 and in a way can have a long-term effect on their long-term health that is noteworthy(Sheahan et al., 2020). Also, understanding the response and psychological response after emergency situations can help the treatment and care staff to prepare for a social response to a disaster or disaster (Yang et al., 2020). Based on the results of the presented studies and the severe effects of exposure to infectious infectious disease as well as Covid 19 disease on the physical and mental health of health workers and its direct and indirect effects on community health, attention to maintaining and promoting mental health of medical care workers is very important(Hall et al., 2008).

Because the Covid 19 epidemic is a public health emergency of international concern, it poses a challenge to psychological resilience. According to the evidence, ordinary people, patients, staff and family members of patients and health workers are at risk of psychological damage due to the epidemic of the virus. Understanding the mental state of people at risk for psychological disorders can help specialists in diagnosing these problems to provide targeted psychological interventions to improve the patient's mental health (Sheahan et al., 2020). With the onset of the Covid 19 epidemic in China, various studies have been conducted on mental disorders in different segments of society (Yang et al., 2020; Gao et al., 2020), but at present, limited information on the psychological impact and mental health of the general public at the height of the Covid 19 epidemic in Iran is available. Therefore, considering the prevalence of Covid 19 disease in Iran and the high population of hospitalization and care in all hospitals in the country as well as medical centers including hospitals and convalescents and the possibility of psychological impact of this epidemic in each community, the aim of this study was to determine perceived stress. Health and non-medical staff affiliated with Baqiyatallah University of Medical Sciences were exposed to Covid-19.

METHODS AND MATERIALS

The present study is a cross-sectional descriptive study that was conducted in April 2016. The study population included health care workers (physician, nurse, assistant nurse and final year medical and nursing students working in hospital) and unhealthy treatment (public and administrative jobs working in hospital such as secretary, nutritionist, recruitment and accounting, etc.) exposed to Covid 19 Were included in the study by available sampling method. The sample size was estimated using the Cochran's formula and the number of samples was calculated to be 508 with 95% confidence interval, so according to the probability of sample loss in this study, a total of 528 samples were studied.

All treatment and non-treatment staff exposed to Covid 19 who had access to a smartphone were included in the study. By asking questions in the demographic and demographic information section, people with a history of mental illness (stress, anxiety, depression, etc.) or who were taking anti-anxiety, anti-depressant, and anti-insane psychiatric medications were excluded from the study(Galal et al., 2014).

The instrument used in the study had two parts; The first part of the demographic and demographic information questionnaire included age, marital status, level of education, employment status, type of occupation (health and non-health treatment), presence or absence of underlying diseases, socio-economic status and drug use. The second part was the Perceived Stress Scale with ten items, the items of which included the negative and positive aspects of stress (Wang et al., 2020). This scale is designed with answering options in five Likert spectrums, in which the order of scores is zero to 4, and the score is calculated in reverse (never = 4, rarely = 3, sometimes = 2, often = 1, always = zero Except for questions 4, 5, 6 and 8, which are positively calculated. A total score of 13 is the usual stress level, but a total score of 20 or higher is considered high stress that requires therapeutic interventions (Wang et al., 2020). The validity of the questionnaire was confirmed by a study. In 2017 and its reliability was confirmed by calculating the Cronbach's alpha coefficient of more than 0.7 (Wang et al., 2020). The online questionnaire was designed using the online website and based on the inclusion of the relevant item in the online questionnaire, individuals were able to complete the questionnaire only once and those who did not complete all the questions in the questionnaire were considered as sample dropouts. A total of 12 samples were removed from the total population of the study participants due to incomplete completion of the questionnaire questions(Chan et al., 2020).

Perceived stress scale questions were provided online in the groups and channels of medical staff (medical and nursing) and non-hospital staff who met the inclusion criteria. Finally, after reaching the desired volume of the sample, the variables in the questionnaire and scale were coded and analyzed using SPSS software version 22. Significance level was considered equal to 0.05. First, demographic variables were described using frequency distribution tables, and then, for the proper use of descriptive indicators and inferential tests, the normality of the distribution of the studied variables was determined by using the Kolmogorov-Smirnov uniform test. Due to the abnormality of the distribution of variables, non-parametric tests were used for analysis. In the descriptive part, the minimum, maximum, median and amplitude indices of changes and in the inferential part, Mann-Whitney and Kruskalovalis non-parametric tests were used to test the research hypotheses(Cohen et al., 2007).

RESULTS AND DISCUSSION

Among 528 participants in the study, 31.8% were single and 68.2% were married, 52.7% were male and 47.3% were female and most of the samples (3.47%) were in the age group of 46-64 years. Occupationally, 57.4% were employed in health care and 42.6% in non-health care. The majority of the samples (50.9%) were official employees and the economic status of most of the samples (68.6%) was moderate, and also most of the people (92.0%) did not use drugs (Table 1)(Arefi & Poursadeqiyan, 2020).

90.2% of the samples had moderate perceived stress and 5.7% had mild or non-pathological stress and only 4.2% of the subjects had pathological and severe stress (Table 2).

Using Mann-Whitney test, stress level was not significantly associated with underlying diseases ($P = 0.65$) and marital status ($P = 0.14$). Also, using Kruskalovalis test, no significant relationship was observed between stress level with age ($P = 0.22$), education level ($P = 0.1$) and socio-economic status ($P = 0.76$). But as shown in Table 3, the relationship between stress level with gender ($P = 0.000$), type of employment ($P <0.000$), job ($P = 0.031$) and drug use ($P=0.019$) was significant, so that by comparing the means, women were more stressed than men, people who were taking drugs and people with medical occupations were more stressed than non-medical occupations, also according to Table 3, individuals Students had more stress than those with formal or contract employment(Yang et al., 2020).

The aim of this study was to investigate the perceived stress of hospital treatment and non-treatment staff in the face of Covid 19. The results of the study showed that the perceived stress level of exposure to Covid 19 in the majority of participants was moderate and about 4.2% was severe and pathological. In a similar study, Wang et al. Found that 8.1 percent of quarantined individuals had moderate to severe stress during the Covid 19 epidemic, with poor personal hygiene (wearing a mask and hand washing) with higher levels of stress (Wang et al., 2020). People who are quarantined at home experience stress and loneliness due to lack of space for physical activity, stress due to limited social interactions, and anxiety due to fear of transmitting the infection to family members, so their mental health needs more attention(Yang et al., 2020). In the United Kingdom and Austria, tallow et al. Rated the perceived stress

Table 1. Frequency distribution of demographic characteristics of the subjects

parameters		Population(Share%)
Age range	20-35	41(7.8%)
	36-46	237(44.9%)
	46-64	250(47.3%)
Gender	male	278(52.7%)
	female	250(47.3%)
Education	Diploma	99(18.8%)
	B.Sc.	237(44.9%)
	M.Sc.	178(33.7%)
	Ph.D.	14(2.7%)
marital status	Single	168(31.8%)
	married	360(68.2%)
Employment status	Full time	269.0(50.9%)
	Part time	120(22.7%)
	intern	139(26.2%)
Job type	Therapeutic	303(57.4%)
	Non-Therapeutic	225(42.6%)
Economic status	Low	103(19.5%)
	Middle	362(68.6%)
	High	63(14.9%)
Drug use	yes	42(8.0%)
	no	486(92.0%)
Total		528(100.0%)

scores of adults in the community as moderate to severe. In Iraq, Kamal and Uthman reported high levels of public stress during the Covid 19 epidemic, with higher levels of stress among those with higher education (Parker, 2021). In other studies in China, one month after the Covid epidemic, 19 levels of acute post-traumatic stress were reported in cities directly and non-directly involved with a prevalence of 7% to 46% (Suryadevara et al., 2020). This suggests that being separate from others can lead to negative emotions (Parker, 2021). In most studies, a high percentage of the general public (97%) were concerned about the prevalence of Covid-19 and 98% had minor disturbances in daily life (Arefi & Poursadeqiyan,

Table 2. Perceived stress of research units in the study group

Stress value	Population(Share%)
Intense	30(5.7%)
Mild	476(90.2%)
Light	22(4.2%)
Total	528(100.0%)

Table 3. Relationship between perceived stress and demographic characteristics

demographic		Mid	Sig.	Test
Gender	Male	254.88	0.000	Mann-Whitney
	Female	276.33		
Job	Therapeutic	270.12	0.031	Kruskalovalis
	Non-Therapeutic	254.99		
Drug use	yes	268.11	0.019	Manovitni Yu
	no	263.94		
Employment type	Full time	271.04	0.000	Mann-Whitney
	Part time	238.88		
	intern	59.287		

2020). Of course, the use of measures such as accurate updating of health information, especially about the number of recovered people, was associated with low stress levels in the Covid 19 epidemic in Chinese society. Additional information about drugs or vaccines, routes of transmission, and updates on the number of infected cases and locations (e.g., real-time, online tracking map) were also associated with lower anxiety levels (Suryadevara et al., 2020), which is important for consideration. Officials in crisis prevention and treatment planning are at the community level.

The results of this study showed that people with therapeutic occupations such as medicine and nursing (57.4%) had higher levels of stress than non-occupational occupations. Other studies in Iran also showed that the level of anxiety and depression of health care workers (physicians and nurses) was higher than the general level of society in the Covid epidemic (Suryadevara et al., 2020). During the CoV - MERS epidemic in Saudi Arabia, among medical staff, nurses became fearful and nervous after experiencing stressful patient care experiences (Rosmond, 2005). The results of a study in China during the Covid epidemic 19 showed that health care workers are highly vulnerable to serious psychological harm in their work environment (Qiu et al., 2020). In a study, Moayed et al. In Iran reported high levels of stress in medical staff, especially nurses, in the face of occupational hazards such as needle sticking (Sheahan et al., 2020). It has been stated that educational interventions according to the model of position stabilization in the occupational hazards of the emergency department and trauma care, are effective in reducing this stress (Qiu et al., 2020). Positive coping strategies with stress have also been found to be effective in reducing the stress of medical staff, so that Jiang et al. In a study on the Covid 19 crisis in China, the most important factor in reducing stress of medical staff was the positive attitude of their colleagues (Yang et al., 2020). As health care providers are at the forefront of dealing with the covid-19 epidemic crisis, they endure a great deal of physical and psychological burden that requires more attention and care from health care providers.

The results of our study showed that women had more stress than men. In most of the internal and external studies, the female population was more vulnerable to psychological disorders such as stress, anxiety and depression (Wang et al., 2020), which is consistent with the results of the present study. Evidence suggests that the higher prevalence of mental disorders in women than men may be more related to women's limitations in social participation, biological factors, and environmental stressors (Xiao et al., 2020). The results of our study also showed that students were more stressed than other medical staff, and that people who were official employees of the organization had more stress in the face of the outbreak of Covid 19. In some studies, younger age groups such as pupils and students were more prone to generalized anxiety and psychological distress (Xiao, 2020). In India, a video study by Adhara et al. Found that 19% of pharmacy students had severe stress on the Covid-19 epidemic (Wang et al., 2020), which could be related to the increased search on virtual networks for epidemic news and their increased stress. Less stress management experiences and appropriate coping skills are also likely to be associated with more interns' stress levels.

According to the results of studies and the stressful effect of Covid 19 disease on different segments of society, quarantined people, the general public, medical staff and their families, timely and effective psychological interventions along with medical care for patients with severe psychological distress, especially patients who need They have serious quarantine, it is mandatory and there is an emphasis on identifying and solving psychological problems in the disease process online (Arefi & Poursadeqiyan, 2020). During the Covid 19 epidemic, psychological counseling services were widely deployed in some countries, including China, using the telephone and the Internet for counseling or intervention programs, and China Provincial Council announced that it was launching online institutions in response to problems.

CONCLUSION

The findings of the present study showed the need for more vulnerable groups in society such as women, students and health care workers in the Covid 19 crisis to prevent and care, which should be reviewed by effective coping strategies and disease epidemic management, access to medical resources and psychiatric services for this group. Be further strengthened. Also, the planning of national strategies and first aid in crises through telemedicine and online services should be emphasized and considered with optimal systems of comprehensive interventions such as monitoring, screening and targeted and referral interventions to reduce psychological distress and prevent mental health problems. In this regard. One of the limitations of the present study is the lack of face sampling due to high risk and critical conditions of the disease and the importance of maintaining physical distance. To overcome this problem with the help of online questionnaire and share it via email and groups and channels, To a large extent this problem was solved. Given that the present study investigated the prevalence of perceived stress in medical and non-medical staff in the face of Covid 19, it is recommended that studies examine the prevalence of various psychological disorders (anxiety, depression, sleep disorders, etc.) or its relationship with quality of life. At different levels of society, especially health care staff in the country to be able to take effective measures in treatment and care planning.

REFERENCES

Arefi, M. F., & Poursadeqiyan, M. (2020). A review of studies on the epidemic crisis of COVID-19 disease with a preventive approach. *Work*, 1-13.

Chan, J. F. W., Yuan, S., Kok, K. H., To, K. K. W., Chu, H., Yang, J., Xing, F., Liu, J., Yip, C. C.-Y., Poon, R. W.-S., Tsoi, H.-W., Lo, S. K.-F., Chan, K.-H., Poon, V. K.-M., Chan, W.-M., Ip, J. D., Cai, J.-P., Cheng, V. C.-C., Chen, H., ... Yuen, K. Y. (2020). A familial cluster of pneumonia associated with the 2019 novel coronavirus indicating person-to-person transmission: A study of a family cluster. *Lancet, 395*(10223), 514–523. doi:10.1016/S0140-6736(20)30154-9 PMID:31986261

Cohen, S., Janicki-Deverts, D., & Miller, G. E. (2007). Psychological stress and disease. *Journal of the American Medical Association, 298*(14), 1685–1687. doi:10.1001/jama.298.14.1685 PMID:17925521

Galal, Y. S., Labib, J. R., & Abouelhamd, W. A. (2014). Impact of an infection-control program on nurses' knowledge and attitude in pediatric intensive care units at Cairo University hospitals. *The Journal of the Egyptian Public Health Association, 89*(1), 22–28. doi:10.1097/01.EPX.0000444562.71691.06 PMID:24717397

Gao, W., Ping, S., & Liu, X. (2020). Gender differences in depression, anxiety, and stress among college students: A longitudinal study from China. *Journal of Affective Disorders, 263*, 292–300. doi:10.1016/j.jad.2019.11.121 PMID:31818792

Hall, R. C., Hall, R. C., & Chapman, M. J. (2008). The 1995 Kikwit Ebola outbreak: Lessons hospitals and physicians can apply to future viral epidemics. *General Hospital Psychiatry, 30*(5), 446–452. doi:10.1016/j.genhosppsych.2008.05.003 PMID:18774428

Hellhammer, D., & Hellhammer, J. (Eds.). (2008). *Stress: the brain-body connection*. Karger Medical and Scientific Publishers. doi:10.1159/isbn.978-3-8055-7969-8

Liu, S., Yang, L., Zhang, C., Xiang, Y. T., Liu, Z., Hu, S., & Zhang, B. (2020). Online mental health services in China during the COVID-19 outbreak. *The Lancet. Psychiatry, 7*(4), e17–e18. doi:10.1016/S2215-0366(20)30077-8 PMID:32085841

Mina, T. H., Lahti, M., & Drake, A. J. (2016). Maternal lipids in pregnancy are associated with. *Psychoneuroendocrinology, 34*, 953–967. PMID:28599146

Parker, R. W. (2021). Why America's Response to the COVID-19 Pandemic Failed: Lessons from New Zealand's Success. *ADMIN L. REV., 73*, 77–77.

Qiu, J., Shen, B., Zhao, M., Wang, Z., & Xie, B. (2020). *A nationwide survey of psychological distress among Chinese people in the COVID-19 epidemic: implications and policy recommendations*. Academic Press.

Rosmond, R. (2005). Role of stress in the pathogenesis of the metabolic syndrome. *Psychoneuroendocrinology, 30*(1), 1–10. doi:10.1016/j.psyneuen.2004.05.007 PMID:15358437

Sheahan, T. P., Sims, A. C., Leist, S. R., Schäfer, A., Won, J., Brown, A. J., Montgomery, S. A., Hogg, A., Babusis, D., Clarke, M. O., Spahn, J. E., Bauer, L., Sellers, S., Porter, D., Feng, J. Y., Cihlar, T., Jordan, R., Denison, M. R., & Baric, R. S. (2020). Comparative therapeutic efficacy of remdesivir and combination lopinavir, ritonavir, and interferon beta against MERS-CoV. *Nature Communications, 11*(1), 1–14. doi:10.103841467-019-13940-6 PMID:31924756

Suryadevara, V., Adusumalli, C., Adusumilli, P. K., Chalasani, S. H., & Radhakrishnan, R. (2020). Mental health status among the south Indian pharmacy students during Covid-19 pandemic quarantine period: A cross-sectional study. medRxiv.

Wang, C., Pan, R., Wan, X., Tan, Y., Xu, L., Ho, C. S., & Ho, R. C. (2020). Immediate psychological responses and associated factors during the initial stage of the 2019 coronavirus disease (COVID-19) epidemic among the general population in China. *International Journal of Environmental Research and Public Health*, *17*(5), 1729. doi:10.3390/ijerph17051729 PMID:32155789

Wong, T. W., Yau, J. K., Chan, C. L., Kwong, R. S., Ho, S. M., Lau, C. C., Lau, F. L., & Lit, C. H. (2005). The psychological impact of severe acute respiratory syndrome outbreak on healthcare workers in emergency departments and how they cope. *European Journal of Emergency Medicine*, *12*(1), 13–18. doi:10.1097/00063110-200502000-00005 PMID:15674079

Xiao, H., Zhang, Y., Kong, D., Li, S., & Yang, N. (2020). Social capital and sleep quality in individuals who self-isolated for 14 days during the coronavirus disease 2019 (COVID-19) outbreak in January 2020 in China. *Medical Science Monitor*, *26*, e923921–e1. doi:10.12659/MSM.923921 PMID:32194290

Yang, X., Yu, Y., Xu, J., Shu, H., Liu, H., Wu, Y., ... Shang, Y. (2020). Clinical course and outcomes of critically ill patients with SARS-CoV-2 pneumonia in Wuhan, China: A single-centered, retrospective, observational study. *The Lancet. Respiratory Medicine*, *8*(5), 475–481. doi:10.1016/S2213-2600(20)30079-5 PMID:32105632

KEY TERMS AND DEFINITIONS

COVID-19: Coronavirus disease 2019 (COVID-19) is a contagious disease caused by severe acute respiratory syndrome coronavirus 2 (SARS-CoV-2). The first known case was identified in Wuhan, China, in December 2019. The disease has since spread worldwide, leading to an ongoing pandemic.

Delusion: A delusion is a fixed belief that is not amenable to change in light of conflicting evidence. As a pathology, it is distinct from a belief based on false or incomplete information, confabulation, dogma, illusion, hallucination, or some other misleading effects of perception, as individuals with those beliefs are able to change or readjust their beliefs upon reviewing the evidence.

Major Depressive Disorder: Major depressive disorder (MDD), also known simply as depression, is a mental disorder characterized by at least two weeks of pervasive low mood, low self-esteem, and loss of interest or pleasure in normally enjoyable activities. Those affected may also occasionally have delusions or hallucinations. Introduced by a group of US clinicians in the mid-1970s, the term was adopted by the American Psychiatric Association for this symptom cluster under mood disorders in the 1980 version of the Diagnostic and Statistical Manual of Mental Disorders (DSM-III) classification, and has become widely used since.

Psychosomatic Medicine: Psychosomatic medicine is an interdisciplinary medical field exploring the relationships among social, psychological, and behavioral factors on bodily processes and quality of life in humans and animals. The academic forebear of the modern field of behavioral medicine and a part of the practice of consultation-liaison psychiatry, psychosomatic medicine integrates interdisciplinary evaluation and management involving diverse specialties including psychiatry, psychology, neurology, psychoanalysis, internal medicine, pediatrics, surgery, allergy, dermatology, and psychoneuroimmunology. Clinical situations where mental processes act as a major factor affecting medical outcomes are areas where psychosomatic medicine has competence.

Stress: Stress, either physiological, biological, or psychological is an organism's response to a stressor such as an environmental condition. Stress is the body's method of reacting to a condition such as a threat, challenge, or physical and psychological barrier. Stimuli that alter an organism's environment are responded to by multiple systems in the body. In humans and most mammals, the autonomic nervous system and hypothalamic-pituitary-adrenal (HPA) axis are the two major systems that respond to stress.

Chapter 3
The Impact of COVID-19 on the Mental Health and Well-Being of Immigrant Healthcare Workers:
Intersectionality Matters

Myia S. Williams
Northwell Health, USA

Vidhi H. Patel
https://orcid.org/0000-0001-9888-8893
Northwell Health, USA

ABSTRACT

The COVID-19 pandemic has placed tremendous strain and presented unprecedented challenges for health systems and healthcare workers (HCW) across the world. Research shows that HCW on the front-line are at higher risk of burnout, anxiety, depression, and symptoms of post-traumatic stress disorder, just to name a few. Traditionally, research on mental health and HCW has predominantly focused on the generalized healthcare professional workforce. Largely missing from this conversation are immigrant HCW. This is surprising given that immigrant workers are crucially important in treating Americans fighting COVID-19 and over-represented in various healthcare occupations and States. Through an intersectionality lens, the authors identify unique factors during the COVID-19 pandemic that can impact the mental health of immigrant HCW. The authors discuss the negative attitudes towards immigrant HCW and mental health outcomes and the unique intersecting factors of race, immigrant status, and class. Recommendations for future interventions, research, and practical implications are provided.

INTRODUCTION

A considerable amount of research has revealed the negative impact of the COVID-19 pandemic on the mental health and well-being of healthcare workers (HCW) (Qiu et al., 2021; Spoorthy, 2020; Tella et

DOI: 10.4018/978-1-7998-8813-0.ch003

al., 2020; Young et al., 2020). Despite the prevalence of mental health challenges of HCW during COVID-19, little attention has been paid to immigrant or foreign-born HCW (Griswold & Salmon, 2020). This is surprising given that immigrant workers are crucially important in treating Americans and fighting COVID-19 (Griswold & Salmon, 2020). For example, at the peak of the COVID-19 pandemic in the United States (U.S), The Migration Policy Institute estimated there were six million immigrant workers on the frontlines of the COVID-19 pandemic keeping Americans safe and fed (Gelatt, 2020), of which 1.7 million were HCW (Bier, 2020; Bureau of Labor Statistics, 2020; Lee et al., 2020). Furthermore, at least two of the developers of the COVID-19 Moderna and Pfizer vaccines were either immigrants or children of immigrants (Kochenderfer, 2021). Immigrant workers are also a large part of the hospital cleaning staff and medical and research scientists (Gelatt, 2020).

So far, research on the mental health challenges of HCW during COVID-19 has focused on identifying and examining high risks groups and evaluating the effectiveness of psychological and organizational-based resources or interventions through a lens of pre-existing COVID-19 factors (Ming & De Jong, 2021). These factors include, but are not limited to demographics such as gender (Tella et al., 2020), living conditions, and established personal relationships (Young et al., 2020), as well as psychological resources that individuals possessed pre-COVID-19 such as resilience (Heath et al., 2020). Recently, studies, commentaries, and other scholarly work have begun to examine the impact of the COVID-19 pandemic on the mental health of immigrant/foreign-born workers (Tiwari et al., 2020). Early findings suggest that COVID-19 has a significant detrimental impact on immigrant HCW and healthcare organizations, including deteriorated psychological well-being (e.g. anxiety, emotional exhaustion/burnout, loneliness/isolation, and anxiety), job withdrawal (e.g. turnover intentions), and negative job attitudes (e.g. job dissatisfaction) (Mahajan, 2020; Mathema, 2020; Tiwari et al., 2020). Despite the significant progress and the potential value that recent studies have made in understanding the consequences of COVID-19 on the mental health and well-being of immigrant/foreign-born and native-born HCW in general (Spoorthy, 2020; Tiwari et al., 2020), more research is needed to provide an understanding of the complex ways in which the COVID-19 may have possibly differentially and disproportionally affected the immigrant HCW and consequently leading to a higher mental health burden and poorer well-being during the pandemic and beyond (Cubrich & Tengesdal, 2021; Maestripieri, 2021).

Specifically, more research that sufficiently investigates how intersections between existing structures of social inequalities of race, class, and immigrant status compound to affect the impact of COVID-19 on the mental health and well-being of immigrant HCW is desperately needed (Cubrich & Tengesdal, 2021). An analysis of the literature on the impact of COVID-19 on mental health has revealed an over-representation and "one size fits all" blanket of high-skilled frontline HCW (e.g. nurses and physicians) with an equivalent underrepresentation of immigrant HCW and other minoritized groups, low-skilled, non-traditional health-related occupations (Vizheh et al., 2020). Irrespective of initial claims, COVID-19 is not an equalizer as it has been noted that worker status (e.g. essential worker vs non-essential worker) does not inevitably affect every psychological process and phenomenon, but there are several unique and complex factors accompanying one's worker status such as race, gender, immigrant status that have clear implications for understanding the mental health effects of the pandemic (Cubrich & Tengesdal, 2021; Maestripieri, 2021).

An examination of the intersections of unique factors is indeed important as only when they are explicitly identified can effective interventions be taken to minimize the negative impact of pandemics on mental health and well-being for immigrant/foreign-born and native-born HCW, as well as members of the general public (Cubrich & Tengesdal, 2021; Maestripieri, 2021; Ming & De Jong, 2021). Hence, there is a need to piece together the many concurrent moving parts occurring during the COVID-19 pandemic that are related to mental health and well-being (Cubrich & Tengesdal, 2021; Maestripieri, 2021; Ming & De Jong, 2021). This is important for two reasons. First, as we detail below immigrant HCW are over-represented in various healthcare-related occupations and states throughout the US, however, there are examined as a monolithic population whose experiences are investigated under the umbrella of the larger racial/ethnic minority populations (Cubrich & Tengesdal, 2021). Second, COVID-19 has brought to the forefront long-existing and well-documented social inequities that are associated with race/ethnicity, class, immigrant status, and gender (Cubrich & Tengesdal, 2021; Lee et al., 2020; Maestripieri, 2021).

It is to this point that there has been a call for more research on this issue to better understand the detrimental impact of mental health challenges during a pandemic, particularly for immigrant/foreign-born workers on the front lines of the COVID-19 pandemic (Clark et al., 2020; Cubrich & Tengesdal, 2021; Maestripieri, 2021; Ming & De Jong, 2021; Spoorthy, 2020). We respond to the call by investigating through an intersectionality lens the unique factors that arise pre and during the COVID-19 pandemic that can impact the mental health and well-being of immigrant HCW. As one of the most widely cited frameworks within the inequality literature in feminist and gender studies, the intersectionality framework evaluates the intersections of multiple factors of inequalities (such as race/ethnicity, immigrant status, class, and gender), which have a multiplying and cumulative effect when historically marginalized identities intersect in the same individual (Cubrich & Tengesdal, 2021; Maestripieri, 2021). The COVID-19 pandemic is a distinct example of an intersectional phenomenon (Maestripieri, 2021), as the disparities experienced by historically minoritized communities and individuals are a result of a plethora of longstanding interrelated social structures of inequality (Cubrich & Tengesdal, 2021; Maestripieri, 2021). Immigrant HCW have multiple intersecting identities which is why it is important to explore the role of intersectionality when examining the impact of COVID-19 on their mental health and well-being.

In this chapter, our aim is two folds. First, we aim to synthesize the evidence of the impact of the COVID-19 pandemic on the mental health of immigrant HCW. Second, we intend to raise awareness of the issues and challenges faced by this population which is often understudied. We will do this by highlighting some of the unique factors that impacted the mental health and well-being of the immigrant HCW during the COVID-19 pandemic. We begin by describing the demographic profile of HCW in the US labor force and immigration experiences. Next, we discuss the negative attitudes towards immigrant HCW and mental health outcomes. Then we discuss the unique intersecting factors of race, immigrant status, and class and conclude by providing considerations for developing future interventions as well as practical implications.

CHARACTERISTICS OF IMMIGRANT HEALTHCARE WORKERS IN THE UNITED STATES LABOR FORCE

Immigrant/foreign-born HCW herein referred to as immigrant HCW, is defined as any healthcare worker who is born outside of the US and/or received their training inside or outside of the US and is currently living and working in healthcare systems in the US. For the purposes of this chapter, we would like to only focus on immigrant HCW who are born outside of the US. Hence, while the term *international medical graduates* (IMG) includes physicians who are US citizens or permanent residents who received training outside of the US and practice in the US (Tiwari et al., 2020), our focus is only on those who are born outside of the US and practice in the US. Similarly, we are aware that there are several foreign-born/

immigrant biomedical and other researchers, biostatisticians, chemists, and others who are working in healthcare industries helping to fight the COVID-19 pandemic, yet for this chapter, we only encompass the experiences of immigrant HCW who are in patient-facing occupations.

According to the Bureau of Labor of Statistics, in 2019, there were 28.4 million (17.4%) immigrant workers in the U.S workforce (Bureau of Labor Statistics, 2020). Many advocates for immigrant workers argue that immigrant HCW can ease the burden of overwhelmed healthcare systems as an efficient immigration system can help increase the supply of immigrant HCW to help fight the COVID-19 pandemic (Bier, 2020; Nowrasteh & Landgrave, 2020; Tiwari et al., 2020). That said, with at least 1 in every 5 HCW being an immigrant, immigrants continue to be overrepresented in both high and low skilled health-related occupations in healthcare fields (Bier, 2020; Lee et al., 2020). For example, in 2018, although legal immigrants over the age of 16 made up 12.1% of the population and undocumented immigrants 4.2%, they were about 15% and 2.3% of all HCW, respectively. This means that legal immigrants were 19% more likely to work in the healthcare field and 72% more likely to be surgeons and physicians compared to native-born individuals in the same age group (Nowrasteh & Landgrave, 2020). Overall, 29% (1 in 4) of physicians, 16% (1 in 6) of registered nurses, 20% (1 in 5) of pharmacists, and 23% (1 in 4) of all nursing, psychiatric, and home health aides are immigrants (Griswold & Salmon, 2020; Patel et al., 2018). Lastly, compared to native-born individuals, immigrant HCW are more likely to be nursing assistants, home healthcare aides, and personal care aids (Batalova, 2020; Bier, 2020; Lee et al., 2020).

Immigrant HCW are also more likely to be overrepresented across the US and within various states. In fact, across 43 states, HCW were more likely to be immigrants than native-born (Nowrasteh & Landgrave, 2020). In states like New York, California, and New Jersey, data from 2018 showed the number of HCW was at least two times higher than the national level, with immigrant workers representing 37%, 35%, and 34% respectively of all HCW. Other states like Florida (30%), Maryland (28%), and Nevada (26%) followed closely behind (Batalova, 2020). Immigrant physicians, surgeons, and nurses were also more likely to be overrepresented across US states. For example, while immigrants were 8% of the population in Michigan, they were 9% of HCW and 28%, or three times more likely, to be physicians and surgeons (Batalova, 2020).

A similar trend was seen across New Jersey (39%), Nevada (38%), Florida and New York (both at 36%), and Massachusetts (34%), whose immigrant population was relatively low compared to the representation of immigrant physicians and surgeons. Likewise, states such as Nevada (36%), California (35%), Maryland (30%), and New York (29%) also had high numbers of immigrant nurses (Batalova, 2020). Lastly, immigrants were also highly represented across various low-skilled healthcare occupations such as health-aides. For example, states such as New York (75%), New Jersey (55%), Florida (52%), Maryland (47%), and Massachusetts (45%) had more immigrant health-aides than native-born individuals (Batalova, 2020).

Immigrant HCW are not a monolith as they come from a wide variety of cultural backgrounds, religions, norms, and values (Bier, 2020). In the US alone, immigrants represent every country in the world, yet there appears to be a higher concentration of immigrant HCW migrating from certain regions compared to others (Budiman, 2020). In 2018, 40% of immigrant HCW were from Asia, 16% from the Caribbean, and 14% from Mexico and Central America making up the top three regions. At least 12% of immigrant HCW came from Africa and Europe, Northern America and Oceania (collectively), and only 6% of immigrant HCW are from South America (Batalova, 2020).

In a related vein, immigrant HCW from various regions are also likely to be more concentrated in various healthcare occupations. Immigrant HCW employed in healthcare support occupations are likely to be from Mexico and Central America (66%), the Caribbean (60%), Africa (48%), and South America (47%). More specifically, certain immigrant HCW are likely to be prevalent in certain healthcare support occupations. For example, at least 28% of personal care aides are Mexico and Central America-born, 24% of registered nurses are likely to be Asia and African-born (each), 23% and 18% of home health aides and nursing assistants, respectively, are Caribbean-born, and 15% of physicians and surgeons are likely to be Asian-born and Europe, Northern America and Oceania-born (each). Of note, at least 33% and 31% of other healthcare practitioners (e.g. family and general practitioners) and technical occupations (e.g. pharmacy technicians) are European, Northern America, and Oceania-born and Asia-born respectively (Batalova, 2020).

Immigration Policies, Procedures, and Attitudes: Immigration as a Gray Area

The high proportion and overrepresentation of immigrant HCW in various states and healthcare-related occupations highlights the specific need to include immigrants in COVID-19 responses and efforts as well as to have interventions specifically tailored towards them. Ironically, despite the importance of immigrant HCW in the fight against COVID-19, immigrant-related issues have halted their ability to maneuver the COVID-19 pandemic particularly as it relates to the working environment (Bier, 2020; Mahajan, 2020; Tiwari et al., 2020). Immigration policies, processes, and procedures around hiring, certifying medical licenses, training, and retaining immigrant HCW are rather multifaceted, complex, and restrictive (Mahajan, 2020; Mathema, 2019). The road to permanent residency or citizenship for immigrant HCW is rather long with many obstacles along the way that depletes the financial and social resources of the immigrant HCW and can take upwards of 10 years post-training (Mathema, 2019). For example, many of the visas under which immigrant HCW practice require them to travel frequently to and from their home countries for renewal and do not have a direct pathway to permanent residency (e.g., green card)(Mahajan, 2020; Tiwari et al., 2020).

Immigrant HCW practice or train in the US under either a J-1 exchange visitor (which allows the immigrant HCW to gain knowledge and skills that are of value to their home country) or an H-1B temporary employment visa (which allows recruitment and subsequential employment to immigrants in specialty occupations such as research) (Mathema, 2019). Under the J-1 visa, after completion of residency training, immigrant HCW are required to return to their home country for 2 years. As an alternative path to permanent residency under the J-1 visa, immigrant physicians, for example, can practice in an underserved region or hospital for three years and then apply for permanent residency (Mahajan, 2020; Tiwari et al., 2020). Hence, many immigrant HCW are located in low-income and underserved regions which were hardest hit by thc COVID-19 pandemic (Lee et al., 2020; Mahajan, 2020; Tiwari et al., 2020).

Conversely, immigrant HCW under the H-1B visa, require an employer to sponsor them after school or training. The H1-B visa is for a 6-year period with renewal required after the first 3 years. Immigrant HCW on an H-1B visa can file for a green card; for immigrant physicians that process can begin after their complete residency (Mathema, 2019; Tiwari et al., 2020). In addition, immigrant HCW (e.g., physicians, surgeons) can apply for permanent residency through an "employment-based" (EB) green card under multiple categories such as EB – 1 (priority workers), EB -2 (professionals holding advance degrees and those of exceptional ability) and EB – 3 (skilled workers, professionals, and unskilled workers/other workers) (U.S. Department of State, n.d.).

One such example of an EB-2 green card is the National Interest Waiver (NIW) which allows highly skilled immigrant HCW to apply for green cards provided that they can prove that it is within national interest that they continue to work and perform their duties in the US (Mathema, 2019; Tiwari et al., 2020). The process for receiving an EB green card is rather prolonged and, in some cases, can be restrictive and difficult to attain for immigrant HCW from certain countries such as India and China. For example, only 7% of EB green cards are allocated per country. Of note, the last EB-2 application for Indian-born and Chinese-born immigrant physicians was in 2009 and 2016, respectively (Tiwari et al., 2020). The COVID-19 pandemic further heightened the legal barriers faced by immigrant HCW, therefore, adding an extra layer that threatens their mental health and well-being.

Negative Attitudes Towards Immigrant Healthcare Workers

Before the COVID-19 pandemic, as the population of immigrant HCW increased to fill the shortage of HCW in the US, native-born individuals' public perceptions and opinions of immigrant HCW, as well as social and political circumstances, determined their experiences (Spilsbury & Cooney, 1998). Rightfully so, throughout the COVID-19 pandemic HCW have been hailed as heroes in the fight against the COVID-19 pandemic; yet, in the same vein, immigrant HCW have often been referred to as subpar healthcare providers (Mahajan, 2020; Spilsbury & Cooney, 1998; Tiwari et al., 2020). In recent years, and even during the COVID-19 pandemic, attitudes towards immigrant HCW and immigrants in general, have become increasingly xenophobic and hostile leading to a significant impact on the mental health and well-being of immigrant HCW (Dhanani & Franz, 2021; Ming & De Jong, 2021; Yellow Horse, 2021).

For example, during the pandemic, there were several reports of Asian American and Pacific Islanders (AAPI) including immigrant HCW of the same racial background having to deal with racist and xenophobic incidents because some members of the general public believed that they were responsible for the COVID-19 virus (Dhanani & Franz, 2021; Ming & De Jong, 2021; Yellow Horse, 2021). This was also fueled when then-President Trump referred to the virus as the "Chinese virus" on Twitter (Budhwani & Sun, 2020). There are also many reports from immigrant HCW of discrimination, racism, ostracism, bullying, and other forms of workplace mistreatment from management, co-workers, and patients alike, resulting in decreased mental well-being and organizational outcomes (e.g. job satisfaction and morale) (Choi et al., 2020; Ming & De Jong, 2021).

Furthermore, the short supply and increasing demand for healthcare jobs have also led to negative attitudes of immigrant HCW and subsequent conservative immigrant laws and policies which have ultimately affected the mental health and well-being of immigrant HCW (Ming & De Jong, 2021; Spilsbury & Cooney, 1998). Initially, HCW were welcomed into the U.S, however, with the lack of HCW in the U.S to fill critical healthcare-related jobs and the increased prevalence of immigrant HCW, native-born HCW perceived them as a threat who was "here to take our jobs" (Spilsbury & Cooney, 1998). As a result, on an interpersonal level, native-born HCW were likely to withhold critical information on resources that are vital for the immigrant HCW to adapt and function adequately in the working environment. On a legal level, U.S Congress passed conservative bills which led to more restrictive immigration laws around visa regulations, work permits, and licensing (Chen et al., 2013; Spilsbury & Cooney, 1998).

Mental Health Outcomes of Immigrant HCW during the COVID-19 Pandemic

Living through the current COVID-19 pandemic, which has been touted as a severe global health disaster by many, is unprecedented in numerous ways, both due to the nature of the disease itself and its long-lasting psychological effects which are still being discovered. A 2020 systematic review on the psychological impact on HCW found that frontline HCW are among the most vulnerable groups at risk of mental health problems (Cabarkapa et al., 2020). For example, in a recent large- study on 1,257 HCW exploring the mental health impact of the COVID-19 pandemic, researchers found high rates of depression, anxiety, and insomnia with over 70% of people reporting psychological distress (Lai et al., 2020).

One of the most visible, but not well understood, are the risks to the mental health and well-being of immigrant HCW during the pandemic. While there is previous literature regarding mental health stressors in the general population and HCW at large, there is a dearth of research focusing on immigrant HCW mental health (depression, anxiety, burnout, traumatic stress being the most common), especially during the COVID-19 pandemic (Chishti & Bolter, 2020; Lee et al., 2020). Considering the over-representation of immigrant HCW in the healthcare occupations, we borrow from the mental health literature on HCW to lend support.

Anxiety and depression were significantly more prevalent in doctors and nurses compared with other occupations on the frontlines of the COVID-19 pandemic (Luceño-Moreno et al., 2020; Shechter et al., 2020). In the US, a cross-sectional study of 657 physicians and nurses indicated that 57% of participants screened positively for acute stress, 48% and 33% for depressive and anxiety symptoms, respectively, with nurses and advanced practice providers more likely to experience psychological distress (Shechter et al., 2020). Similar findings were seen across the globe. For example, in Spain, one of the hardest-hit places in the early outbreak, of the 1,422 health workers surveyed, 56.6% reported feelings of post-traumatic stress disorder, emotional exhaustion, and depersonalization contributing to psychological distress (Luceño-Moreno et al., 2020).

Comparable results were observed in Italy, where 49.3% of respondents reported post-traumatic stress, 21.9% high perceived stress, 19.8% insomnia, 24.7% depression, and 8.2% anxiety (Rossi et al., 2020). Unsurprisingly, results were also no different in the U.S. where Mental Health America (2020) conducted a large-scale study of 1,119 HCW in June- September 2020. Results showed 93% of HCW experienced stress in the last three months, 86% anxiety, 77% frustration, 76% exhaustion/burnout, and 75% feelings of being overwhelmed. Moreover, 39% reported inadequate emotional support with 45% nurses were even less likely to have emotional support. Of note, the largest groups of participants were healthcare staff (30%) and nurses (22%), two occupations where immigrants are overrepresented.

The many risks and factors contributing to the well-being of immigrant HCW are not well understood as these vary from immigrant HCW contracting COVID-19 virus, fear, uncertainty, transmitting the virus to others, loss of family and/or friends, social isolation, loneliness, suicidal thoughts, and stigma while working at the frontlines (Chishti & Bolter, 2020; Lee et al., 2020; Mahajan, 2020). The situations faced by immigrant HCW during the pandemic have been compared to nothing short of a war zone as they have been forced to play both a victim and a service provider (Brooks et al., 2020). These findings echo research during the Severe Acute Respiratory Syndrome (SARS) epidemic (Lancee et al., 2008)

However, there is a scarcity of information about the impact on mental health outcomes during a pandemic of this proportion and how to best address this psychological distress (Lee et al., 2020). Although previous studies have shown that any epidemic or outbreak can lead to psychological distress or adverse reactions, these are dependent on both individual as well as contextual and environmental factors (Brooks et al., 2016). For instance, studies have illustrated that immigrants tend to use mental health services or resources at lower rates than non-immigrants, despite an equal or greater need for these services (Bauldry & Szaflarski, 2017). Structural barriers such as lack of insurance, high cost, and language are some of the key factors that drive this discrepancy which forces immigrants to rely on family, friends, or local community leaders for help (Derr, 2015). Furthermore, countless immigrants were excluded from government stimulus packages or financial relief which was designed to mitigate the effect of COVID-19, adding additional stress on these individuals during the COVID-19 pandemic (Amandolare et al., 2020; Chishti & Bolter, 2020).

As evidenced by the findings of various studies that have been published regarding the mental health outcomes and by combining the statistics of immigrants in the health care workforce, we can extrapolate these findings to immigrant HCW, as this category of HCW are likely to experience more of these stressors than their non-immigrant HCW counterparts. In the next section, we discuss how the intersection of factors such as race, immigrant status, and class adds an additional layer to the mental health effects.

OVERVIEW OF WORKPLACE EXPERIENCES OF IMMIGRANT HCW DURING COVID-19 PANDEMIC AT THE INTERSECTION OF RACE, CLASS, AND IMMIGRANT STATUS

In this section, we provide evidence to support *why the COVID-19 pandemic is likely to disproportionately affect the mental health and well-being of immigrant healthcare workers.* Immigrant HCW are more susceptible to worse mental health and well-being because their vulnerability lies at the intersection of race, class, and immigrant status (Cubrich & Tengesdal, 2021; Guadagno, 2020). Coined by Kimberly Crenshaw, intersectionality means an individual with two or more protected classes (e.g., race and national origin) are affected by several discriminations and disadvantages. Intersectionality provides a useful framework for understanding the impact of COVID-19 on immigrant HCW as it shows how intersecting identities (e.g., race, immigrant status, and class) and systems (e.g., healthcare, anti-immigrant policies, and society) intertwine to create an added layer of disadvantage and harm which contributes to cumulative adverse mental health effects (Cubrich & Tengesdal, 2021).

Acculturation and Acculturative Stress

We wanted to first briefly touch on the acculturation process and acculturative stress which may have existed before the COVID-19 pandemic for many immigrant HCW. Historically, the process of acculturation and migration is a significant life event that presents chronic stressors that adversely affect an immigrant's mental health (Berry, 1997). Acculturation is defined as "the process of psychological and behavioral change individuals and groups undergo as a consequence of long-term contact with another culture" (Zea et al., 2003, p. 108). For an immigrant, being a "stranger in a strange land" can result in several changes from resource loss during migration that can affect their mental health and well-being. For example, immigrant HCW can experience feelings of homesickness, alienation, and nuances in learning new cultural norms and languages that make it difficult to adjust to the host culture (Cohen et al., 2018; Mehta, 2014). These changes can lead to stress which constitutes the negative side of the acculturation process that, although frequent, are not necessarily inevitably present (Williams & Berry, 1991). More specifically, *acculturative stress* arises from the stressors that are tied specifically to the acculturation process.

Acculturative stress leads to outcomes such as anxiety, depression, feelings of alienation and marginality, identity confusion, and psychosomatic symptoms which results in a reduction of the mental health and well-being of the immigrant (Berry, 1997; Williams & Berry, 1991). Hence, the addition of stressors from the COVID-19 pandemic will only serve to exacerbate anxiety and depression. Similarly, in research on traumatic life events (e.g., chronic death) and immigrants, Ward et al., (2018) found that immigrants who had witnessed traumatic events such as violence and excess death reported higher levels of depression.

Work and Working Conditions (Class)

As noted earlier, an immigrant HCW comprised a disproportionate share of the workers on the frontlines, particularly in communities with high COVID-19 infection rates, placing them at a higher risk of contracting the COVID-19 virus and dying from it (Lee et al., 2020). Immigrant HCW, such as health-aids at various health facilities were more likely to fill in for staff shortages, work non-traditional shifts, and risk death for a paycheck irrespective of on-the-job risks and despite not qualifying for hazard pay, lack of proper compensation, sick leave options, testing, inability to social distance in the workplace, language barriers, fear of deportation, and lack of proper protective equipment (PPE) (Griswold & Salmon, 2020; Lee et al., 2020). Furthermore, as front-line workers, immigrant HCW were unable to work from home and were near infected co-workers and patients without adequate PPE, all of which created intense fear and anxiety about infecting family members and friends.

Alternatively, family and friends also feared that immigrant HCW would infect them (Bhandari et al., 2021). Despite these work-related constraints, a high risk of the possibility of COVID-19 infection, and showing COVID-19 symptoms, immigrant HCW still had to come to work out of fear of deportation and reduced income insecurity and loss (Clark et al., 2020; Guadagno, 2020; Tiwari et al., 2020). Across the board, there is empirical support that a lack of proper protective gear, testing, and being on the frontlines have left HCW with severe mental health problems (Arnetz et al., 2020); for immigrant HCW, this is exacerbated due to their inability to get social support from family members who might be thousands of miles away and/or having to face immigration-related issues such as those implemented by the Trump administration (e.g. restricting temporary work visas such as H1B visa for skilled immigrant workers and barring of grant relief for international and undocumented students including Deferred Action for Childhood Arrival, DACA student of which some immigrant HCW were part of (e.g. medical students)) (Mahajan, 2020; Tiwari et al., 2020).

Again, due to anti-immigration policies, immigrant HCW may become underemployed or unemployed which resulted in abrupt loss of income particularly for those who had lower incomes and limited access to savings which led to financial and food insecurity (Guadagno, 2020). Despite paying their fair share of taxes, immigrant HCW were also likely to be excluded from certain government programs (e.g., welfare programs) that protect individuals who lose their jobs or had reduced hours due to pandemic relatedlated lockdowns. Similarly, in some occupations, immigrant HCW may be unable to get paid time off (were also unable to take time off because of financial insecurity) or have paid sick time and unemployment benefits. As a result, they were at times excluded from organizational and government financial aids provided during the COVID-19 pandemic or failed to be included and prioritized when assistance was provided and resources were limited (Clark et al., 2020; Gelatt, 2020; Guadagno, 2020).

For example, in a report on New York City's immigrant population, Amandolare et al., (2020) found that non-profit organizations that catered to immigrant individuals reported at least 95 to 100% of their immigrant clients did not receive the $1,200 stimulus package during the COVID-19 pandemic. Of note, New York City was once the epicenter of the pandemic and, as reported earlier, has a large proportion of immigrant HCW (Batalova, 2020). Not surprising, immigrants in this report also indicated high levels of mental health challenges and impact on their overall well-being; however, there was limited access to mental health services and in the event they were available, immigrants were placed on a long waiting list (Amandolare et al., 2020).

Before the COVID-19 pandemic immigrant HCW may have been working in toxic and exploitative conditions which impacted their mental health (Schilgen et al., 2020; Tiwari et al., 2020). COVID-19 stressors such as lockdowns and the threat of income loss may have intensified such conditions and its subsequent effects (Guadagno, 2020; Ming & De Jong, 2021). In addition to work-related visa restrictions (e.g. H1-B visas allow for immigrant workers to work for one specific company and need to be sponsored to work for another company), the COVID-19 pandemic may have made it even more difficult and provided limited options to job opportunities, job search, or move to another job both internally and externally. Additionally, immigrant HCW may have had limited savings to cope with hardship due to a loss of employment for the household breadwinner or other source of income in the household (Clark et al., 2020; Guadagno, 2020). For immigrant HCW on employment-based visas, it was even more difficult to leave the employer, plus there were fears of being laid off and subsequent deportation, as well as an inability to pay to renew work permits/visas if income is reduced or lost and U.S embassies are closed with lockdowns instituted worldwide (Griswold & Salmon, 2020; Mahajan, 2020; Tiwari et al., 2020). Ultimately, such conditions affect the mental health and well-being of immigrant HCW with the possibility of limited mental health services available through work to help buffer the effects of both COVID-19 related and non-related risks.

The Risk From the Enforcement of Immigrant Policies (Immigration Status)

Despite the presence and importance of immigrant HCW in the U.S workforce, policies by the Trump administration on H1-B visas and international students (including IMG students) have left immigrant HCW vulnerable and anxious (Griswold & Salmon, 2020). During the COVID-19 pandemic, many IMG students, physicians, postdocs, research scientists in health systems, and others on the frontline also feared violation of various visa rules. For example, certain visas mandate that an immigrant HCW can only work at a given location for a particular number of hours. For F1 students on optional practicum training (OPT), that meant that if they lost their job during the pandemic, they had 30-60 days to get another job or face deportation (Mahajan, 2020; Tiwari et al., 2020).

Certain visa restrictions also bar immigrants from holding two jobs or a job outside of their area of study even when wages are lost and industries are suffering (Guadagno, 2020). While various governors such as Andrew Cuomo in New York and Phil Murphy in New Jersey, passed various laws which allowed IMG and other HCW professionals on visas to work during the pandemic, more should and also can be done (Bier, 2020; Griswold & Salmon, 2020). In addition to all the stressors of the COVID-19 pandemic which affected the mental health of HCW, having to deal with immigrant law-related stressors only served to exacerbate the mental health issues that immigrant HCW faced (Bier, 2020; Griswold & Salmon, 2020; Guadagno, 2020).

Consequently, it is because of working visas that most immigrants cannot leave toxic working environments or speak up about the mistreatment and microaggressions which are experienced in the workplace out of fear of retaliation in either losing their visa or not being reinstated a visa (Mahajan, 2020; Painter, 2020; Tiwari et al., 2020). The current political climate also means that organizations are reluctant to sponsor and hire immigrant workers partly because they do not understand the visa process and do not want to pay for the process. For others, qualifications from their home country cannot be transferred to the American working system, which means having to settle for a low-skilled job to make ends meet (Bier, 2020; Griswold & Salmon, 2020; Tiwari et al., 2020).

Even at the height of the COVID-19 pandemic, immigrant HCW were still required to comply with visa-based requirements such as status determination and visa renewals. Before the COVID-19 pandemic, such procedures were often nuanced and expensive, however, with worldwide lockdowns and limited working hours for US embassies across the world, fear of financial loss, and closed borders made the scheduling of visa appointments even more challenging and delayed (Guadagno, 2020). Many violations such as protesting, breaking curfew, or an inability to wear a mask increased the number of arrests and fear of deportation particularly if immigrant HCW violated their visa status. As is evidenced by other immigrant groups, this may have a detrimental impact on the mental health and well-being of immigrant HCW (Guadagno, 2020).

At times, immigrant HCW on employment-based visas may have family members tied to visas as dependents. In the event the immigrant HCW loses their job or lost their life to COVID-19, then those family members were left without financial support and at times faced deportation. Having such responsibility often weighs heavily on the minds of immigrant HCW further adding to the mental health challenges that they encounter during the COVID-19 pandemic (Bhandari et al., 2021; Mahajan, 2020; Tiwari et al., 2020). For example, in a recent feature in The BMJ journal, Painter (2020) highlighted the concerns of Dr. Karthik Karanam, a nephrologist from India on a temporary working visa. Dr. Karanam reported feeling fear and anxiety that if he were to die, lost his job, or gotten seriously ill from COVID-19, his wife would lose her spousal visa and his entire family would be deported immediately. Dr. Karanam also reported concerns over what that would do to his children as the US was the "only country that they had ever known." (Painter, 2020). Similarly, in a quantitative study on COVID-19 challenges faced by Nepalese immigrants in Japan, a majority of participants reported feelings of stress, worry, anxiety, and fear over an inability to support family members if they got infected with the COVID-19 virus (Bhandari et al., 2021).

Impact of Border Closures (Immigration)

With COVID-19 dubbed a global pandemic, a majority of countries the world over closed their borders and heightened immigration-related policies such that borders were closed to even citizens outside of their home country (Guadagno, 2020). This created heightened stressful situations for many immigrant HCW who already faced nuances and challenges when traveling on working visas before the COVID-19 pandemic. First, depending on where in the world home countries were located for the immigrant HCW, those who went home for thc holidays were stranded in countries that like China, Italy, and the United Kingdom instituted lockdowns during the early start of the global pandemic (e.g., December 2019 and January/February 2020; (Guadagno, 2020). Similarly, many others who were trying to return to the US from their home countries were also stranded in countries for which they had connecting flights and layovers. Such a situation was stressful for immigrant HCW who had to return to the US to resume work and studies according to requirements of their employment-based visa and financial and mental stress incurred as a result of the possibility of lack of financial resources to cover being in a foreign country and out of work.

Second, for immigrant HCW in the US on employment-based visas, there was uncertainty about their future in the US as well as the issue of deportation once the visa officially expired. In addition, immigrant HCW also have family abroad that they visited yearly at times; yet, with borders closed there was also uncertainty around the possibility of seeing family members in the future (Guadagno, 2020). Closure of borders resulted in a lack of social and financial support from family members which insinuated feelings of loneliness, isolation, and limited resources to be able to cope with those feelings (Ming & De Jong, 2021). In several studies assessing mental health challenges during the lockdown, immigrant workers screened positively for anxiety and depression, suggesting high co-morbidity. Immigrant workers also reported significant increases in negative emotions and feelings such as frustration, tension, fear of death, fear, isolation, irritability, low mood, and loneliness (Kumar et al., 2020; Srivastava et al., 2021). Noticeably, these feelings were also recorded in HCW (Qiu et al., 2021), in various countries (Rossi et al., 2020), and the world over (Sameer et al., 2020).

Third, not all countries have the resources to be able to handle the COVID-19 pandemic with some countries such as India, Italy, China, and the United Kingdom at one point being the epicenter of the COVID-19 pandemic (Guadagno, 2020). As a result, immigrant HCW were also worried about their family members and feared that perhaps if family members got infected and seriously ill from the COVID-19 virus they would be unable to pay their respects and say goodbye (Bhandari et al., 2021; Ming & De Jong, 2021). Furthermore, immigrant HCW financially support their family members abroad; however, with country-wide lockdowns and financial institutions closed both in the home and host countries it was challenging to provide this financial support. Ultimately, all of this exacerbated and created mental health challenges and affected the well-being of immigrant HCW (Bhandari et al., 2021; Guadagno, 2020; Ming & De Jong, 2021).

In January 2021, about a year into the pandemic, the COVID-19 vaccine brought renewed hope for many immigrant HCW. Many countries have begun to re-open their borders and allow for citizens to return to their home countries. Initially, certain countries loosened restrictions by allowing quarantine of visitors (including where safe, home quarantine for returning nationals) for 7-14 days. However, with the COVID-19 vaccine, some countries removed quarantine restrictions for fully vaccinated individuals. Immigrant HCW can reunite with their families in their home countries, and while life might appear different before COVID-19, at least being able to travel and see family reduced the mental health burdens imposed by lockdowns.

Discrimination, Stigmatization, and Xenophobia (Race)

In 2020, there was a rise in social justice movements during the COVID-19 pandemic. Antecedents to such social uprising (e.g., killings of unarmed Black individuals, hate crimes against AAPI) could also serve to exacerbate the mental health stressors of immigrant HCW (Choi et al., 2020; Cubrich & Tengesdal, 2021; Maestripieri, 2021). Not surprisingly, groups and individuals against immigration profited the opportunity to spew anti-immigrant rhetoric during the COVID-19 pandemic, such as immigrants were draining the country of its resources to fight the COVID-19 pandemic, and immigrants were the ones responsible for bringing the virus into the country. At times such stances were targeted at specific immigrant groups such as members of the AAPI community.

According to the Pew Research Center (2020), a majority of immigrants are likely to be from racial and ethnic minority groups (e.g., Asians, Hispanic/Latino) and for the first time have to contend with racial and ethnic discrimination (Budiman, 2020). At the beginning of the pandemic as COVID-19 spread across the U.S so too did xenophobia and discrimination against Asian Americans (Le et al., 2020). According to a report by the New American Economy (2020), AAPI makes up 1.4 million (about 8.5%) of healthcare workers, with almost one million of them being frontline HCs. To borrow from research on other immigrant groups, in a study on discrimination and coping mechanisms of Korean immigrants in the US, Choi et al. (2020) reported an increase in distress in the mental health and well-being of Korean immigrants due to an uptick in racial discrimination directed at Asian Americans during the COVID-19 pandemic.

By May 2020, the senseless killings of unarmed black individuals - George Floyd, Ahmaud Arbery, and Breonna Taylor – left black individuals including black immigrants worrisome (South et al., 2020). While companies have implemented several policies to protect minority groups (e.g., race, gender, age) against open workplace mistreatments such as discrimination, the success of such policies have often meant that individuals who belong to hidden minority groups (e.g., immigrants based on immigrant status) are more exposed to more subtle forms of workplace mistreatment or unprotected and helpless by various laws and policies (Carter-Sowell et al., 2020). One of the underlying reasons for this is due to intersectionality. Being an immigrant HCW, especially an immigrant worker on a working visa or undocumented exacerbates the experiences of racism and discrimination. For racial/ethnic minority immigrants, in addition to dealing with racism, one also must deal with immigration-related issues such as work permits and visas, language discrimination, and ostracism. Even while on the frontlines, immigrant HCW face widespread hate speech, stigmatization, discrimination, and xenophobic remarks from both their co-workers and patients (Carter-Sowell et al., 2020).

Immigrant HCW may experience doubt and uncertainty regarding what is expected from them in the host culture and in health systems with norms and policies that deviate from what they are used to. Immigrant HCW experience anxiety about the lack of predictability in the work setting and with the realization that their cultural and ethnic identity is different from that of the host society (Schilgen et al., 2020; Spilsbury & Cooney, 1998). Research has found that immigrant HCW are judged based on their ethnic group membership rather than their attributes, personalities, and performance. As such, anxiety emerges from unease and worry of being perceived as unqualified, lacking workplace initiative, and missing out on career development and advancement opportunities (Schilgen et al., 2020; Spilsbury & Cooney, 1998). Kirkcaldy et al., (2006) found that compared to native-born individuals, immigrants suffer from chronic anxiety and depression for a much longer period due to the challenges of racism, stigmatization, and xenophobia that they face and compounded by their intersecting identities.

On the other hand, immigrants HCW who returned to their home country also faced discrimination and stigmatization from citizens in the home country (Bhandari et al., 2021; Guadagno, 2020; Ming & De Jong, 2021). In a mixed-methods study exploring anxiety and depression levels in individuals in quarantine centers in Nepal, immigrants returning to Nepal reported being ostracized and "treated like dogs" from employees at quarantine centers as well as family members because individuals feared that they brought the COVID-19 virus back to the country with them. Additionally, the immigrants reported experiencing high levels of depression and anxiety as a result of how they were treated (Bhandari et al., 2021). Research shows that such circumstances were often amplified when immigrants returned to countries that were inadequately prepared to handle the COVID-19 pandemic due to a lack of testing and screening as well as effective COVID-19 guidelines and protocols (Bhandari et al., 2021; Guadagno, 2020; Ming & De Jong, 2021).

MODERATORS THAT CAN EITHER BUFFER OR AGGRIVATE MENTAL HEALTH OUTCOMES AND WELL-BEING FOR IMMIGRANT HCW

In this section, we identify moderating factors that either exacerbate or mitigate the effects of COVID-19 on the mental health of immigrant HCW. We explore these moderators along three dimensions: organizational, institutional, and individual.

Organizational Moderators

Occupational Role

Earlier we mentioned that the work and working environment can create undue stress on the immigrant particularly if it was toxic before the COVID-19 pandemic. In addition, fear of and increased risk of contracting the COVID-19 virus depends on the individual's occupational role, which will also affect the impact on the immigrant HCW mental health and well-being (Hamouche, 2020). For example, during the pandemic, several immigrant HCW were deployed. Research shows that nurses and physicians, particularly those deployed on the frontlines, reported higher negative mental health outcomes and stress (Qiu et al., 2021). Similar findings were found in immigrant HCW deployed in areas most significantly impacted by the COVID-19 pandemic, which were more likely to be underserved and low-income communities with high rates of racial/ethnic minorities including immigrants or long term health care facilities (e.g., nursing homes) (Gold, 2020; Lee et al., 2020).

Of note, during the lockdown, many organizations resorted to working from home or telework to control the spread of COVID-19. However, the downside of telework is that it increased feelings of isolation, depression, and other forms of psychological distress (Hamouche, 2020). For example, physicians with dual roles in practice and research still had to go home to ensure that their research commitments were met even after working on the frontlines. Thus, telework can increase workload and working hours. Telework also blurred the lines between personal and private lives and further intensified role conflict particularly if immigrant HCW also had to perform caregiving responsibilities for the elderly and children (Hamouche, 2020).

Occupational Safety and Health Management

Although the COVID-19 pandemic created challenges for all organizations across the world, healthcare systems were particularly tested as their employees were at the center of the fight against the COVID-19 pandemic. The COVID-19 pandemic brought to light long-standing health disparities created by the system. As such, healthcare systems serving low-income and underserved racial and ethnic minority and immigrant communities were likely to have fewer resources such as testing, screening, and later vaccine access for this population (Kim et al., 2020; Yancy, 2020). As we have consistently mentioned before, immigrant HCW were more likely to be serving on the frontlines in these institutions (Batalova, 2020). As a result, they were more likely to have higher negative mental health outcomes than immigrant HCW who served at health systems that were well equipped with PPE and saw fewer severely ill COVID-19 patients (Arnetz et al., 2020).

Similarly, immigrant HCW at health care institutions that were quick to implement and follow guidelines set out by the Centers for Disease Control and Prevention (CDC) and World Health Organization

(WHO; e.g., enforcing social distance, providing hand sanitizers and masks, etc.), as well as providing and encouraging access to mental health services, had lower mental health stress and better well-being (Hamouche, 2020). By implementing clear preventative measures, providing a safe working environment, and making mental health a priority organizations were able to build trust and make employees feel supported and protected, which ultimately increased employee outcomes (e.g., job satisfaction), well-being, and reduced mental health stress (Hamouche, 2020).

Institutional Moderators

Government Financial Aid Packages (e.g. Stimulus Packages)

During the COVID-19 pandemic, the US government gave stimulus packages to individuals. However, the government instituted guidelines that determined who received the stimulus packages, and often immigrant workers were left out from government financial relief packages (Amandolare et al., 2020; Chishti & Bolter, 2020). While immigrant HCW with green cards may have received the stimulus package, others on employment-based visas and within various income brackets may have been left out. Therefore, for immigrants who did receive the stimulus package, it may have provided some form of financial security and relief. However, some argue that with the economic impact of the COVID-19 pandemic this may not have been enough and may have only lessened the mental health impact only slightly (Bier, 2020; Chishti & Bolter, 2020; Griswold & Salmon, 2020).

Bi-Partisan Bills and State-Wide Immigrant Policies

In certain states like New York and New Jersey which were heavily hit by the pandemic and once epicenters, governors passed laws that lessened the immigrant policies allowing immigrant HCW on visas from working freely. For immigrant HCW in these states, this lessened the immigrant-related stressors, yet, uncertainty still lingered as to what happened legally once the pandemic was over (Bier, 2020; Griswold & Salmon, 2020; Mathema, 2020). In addition, as a response to the shortage of HCW in the US during the COVID-19 pandemic, a bipartisan group of senators introduced The Healthcare Workforce Resilience Act, S. 3599, 116, which recaptured at least 40,000 unused green-cards and offered them to medical front line workers, namely physicians and nurses (Leviyeva, 2021). While this offers some sort of relief, again for other immigrant HCW in low-skilled high-risk frontline jobs (e.g., health aids in long-term care facilities) this does not provide any relief from immigrant-related stressors and the subsequent reduction in psychological distress that such a bill can provide.

Mental Health Systems

Traditionally, due to stigma, cultural differences, lack of access, and mental health-related disparities, immigrants and racial/ethnic minorities have lower rates of mental health services utilization compared to White individuals (Bauldry & Szaflarski, 2017; Derr, 2015). Noticeably, with increases in xenophobia, racial discrimination, and stigmatization during the COVID-19 pandemic, racial/ethnic minority groups, including immigrants reported higher rates of mental health distress and decreased well-being than their White counterparts (Choi et al., 2020; Gibbs et al., 2020).

Yet, the availability of mental healthcare services and access to those services has been under-addressed and understudied particularly for immigrant HCW (Hamouche, 2020). With that being said, previous research on the Ebola outbreak show immigrant HCW in areas with zero to limited mental health services and access, psychosocial support systems, and absence of well-trained culturally sensitive mental health professionals saw an increased risk of psychological distress compared with immigrant HCW who had such services available (Alegría et al., 2013; Mukumbang et al., 2020; Qiu et al., 2021; Rabelo et al., 2016).

Individual Moderators

Sociodemographic Factors

Research on the moderating role of sociodemographic factors such as race, age, and gender on the relationship between COVID-19 stressors and mental health is scant (Hamouche, 2020). Research on depression shows that women, more so than men, are prone to depression and have a greater vulnerability to stress (Hamouche, 2020). These findings are similar in research that explores the negative effects of traumatic events (e.g. chronic death) on immigrants (Böttche et al., 2016; Starck et al., 2020). Immigrant households are multi-generational households. Hence, at the intersection of race, gender, and immigrant status, immigrant women are significantly more likely to bear the brunt of these responsibilities due to the historical structural inequities. A recent poll showed that since the COVID-19 pandemic hit, women engaged in 31 more hours of housework each week. Additionally, compared to an overall 37% of white women, at least 57% of Latinx women struggled to manage both work and family burdens (Rajai & Jackson, 2020). Naturally, women with children and those who were pregnant, compared to those without, reported higher levels of anxiety from fear of contracting the disease and spreading it to their young children and elderly parents (Hamouche, 2020).

Acculturation Strategies and Social Support

Berry (1997) developed four acculturation strategies

1. *Assimilation,* the immigrant does not wish to maintain or have contact with individuals from the heritage culture and so adopts aspects of and fosters strong relationship in the host culture.
2. *Integration,* the immigrant maintains the heritage culture and adopts aspects of the host culture while keeping and establishing relationships in both cultures.
3. *Separation,* the immigrant maintains their relationships and cultural aspects from the heritage culture and minimizes contact and adopting aspects of the host culture.
4. *Marginalization,* the immigrant maintains neither the heritage culture nor the host culture and does not seek to keep or establish relationships in either culture.

To our knowledge there is no research on the moderating effect of acculturation strategies on mental health and well-being of immigrant healthcare workers during the COVID-pandemic, however, previous research on acculturation strategies, social support, and mental health have shown that immigrant workers, including immigrant HCW who adopt integration strategy, have more social support and better mental health outcomes than immigrants who adopt the other acculturation strategies. Immigrants who adopted the marginalization strategy had the worst mental health outcomes.

SUGGESTIONS AND RECOMMENDATIONS TO HELP IMMIGRANT HCW COPE WITH COVID-19 STRESSORS

Immigration Policy Changes

Perhaps the biggest source of stress for immigrant HCW workers was immigrant-related. Hence, we suggest that, where possible, governments and organizations help facilitate a more efficient immigration system to help reduce the burden. Bipartisan bills such as The Healthcare Workforce Resilience Act, S. 3599, 116 are a step in the right direction, however, bills such as that should also include other healthcare frontline workers such as healthcare aides in long-term care facilities (Lee et al., 2020). Immigrant HCW also dedicate a significant portion of their training in the US and dedicate their time to serving historically minoritized populations that are disproportionally affected by health outcomes across the board (Mahajan, 2020). Therefore, policy changes that support a smoother pathway to American citizenship are also suggested (Tiwari et al., 2020).

Prevention of Stigma Through Anti-Racism Policies

With the increase in social justice movement and advocacy in 2020, some healthcare systems pledged their commitment to creating more anti-racist and inclusive cultures. Many trainings and interventions in this area are targeted at unconscious bias, microaggressions, and reducing racist/biased interpersonal interactions between providers and patients (South et al., 2020). Hence, we suggest that additional programs and training focused on cultural humility and interactions around cross-cultural teams should also be implemented. In addition, zero-tolerance policies around xenophobia should also be reinforced or implemented to help reduce stigma around the COVID-19 pandemic and enhance well-being and mental health outcomes for immigrant HCW.

Cultural Tailored/Sensitive Mental Health Programs

The intersectionality of race, immigrant status, and class add an extra layer that immigrant HCW have to contend with before, during, and after the COVID-19 pandemic. We cannot stress enough how important it is that immigrant status is taken into consideration when developing interventions and mental health policies and that interventions should be culturally tailored to help immigrant HCW cope with their mental health challenges. We say that because even when generic mental health interventions are developed, cultural backgrounds, stigmatization, and beliefs in addition to limited access and fear hinder immigrant HCW from making use of these services. Mental health professionals who are employed to serve this population should also be trained to be culturally sensitive.

Open Communication, Transparency, and Social Support

The COVID-19 pandemic brought along with it many uncertainties and unknowns around the virus, treatment options, and, for immigrant HCW, uncertainty around their immigrant status. While healthcare organizations were learning as the COVID-19 virus unfolded, clear continuous communication, transparency, and provision of up-to-date information around workplace policies, treatment options, and immigrant-related factors should be provided to help reduce stress and uncertainty. Furthermore, the management of healthcare systems should actively involve frontline workers in the recovery efforts and plans to fight the COVID-19 pandemic. Inclusion into such matters will help them feel valued and involved as decisions are being made that affect them. In addition to communication, health care systems should also provide immigrant HCW with social support such as childcare services, legal assistance, adequate PPE, organizational bonuses (since they were unable to get government assistance), and other work-related resources to help reduce stresses in the working environment.

PRACTICAL IMPLICATIONS AND FUTURE RESEARCH

We have attempted to provide a comprehensive, though not exhaustive, account of the impact of the COVID-19 pandemic on the mental health and well-being of immigrant HCW by providing factors that intersect along with race, immigrant status and class, moderators, and suggestions to develop interventions for HCW. The information presented here will help raise awareness of the experiences of immigrant HCW both from a societal and organizational perspective. Plus, it will help healthcare institutions be mindful of how to culturally tailor and target interventions and workplace policies to reduce the negative mental health challenges and increase the well-being of immigrant HCW. As stated earlier, we strongly recommend that mental health intervention be designed from an intersectionality lens given the fact that immigrant status adds an extra layer that native-born HCW, even those from the same racial/ethnic and gender group, may not necessarily encounter. Future empirical research should also examine the impact of COVID-19 on the mental health and well-being of immigrant HCW from an intersectionality framework, and explore moderators such as acculturation strategies.

CONCLUSION

The global COVID-19 pandemic has brought into the forefront pre-existing inequities and injustices faced by racial/ethnic minorities including immigrants in the US and threatens to make permanent the inequities and disparities in the mental health outcomes of traditionally marginalized groups such as immigrant workers. Specifically, immigrant HCW are over-represented in healthcare occupations and areas hardest hit by the pandemic. They are required to continue working without the proper PPE, financial security, and uncertainty over their future in the US because of immigrant-related challenges which have taken a heavy toll on their mental health and well-being. Yet, immigrants HCW experiences and mental health outcomes are lumped under the umbrella of the experiences of racial/ethnic minorities and as such are considered low-priority, or their unique needs are ignored when designing mental health services and interventions.

The COVID-19 pandemic has created both intentional and non-intentional circumstances that severely impact the mental health and well-being of immigrant HCW. However, the COVID-19 pandemic also brought an uprise of social justice and advocacy and changing workplace dynamics which creates a golden opportunity for changes in policy and workplace conditions and allows for the inclusion of an often forgotten and underserved minority population.

REFERENCES

Alegría, M., Fortuna, L. R., Lin, J. Y., Norris, F. H., Gao, S., Takeuchi, D. T., Jackson, J. S., Shrout, P. E., & Valentine, A. (2013). Prevalence, risk, and correlates of posttraumatic stress disorder across ethnic and racial minority groups in the United States. *Medical Care*, *51*(12), 1114–1123. doi:10.1097/MLR.0000000000000007 PMID:24226308

Amandolare, S., Gallagher, L., Bowles, J., & Dvorkin, E. (2020). *Under Threat & Left Out: NYC's Immigrants and the Coronavirus Crisis.* Academic Press.

Udaya, B. B., Pokharel, S., Munikar, S., Wagle, C. N., Adhikary, P., Shahi, B. B., Thapa, C., Bhandari, R. P., Adhikari, B., & Thapa, K. (2021). Anxiety and depression among people living in quarantine centers during COVID-19 pandemic: A mixed-method study from western Nepal. *PLoS One*, *16*(7), e0254126. doi:10.1371/journal.pone.0254126 PMID:34242319

Arnetz, J. E., Goetz, C. M., Sudan, S., Arble, E., Janisse, J., & Arnetz, B. B. (2020). Personal protective equipment and mental health symptoms among nurses during the COVID-19 pandemic. *Journal of Occupational and Environmental Medicine*, *62*(11), 892–897. doi:10.1097/JOM.0000000000001999 PMID:32804747

Batalova, J. (2020). *Immigrant Health-Care Workers in the United States*. Academic Press.

Bauldry, S., & Szaflarski, M. (2017). Immigrant-based disparities in mental health care utilization. *Socius: Sociological Research for a Dynamic World*, *3*. doi:10.1177/2378023116685718 PMID:28845455

Berry, J. (1997). Immigration, acculturation, and adaptation. *Applied Psychology*, *46*(1), 5–34.

Bhandari, D., Kotera, Y., Ozaki, A., Abeysinghe, S., Kosaka, M., & Tanimoto, T. (2021). COVID-19: challenges faced by Nepalese migrants living in Japan. *BMC Public Health, 21*(1), 1–14.

Bier, D. J. (2020). Immigrants aid America during COVID-19 crisis. Cato Institute.

Böttche, M., Stammel, N., & Knaevelsrud, C. (2016). Psychotherapeutic treatment of traumatized refugees in Germany. *Der Nervenarzt*, *87*(11), 1136–1143. doi:10.100700115-016-0214-x PMID:27649983

Brooks, S. K., Dunn, R., Amlôt, R., Greenberg, N., & Rubin, G. J. (2016). Social and occupational factors associated with psychological distress and disorder among disaster responders: a systematic review. *BMC Psychology, 4*(1), 1–13. doi:10.1186/s40359-016-0120-9

Brooks, S. K., Webster, R. K., Smith, L. E., Woodland, L., Wessely, S., Greenberg, N., & Rubin, G. J. (2020). The psychological impact of quarantine and how to reduce it: Rapid review of the evidence. *Lancet*, *395*(10227), 912–920. doi:10.1016/S0140-6736(20)30460-8 PMID:32112714

Budhwani, H., & Sun, R. (2020). Creating COVID-19 stigma by referencing the novel coronavirus as the "Chinese virus" on Twitter: Quantitative analysis of social media data. *Journal of Medical Internet Research, 22*(5), e19301. doi:10.2196/19301 PMID:32343669

Budiman, A. (2020, August 20). *Key findings about U.S. immigrants*. Pew Research Center.

Bureau of Labor Statistics. (2020). *Foreign-born workers: Labor force characteristics - 2019*. Author.

Cabarkapa, S., Nadjidai, S. E., Murgier, J., & Ng, C. H. (2020). The psychological impact of COVID-19 and other viral epidemics on frontline healthcare workers and ways to address it: A rapid systematic review. *Brain, Behavior, & Immunity - Health, 8*, 100144.

Chen, P. G., Auerbach, D. I., Muench, U., Curry, L. A., & Bradley, E. H. (2013). Policy solutions to address the foreign-educated and foreign-born health care workforce in the United States. *Health Affairs, 32*(11), 1906–1913. doi:10.1377/hlthaff.2013.0576 PMID:24191079

Chishti, M., & Bolter, J. (2020, April 24). *Vulnerable to COVID-19 and in frontline job, immigrants are mostly shut out of U.S. relief*. Migration Policy Institute.

Choi, S., Hong, J. Y., Kim, Y. J., & Park, H. (2020). Predicting psychological distress amid the COVID-19 pandemic by machine learning: Discrimination and coping mechanisms of Korean immigrants in the U.S. *International Journal of Environmental Research and Public Health, 17*(17), 1–14. doi:10.3390/ijerph17176057 PMID:32825349

Clark, E., Fredricksid, K., Woc-Colburn, L., Bottazzi, M. E., & Weatherheadid, J. (2020). Disproportionate impact of the COVID-19 pandemic on immigrant communities in the United States. *PLoS Neglected Tropical Diseases, 14*(7), 1–9. doi:10.1371/journal.pntd.0008484 PMID:32658925

Cohen, C. I., Lo, P., Nzodom, C., & Sahlu, S. (2018). Culture, heritage, and diversity in older adult mental health care. In Migration, acculturation, and mental health (pp. 53–180). Academic Press.

Cubrich, M., & Tengesdal, J. (2021). Precarious work during precarious times: Addressing the compounding effects of race, gender, and immigration status. *Industrial and Organizational Psychology: Perspectives on Science and Practice, 14*(1–2), 133–138. doi:10.1017/iop.2021.42

Derr, A. S. (2016). Mental health service use among immigrants in the United States: A systematic review. *Psychiatric Services (Washington, D.C.), 67*(3), 265–274. doi:10.1176/appi.ps.201500004 PMID:26695493

Dhanani, L. Y., & Franz, B. (2021). Why public health framing matters: An experimental study of the effects of COVID-19 framing on prejudice and xenophobia in the United States. *Social Science & Medicine, 269*, 113572. doi:10.1016/j.socscimed.2020.113572 PMID:33321405

Di Tella, M., Romeo, A., Benfante, A., & Castelli, L. (2020). Mental health of healthcare workers during the COVID-19 pandemic in Italy. *Journal of Evaluation in Clinical Practice, 26*(6), 1583–1587. doi:10.1111/jep.13444 PMID:32710481

Gelatt, J. (2020). *Immigrant Workers: Vital to the U.S. COVID-19 Response, Disproportionately Vulnerable*. Migration Policy Institute.

Gibbs, T., Pauselli, L., Vieux, U., Solan, M., & Rosenfield, P. (2020). Mental Health Disparities Among Black Americans During the COVID-19 Pandemic. *Psychiatric Times.*

Gold, J. A. (2020). Covid-19: Adverse mental health outcomes for healthcare workers. *BMJ (Clinical Research Ed.)*, 369. doi:10.1136/bmj.m1815 PMID:32371465

Griswold, D. T., & Salmon, J. (2020). Lower Barriers to Immigrant Healthcare Workers to Help Combat the COVID-19 Pandemic. SSRN *Electronic Journal*. doi:10.2139/ssrn.3592978

Guadagno, L. (2020). *Migrants and the COVID-19 pandemic: An initial analysis*. International Organization for Migration.

Hamouche, S. (2020). COVID-19 and employees' mental health: Stressors, moderators and agenda for organizational actions. *Emerald Open Research*, *2*, 15. doi:10.35241/emeraldopenres.13550.1

Heath, C., Sommerfield, A., & von Ungern-Sternberg, B. S. (2020). Resilience strategies to manage psychological distress among healthcare workers during the COVID-19 pandemic: A narrative review. *Anaesthesia*, *75*(10), 1364–1371. doi:10.1111/anae.15180 PMID:32534465

Kim, E. J., Marrast, L., & Conigliaro, J. (2020). COVID-19: Magnifying the Effect of Health Disparities. *Journal of General Internal Medicine*, *35*(8), 2441–2442. Advance online publication. doi:10.100711606-020-05881-4 PMID:32394141

Kirkcaldy, B., Wittig, U., Furnham, A., Merbach, M., & Siefen, R. G. (2006). Health and migration. Psychosocial determinants. *Bundesgesundheitsblatt, Gesundheitsforschung, Gesundheitsschutz*, *49*(9), 873–883. doi:10.100700103-006-0021-9 PMID:16953359

Kochenderfer, A. (2021, February 11). *Immigrant Healthcare Workers Are Essential to the U.S. Comeback*. Think Immigration.

Kumar, K., Mehra, A., Sahoo, S., Nehra, R., & Grover, S. (2020). The psychological impact of COVID-19 pandemic and lockdown on the migrant workers: A cross-sectional survey. *Asian Journal of Psychiatry*, *53*, 102252. doi:10.1016/j.ajp.2020.102252 PMID:32593970

Lai, J., Ma, S., Wang, Y., Cai, Z., Hu, J., Wei, N., Wu, J., Du, H., Chen, T., Li, R., Tan, H., Kang, L., Yao, L., Huang, M., Wang, H., Wang, G., Liu, Z., & Hu, S. (2020). Factors associated with mental health outcomes among health care workers exposed to coronavirus disease 2019. *JAMA Network Open*, *3*(3), e203976–e203976. doi:10.1001/jamanetworkopen.2020.3976 PMID:32202646

Lancee, W. J., Maunder, R. G., & Goldbloom, D. S. (2008). Prevalence of psychiatric disorders among Toronto hospital workers one to two years after the SARS outbreak. *Psychiatric Services (Washington, D.C.)*, *59*(1), 91–95. doi:10.1176/ps.2008.59.1.91 PMID:18182545

Le, T. K., Cha, L., Han, H. R., & Tseng, W. (2020). Anti-asian xenophobia and Asian American COVID-19 disparities. In American Journal of Public Health (Vol. 110, Issue 9, pp. 1371–1373). American Public Health Association Inc. doi:10.2105/AJPH.2020.305846

Lee, C., Podury, A., Kaduthodil, J., & Graham, L. (2020). Long-term care facilities must prioritize immigrant workers' needs to contain COVID-19. *Health Affairs Blog*.

Leviyeva, E. (2021, April 13). *Proposed bipartisan bill to recapture 40,000 visas for physicians and nurses to remedy ongoing shortage, id Onogoing COVID-19 health response*. Inside Business Immigration.

Luceño-Moreno, L., Talavera-Velasco, B., García-Albuerne, Y., & Martín-García, J. (2020). Symptoms of posttraumatic stress, anxiety, depression, levels of resilience and burnout in Spanish health personnel during the COVID-19 pandemic. *International Journal of Environmental Research and Public Health, 17*(15), 5514. doi:10.3390/ijerph17155514 PMID:32751624

Maestripieri, L. (2021). The Covid-19 pandemics: Why intersectionality matters. *Frontiers in Sociology, 6*, 52. doi:10.3389/fsoc.2021.642662 PMID:33869589

Mahajan, A. (2020, December 12). *Heroes or aliens: The hidden dichotomy of immigrant physicians*. The Hill.

Mathema, S. (2019). Immigrant Doctors Can Help Lower Physician Shortages in Rural America. Center for American Progress.

Mathema, S. (2020, April 2). *Removing Barriers for Immigrant Medical Professionals Is Critical To Help Fight Coronavirus*. Center for Immigrant Progress.

Mehta, S. (2014). *Acculturation and mental health: Asian Indian immigrants in the United States*. Academic Press.

Mental Health America. (2020). *The Mental Health of Healthcare Workers in COVID-19*. Mental Health America.

Ming, X., & De Jong, M. D. T. (2021). Mental well-being of Chinese immigrants in the Netherlands during the covid-19 pandemic: A survey investigating personal and societal antecedents. *Sustainability (Switzerland), 13*(8), 4198. doi:10.3390u13084198

Mukumbang, F. C., Ambe, A. N., & Adebiyi, B. O. (2020). Unspoken inequality: how COVID-19 has exacerbated existing vulnerabilities of asylum-seekers, refugees, and undocumented migrants in South Africa. *International Journal for Equity in Health, 19*(1), 1–7.

New American Economy. (2020). *Asian Americans and Pacific Islander Americans on the Frontlines*. Author.

Nowrasteh, A., & Landgrave, M. (2020). *Immigrant Health Care Workers by Occupation and State*. Academic Press.

Painter, K. (2020). Work visas: Foreign doctors in the US have more than covid-19 to fear. *BMJ (Clinical Research Ed.)*, 370. doi:10.1136/bmj.m3172 PMID:32816818

Patel, Y. M., Ly, D. P., Hicks, T., & Jena, A. B. (2018). Proportion of non-US-born and noncitizen health care professionals in the United States in 2016. *Journal of the American Medical Association, 320*(21), 2265–2267. doi:10.1001/jama.2018.14270 PMID:30512091

Qiu, X., Lan, Y., Miao, J., Wang, H., Wang, H., Wu, J., Li, G., Zhao, X., Cao, Z., Mei, J., Sun, W., Zhu, Z., Zhu, S., & Wang, W. (2021). A Comparative study on the psychological health of frontline health workers in Wuhan under and after the lockdown. *Frontiers in Psychiatry*, •••, 12.

Rabelo, I., Lee, V., Fallah, M. P., Massaquoi, M., Evlampidou, I., Crestani, R., ... Severy, N. (2016). Psychological distress among Ebola survivors discharged from an Ebola treatment unit in Monrovia, Liberia–a qualitative study. *Frontiers in Public Health*, •••, 142.

Rajai, P., & Jackson, M. (2020). *How to support women of color during COVID-19 - Culture Amp Blog*. Culture Amp - Blog. https://www.cultureamp.com/blog/how-to-support-women-of-color-during-covid-19/

Rossi, R., Socci, V., Talevi, D., Mensi, S., Niolu, C., Pacitti, F., Di Marco, A., Rossi, A., Siracusano, A., & Di Lorenzo, G. (2020). COVID-19 pandemic and lockdown measures impact on mental ealth among the general population in Italy. *Frontiers in Psychiatry*, *11*, 790. doi:10.3389/fpsyt.2020.00790 PMID:32848952

Sameer, A. S., Khan, M. A., Nissar, S., & Banday, M. Z. (2020). Assessment of mental health and various coping strategies among general population living under imposed COVID-lockdown across world: A cross-sectional study. *Ethics, Medicine, and Public Health*, *15*, 100571. doi:10.1016/j.jemep.2020.100571 PMID:32838000

Schilgen, B., Nienhaus, A., & Mösko, M. (2020). The extent of psychosocial distress among immigrant and non-immigrant homecare nurses—A Comparative cross sectional survey. *International Journal of Environmental Research and Public Health*, *17*(5), 1635. doi:10.3390/ijerph17051635 PMID:32138277

Shechter, A., Diaz, F., Moise, N., Anstey, D. E., Ye, S., Agarwal, S., Birk, J. L., Brodie, D., Cannone, D. E., Chang, B., Claassen, J., Cornelius, T., Derby, L., Dong, M., Givens, R. C., Hochman, B., Homma, S., Kronish, I. M., Lee, S. A. J., ... Abdalla, M. (2020). Psychological distress, coping behaviors, and preferences for support among New York healthcare workers during the COVID-19 pandemic. *General Hospital Psychiatry*, *66*, 1–8. doi:10.1016/j.genhosppsych.2020.06.007 PMID:32590254

South, E. C., Butler, P. D., & Merchant, R. M. (2020). Toward an equitable society: Building a culture of antiracism in health care. *The Journal of Clinical Investigation*, *130*(10), 5039–5041. Advance online publication. doi:10.1172/JCI141675 PMID:32692730

Spilsbury, J. C., & Cooney, M. C. (1998). Immigrant Health Care Providers in the United States. Handbook of Immigrant Health, 607–627. doi:10.1007/978-1-4899-1936-6_29

Spoorthy, M. S., Pratapa, S. K., & Mahant, S. (2020). Mental health problems faced by healthcare workers due to the COVID-19 pandemic–A review. *Asian Journal of Psychiatry*, *51*, 102119. doi:10.1016/j.ajp.2020.102119 PMID:32339895

Srivastava, A., Arya, Y. K., Joshi, S., Singh, T., Kaur, H., Chauhan, H., & Das, A. (2021). Major stressors and coping strategies of internal migrant workers during the COVID-19 pandemic: A qualitative exploration. *Frontiers in Psychology*, *12*, 12. doi:10.3389/fpsyg.2021.648334 PMID:34093333

Starck, A., Gutermann, J., Schouler-Ocak, M., Jesuthasan, J., Bongard, S., & Stangier, U. (2020). The relationship of acculturation, traumatic events and depression in female refugees. *Frontiers in Psychology*, *11*, 906. doi:10.3389/fpsyg.2020.00906 PMID:32528358

Tiwari, V., Bhardwaj, A., Sonani, B., & Mehta, A. C. (2020). Urgent issues facing immigrant physicians in the United States in the COVID-19 era. In Annals of internal medicine (Vol. 173, Issue 10, pp. 838–839). NLM (Medline). doi:10.7326/M20-4103

U.S. Department of State. (n.d.). *Employment-Based Immigrant Visas*. Retrieved July 5, 2021, from https://travel.state.gov/content/travel/en/us-visas/immigrate/employment-based-immigrant-visas.html

Vizheh, M., Qorbani, M., Arzaghi, S. M., Muhidin, S., Javanmard, Z., & Esmaeili, M. (2020). The mental health of healthcare workers in the COVID-19 pandemic: A systematic review. *Journal of Diabetes and Metabolic Disorders*, *19*(2), 1967–1978. doi:10.100740200-020-00643-9 PMID:33134211

Ward, K. P., Shaw, S. A., Chang, M., & El-Bassel, N. (2018). Social support moderates the association between traumatic life events and depression among migrant and nonmigrant men in Almaty, Kazakhstan. *Journal of Traumatic Stress*, *31*(5), 698–707. doi:10.1002/jts.22324 PMID:30338586

Williams, C. L., & Berry, J. W. (1991). Primary prevention of acculturative stress among refugees: Application of psychological theory and practice. *The American Psychologist*, *46*(6), 632–641. doi:10.1037/0003-066X.46.6.632 PMID:1952422

Yancy, C. W. (2020). COVID-19 and African Americans. *Journal of the American Medical Association*. doi:10.1001/jama.2020.6548

Yellow Horse, A. J. (2021). Anti-Asian racism, xenophobia, and Asian American health during COVID-19. *The COVID-19 Crisis: Social Perspectives*, 195–206. doi:10.4324/9781003111344-21

Young, K. P., Kolcz, D. L., O'Sullivan, D. M., Ferrand, J., Fried, J., & Robinson, K. (2020). Health Care Workers' Mental Health and Quality of Life During COVID-19: Results From a Mid-Pandemic, National Survey. *Psychiatric Services (Washington, D.C.)*, *72*(2), 122–128. doi:10.1176/appi.ps.202000424 PMID:33267652

Zea, M. C., Asner-Self, K. K., Birman, D., & Buki, L. P. (2003). The abbreviated multidimensional acculturation scale: Empirical validation with two Latino/Latina samples. *Cultural Diversity & Ethnic Minority Psychology*, *9*(2), 107–126. doi:10.1037/1099-9809.9.2.107 PMID:12760324

Chapter 4
Pediatric Healthcare Providers: Unique Challenges and Strategies to Improve Wellness

Janelle M. Mentrikoski
Department of Behavioral Medicine and Psychiatry, West Virginia University School of Medicine, Morgantown, USA & Rockefeller Neuroscience Institute, Morgantown, USA

Stephany Lora
Department of Behavioral Medicine and Psychiatry, West Virginia University School of Medicine, Morgantown, USA & Rockefeller Neuroscience Institute, Morgantown, USA

Claire Baniak
Department of Pediatrics, West Virginia University School of Medicine, Morgantown, USA & Department of Behavioral Medicine and Psychiatry, West Virginia University School of Medicine, Morgantown, USA

Jennifer Ludrosky
Department of Behavioral Medicine and Psychiatry, West Virginia University School of Medicine, Morgantown, USA & Rockefeller Neuroscience Institute, Morgantown, USA

Jonathan G. Perle
Department of Behavioral Medicine and Psychiatry, West Virginia University School of Medicine, Morgantown, West Virginia, USA & Rockefeller Neuroscience Institute, Morgantown, West Virginia, USA

ABSTRACT

Healthcare providers are at risk for stress-related illness (e.g., burnout, compassion fatigue, and secondary traumatic stress) due to the nature of their jobs. Healthcare providers who work in pediatrics face unique challenges compared to those who work in adult healthcare. This chapter reviews three common challenges pediatric healthcare providers face, including working with children who may die or may be facing death, managing difficult family dynamics, and responding to cases of suspected child abuse and neglect. In addition, pediatric providers face additional challenges during public health crises (e.g., natural disasters and the COVID-19 pandemic), including specific challenges related to telehealth, navigating a lack of services and mental health programs and managing adverse childhood events. Several recommendations are made throughout this chapter to assist pediatric providers with these challenges.

DOI: 10.4018/978-1-7998-8813-0.ch004

INTRODUCTION

Regular exposure to others' traumas, heavy workload, high-pressure situations, and generally stressful work-related activities are all hallmarks of working in healthcare. Unfortunately, each remains a significant risk factor for stress-related illness (Koinis et al., 2015). Stress-related illness in healthcare providers has been studied under many names: burnout, compassion fatigue, secondary traumatic stress, vicarious or primary traumatization, and occupational stress (Meadors et al., 2010). These constructs are related and share some overlap, but they also have unique features and represent slightly different conceptualizations. Most of the literature on stress-related illness related to employment focuses on the major constructs of burnout, compassion fatigue, and secondary traumatic stress. These are not distinct constructs, as burnout and secondary traumatic stress are believed to be symptoms of compassion fatigue and burnout is believed to be a risk factor for the development of secondary traumatic stress (Figley, 1995). However, each construct is valuable for its unique contribution to the broad domain of stress-related illness in healthcare providers. Regardless of name, these constructs try to capture the negative consequences of working in caring professions

Burnout is defined as a "defensive response to prolonged occupational exposure to demanding interpersonal situations that produce psychological strain and provide inadequate support" (Jenkins & Baird, 2002). It is characterized by emotional exhaustion, depersonalization, irritability and emotional instability, disrupted relationships with coworkers, disrupted physical health behaviors (e.g., sleeping and eating), and a decreased sense of personal accomplishment (Embriaco et al., 2007; MacKinnon & Murray, 2017). Physicians and nurses have been identified as experiencing burnout at nearly twice the rate of providers in other fields, and greater than 50% of physicians and nurses experience burnout at any given time (e.g., Colville & Smith, 2017; Shanafelt et al., 2015). Psychologists may experience burnout at rates of 20–70%, depending on the study (Morse et al., 2012). Consequences of burnout for healthcare providers include impaired work performance (Rabatin et al., 2016), lower patient quality of care (e.g., Shanafelt et al., 2010), and job turnover (Waldman et al., 2004).

Compassion fatigue is described as a consequence of working with a significant number of traumatized individuals (i.e., medical or psychological trauma), in combination with having a strong empathic orientation (Figley, 1995). In other words, empathic individuals are affected by others' traumas, resulting in them experiencing their own corresponding traumatic symptoms. Compassion fatigue is characterized by emotional exhaustion, cynicism, and a low sense of personal accomplishment (Maslach et al., 2001). Prolonged compassion fatigue can lead to burnout in healthcare providers (Zadeh et al., 2012).

Secondary traumatic stress is defined as emotional stress related to hearing or witnessing the trauma of someone else (National Traumatic Stress Network, 2021; Clay, 2020). Secondary traumatic stress is believed to share significant overlap with compassion fatigue and may, in fact, describe the same construct (Figley, 1995). In one study of 274 pediatric providers, 25.1% were found to be at high risk for compassion fatigue, while 30.9% were at high risk for burnout and 26.9% were at high risk for secondary traumatic stress (Branch & Klinkenberg, 2015), suggesting that about a quarter of the pediatric healthcare workforce may be at risk for developing a stress-related illness, regardless of the name or construct used.

Numerous variables have been linked to the development of burnout, compassion fatigue, and secondary traumatic stress for healthcare providers. It is important to note that these variables are consistently identified across healthcare specialties (e.g., physicians, nurses, psychologists, social workers, counselors, and child life specialists). Factors influencing burnout may be characterized into those related to the work setting and those related to the individual. Individual factors related to burnout include younger age and less work experience (Buckley et al., 2020), sadness and depression, recent negative life events, and poor health status (Starmer et al., 2016). Work factors are believed to be strongly related to burnout, including a lack of job control or reduced autonomy, low social support among colleagues, poor supervisory relationships, poor work environment, high work stress, and job demands (e.g., hours of work and workload; Yang & Hayes, 2020; Kim et al., 2018). Meanwhile, factors relating to compassion fatigue include burnout, empathic orientation towards patients, and more years in direct care, suggesting a cumulative effect of the exposure of trauma over time (Robins et al., 2009; Figley, 1995). Finally, factors such as a large caseload of trauma patients and having a personal history of trauma are associated with developing secondary traumatic stress (Hensel et al., 2015).

A common factor in conceptualizations of healthcare provider stress-related illness is the concept of moral distress and moral injury. Moral distress occurs when an individual knows the right thing to do but cannot do it due to environmental or situational constraints (Williams et al., 2020), whereas moral injury is the damage done to the psyche or conscience when that person witnesses, perpetrates, or fails to prevent an outcome that violates one's moral beliefs or moral code (The Moral Injury Project, 2021). In essence, moral injury occurs for healthcare providers when they are unable to provide appropriate or optimal care for their patients due to systemic or administrative factors. Contributors can include having low or no access to appropriate referrals for patients, having ever-increasing clinical productivity standards, and having to provide care outside of the training comfort zone (Houtrow, 2020). Healthcare providers are at significant risk for moral distress and moral injury, especially during public health crises, such as for providers addressing the ongoing opioid epidemic, as well as those providing services throughout the COVID-19 pandemic. Using the pandemic as an example, resources (e.g., medical equipment) may be limited, healthcare providers may place family members at risk for disease transmission, and both rational and ethical decision-making may be comprised, all of which may contribute to moral distress (Williams et al., 2020). Moral distress can lead to similar physical ailments as burnout, including physical symptoms (e.g., muscle tension, headaches), exhaustion, and feelings of helplessness (Williams et al., 2020), and may ultimately lead to burnout and leaving the healthcare field entirely (Trotochaud et al., 2015).

UNIQUE CHALLENGES IN PEDIATRIC POPULATIONS

While healthcare providers (e.g., physicians, nurses, psychologists, social workers, counselors, child life specialists, and occupational therapists) are at significant risk for stress-related illness due to the intense, high pressure, and emotional nature of their work, pediatric providers may be at an increased risk of stress-related illness due to the unique factors of working with children. Although previous research has been mixed in determining whether the rates of burnout and compassion fatigue in pediatric providers are similar to or greater than adult providers, enough evidence suggests that pediatric providers are at least at a similar risk compared to adult providers, and possibly at greater risk of burnout and compassion fatigue compared to adult providers (Robins et al., 2009; Cull et al., 2018; Park et al., 2020). In order to effectively work with children, providers must be highly skilled in empathy, compassion, and enhanced communication in order to be able to relate to and care for patients at various stages of life (McKinley et al., 2017). While these traits are especially valued in pediatric providers, they also predispose them to stress-related illness in healthcare settings.

Inherent to the roles, pediatric healthcare providers often have first-hand access to a child's history and ongoing challenges. Unfortunately, this also allows them insight into negative events in a child's life.

For example, being exposed to children with serious illnesses who may be facing death can significantly impact the well-being of pediatric providers (Zadeh et al., 2012). While any death can be viewed as traumatic, child-related death may be especially impactful for pediatric providers, given the social value placed upon protecting and caring for children (Robins et al., 2009). In addition, direct work with family members can create challenges, such as the need to address family- or caregiver-related difficulties that arise from a child's injury or behaviors (Robins et al., 2009). Additionally, family members or caregivers may have their own mental health concerns that cannot be ignored if attempting to help the child (Robins et al., 2009). Furthermore, pediatric providers who have to evaluate reports of abuse or trauma and address or "repair" the issues resulting from abuse or trauma can be difficult and emotionally taxing. Given the value in protecting and caring for children, evaluating and addressing cases of suspected abuse in children might be more impactful for the pediatric provider (Robins et al., 2009). While there are certainly other challenges related to pediatric healthcare, a pediatric patient dying, difficult family dynamics, and caring for children with suspected abuse and neglect are some of the more common challenges that pediatric healthcare providers experience during their careers (e.g., Weiss & Ludwig, 2019).

Grief and Bereavement After Losing a Patient

Discussion

While grief in losing a patient is not unique to pediatric populations, the death of a child may carry additional weight due to the child losing their potential for a bright future and long life (Weiss & Ludwig, 2019). Historically, about one-third of physicians endorsed feelings of guilt after a patient's death, and about half of physicians reported experiencing a sense of failure (Rabow et al., 2021). This notion became increasingly complicated with the recognition of specific types of provider-focused grief, such as incomplete grief or disenfranchised grief. While *incomplete grief* is most often associated with families being unable to stay goodbye or engage in other rituals associated with dying (Rabow et al., 2021), providers themselves can experience the family's sorrow, stress, and feeling of incompleteness. Contrastingly, *disenfranchised grief*, or grief that is not openly acknowledged, sanctioned, or mourned, can also lead to healthcare provider distress through a provider feeling unable to express themselves or process the grief in a healthy manner (Rabow et al., 2021). Further compounding grief are factors such as staff feeling unprepared for the settings and types of deaths, logistics such as lack of time or equipment, understaffing, impotency of treatment and care, and having to say goodbyes to patients for their families due to families being unable to be with patients (Rabow et al., 2021). Pediatric healthcare providers may experience additional distress when having to make decisions regarding visitor policies when a pediatric patient is nearing the end of life, which comes along with significant feelings of moral distress (Wiener et al., 2021). While primary treatment responsibilities can be challenging enough, healthcare providers face additional challenges with defining goals (i.e., curative treatment versus palliative care), especially when a family is insisting on medically futile treatments that are either against the provider's recommendations or even against the patient's prior wishes (Bergsträsser et al., 2017; Dzeng et al., 2016).

Pediatric palliative care clinicians (e.g., physicians, nurses, chaplains, social workers, child life, and psychologists) may be at particular risk for experiencing moral distress and burnout associated with their job roles. For example, in a sample of Canadian palliative care physicians, results suggested that 36.4% of palliative care physicians endorsed high emotional exhaustion, 15.1% endorsed high depersonalization, 7.9% endorsed low personal accomplishments, and 38.2% of physicians reported a high degree of burnout (Wang et al., 2020). Although results may be similar to health care providers in other areas of practice, there are specific experiences in palliative and end of life (EOL) care that provide additional challenges. For instance, palliative care providers may experience high emotional involvement in their work and may find it difficult to create trusting relationships with colleagues, patients, and families, as well as maintain contact with the family after death (Bergsträsser et al., 2017). In addition, palliative care providers may experience difficulties due to high workloads and misconceptions about the role of palliative care in acute settings (Grauerholz et al., 2020).

Recommendations for Managing Stress-Related Illness Related to Grief and Bereavement

Several recommendations have been made to improve resilience and career satisfaction in healthcare providers who experience pediatric patient death. For example, comprehensive and interdisciplinary bereavement care training, formal and informal debriefing after death, and individual self-care measures may be beneficial (Grauerholz et al., 2020). Individual self-care strategies, such as faith, seeking support from friends and family, rest and distraction, and acceptance of death have been found to be helpful (Wenzel et al., 2011; Kitao et al., 2018). Of note, healthcare providers acknowledge that close relationships with patients both exacerbate grief and help with feelings of loss (Wenzel et al., 2011).

Recommendations to address pediatric healthcare provider burnout in palliative care includes developing effective and supportive leaders, cultivating community and a culture of wellness, improving practice efficiency, and improving administrative policies (Tawfik et al., 2019). Time for reflection and institutional recognition of losses has also been helpful in addressing grief and bereavement (Rabow et al., 2021). Additionally, an institutional culture of open discussion and reflection around deaths and normalization of emotional reactions may be beneficial (Dzeng et al., 2016). Regarding training, education in communication strategies for discussing poor prognosis and withdrawing life support is likely needed (Bergsträsser et al., 2017). As an example, neonatal intensive care unit (NICU) nurses who attended a day-long bereavement seminar reported increased comfort level and less moral distress around end-of-life and palliative care in comparison to those who did not attend (Zhang & Lane, 2013).

Family Dynamics

Discussion

Unique aspects of pediatric healthcare include the need to balance developmentally appropriate healthcare with the identified patient and the inclusion of and support from the patient's family, who may present with their own complexity (e.g., need for resources) or pathology (Weiss & Ludwig, 2019). Not only will pediatric providers face difficult patients with their own concerns (e.g., oppositionality and anxiety), but they might also face difficult caregivers who contribute to or exacerbate provider stress related to the care of the patient. Caregivers presenting with difficult or disruptive behaviors (e.g., threatening or cursing at staff, making changes to medical equipment, and perceived disrespect or hostility towards staff and hospital rules) can have a significant impact on medical care, such as interfering with medical care or increasing child distress. Indeed, a medical simulation conducted in a NICU demonstrated that medical care was negatively impacted when parents made rude comments to medical providers (Riskin et al., 2015). The disruptive behaviors of some families may even lead to serious safety concerns for pediatric healthcare providers, such as verbal or physical aggression towards staff. It is difficult to estimate the prevalence of physical aggression towards staff, as often, these instances are underreported (Phillips, 2016). However, while not specific to pediatric healthcare, a recent review found the one-year prevalence of physical violence by patients or visitors against healthcare providers to be 19.33% (Li et al., 2020), highlighting the risk healthcare providers might face as part of their jobs. In another study, 118 out of 410 pediatricians (42.5%) reported experiencing aggressive behavior from parents of their patients (Esmee van Steijn et al., 2019).

By taking care of multiple patients and families with disruptive behaviors, healthcare providers may place themselves at a higher risk for burnout and job dissatisfaction, in addition to feeling unsafe at work (Phillips, 2016). Unlike adult healthcare providers, pediatric providers will likely have to work with difficult families throughout the entirety of the patient's hospitalization or throughout the child's life, further compounding their stress. On the other hand, patients and families who are labeled as "difficult" by the medical team might experience negative outcomes, including less satisfaction and trust with their medical providers, worsening physical symptoms, and increased healthcare utilization (Hinchey & Jackson, 2011).

Recommendations for Managing Stress-Related Illness Related to Family Dynamics

Managing difficult family dynamics in a hospital or office setting is often demanding and stressful for pediatric healthcare workers; however, effectively addressing difficult family relationships will likely reduce providers' overall stress and improve their job satisfaction. One way to improve family dynamics is to ensure that *patient- and family-centered* (PFCC) care is part of daily practice. PFCC involves collaboration and a working relationship among patients and their families with all members of the treatment team (American Academy of Pediatrics, 2012). PFCC is considered the gold standard of care in pediatric healthcare (Baird et al., 2015). Studies have demonstrated that PFCC is associated with positive outcomes, including greater patient and family satisfaction, decreased distress during medical procedures, improved adherence to treatment recommendations, and improved patient safety (American Academy of Pediatrics, 2012). PFCC also improves outcomes for providers, including increased professional satisfaction, improved efficiency and better time management, and improved communication (American Academy of Pediatrics, 2012). By adopting a collaborative framework for engaging with patients and their families, pediatric healthcare providers may reduce or avoid conflict that can arise when working with patients and their families.

Despite the well-known benefits and wide endorsement of PFCC, achieving PFCC in pediatric hospital settings can be challenging, particularly in pediatric intensive care units (Baird et al., 2015). While pediatric hospitals strive towards PFCC, pediatric healthcare providers can incorporate aspects of PFCC into their daily work. Preventative strategies, such as effective and clear communication, might improve interactions with patients and their families (Curtis et al., 2014). For example, healthcare providers can invite family members to contribute to patient discussions and may even consider weekly family-centered rounds during hospitalizations to facilitate communication and decision-making. When confronted with hostility or anger from families, it is recommended that providers use empathy, try to approach the situation in a non-defensive manner, and validate families' frustrations while reminding them of the shared goal to help their child (Perle, 2015).

Another effective model used to address disruptive family behavior is called the SAFTeam (Strengthening Alliances with Families Team), which was developed by a psychiatry inpatient medical team with the goal to improve communication among the medical team and families and develop interventions to address disruptive family behaviors (see Judd-Glossy & Twohy, 2020, for more details). Regardless of the setting or available organization resources, all medical providers can manage difficult family dynamics by utilizing some of the following recommendations: engaging a multidisciplinary team (e.g., risk management and ethics), utilizing security to maintain staff safety, creating behavioral expectations and contracts for families, maintaining a consistent standard of care (i.e., not changing medical care to accommodate a challenging family), increasing psychosocial support for families and medical providers, and empowering team members to address challenging behaviors when they occur (Judd-Glossy & Twohy, 2020). While requiring some effort upfront, these strategies can greatly impact patient care and may prevent difficult family interactions, which in turn may reduce conflicts and ultimately decrease burnout in staff.

Child Abuse and Neglect

Discussion

Pediatric healthcare providers can experience significant stress and secondary trauma when providing care for pediatric patients who present with concerns related to physical or sexual abuse or neglect. It is estimated that approximately one in seven children in the United States experiences child abuse (Centers for Disease Control, 2021). In 2019, an estimated 656,000 children experienced abuse or neglect in the United States (Child Welfare Information Gateway, 2021). While not all cases of child abuse or neglect result in the child needing medical care or hospitalizations, often these cases present to local hospitals or doctor's offices in a variety of circumstances, thus making it likely that pediatric providers will witness or care for a child with suspected or confirmed child abuse or neglect. For example, caregivers may seek out medical care for injuries or symptoms and be unaware that the symptoms are related to child abuse, while abusers may seek out medical care when the injury is severe (Christian et al., 2015).

As healthcare providers are likely to witness or care for a child presenting with suspected or confirmed child abuse or neglect, it is no surprise that they might experience stress-related illnesses such as secondary traumatic stress and burnout. Indeed, out of 410 healthcare providers surveyed in one study, 202 (49.3%) cited suspicion of child abuse as a significant stressor (Esmee van Steijn et al., 2019). Beyond the general stress of hearing or observing outcomes of the abuse itself, healthcare providers are faced with managing their own emotional responses to the trauma while at the same time providing care to these patients (Weiss & Ludwig, 2019). While providing treatment (e.g., completing a physical exam) may be challenging given the circumstances, it is often necessary to provide appropriate care to the child. In addition, pediatric providers will likely have to manage strong emotional reactions when interacting with members of the child's family, who may or may not have had a role in the abuse of the child (Weiss & Ludwig, 2019). Regarding the patient–physician relationship, some providers might experience adverse family relationships due to mandatory reporting laws that result in termination of parental rights or imprisonment (Flaherty et al., 2012). In addition, pediatricians who specialize in treating children who have experienced child abuse, known as *child abuse pediatricians*, are at particular risk for conflictual family interactions, as well as threats to their personal and professional well-being through lawsuits and complaints to licensing boards (Flaherty et al., 2012).

Recommendations for Managing Stress-Related Illness Related to Child Abuse and Neglect

Several interventions have been developed to mitigate some of the risks for secondary trauma in medical providers who care for children with suspected or confirmed abuse or neglect. Both individual interventions (e.g., improved coping) and organizational interventions (e.g., mandatory group sessions) are likely needed to address symptoms of things such as secondary trauma and burnout in healthcare providers working with children who experienced abuse or neglect. At an individual level, healthcare providers working with children with child abuse will likely benefit from strategies such as setting appropriate limits, engaging in positive coping strategies (e.g., physical activity, distraction through fun activities), engaging with social support networks (both internally within the organization and externally through national organizations), and holding debriefing meetings for staff involved in caring for patients with suspected child abuse (Flaherty et al., 2012; O'Hara et al., 2020). While improved communication between providers and families might mitigate the risk for conflictual family relationships, it is often difficult to achieve a strong partnership between providers and families when the providers believe a child might be maltreated (Flaherty et al., 2012). Nonetheless, open and honest communication with families is important. In addition, finding meaning in one's work and higher levels of hope may reduce the effects of secondary traumatic stress (Passmore et al., 2020).

At an organizational level, increased flexibility in caseloads (i.e., redistributing child abuse cases among providers) and bereavement leave for difficult cases can be beneficial in decreasing the risk of secondary traumatic stress (O'Hara et al., 2020). An example of an organizational intervention is one that involved mandatory monthly sessions for child abuse pediatrician trainees, with topics ranging from mindfulness and effective coping strategies and sharing of impactful work experiences (Smith et al., 2021). Results from this study demonstrated improved secondary trauma symptoms and improved resiliency (Smith et al., 2021), thus demonstrating the value of organizational and peer support.

UNIQUE CHALLENGES DURING PUBLIC HEALTH CRISES

From work-related challenges, such as staffing and equipment shortages, to personal difficulties, such as managing changes to daycare or school schedules, healthcare providers are faced with a multitude of challenges during public health crises. Public health crises, such as natural disasters and mass causality events, as well as healthcare crises including the opioid epidemic and the COVID-19 pandemic, present unique challenges for the pediatric healthcare provider. While there are likely many challenges faced by pediatric healthcare providers during public health crises, the next section reviews some common challenges, including changing to a telehealth format, providing care with limited available school and outpatient and inpatient programming, and mitigating the effects of adverse childhood events.

Telehealth

Discussion

The use of telehealth brings a range of new evidence-informed possibilities to reach children and families while overcoming common barriers to care (e.g., lack of local providers, transportation issues, financial challenges, and scheduling conflicts); however, utilization also creates novel stressors that can affect a provider's well-being and subsequent practice (Myers et al., 2017; Langarizadeh et al., 2017). For instance, logistical considerations, such as referring patients to local clinics for specific services (e.g., vital signs, physical examination, and bloodwork) or utilizing available technological devices to collect data (e.g., smartphone heartbeat counter), requires additional planning. The telehealth modality chosen can also create challenges for the provider. For example, if videoconferencing, not all internet connections are equally high-speed or stable, and as such, connection issues may require the provider and family (or coordinating distant clinic) to spend additional time problem-solving (Myers et al., 2017).

In addition to logistical considerations, work with children and families requires extra provider attention and energy that likely was not required for face-to-face care. During telehealth visits, a child now has all of their toys and electronics at their disposal, can leave the room at any time in the session, can turn off the audio or video at will, or can leave the session if significantly agitated. Such situations may be especially problematic for children with specific pathology (e.g., inattention, impulsivity, hyperactivity, and oppositionality) or for those who recently arrived home from school and are tired, hungry, and want to play instead of sitting in one location and engaging with a healthcare provider. This is further compounded by caregivers also being tired and potentially having less patience for managing their child's behavior during the visit, meaning it may be up to the provider to assist some families in managing the child. As this level of management likely was not necessary for many providers during face-to-face visits, it can be viewed as mentally taxing.

While many telehealth methods exist (e.g., telephone and email), the common use of videoconferencing creates a subset of unique challenges. For example, the significant increase in video usage prompts providers to sit in one place while staring at a screen for extended periods. Referred to as *Zoom fatigue* or more generally as *screen fatigue*, the extended exposure can create both physical (e.g., body pains and posture issues; Shikdar & Al-Kindi, 2007) and ocular issues (Perle, 2021a). One ocular issue that results from prolonged digital screen exposure, known as *computer vision syndrome* (CVS), results in symptoms such as eyestrain, headache, blurred vision, eye redness, eye burning, eye pain, and dry eyes (Agarwal et al., 2018; Turgut, 2018).

Regardless of modality, telehealth's ability to allow providers to easily reach families where they are can be viewed as a double-edged sword. On the one hand, allowing a provider to see what naturally occurs within a patient's home can provide a wealth of real-world diagnostic information relevant to the environment and child management. On the other hand, healthcare providers can see problematic aspects that they may otherwise not observe if reserved to a face-to-face setting, such as seeing drug paraphernalia or witnessing either questionable living conditions or abusive behavior management strategies, all of which may require the provider to make an abuse report to the local child protection team for further investigation.

Just as telehealth increases a provider's access to the family, it also increases the family's access to the provider. Due to this, providers may be faced with boundary issues that can create undue strain on the provider's ability to manage their practice. Increased availability and flexibility of the technological mediums may motivate some providers to begin having visits outside of typical business hours; however, some providers may become overly flexible, leading to insidious stress to develop from a lack of self-care.

Recommendations for Managing Challenges Related to Telehealth

To manage stressors related to telehealth utilization, providers can seek telehealth-focused education to prevent stress related to technology issues (e.g., patient not responding to treatment-as-usual approaches when conducted remotely, difficulty holding the attention of child patient through a virtual format). Education should review several key competencies outlined in the literature, including, but not limited to, the basics of efficacy and effectiveness (e.g., types of treatments and methods most effective or least effective for different populations), methods of adapting face-to-face approaches for telehealth delivery, ethical factors (e.g., informed consent), legal considerations (e.g., cross-state practice), safety and crisis planning, data security (e.g., encryption standards and business associates agreements), and technology selection and troubleshooting (Galpin et al., 2020; Gifford et al., 2012; Gustin et al., 2020; Maheu et al., 2020; McCord et al., 2020; Perle, 2021b). Methods of engaging children, as well as managing family turmoil from a distance, can also be viewed as essential for the pediatric telehealth provider.

From a practice standpoint, providers should create structures that foster success for both themselves and the families, such as creating handouts detailing the types of rooms that families should use, with an emphasis on a quiet, private, and predominantly distraction-free area that is ideally as similar to a provider's office (Myers et al., 2017). The provider should also plan ahead to maintain the child's engagement, with online shared games (e.g., Connect4, Battleship), online coloring or block building programs, or video clips from websites cued up to balance clinical processes and fun. Ultimately, a child who enjoys meeting with a provider will remain more engaged and exhibit fewer behavioral issues. Use of between-session mobile applications and technology to monitor symptoms, medication taking, psychological factors, or physiological indicators (e.g., blood pressure and glucose) can also make a patient's care (or family's monitoring) more engaging and accurate, reducing the need for providers to take extra time to follow up. As crisis (e.g., imminent harm situations) often lead to high stress for providers, pediatric telehealth providers should gather emergency contact information (e.g., nearest medical and law enforcement offices) up front in case there are any issues that require a higher level of care (Perle, 2021a). To further ensure a smooth process, providers are recommended to adhere to their usual boundary standards to maintain work–life balance, even though they can be more flexible. As an example, providers should create policies for the average turnaround time for responses to phone calls, emails, or other messages sent and avoid scheduling patients off-hours.

To avoid physical and eye-related issues, providers should enact several self-care activities. As screens are often necessary for both the telehealth visits and the subsequent documentation (Occupational Safety and Health Administration [OSHA], n.d.), providers should create a schedule that allows for motion breaks (e.g., getting a drink of water and using the restroom) to reduce the amount of continuous time spent in front of the screens. When sitting, providers should attempt to frequently adjust how they are sitting, keep the screen at approximate eye level, and have a chair with appropriate lumbar support (Cook & Burgess-Limerick, 2003; OSHA, n.d.; Woo et al., 2015).

Access to Services and Mental Health Programs

Discussion

While access to services is a challenge for both adult and pediatric populations, it is particularly relevant for pediatric healthcare providers who might feel powerless to help (Weiss & Ludwig, 2019). During public health crises (e.g., natural disasters), access to services may become even more challenging. Public health crises often negatively impact access to school and educational services, including loss of learning milestones, nutritional access, structure, positive role models, and exercise (Brandenburg et al., 2020; Bylander, 2020; Imboden et al., 2021). For example, public health crises might cause many schools and childcare centers to close, which leads to food insecurity and decreased access to educational supports. Children receiving special education supports are directly impacted by limited access to educational supports, especially if schools move to a virtual learning format or close for extended periods of time. Many children in special education receive not only direct academic supports at school but also therapeutic supports, such as speech, occupational, or physical therapies. These services are challenging to provide in alternate learning environments, and schools might rely on the capacity of parents and caregivers to assist teachers with delivering those supports (United States Government Accountability Office, 2020). As these examples demonstrate, children and adolescents often have little control over their environments and social determinants of health (e.g., access to food and school) during public health crises, further contributing to the stress felt by pediatric healthcare providers who must not only consider such factors in their care but potentially feel compelled to intervene whether part of the treatment plan or not (Weiss & Ludwig, 2019). For example, pediatric providers, such as pediatricians, might be tasked with supporting patients and families who are frustrated and struggling due to a lack of services. Furthermore, healthcare providers with families of their own might experience additional stressors with trying to balance their work schedules when services become unavailable (e.g., daycare, schools).

Not only do public health crises impact school services for the general public, but they can be especially impactful for children with developmental delays who require early intervention. Early childhood is a crucial time for development that has direct implications for children's futures. Approximately one in six children ages 3–17 has developmental delays, with increases in prevalence over the last couple of decades (Zablotsky et al., 2019). Early intervention for children with developmental delays is critical for later success in life and is linked to more positive health, language, communication, cognitive, and social-emotional development and outcomes (Goode et al., 2011). Unfortunately, during public health crises, access to care can be limited. Using the COVID-19 pandemic as an example, children with developmental delays saw a significant decrease in access to services, with one study finding that 77.9% of parents reported a decrease in services (Neece et al., 2020). A lack of access to services, both through early intervention and early school-based supports, is associated with regression in both skills and development in children with developmental delays (Bylander, 2020). In addition, families might miss well-child checks during public health crises, which are crucial in identifying early delays in development and coordinating access to early intervention supports (Paulauskaite et al., 2021; Center for Translational Neuroscience, n.d.; Imboden et al., 2021). Pediatric providers might once again find themselves feeling frustrated and stressed with the lack of resources and feeling powerless to help some of their patients who need crucial services. Furthermore, some providers might find themselves trying to make up for the lack of services by providing more frequent visits or overbooking patients, thus contributing to feelings of burnout.

Along with the lack of school services, public health crises may also worsen access to mental health care. While access to mental health care is a longstanding public health concern for both adults and children, a lack of inpatient and outpatient mental health facilities for pediatric patients has led to hospitals facing the additional burden of providing services for which they are not well equipped (Nolan et al., 2015), thus exacerbating pediatric provider work-related illness. For instance, the overall emergency department visits for psychiatric and behavioral emergencies have doubled since 2001, while hospital beds in psychiatric units have decreased (Becker et al., 2020). More recently, in 2020, mental health emergency department visits increased by 31% in comparison to 2019 (Yard et al., 2021).

Due to emergency departments being unable to provide long-term services, patients often are placed on the inpatient medical floors (Becker et al., 2020). Patients who are admitted to the hospital with self-harm and/or suicidal ideation who are waiting for transfer to another hospital or psychiatric unit may be boarded in the hospital for twice as long compared to other patients (Smith et al., 2019). "Boarders," or patients who experience extended stays in the emergency department or medical floors due to a lack of inpatient or outpatient mental health services, are more likely to carry a diagnosis of a neurodevelopmental or neurocognitive disorder (Nolan et al., 2015). More specifically, children with a diagnosis of autism spectrum disorder (ASD) or other developmental delays are particularly difficult to place in mental health facilities due to lack of services, which results in a higher health care utilization and a 50% greater chance of a longer length of stay than the general population (Becker et al., 2020). These boarders create significant challenges for hospital staff. As a significant portion of boarders are children with ASD and developmental delays, these children often experience increased stress due to sensory sensitivities, routine disruption, and communication difficulties (Becker et al., 2020. In addition, patient agitation while boarding in the emergency department and inpatient medical floors can be a source of stress and risks to both patients and health care providers, including increased risk of injury to patients and staff, increased use of restraints, and disruption in care (Gerson et al., 2018). Meanwhile, healthcare providers and hospitals face their own challenges in managing boarders, including lack of education and training, lack of physical and therapeutic support, greater access to potential causes of injuries, and less supervision than would be found in community resources (Becker et al., 2020). In addition, when addressing agitation with restraints or psychopharmacologic medications, staff may experience moral or ethical distress (Carubia et al., 2016).

Recommendations for Managing Challenges Related to Lack of Services

To fully address the lack of services (i.e., food, school, and early intervention services) during public health crises, governmental supports are likely required. For example, federal support for free school meals for all children, meal delivery, or grab-and-go meals might be beneficial. Pediatric healthcare providers are in a unique position to advocate for such programs or services. Healthcare providers might also coordinate services with schools, such as providing supervised locations for children to attend virtual school. As parents might look to their healthcare providers for support during public crises, pediatric providers should familiarize themselves with available resources to provide to families.

For concerns related to hospital boarders and lack of mental health services, several strategies can be employed. For example, pediatric patients with agitation should be addressed via early recognition and assessment for triggers and sensory sensitivities (Gerson et al., 2018). Use of distraction or sensory tools, effective communication (e.g., repetition and reflective statements), cue boards, use of neutral speaking tone, offering appropriate choices, having family members present to provide comfort, praising adaptive and positive behaviors are all strategies that can be effective at managing agitation and behavioral concerns for patients who are boarding or who present with neurodevelopmental disorders (Gerson et al., 2018). Restraints via physical restraints, psychopharmacologic medication, or seclusion should only be used when the possibility of harm to self or others and other non-pharmacological strategies have not been effective (Gerson et al., 2018). Healthcare providers might also find it beneficial to network and consult with other hospital systems to learn additional strategies for managing boarders and lack of mental health resources.

Adverse Childhood Events

Discussion

Adverse childhood events (ACEs) are defined as potentially traumatic events that occur during childhood, which can occur in the child's family or social environment (Centers for Disease Control, 2021; Kalmakis & Chandler, 2013). Common ACEs include things such as experiencing abuse or neglect, witnessing violence, or substance use problems in the home (Centers for Disease Control, 2021). ACEs are often associated with poor outcomes in adulthood, including increased risk for chronic health problems and mental health concerns (Felitti et al., 1998). More specifically, research shows that more ACEs are associated with speech delays; behavior challenges, such as inattention, hyperactivity, and impulsivity; decreased cognitive flexibility; mood and anxiety disorders; decreased school readiness; poor coping skills; unhealthy lifestyles; and increased risk of heart disease, diabetes, mental illness, and substance abuse (Berken et al., 2021; Marie-Mitchell & O'Connor, 2013). When further considering the impact of ACEs and their link to poorer health and developmental outcomes for children (Dowd, 2019), it is especially important that ACEs not be overlooked by pediatricians and other medical or mental health providers, as ACEs are known to be cumulative and lifelong (Berken et al., 2021).

Public health crises, and the associated negative sequelae, can be another adverse event that contributes to long-term concerns in adulthood. Indeed, the risk for ACEs considerably increases during public health crises, natural disasters, humanitarian crises, and conflicts (Araujo et al., 2020; Bryce, 2020). These experiences may lead to ACEs for children who were previously at very low risk and compound ACEs for children previously at high risk. Public health crises, such as the more recent COVID-19 pandemic, can put many children and families at a disadvantage socially and financially, which compounds the risk of ACEs (Bryant et al., 2020; Bryce, 2020). Additionally, social isolation and parental stress increase the risk of physical and emotional violence, and increased time spent online increases the risk of virtual and online child abuse (Bryce, 2020). Coupled with decreased access to mandated reporters, such as teachers and healthcare providers, many ACEs may go unchecked during public health crises (Bryce, 2020).

Recommendations for Managing Challenges Related to ACEs

In general, the literature supports the need for ACEs screenings during regular well-child visits or other visits with a child's pediatrician or primary care physician (Bright et al., 2015; Kerker et al., 2016; Marie-Mitchell et al., 2016). ACEs screenings become especially important during public health crises, given the increased need for referrals and social and systemic supports (Berken et al., 2021; Bryant et al., 2020; Bryce, 2020). Unfortunately, many pediatricians do not routinely survey children and families for ACEs, as they may lack training and understanding of ACEs or do not know ACEs screening tools exist (Bright et al., 2015; Kerker et al., 2016). It is crucial that healthcare providers working with children and families have adequate training and resources to help combat ACEs and increase protective factors, as they are often the first line of defense in ACEs protection for their patients.

CONCLUSION

Pediatric healthcare providers have an undeniable passion for helping children; however, they also face distinctive challenges that put them at risk for things such as burnout, compassion fatigue, or secondary traumatic stress. Managing grief and bereavement, navigating difficult family dynamics, and working with children with suspected or confirmed child abuse or neglect can be trying for any pediatric provider. On top of these challenges, public health crises, such as natural disasters or the COVID-19 pandemic, can introduce additional challenges, including navigating telehealth and handling a shortage of services for children in inpatient hospital settings and developmental disabilities. Future studies should continue to explore the concepts outlined in this chapter and further expand upon the unique challenges pediatric healthcare providers face in their field, as there are likely additional challenges that were not included in this review.

Studies have suggested a variety of strategies to mitigate the negative consequences of these challenges. Some researchers have found that working in multidisciplinary teams (Zubatsky et al., 2020) and having a high-quality relationship with a supervisor, peers, and other medical staff (Hoelscher & Ravert, 2021) are protective against burnout. Relaxation strategies, stress management techniques, and mindfulness (e.g., mindful breathing) are effective individual or person-directed interventions, while primary nursing and mandatory educational sessions are effective organizational strategies (Van Moi et al., 2015). Recently, there has been a call to address the systemic factors related to burnout and compassion fatigue, as some suggest that focusing on burnout implies that healthcare providers have the problem and should be the focus of the intervention, insinuating that if providers were better and more successful at coping, or more mindful, or more resilient, they would not have a problem (Houtrow, 2020). Instead, interventions should focus on addressing the systemic factors influencing burnout and compassion fatigue, such as ever-increasing workloads and clinical productivity standards, low institutional support, and systemic inequities (Houtrow, 2020). Ultimately, it is recommended that a combination of individual and organizational strategies be utilized to produce the best outcomes and support for pediatric healthcare providers (Van Moi et al., 2015).

More specifically, "psychological first aid" has been recommended to address moral distress and injury in healthcare providers during a public health crisis such as the COVID-19 pandemic (National Traumatic Stress Network, 2021; Williams et al., 2020). Psychological first aid addresses the emotional and physical needs of providers by promoting positive health behaviors, such as sleep hygiene, regular exercise, problem-solving, self-compassion, and mindfulness. Psychological first aid also offers a variety of additional recommendations for individuals and organizations, including creating quiet spaces for staff to relax, improving connectedness through showing appreciation for all staff, acknowledging the stress and fatigue felt by all, and offering peer support groups (Williams et al., 2020). In addition, psychological first aid helps healthcare providers to focus on what they can control, while reminding them of their personal values and mission, which can be especially helpful during a public health crisis (Williams et al., 2020). Finally, having accessible mental health providers for staff can help staff learn and utilize effective coping strategies. Mental health providers can also help to advocate for the needs of healthcare providers at the organizational level.

In order to fully address healthcare providers' well-being, changes will likely need to be made at the organizational level. Shanafelt and Noseworthy (2017) outlined nine strategies that organizations can utilize to promote physician well-being and reduce burnout, including acknowledging the problem through townhalls, video interviews, or weekly newsletters and assessing the problem as part of a routine annual institution-wide assessment. Organizational strategies such as choosing effective leaders, implementing targeted interventions that are salient to staff, creating spaces for providers to feel a sense of community and connection with other staff, and using incentives for productivity or quality metrics can address provider burnout (Shanafelt & Noseworhty, 2017). Finally, evaluation of values and culture, fostering flexibility and work–life balance, providing self-care and resiliency resources to staff, and developing a program focused on reducing burnout and improving well-being can also be worthwhile efforts made by organizations to address the needs of its' providers (Shanafelt & Noseworthy, 2017).

While most of this review focused on the challenges faced by providers in pediatric healthcare, it is worth noting the positive aspects that often draw providers into working with children. For example, witnessing the resiliency of children and adolescents and watching them grow throughout the years can help healthcare providers find joy in their work, which in turn may buffer the effects of stress-related illness (Weiss & Ludwig, 2019; Passmore et al., 2020). During challenging times, such as during a worldwide pandemic, reminding oneself of this passion and joy is critical to preserving and thriving in the field of pediatric healthcare.

REFERENCES

Agarwal, S., Goel, D., & Sharma, A. (2013). Evaluation of the factors which contribute to the ocular complaints in computer users. *Journal of Clinical and Diagnostic Research: JCDR*, *7*(2), 331–335. doi:10.7860/JCDR/2013/5150.2760 PMID:23543722

American Academy of Pediatrics. (2012). Patient- and family-centered care and the pediatrician's role. *Pediatrics*, *129*(2), 394–404. doi:10.1542/peds.2011-3084 PMID:22291118

Araujo, L. A., Veloso, C. F., Souza, M. C., Azevedo, J. M. C., & Tarro, G. (2021). The potential impact of the COVID-19 pandemic on child growth and development: A systematic review. *Jornal de Pediatria*, *97*(4), 369–377. doi:10.1016/j.jped.2020.08.008 PMID:32980318

Baird, J., Davies, B., Hinds, P. S., Baggott, C., & Rehm, R. S. (2015). What impact do hospital and unit-based rules have upon patient- and family-centered care in the pediatric intensive care unit? *Journal of Pediatric Nursing*, *30*(1), 133–142. doi:10.1016/j.pedn.2014.10.001 PMID:25450441

Becker, J. E., Smith, J. R., & Hazen, E. P. (2020). Pediatric consultation-liaison psychiatry: An update and review. *Psychosomatics*, *61*(5), 467–480. doi:10.1016/j.psym.2020.04.015 PMID:32482345

Bergsträsser, E., Cignacco, E., & Luck, P. (2017). Health care professionals' experiences and needs when delivering end-of-life care to children: A qualitative study. *Palliative Care*, *10*. Advance online publication. doi:10.1177/1178224217724770 PMID:28835736

Berken, J. A., Heard-Garris, N., & Wakschlag, L. S. (2021). Guardians at the gate: Early adversity, neurocognitive development, and the role of the pediatrician in the era of COVID-19. *Frontiers in Pediatrics*, *9*, 1–6. doi:10.3389/fped.2021.665335 PMID:33937157

Branch, C., & Klinkerberg, D. (2015). Compassion fatigue among pediatric healthcare providers. *The American Journal of Maternal/Child Nursing*, *40*(3), 160–166. doi:10.1097/NMC.0000000000000133

Brandenburg, J. E., Holman, L. K., Apkon, S. D., Houtrow, A. J., Rinaldi, R., & Sholas, M. G. (2020). School reopening during COVID-19 pandemic: Considering students with disabilities. *Journal of Pediatric Rehabilitation Medicine: An Interdisciplinary Approach*, *13*(3), 425–431. doi:10.3233/PRM-200789 PMID:33136082

Bright, M. A., Thompson, L., Esernio-Jenssen, D., Alford, S., & Shenkman, E. (2015). Primary care pediatricians' perceived prevalence and surveillance of adverse childhood experiences in low-income children. *Journal of Health Care for the Poor and Underserved*, *26*(3), 686–700. doi:10.1353/hpu.2015.0080 PMID:26320905

Bryant, D. J., Oo, M., & Damian, A. J. (2020). The rise of adverse childhood experiences during the COVID-19 pandemic. *Psychological Trauma: Theory, Research, Practice, and Policy*, *12*(S1), S193–S194. doi:10.1037/tra0000711 PMID:32551773

Bryce, I. (2020). Responding to the accumulation of adverse childhood experiences in the wake of the COVID-19 pandemic: Implications for practice. *Children Australia*, *45*(2), 80–87. doi:10.1017/cha.2020.27

Buckley, L., Berta, W., Cleverley, K., Medeiros, C., & Widger, K. (2020). What is known about paediatric nurse burnout: A scoping review. *Human Resources for Health*, *18*(1), 1–23. doi:10.118612960-020-0451-8 PMID:32046721

Bylander, J. (2020). How COVID-19 threatens the safety net for US children. *Health Affairs*, *39*(10), 1668–1671. doi:10.1377/hlthaff.2020.01576 PMID:33017239

Carubia, B., Becker, A., & Levine, B. H. (2016). Child psychiatric emergencies: Updates on trends, clinical care, and practice challenges. *Current Psychiatry Reports*, *18*(4), 41. doi:10.100711920-016-0670-9 PMID:26932516

Center for Translational Neuroscience. (n.d.). *Rapid assessment of pandemic impact on development–early childhood (RAPID-EC)*. University of Oregon. https://www.uorapidresponse.com/latest-data-and-trends

Centers for Disease Control. (2021). *Preventing child abuse and neglect.* https://www.cdc.gov/violenceprevention/childabuseandneglect/fastfact.html

Child Welfare Information Gateway. (2021). Child maltreatment 2019: *Summary of key findings*. U.S. Department of Health and Human Services. https://www.childwelfare.gov/pubs/factsheets/canstats/

Christian, C. W., Crawford-Jakubiak, J. E., Flaherty, E. G., Leventhal, J. M., Lukefahr, J. L., Sege, R. D., MacMillan, H., Nolan, C. M., Valley, L. A., & Hurley, T. P. (2015). The evaluation of suspected child physical abuse. *Pediatrics*, *135*(5), e1337–e1354. doi:10.1542/peds.2015-0356 PMID:25917988

Clay, R. A. (2020, June 11). *Are you experiencing compassion fatigue?* American Psychological Association. http://www.apa.org/topics/covid-19/compassion-fatigue

Colville, G. A., & Smith, J. G. (2017). The overlap between burnout and depression in ICU staff. *Critical Care Medicine*, *45*(10), e1102–e1103. doi:10.1097/CCM.0000000000002546 PMID:28915199

Cook, C., & Burgess-Limerick, R. (2003). Guidelines for computer workstations. *Ergonomics Australia*, *17*(1), 19–37. doi:10.1080/00140139.2015.1076528

Cull, W. L., Frintner, M. P., Starmer, A. J., & Leslie, L. K. (2019). Longitudinal analyses of pediatrician burnout. *Academic Pediatrics, 19*(3), 256–262. doi:10.1016/j.acap.2018.11.006 PMID:30412766

Curtis, J. R., Sprung, C. L., & Azoulay, E. (2014). The importance of word choice in the care of critically ill patients and their families. *Intensive Care Medicine, 40*(4), 606–608. doi:10.100700134-013-3201-8 PMID:24441669

Dowd, M. D. (2019). The relevance of parental adverse childhood experiences in pediatric patients. *Pediatric Annals, 48*(12), e463–e465. doi:10.3928/19382359-20191118-03 PMID:31830283

Dzeng, E., Colaianni, A., Roland, M., Levine, D., Kelly, M. P., Barclay, S., & Smith, T. J. (2016). Moral distress amongst American physician trainees regarding futile treatments at the end of life: A qualitative study. *Journal of General Internal Medicine, 31*(1), 93–99. doi:10.100711606-015-3505-1 PMID:26391029

Embriaco, N., Papazian, L., Kentish-Barnes, N., Pochard, F., & Azoulay, E. (2007). Burnout syndrome among critical care healthcare workers. *Current Opinion in Critical Care, 13*(5), 482–488. doi:10.1097/MCC.0b013e3282efd28a PMID:17762223

Esmee van Steijn, M., Scheepstra, K. W. F., Yasar, G., Olff, M., Charlotte de Vries, M., & Gabriel van Pampus, M. (2019). Occupational well-being in pediatricians: A survey about work-related posttraumatic stress, depression, and anxiety. *European Journal of Pediatrics, 178*(5), 681–693. doi:10.100700431-019-03334-7 PMID:30783762

Felitti, V. J., Anda, R. F., Nordenberg, D., Williamson, D. F., Spitz, A. M., Edwards, V., Koss, M. P., & Marks, J. S. (1998). Relationship of childhood abuse and household dysfunction to many of the leading causes of death in adults: The adverse childhood experiences (ACS) study. *American Journal of Preventive Medicine, 14*(4), 245–258. doi:10.1016/S0749-3797(98)00017-8 PMID:9635069

Figley, C. R. (1995). Compassion fatigue: Toward a new understanding of the costs of caring. In B. H. Stamm (Ed.), *Secondary traumatic stress: Self-care issues for clinicians, researchers, and educators* (pp. 3–28). The Sidran Press.

Flaherty, E. G., Schwartz, K., Jones, R. D., & Sege, R. D. (2012). Child abuse physicians: Coping with challenges. *Evaluation & the Health Professions, 36*(2), 163–173. doi:10.1177/0163278712459196 PMID:22960291

Galpin, K., Sikka, N., King, S. L., Horvath, K. A., & Shipman, S. A.AAMC Telehealth Advisory Committee. (2021). Expert consensus: Telehealth skills for health care professionals. *Telemedicine Journal and e-Health, 27*(7), 820–824. doi:10.1089/tmj.2020.0420 PMID:33236964

Gerson, R., Malas, N., & Mroczkowski, M. (2018). Crisis in the emergency department: The evaluation and management of acute agitation in children and adolescents. *Child and Adolescent Psychiatric Clinics of North America, 27*(3), 367–386. doi:10.1016/j.chc.2018.02.002 PMID:29933788

Gifford, V., Niles, B., Rivkin, I., Koverola, C., & Polaha, J. (2012). Continuing education training focused on the development of behavioral telehealth competencies in behavioral healthcare providers. *Rural and Remote Health, 12*, 1–15. doi:10.22605/RRH2108 PMID:23240871

Goode, S., Diefendorf, M., & Colgan, S. (2011). *The importance of early intervention for infants and toddlers with developmental disabilities and their families*. National Early Childhood Technical Assistance Center. https://ectacenter.org/~pdfs/pubs/importanceofearlyintervention.pdf

Grauerholz, K. R., Fredenburg, M., Jones, P. T., & Jenkins, K. N. (2020). Fostering vicarious resilience for perinatal palliative care professionals. *Frontiers in Pediatrics*, *8*, 572933. Advance online publication. doi:10.3389/fped.2020.572933 PMID:33134232

Gustin, T. S., Kott, K., & Rutledge, C. (2020). Telehealth etiquette training: A guideline for preparing interprofessional teams for successful encounters. *Nurse Educator*, *45*(2), 88–92. doi:10.1097/NNE.0000000000000680 PMID:31022072

Hensel, J. M., Ruiz, C., Finney, C., & Dewa, C. S. (2015). Meta-analysis of risk factors for secondary traumatic stress in therapeutic work with trauma victims. *Journal of Traumatic Stress*, *28*(2), 83–91. doi:10.1002/jts.21998 PMID:25864503

Hinchey, S. A., & Jackson, J. L. (2011). A cohort study assessing difficult patient encounters in a walk-in primary care clinic: Predictors and outcomes. *Journal of General Internal Medicine*, *26*(6), 588–594. doi:10.100711606-010-1620-6 PMID:21264521

Hoelscher, L., & Ravert, R. (2021). Workplace relationships and professional burnout among certified child life specialists. *The Journal of Child Life: Psychosocial Theory and Practice*, *2*(1), 15–25. doi:10.55591/001c.22523

Houtrow, A. J. (2020). Addressing burnout: Symptom management versus treating the cause. *The Journal of Pediatrics*, *224*, 18–19. doi:10.1016/j.jpeds.2020.04.068 PMID:32370952

Imboden, A., Sobczak, B. K., & Griffin, V. (2021). The impact of the COVID-19 pandemic on infant and toddler development. *Journal of the American Association of Nurse Practitioners*, 1–11. doi:10.1097/JXX.0000000000000653 PMID:34519673

Jenkins, S. R., & Baird, S. (2002). Secondary traumatic stress and vicarious trauma: A validational study. *Journal of Traumatic Stress: Official Publication of The International Society for Traumatic Stress Studies*, *15*(5), 423–432. doi:10.1023/A:1020193526843 PMID:12392231

Judd-Glossy, L., & Twohy, E. (2020). Distress parents and family issues. In B. D. Carter & K. A. Kullgren (Eds.), *Clinical Handbook of Psychological Consultation in Pediatric Medical Settings* (pp. 401–412). Springer Nature. doi:10.1007/978-3-030-35598-2_30

Kalmakis, K. A., & Chandler, G. E. (2013). Adverse childhood experiences: Towards a clear conceptual meaning. *Journal of Advanced Nursing*, *70*(7), 1489–1501. Advance online publication. doi:10.1111/jan.12329 PMID:24329930

Kerker, B. D., Storfer-Isser, A., Szilagyi, M., Stein, R. E. K., Garner, A. S., O'Connor, K. G., Hoagwood, K. E., & Horwitz, S. M. (2016). Do pediatricians ask about adverse childhood experiences in pediatric primary care? *Academic Pediatrics*, *16*(2), 154–160. doi:10.1016/j.acap.2015.08.002 PMID:26530850

Kim, J. J., Brookman-Frazee, L., Gellatly, R., Stadnick, N., Barnett, M. L., & Lau, A. S. (2018). Predictors of burnout among community therapists in the sustainment phase of a system-driven implementation of multiple evidence-based practices in children's mental health. *Professional Psychology, Research and Practice*, *49*(2), 131–142. doi:10.1037/pro0000182 PMID:30270968

Kitao, M., Setou, N., Yamamoto, A., & Takada, S. (2018). Associated factors of psychological distress among Japanese NICU nurses in supporting bereaved families who have lost children. *The Kobe Journal of Medical Sciences*, *64*(1), E11–E19. PMID:30282893

Koinis, A., Giannou, V., Drantaki, V., Angelaina, S., Stratou, E., & Saridi, M. (2015). The impact of healthcare workers job environment on their mental-emotional health. Coping strategies: The case of a local general hospital. *Health Psychology Research*, *3*(1). Advance online publication. doi:10.4081/hpr.2015.1984 PMID:26973958

Langarizadeh, M., Tabatabaeim, M. S., Tavakol, K., Naghipour, M., Rostami, A., & Moghbeli, F. (2017). Telemental health care, an effective alternative to conventional mental care: A systematic review. *Acta Informatica Medica*, *25*(4), 240–246. doi:10.5455/aim.2017.25.240-246 PMID:29284913

Li, Y.-L., Li, R.-Q., Qiu, D., & Xiao, S.-Y. (2020). Prevalence of workplace physical violence against healthcare professionals by patients and visitors: A systematic review and meta-analysis. *International Journal of Environmental Research and Public Health*, *17*(1), 299. doi:10.3390/ijerph17010299 PMID:31906306

MacKinnon, M., & Murray, S. (2018). Reframing physician burnout as an organizational problem: A novel pragmatic approach to physician burnout. *Academic Psychiatry*, *42*(1), 123–128. doi:10.100740596-017-0689-1 PMID:28247366

Maheu, M., Callan, J., & Hilty, D. M. (2020). *Telebehavioral health: foundations in theory and practice for graduate learners*. Cognella.

Marie-Mitchell, A., & O'Connor, T. (2013). Adverse childhood experiences: Translating knowledge into identification of children at risk for poor outcomes. *Academic Pediatrics*, *13*(1), 14–19. doi:10.1016/j.acap.2012.10.006 PMID:23312855

Marie-Mitchell, A., Studer, K. R., & O'Connor, T. G. (2016). How knowledge of adverse childhood experiences can help pediatricians prevent mental health problems. *Families, Systems & Health*, *34*(2), 128–135. doi:10.1037/fsh0000179 PMID:26950476

Maslach, C., Schaufeli, W. B., & Leiter, M. P. (2001). Job burnout. *Annual Review of Psychology*, *52*(1), 397–422. doi:10.1146/annurev.psych.52.1.397 PMID:11148311

McCord, C., Bernhard, P., Walsh, M., Rosner, C., & Console, K. (2020). A consolidated model for telepsychology practice. *Journal of Clinical Psychology*, *76*(6), 1060–1082. doi:10.1002/jclp.22954 PMID:32285940

McKinley, T. F., Boland, K. A., & Mahan, J. D. (2017). Burnout and interventions in pediatric residency: A literature review. *Burnout Research*, *6*, 9–17. doi:10.1016/j.burn.2017.02.003

Meadors, P., Lamson, A., Swanson, M., White, M., & Sira, N. (2010). Secondary traumatization in pediatric healthcare providers: Compassion fatigue, burnout, and secondary traumatic stress. *Omega*, *60*(2), 103–128. doi:10.2190/OM.60.2.a PMID:20222232

Morse, G., Salyers, M. P., Rollins, A. L., Monroe-DeVita, M., & Pfahler, C. (2012). Burnout in mental health services: A review of the problem and its remediation. *Administration and Policy in Mental Health*, *39*(5), 341–352. doi:10.100710488-011-0352-1 PMID:21533847

Myers, K., Nelson, E. L., Rabinowitz, T., Hilty, D., Baker, D., Barnwell, S. S., Boyce, G., Bufka, L. F., Cain, S., Chui, L., Comer, J. S., Cradock, C., Goldstein, F., Johnston, B., Krupinski, E., Lo, K., Luxton, D. D., McSwain, S. D., McWilliams, J., ... Bernard, J. (2017). American telemedicine association practice guidelines for telemental health with children and adolescents. *Telemedicine Journal and e-Health*, *23*(10), 779–804. doi:10.1089/tmj.2017.0177 PMID:28930496

National Traumatic Stress Network. (2021). https://www.nctsn.org

Neece, C., McIntyre, L. L., & Fenning, R. (2020). Examining the impact of COVID-19 in ethnically diverse families with young children with intellectual and developmental disabilities. *Journal of Intellectual Disability Research*, *64*(10), 739–749. doi:10.1111/jir.12769 PMID:32808424

Nolan, J. M., Fee, C., Cooper, B. A., Rankin, S. H., & Blegen, M. A. (2015). Psychiatric boarding incidence, duration, and associated factors in United States emergency departments. *Journal of Emergency Nursing: JEN*, *41*(1), 57–64. doi:10.1016/j.jen.2014.05.004 PMID:25034663

O'Hara, M. A., McCann, T. A., Fan, W., Lane, M. M., Kernie, S. G., & Rosenthal, S. L. (2020). Child abuse taking its toll on the emotional well-being of pediatricians. *Clinical Pediatrics*, *59*(4–5), 450–457. doi:10.1177/0009922820905865 PMID:32070135

Occupational Safety and Health Administration. (n.d.). *Computer workstations eTool*. United States Department of Labor. https://www.osha.gov/SLTC/etools/computerworkstations/positions.html

Park, E., Meyer, R. M., & Gold, J. I. (2020). The role of medical specialization on posttraumatic symptoms in pediatric nurses. *Journal of Pediatric Nursing*, *53*, 22–28. doi:10.1016/j.pedn.2020.03.019 PMID:32339973

Passmore, S., Hemming, E., McIntosh, H. C., & Hellman, C. M. (2020). The relationship between hope, meaning in work, secondary traumatic stress, and burnout among child abuse pediatric clinicians. *The Permanente Journal*, *24*. Advance online publication. doi:10.7812/TPP/19.087 PMID:31852051

Paulauskaite, L., Farris, O., Spencer, H. M., & Hassiotis, A.EPICC-ID Group. (2021). My son can't socially distance or wear a mask: How families of preschool children with severe developmental delays and challenging behavior experienced the COVID-19 pandemic. *Journal of Mental Health Research in Intellectual Disabilities*, *14*(2), 225–236. doi:10.1080/19315864.2021.1874578

Perle, J. G. (2015). Avoiding the clash of the titans: A literature- and experience-based discussion of considerations for preventing and managing challenging caregiver behaviors throughout child-focused family therapy. *Professional Psychology, Research and Practice*, *46*(5), 366–374. doi:10.1037/pro0000028

Perle, J. G. (2021a). *A mental health provider's guide to telehealth: Providing outpatient videoconferencing services*. Routledge. doi:10.4324/9781003150473

Perle, J. G. (2021b). Training psychology students for telehealth: A model for doctoral-level education. *Journal of Technology in Behavioral Science*, *6*(3), 456–459. doi:10.100741347-021-00212-8

Phillips, J. P. (2016). Workplace violence against health care workers in the United States. *The New England Journal of Medicine*, *374*(17), 1661–1669. doi:10.1056/NEJMra1501998 PMID:27119238

Rabatin, J., Williams, E., Baier Manwell, L., Schwartz, M. D., Brown, R. L., & Linzer, M. (2016). Predictors and outcomes of burnout in primary care physicians. *Journal of Primary Care & Community Health*, *7*(1), 41–43. doi:10.1177/2150131915607799 PMID:26416697

Rabow, M. W., Huang, C. S., White-Hammond, G. E., & Tucker, R. O. (2021). Witnesses and victims both: Healthcare workers and grief in the time of COVID-19. *Journal of Pain and Symptom Management*, *62*(3), 647–656. doi:10.1016/j.jpainsymman.2021.01.139 PMID:33556494

Riskin, A., Erez, A., Foulk, T. A., Kugelman, A., Gover, A., Shoris, I., Riskin, K. S., & Bamberger, P. A. (2015). The impact of rudeness on medical team performance: A randomized trial. *Pediatrics*, *136*(3), 487–495. doi:10.1542/peds.2015-1385 PMID:26260718

Robins, P. M., Meltzer, L., & Zelikovsky, N. (2009). The experience of secondary traumatic stress upon care providers working within a children's hospital. *Journal of Pediatric Nursing*, *24*(4), 270–279. doi:10.1016/j.pedn.2008.03.007 PMID:19632504

Shanafelt, T. D., Balch, C. M., Bechamps, G., Russell, T., Dyrbye, L., Satele, D., Collicott, P., Novotny, P. J., Sloan, J., & Freischlag, J. (2010). Burnout and medical errors among American surgeons. *Annals of Surgery*, *251*(6), 995–1000. doi:10.1097/SLA.0b013e3181bfdab3 PMID:19934755

Shanafelt, T. D., Hasan, O., Dyrbye, L. N., Sinsky, C., Satele, D., Sloan, J., & West, C. P. (2015). Changes in burnout and satisfaction with work–life balance in physicians and the general US working population between 2011 and 2014. *Mayo Clinic Proceedings*, *90*(12), 1600–1613. doi:10.1016/j.mayocp.2015.08.023 PMID:26653297

Shanafelt, T. D., & Noseworthy, J. H. (2017). Executive leadership and physician well-being: Nine organizational strategies to promote engagement and reduce burnout. *Mayo Clinic Proceedings*, *92*(1), 129–146. doi:10.1016/j.mayocp.2016.10.004 PMID:27871627

Shikdar, A. A., & Al-Kindi, M. A. (2007). Office ergonomics: Deficiencies in computer workstation design. *International Journal of Occupational Safety and Ergonomics*, *13*(2), 215–223. doi:10.1080/10803548.2007.11076722 PMID:17599795

Smith, J., Cho, R., Martin, C., Cory, E., Smith, T., & Shouldice, M. (2021). Building skills and resilience in child abuse pediatricians: A novel program to address secondary traumatic stress. *Child Abuse & Neglect*, *117*, 105082. doi:10.1016/j.chiabu.2021.105082 PMID:33930661

Smith, J. L., De Nadai, A. S., Petrila, J., & Storch, E. A. (2019). Factors associated with length of stay in emergency departments for pediatric patients with psychiatric problems. *Pediatric Emergency Care*, *35*(10), 716–721. doi:10.1097/PEC.0000000000001651 PMID:31593981

Starmer, A. J., Frintner, M. P., & Freed, G. L. (2016). Work–life balance, burnout, and satisfaction of early career pediatricians. *Pediatrics, 137*(4), e20153183. Advance online publication. doi:10.1542/peds.2015-3183 PMID:27020792

Tawfik, D. S., Profit, J., Webber, S., & Shanafelt, T. D. (2019). Organizational factors affecting physician well-being. *Current Treatment Options in Pediatrics, 5*(1), 11–25. doi:10.100740746-019-00147-6 PMID:31632895

The Moral Injury Project. (2021). *What is moral injury*? Syracuse University. https://moralinjuryproject.syr.edu/about-moral-injury/

Trotochaud, K., Coleman, J. R., Krawiecki, N., & McCracken, C. (2015). Moral distress in pediatric healthcare workers. *Journal of Pediatric Nursing, 30*(6), 908–914. doi:10.1016/j.pedn.2015.03.001 PMID:25869472

Turgut, B. (2018). Ocular ergonomics for the computer vision syndrome. *Journal of Eye and Vision, 1*(2), 1–2. https://www.imedpub.com/articles/ocular-ergonomics-for-the-computer-vision-syndrome.php?aid=22200

United States Government Accountability Office. (2020). *Distance learning: Challenges providing services to K-12 English learners and students with disabilities during COVID-19*. https://www.gao.gov/assets/gao-21-43.pdf

Van Moi, M. M. C., Kompanje, E. J. O., Benoit, D. D., Bakker, J., & Nijkamp, M. D. (2015). The prevalence of compassion fatigue and burnout among healthcare professionals in intensive care units: A systematic review. *PLoS One, 10*(8), e0136955. doi:10.1371/journal.pone.0136955 PMID:26322644

Waldman, J. D., Kelly, F., Aurora, S., & Smith, H. L. (2004). The shocking cost of turnover in health care. *Health Care Management Review, 29*(1), 2–7. doi:10.1097/00004010-200401000-00002 PMID:14992479

Wang, C., Grassau, P., Lawlor, P. G., Webber, C., Bush, S. H., Gagnon, B., Kabir, M., & Spilg, E. G. (2020). Burnout and resilience among Canadian palliative care physicians. *BMC Palliative Care, 19*(1), 169. doi:10.118612904-020-00677-z PMID:33158428

Weiss, A. K., & Ludwig, S. (2019). Physician well-being: Special considerations in pediatrics. *Current Problems in Pediatric and Adolescent Health Care, 49*(11), 100657. Advance online publication. doi:10.1016/j.cppeds.2019.100657 PMID:31542326

Wenzel, J., Shaha, M., Klimmek, R., & Krumm, S. (2011). Working through grief and loss: Oncology nurses' perspectives on professional bereavement. *Oncology Nursing Forum, 38*(4), E272–E282. doi:10.1188/11.ONF.E272-E282 PMID:21708522

Wiener, L., Rosenberg, A. R., Pennarola, B., Fry, A., & Weaver, M. (2021). Navigating the terrain of moral distress: Experiences of pediatric end-of-life care and bereavement during COVID-19. *Palliative & Supportive Care, 19*(2), 129–134. doi:10.1017/S1478951521000225 PMID:33648612

Williams, R. D., Brundage, J. A., & Williams, E. B. (2020). Moral injury in times of COVID-19. *Journal of Health Service Psychology, 46*(2), 65–69. doi:10.100742843-020-00011-4 PMID:32363349

Woo, E. H. C., White, P., & Lai, C. W. K. (2015). Ergonomics standards and guidelines for compute workstation design and the impact on users' health: A review. *Ergonomics*, *59*(3), 464–475. doi:10.1080/00140139.2015.1076528 PMID:26224145

Yang, Y., & Hayes, J. A. (2020). Causes and consequences of burnout among mental health professionals: A practice-oriented review of recent empirical literature. *Psychotherapy (Chicago, Ill.)*, *57*(3), 426–436. doi:10.1037/pst0000317 PMID:32463274

Yard, E., Radhakrishnan, L., Ballesteros, M. F., Sheppard, M., Gates, A., Stein, Z., Hartnett, K., Kite-Powell, A., Rodgers, L., Adjemian, J., Ehlman, D. C., Holland, K., Idaikkadar, N., Ivey-Stephenson, A., Martinez, P., Law, R., & Stone, D. M. (2021). Emergency department visits for suspected suicide attempts among persons aged 12–25 years before and during the COVID-19 pandemic: United States, January 2019–May 2021. *Morbidity and mortality weekly report*, *70*(24), 888–894. doi:10.15585/mmwr.mm7024e1 PMID:34138833

Zablotsky, B., Black, L. I., Maenner, M. J., Schieve, L. A., Danielson, M. L., Bitsko, R. H., Blumberg, S. J., Kogan, M. D., & Boyle, C. A. (2019). Prevalence and trends of developmental disabilities among children in the United States: 2009–2017. *Pediatrics*, *144*(4), 1–21. doi:10.1542/peds.2019-0811 PMID:31558576

Zadeh, S., Gamba, N., Hudson, C., & Wiener, L. (2012). Taking care of care providers: A wellness program for pediatric nurses. *Journal of Pediatric Oncology Nursing*, *29*(5), 294–299. doi:10.1177/1043454212451793 PMID:22907685

Zhang, W., & Lane, B. S. (2013). Promoting neonatal staff nurses' comfort and involvement in end of life and bereavement care. *Nursing Research and Practice*, *365329*, 1–5. Advance online publication. doi:10.1155/2013/365329 PMID:23606955

Zubatsky, M., Runyan, C., Gulotta, S., Knight, J. R., & Pettinelli, J. D. (2020). Burnout among behavioral health providers in integrated care settings. *Families, Systems & Health*, *38*(1), 74–82. doi:10.1037/fsh0000456 PMID:31789532

KEY TERMS AND DEFINITIONS

Burnout: When individuals experience significant occupational stress that it leads to physical and emotional symptoms.

Compassion Fatigue: When empathetic individuals experience trauma symptoms due to their work with traumatized individuals.

Moral Distress: The conflict felt by individuals when they know the right thing to do but cannot do it because of a lack of resources or time.

Moral Injury: Damage to an individual's emotional state after experiencing a situation that goes against his or her moral beliefs or ethics.

Psychological First Aid: A set of strategies that were developed to specifically manage and address emotional and physical stress related to public health crises.

Public Health Crises: Local, national, or international events that significantly disrupt the daily lives of a large group of people. Examples include natural disasters, mass causality events, the opioid epidemic, and the COVID-19 pandemic.

Secondary Traumatic Stress: When individuals experience emotional stress due to hearing about the trauma of others or witnessing trauma of someone else.

Stress-Related Illness: Physical or emotional symptoms associated with increased stress perceived by individuals. Increased stress can be associated with one's occupation, living situation, or environment.

Chapter 5
Barriers to Healthy Nutrition and Exercise Behaviors Among Healthcare Workers

Joseph J. Mazzola
Meredith College, USA

ABSTRACT

Healthcare workers often struggle with being able to complete healthy eating and exercise behaviors, and this can lead to issues like obesity and chronic illness. The focus of this chapter is on the healthy nutrition and exercise behaviors of healthcare workers, specifically workplace barriers encountered that hinder those behaviors. The major barrier categories discussed in this chapter are time and shiftwork issues, job demands/work stress, absence of healthy options, lack of health knowledge, the work environment, social barriers, and personal factors. Potential facilitators to health behavior and initiatives organizations can implement to improve the health of healthcare employees are also included.

INTRODUCTION

Most employees can relate to the persistent struggle of trying to fit healthy eating and regular physical activity into our busy schedules, as part of their efforts to maintain or improve their overall physical health. In fact, often the directives to improve eating and exercise behaviors, and how to do so, come directly from healthcare workers (HCWs) themselves, but we do not often think about the difficulty those workers have maintaining their own health and health behaviors. When the often challenging and hectic work environment of HCWs is factored in, that task becomes incredibly difficult for the average healthcare employee. This puts HCWs in a particularly tough situation, since many of them work long hours, experience larger than average overall and workload stress, and often have relative uncertainty about what they will do that day or when they will get a break (e.g., Kakunje, 2011; Piko, 2006). These factors, among many others discussed in this chapter, are consistently shown as barriers to proper nutrition and exercise habits (Mazzola et al., 2019).

DOI: 10.4018/978-1-7998-8813-0.ch005

The focus of this chapter is the healthy nutrition and exercise behaviors of HCWs, and within this context, HCWs include doctors, nurses, residential care workers, and those who work in hospitals and medical facilities in an administrative or support staff capacity. This both creates a large umbrella under which to consider these individuals (14% of employees in the United States are working population in the healthcare industry; U.S. Census Bureau, 2019), while also accentuating important distinctions among different subtypes of workers that often affect both health indicators and health behaviors, such as between blue-collar (e.g., many nurses, some support staff) and white-collar workers (e.g., doctors, most administrative staff).

Data supports the idea that HCWs as a whole are actually unhealthier than the average person and often are not able to follow guidelines for proper nutrition and exercise behaviors. A recent study of healthcare workers in South Africa found that the majority of staff were overweight/obese (73.5%; Skaal & Pengpid, 2011), above the typical average of around 2/3rds (Wang et al., 2020), and almost all of them had low fitness levels (81.5%). A study using data from 2008-2012 found that 61% of nurses in England were obese or overweight (Kyle et al. 2017), which while not much different from the overall prevalence in the population, still illustrates the high risk of obesity for this population. Interestingly, other healthcare professionals in this sample (e.g., medical practitioners, pharmacists, dentists) had only a 49% prevalence rate, which while still high enough for concern and study, emphasizes the differences of these populations from nurses that suggests they possess protective factors, potentially related to socio-economic and white-collar worker statuses. Obesity is a major indicator of poor health and is related to higher morbidity for hypertension, coronary heart disease, type 2 diabetes, stroke, sleep apnea, and complications with pregnancy, just to name a few (National Heart, Lung, and Blood Institute, 1998). Extreme obesity is associated with a 6.5 to 13.7-year lowered life expectancy depending on the specific BMI ratio of the individual (Kitahara et al., 2014).

Meanwhile, as it relates specifically to health behaviors themselves, Malik and colleagues (2011) found 64.8% of U.K. hospital nurses reported not consuming 5 servings of fruits and vegetables per day, but 42.5% ate food high in sugar and fat daily. In Australia, almost all of the hospital nurses surveyed (94.5%) by Perry and colleagues (2015) failed to meet the fruits and vegetables recommendation. In a survey of Irish hospital doctors, only 36.9% reported going for a run or taking part in another form of exercise (Feeney et al., 2016).

Given the importance and ubiquity of the workplace in the lives of HCWs, it is vital that the work environment is supportive of healthy behaviors. In a survey of National Health Service (NHS) hospital doctors, only 12% felt the organization supported healthy eating (Winston et al., 2008). This might help explain why despite their medical training specifically directed towards keeping people healthy and seeing the effects of an unhealthy lifestyle on their patients on a daily basis, many healthcare workers still have issues practicing these healthy habits themselves. It is important for researchers and practitioners to understand and mitigate the potential barriers to healthy nutrition and exercise behaviors, in the workplace and their regular lives. These barriers are shown to significantly relate to whether proper eating and exercise behaviors themselves occur (Mazzola et al., 2017), which ultimately will lead to unhealthier HCWs.

The reason barriers can potentially prevent healthy behaviors is explained by the Theory of Planned Behavior (TPB; Ajzen, 1991), which states that individuals create intentions towards behaviors based on various factors (e.g., the social norms towards exercise of their family/friends/coworkers) and then the factors/barriers around them, such as time restrictions and social support, help influence if they enact the actual behavior. Put simply, barriers inhibit the individual's ability to translate planned behaviors into actual ones. Additionally, some barriers also affect the cultural norms for healthy behaviors the employees identify around them, and their perceived control over whether they can complete the behaviors, falling into line with other tenets of the TPB and further reducing the chance of successfully eating healthy and exercising. Given the well-established literature regarding how proper nutrition and exercise habits help to prevent obesity and decrease risk for ailments like heart disease, diabetes, and cancer (healthypeople.gov), barriers to healthy behaviors become particularly problematic. As indicated by the obesity and health behavior adherence numbers presented above, there is ample opportunity to find ways to support HCW's health and institute targeted organizational efforts that could make a real difference in their overall lives.

Recent studies have found that performing physical exercise with colleagues at the workplace helped "prevent deterioration of work ability among female healthcare workers" (Jakobsen et al., 2015, pg. 1) and improve low back and foot pain (Jakobsen et al., 2018). Another intervention focused on nutrition found that HCWs lost an average of 13 pounds after a 16-week program and that the extreme obesity rates had dropped from 36.6% to 17.1% (Nepper et al., 2021). Albert and colleagues (2014) found that a healthy diet in nurses was related to higher self-efficacy and more confidence in body image. These findings illustrate both the importance of these behaviors and the potential for positive effects when they are promoted and supported by healthcare organizations. However, to do so effectively, it is necessary for decision makers to understand the obstacles to proper nutrition and exercise behavior that exist in the typical healthcare employment setting, in order to eliminate those barriers and create facilitators that aid employees in reaching their health goals.

This chapter will focus on those barriers that research has shown affect employees' ability to successfully eat healthy meals and get physical activity with a special focus on any research specific to nurses, doctors, or other HCWs. As you might expect, most of the barriers that affect healthcare workers are similar to those that affect the working population as a whole, but when possible, research specific to HCW is provided (e.g., Cheong et al., 2021). For example, overall barriers to healthy nutrition and exercise decisions found in the general working population include deficiencies in access to healthy food options and/or exercise facilities, workload/job demands, and poor workplace culture and norms towards these behaviors (Mazzola et al., 2019), all of which can certainly affect HCWs. Meanwhile, some other barriers that have come specifically out of the HCW research are inadequate food storage and preparation areas, long working hours, and lack of self-efficacy and motivation (Nicholls et al., 2016).

The barriers will be discussed in the upcoming sections, and for the most part, the nutrition and exercise barriers are presented together, as they typically affect both (e.g., having inadequate time due to long shifts or a high workload would very likely affect both one's ability to eat healthy and fit exercise into the day). Where findings are available specific to nutrition or exercise though, they will be presented to accentuate barriers related to specific types of health behaviors. Further, how these barriers can be mitigated by employees and organizations is discussed throughout the chapter, and where applicable, even how facilitators could be created for health behaviors through proper training, interventions, and programs. But first, both nutrition and exercise behaviors are operationally defined, as well as what is meant by "organizational barriers" to these behaviors.

DEFINING ORGANIZATIONAL BARRIERS TO NUTRITION AND EXERCISE

In this chapter, nutrition behaviors are mainly focused on eating a diet that includes fruits and vegetables and whole grains, limiting fats and sodium, including lean protein, and staying within the daily calorie needs for that individual (U.S. Department of Agriculture, 2020). Other dietary behaviors that might be specific to an individual (e.g., avoiding gluten, maintaining an insulin balance) are also important, but research, policy, and interventions typically focuses on the behaviors that are most effective for losing or maintaining weight for the majority of healthy adults. Similarly, exercise behaviors are related to participating in physical activity that elevates the heart rate, increases joint movement and flexibility, and/or builds muscle (cdc.gov, 2021). Specifically, the CDC in the United States suggests 150 minutes each week of moderate-intensity aerobic activity (i.e., something that "gets your heart beating faster") and 2 days a week of muscle-strengthening activity.

Whenever the general term "healthy behaviors" is used in this chapter, it is referring specifically to these nutrition and exercise definitions, and not to other important behaviors like refraining from smoking, getting proper sleep, or staying mindful that are not part of this specific discussion but are often still important to maintaining one's health. Overall, healthy nutrition and exercise habits have been shown to lower obesity risk (healthypeople.gov), and thus lower the negative consequences of obesity itself (e.g., Kitahara et al., 2014). Mental health is discussed at points in this chapter because of its overall importance to someone's overall well-being and its strong relations to physical health (e.g., exercise is frequently shown to reduce anxiety and depression; de Moor et al., 2006), but given the limited time and scope of this chapter, the main focus is on physical health behaviors and their barriers.

Since this chapter is specific to HCWs and healthcare organizations, it will focus on "organizational barriers" to these healthy behaviors, meaning a factor that makes it harder to eat healthy or exercise that in some way relates to the work environment. However, given the nature of healthy behaviors and how individuals improve their health, it is impossible for all barriers to be strictly in the workplace, and so they will often transcend multiple life domains. The organization may support nutrition by providing information about how to cook and incorporate healthy meals, but much of the actual behavior will occur outside work hours, when the individual decides whether to cook those meals and/or is making their eating choices. One additional concept to recognize is that a "barrier" in this context only needs to make it more difficult or less likely that someone will complete a healthy behavior, but does not need to stop someone from performing the behavior. A person may intend to exercise, but have a particular busy day at work that makes it difficult for them to find the time to meet their daily physical activity goals. If that employee stops at the gym on the way home anyway, they have still encountered a difficult barrier but have overcome it to still accomplish their goal behavior.

The upcoming sections will break down these barriers into several important categories to help conceptualize overarching themes and obstacles that relate to one another. The major barrier categories discussed in this chapter are: time and shiftwork issues, job demands/work stress, absence of healthy options, lack of health knowledge, the work environment, social barriers, and personal factors.

Specific Organizational Barriers to Healthy Behaviors

Time and Shiftwork Issues

Understaffing is common in nursing and other healthcare professions (Shang et al., 2019). This issue can lead to HCWs having to work long hours, which will significantly reduce the chance of exercising and/or being able to plan and execute health meals. Workload was associated with an increased risk of obesity in a sample of nurses (OR = 1.23, $p < .01$; Han et al., 2011). Even "regular" shifts for some HCWs like nurses and doctors are often 10-12 hours or more, and when nurses and health care assistants work most of their shifts as long shifts (>12 hours), it was associated with more absence due to both short-term and long-term sickness (Dall'Ora et al., 2018). This is likely partially attributable to worse health behaviors stemming from a lack of time to plan and complete them. Sixty percent of doctors in one study said they were not able to take time off when they were sick (Feeney et al., 2016). These working conditions and expectations can also lead to presenteeism (i.e., working even when one is ill), which has numerous negative consequences for employees and employers (Howard et al., 2012), and potentially even societies, as recently seen with COVID.

Because around the clock care and working hours are often required in the healthcare sector, the shiftwork often inherent in these jobs may pose a particular problem for HCWs. Research generally shows people employed in shiftwork have lower quality diets and irregular eating patterns (Nea et al., 2015), and among nurses working in hospitals, shift duties relate to more abnormal emotional and restraint eating behavior (Wong et al., 2010). Night shift nurses in one study specifically mentioned weight as a personal health concern, with participants in general further indicating "pressure from colleagues to eat unhealthy" and "unavailability of healthy foods in cafeteria" (two themes that will be prominent later in this chapter) as barriers to health behaviors (Phiri et al., 2014). In a separate qualitative study on night shift nurses, some of the most commonly mentioned themes were preferring fast food due to lack of time, refraining from exercise due to fatigue, and cravings for sweet/unhealthy food (Persson & Martensson, 2006). These types of shifts seem to be especially problematic for healthy behaviors, and often further disrupt circadian rhythms, which creates further health risks like cardiovascular disease, cancer, and reproductive issues (Smith et al., 2003), as well as mental health problems (Vogel et al., 2012).

Case in point, workload and inadequate break time were specifically identified as reasons HCWs adopt unhealthy diet behaviors, which also ultimately negatively affects their work performance and well-being (Al Hazmi et al., 2018). Both time and shiftwork were key barriers to healthy eating and physical activity in new graduate nurses (Brogan et al., 2021), and National Health Service doctors perceived lack of breaks as one of the barriers to their healthy eating behaviors (Winston et al., 2008). Further, lack of time has been found to be a barrier to physical activity among military hospital employees (65%, Hearn et al., 2018). A study in the general population (Wardle et al., 2000) found those working a higher number of hours (average of 47 hrs/week) ate more saturated fat and sugar than those with lower hours (32 hrs/week). Mazzola et al. (2017) investigated organizational barriers to healthy behaviors through open-ended questions, and workload and time constraints were the 1st and 4th most prevalent barrier responses for nutrition (19.92% and 10.34%, respectively) and the 1st and 3rd most prevalent responses for barriers to exercise behaviors (26.79% and 15.58%, respectively).

These findings support the ego depletion theory, such that employees do not have enough physical and mental energy left after a long or stressful work day to successfully finish their healthy behaviors

(Baumeister, 2014). Thus, fatigue itself can also be a barrier to healthy eating and exercise choices for HCWs to cook healthy meals or participate in physical activity (Atkinson et al., 2009, Phiri et al., 2014).

Despite these problems with long shifts, parts of the healthcare sector are increasingly utilizing them, particularly as the industry sees continued staff shortages (Merrifield, 2017). It is vital for healthcare organizations to recognize workload and shiftwork as important issues regarding employee health, and create time availability for their employees to live a healthy lifestyle. Time availability was one of the three most prevalent facilitators indicated by employees in a qualitative study (Mazzola et al., 2017), and finding ways to create time for either meal planning or physical activity could lead to employees making healthier choices and reducing obesity risk. Research has called for more health promotional efforts specifically aimed at healthier eating habits for hospital workers that require frequent night shifts, (Wong et al., 2010). This support from healthcare organizations should ultimately yield positive health outcomes for employees (e.g., Proper & van Oostrom, 2019), even if it may mean a slight initial dip in productivity or a need for more employees.

Job Demands and Work Stress

As one would expect, this category is heavily intertwined with the aspects of workload and time constraints discussed above. An employee that works long hours and hard shifts has a lot of job demands and is inherently more stressed. However, work stress is a very broad concepts in the workplace literature (Cooper et al., 2001) and has such an effect on these health behaviors and overall health, even beyond simply the number of hours or amount of work an employee has. Work stress and was related to being sick more often and binge eating in doctors (Medisauskaite & Kamau, 2019). In a 2011 survey, the acute or chronic effects of stressors were the most common health and safety concern among nurses (74% of respondents; American Nurses Association, 2011). Work demands were cited as a barrier to healthy behaviors by white-collar HCWs (Leslie et al., 2013), as well as to healthy eating specifically among nurses (Cheong et al., 2021). Finally, higher work stress was related to a more irregular meal schedule among nurses (Nahm et al., 2012).

Further, workplace stress often leads to burnout, a psychological syndrome where work becomes debilitating and emotionally fatiguing and is characterized by depersonalization, emotional exhaustion, and low sense of personal accomplishment (Maslach & Jackson, 1981). Research also shows that HCWs have some of the highest levels of stress and burnout, being specifically shown in nurses (53%, Laschinger & Leiter., 2006), doctors (54.4%, Shanafelt et al., 2015), and ICU HCWs (Embriaco et al., 2007). Burnout was associated with lower psychological well-being and difficulties outside of work in doctors (Yates & Samuel, 2019) and was positively related to infrequent exercise and fast food consumption in a sample of HCWs in Europe (Alexandrova-Karamanova et al., 2016). All these findings illustrate the importance of lowering stress and burnout in HCWs in order to promote healthy behaviors.

Being stressed from work can lead to fatigue and feeling one has less opportunities to make healthy nutrition and exercise choices, ultimately leading them to have less behavior intention and lowered actual health behaviors in the long run (Azjen, 1991). For instance, the results of a daily diary study found the number of daily hassles a person encountered was related to an increase in consumption of high fat and high sugar food and a decrease in vegetable consumption (Conner et al., 2008). A separate diary study showed that daily job demands lowered an employees' physical activity on the day the demands occurred (Payne et al., 2010). Further, these organizational demands can lead to employees not reaching the recommended amounts of daily physical activity (Salmon et al., 2003) and lacking the resources for putting effort into sporting activities (Sonnentag & Jelden, 2009). These findings show that both healthy nutrition and exercise behaviors are affected by stress, an effect that can be compounded by the negative biological effects that stress has on the human body (Nixon et al., 2011).

Control has frequently been shown to buffer the relationship between stress and strains such as burnout, through the Job-Demands-Control Model (Gameiro et al., 2020). This was also found specifically among nurses (Laschinger & Leiter., 2006), so creating more autonomy in the jobs of HCWs may alleviate some of the stress and burnout and act as a facilitator towards healthy behaviors. In a study of self-leadership among HCWs, job autonomy was found to related to work engagement and general health (van Dorssen-Boog et al., 2020), making it an ideal way to potentially increase time availability for healthy behaviors and, ultimately, improve employee health.

Organizations can do more to lower workload and stress for their employees. This can be difficult given that the necessary work needs to be done, and the bottom line is often going to inform how many workers are employed and how much work they need to each complete. However, research consistently finds that lowered stress leads to not only to better health behaviors by employees (e.g. Albertson et al., 2001), but also greater productivity overall (Donald et al., 2005). Further, a job that is moderately enriching (enough "stress" to be challenging and interesting, but not create burnout) lowers indicators of abdominal obesity over time (Fried et al., 2013). Therefore, creating healthcare workplaces that are engaging and interesting, allow employee autonomy, and limit the stressors present, will have positive consequences for the employees and the organizations in the long run.

Absence of Healthy Food or Exercise Options

Previous research shows that the presence of and/or access to unhealthy food options is very commonly mentioned as a barrier and can have a profound effect on what employees eat (Chang et al., 2008; Leslie et al., 2013). A sample of Western Australian employees had 30.6% of employees report the presence of unhealthy food in the office and 28.8% report the lack of healthy choices near the workplace as barriers to eating healthy (Blackford et al., 2013) Similarly, vending machines encourage employees to snack on unhealthy food options (Pridgeon & Whitehead, 2013), which many HCWs, particularly those on the night shift, often rely on for their snacks or even meals. Hospital cafeterias were also cited as an organizational barrier to wholesome healthy eating by nurses (Cheong et al., 2021). On the positive end of the spectrum, one study showed white-collar HCWs found the highest support for their healthy eating and physical activity through the availability of healthy food and fitness opportunities (Leslie et al., 2013), however, there is not similar research to indicate this is the case for blue-collar HCWs. All of these findings together suggest that how an organization provides food options for its employees will likely affect their eating habits, obesity levels, and overall physical and mental health.

Therefore, the availability of healthy food options affects employees' ability to eat nutritiously, especially while at work. In a study examining how cafeteria options affected food choice, Jeffery and colleagues (1994) found that increasing the amount of vegetable and fruit options in the cafeteria (and making them more affordable) created an increase in the number of fresh items purchased. Unfortunately though, this indicator returned to baseline once the intervention was removed. Additionally, another study showed that by including nutrition labels on cafeteria and vending machine foods, in addition to changing catering policies to emphasize healthier options, there were significant increases in fruit and vegetable consumption (Emmons et al., 1999). Finally, a more recent study found that restricting high calorie options in vending machines was a helpful way to increase healthy eating habits (Bos et al., 2018).

Therefore, creating more availability and opportunity for health food and physical activity can have a positive effect on the behaviors and health of HCWs. Many hospitals work to maintain healthy options in their cafeterias, but it is important to label these choices in a way that encourages and supports healthy decisions, as well as making sure these options are available consistently, including for overnight and on-call health-care workers.

Similarly, lack of access to exercise facilities and equipment was reported as a barrier to physical activity (Mazzola et al., 2017). Accessibility and opportunity have been shown significantly related to actual physical activity (Humpel et al., 2002), and Emmons and colleagues (1999) found that adding space and equipment for exercise increased actual exercise behaviors. Even when exercise options are present in the workplace, the fact that some employees may get sweaty during their exercising can further act as a barrier (Bredahl et al., 2015), and the lack of shower access at some healthcare institutions might make it difficult to turn exercise intentions into action. Organizations can and should work to provide gym space, workout classes, and/or shower facilities, in order to promote more physical activity in their employees. However, there is some research showing that people who are already regularly exercising may be the primary utilizers of these resources (Abraham et al., 2011), so organizations should further seek to target specific health promotions among currently sedentary individuals to maximize the benefits of their program. Conducting a needs assessment that gets input and buy-in from HCWs at all stages of health behavior adherence/adoption is an excellent start for any nutrition and/or physical activity intervention.

Safety can also be an issue, particularly for physical activities that would take place outside. Employees who work and/or live in unsafe areas are less likely to want to walk or run outdoors, especially in the night time and dark hours. Research found that physical environment factors directly impact physical activity, such that individuals were more likely to take walks if they felt they were in a secure environment (McNeill et al., 2006). Moreover, Nies and colleagues (1996) found that neighborhood safety was a major barrier preventing African-American women from engaging in physical exercise. For health care workers who might work unusual shifts and need to fit their physical activity during the night time hours (or want to bike/walk to work), or in cases where the hospital is located in areas that are perceived less safe, this could be particularly salient for employees in deciding if, how, and where to complete physical activity.

Additionally, many studies reported financial cost as a barrier to physical activity, making individuals more likely to participate in a variety of sedentary behaviors (e.g., Hammerback et al., 2015; Salmon et al., 2003). This is further an issue for food choices as many people who live in poorer or less affluent neighborhoods may reside in what is known as a food desert, which is a neighborhood or community that has limited to no access to healthy *and* affordable food (Wright et al., 2016). Hospitals and healthcare institutions may themselves be situated in one, making it difficult for HCW to find the healthy food options they need while at work, and proximity to a food desert is related to obesity status (Chen et al., 2016). Further, many healthcare workers such as nurses and support staff might be of blue-collar or lower socioeconomic statuses, which limits their ability to find and purchase health food and find safe and secure exercise options.

While it is not necessarily the responsibility of organizations to provide access to healthy food options or exercise/shower facilities, this lack of access to healthy options can be enough to prevent employees from engaging in healthy behavior (Mazzola et al., 2017). This follows the TPB, such that turning intended health behaviors into actual ones is much more likely when access to the necessary resources is easy for the employee (Azjen, 1991). But organizations should care about providing these opportunities to their employees because beyond the health consequences for the employees, it potentially has some for the company as well, including lost productivity and less engagement (e.g., Tryon, 2014). Therefore, providing access to healthy food choices and exercise facilities *helps* HCWs make important healthy choices, but certainly is not the only factor involved in these decisions. To wit, employees may not know what are the right choices in regards to making healthy eating and exercise decisions.

Lack of Nutrition and Exercise Knowledge

Another common barrier is a lack of knowledge of the proper eating and exercise behaviors that would aid the individual in reaching their health goals (Tessaro et al., 1998). Employees sometimes worry that they will hurt themselves if they exercise without the proper instruction and knowledge, potentially even leading to a "fear" of certain types of exercise (Zunker et al., 2008), which was explicitly reported as a barrier to exercise adoption in older women in the early stages of exercise adoption (Heesch et al., 2000). Participants who are asked about health behaviors also complained of mixed signals, such as research constantly changing what foods should and should not be eaten, in what combination/quantity, and/or just having the wrong perceptions of what constitutes "healthy food" (Shrestha et al., 2017). In a study examining nurses and community HCWs in Brazil, more than 95% reporting needing "additional information on physical activity guidelines" (Burdick et al., 2015, p. 467) (it was 80% among physicians), and many incorrectly identified how many minutes of exercise were recommended for adults to complete weekly. A study involving a stretching exercise program in Taiwanese nurses showed that not only did it reduce back pain, but it increased exercise self-efficacy, giving them the knowledge and confidence to potentially be more active on their own after the program ends (Chen & Hu, 2019).

Further, workers are often not aware of the need to change their behaviors. One study found that 57% of the obese participants in their study misclassified their bodyweight as normal (Skaal, 2011), and this was in a healthcare sample who generally would have better knowledge of health status and behaviors! In order to make health behavior knowledge a facilitator, it is important to identify and design interventions that help HCWs make the right choices to both reach their goals and remain safe in these efforts. Research found that a combined intervention focused on education and environmental changes showed the largest improvements in nutrition knowledge (Geaney et al., 2016), while other studies have found nutrition education to help increase fruit and vegetable consumption (e.g., Geaney et al., 2013). Similarly, a workplace exercise intervention that included educational lectures showed a significant decrease in body fat, flexibility, and exercise performance in the experimental group after 4 months (compared to no significant changes in the control group, Lima Vilela et al., 2015). Oenema and colleagues (2001) examined how a computer-tailored nutrition education program could improve healthy eating behaviors, which showed increased awareness and intention to change behaviors related to fat and fruits and vegetable intake. Given the long hours and unpredictable schedules that healthcare professionals work, this could be a great avenue to get important information about healthy nutrition and exercise out to employees, and create a facilitator to those behaviors.

Studies further show that it often takes planning to effectively eat a healthy diet (Stankevitz et al., 2017), which healthcare organizations can both a) help train their employees to do and b) make it easier by providing affordable and convenient health food options. In the Mazzola and colleagues study (2017), planning was by far the most common facilitator to nutrition (45% of all responses), including behaviors like being able to prepare meals beforehand and bring them to work, something likely to be important for HCWs that work long or unusual shifts. Healthcare organizations could hold sessions that instruct employees on a variety of healthy behavior information such as proper meal planning, recipes and food prep, safe and effective exercise behaviors, and/or where and how to fit in healthy behaviors. Further, some health insurance providers already include these classes, videos, and additional services (e.g. personal trainers and health consultants), which organizations and employees can leverage without having to invest in new interventions or initiatives.

Work Environment

Jobs in healthcare often include a fair amount of physical movement. Nurses' jobs, for example, have been shown to consist of light-intensity physical activity mixed with occasional moderate-intensity moments (Chappel et al., 2017). On one hand, this can be a positive in that they get vital physical activity throughout the day that may contribute to their health. Blue-collar healthcare workers, for example, have cited the physical activity of their jobs as supporting their healthy behaviors (Leslie et al., 2013). Conversely, this can also leave them too exhausted after work for more targeted exercise and making/eating healthy meals. This further shows the importance of facilitators like planning/cooking meals beforehand and having social support, such as from a spouse who makes meals and/or is active with them. Ironically, in one study, nurses who had more job stress actually reported eating more servings of fruits and vegetables and burning more work-related calories (including more flights of stairs climbed) (Zapka et al., 2009), however, the effects of these behaviors are likely to be counteracted by the issues with burnout previously discussed.

Organizations can further find ways to incorporate physical activity throughout the day both for improved health and coping with stress. One study found that even short bouts of physical activity during the work day can have positive effects on work performance, mood, and body mass index (Barr-Anderson et al., 2011). As mentioned, some HCW jobs inherently contain physical activity, but further interventions could look to create small breaks for walks/exercise or encourage HCWs to take the stairs when traveling between floors (probably particularly salient for some HCWs, like those that work in hospitals).

Organizational policies and environment further have an affect health behavior. One such policy is workplace flexibility, which may make it easier for employees to prepare healthy meals, choose healthy food options, and/or create daily exercise routines. Perceived workplace flexibility is related to physical activity frequency and sleep hours (Grzywacz et al., 2007). Survey results from over 500 companies found that health culture and policies help create supportive leadership and ultimately lead to reduced health risks for employees (Aldana et al., 2012). It can be difficult to increase flexibility for some jobs within healthcare (such as nurses), but even small interventions that could affect the perceptions of autonomy and flexibility could have profound effects. This is especially important in the post-COVID world where work from home and increased choices in how/where individual work have become the norm as opposed to the exception. One study of an organizational intervention to promote more control over work time showed that over 12 months, employees showed reduced burnout, lowered stress, and higher job satisfaction (Moen et al., 2006). While the study did not look at health behaviors specifically, based on previously discussed barriers like stress, it is very possible such an intervention would also increase exercise and healthy eating.

Research shows managerial and organizational support are vital factors for health promotion to be effective (Pelletier, 2001), and leadership was found to be one of the most important facilitators for engaging in a workplace exercise intervention (Bredahl et al., 2015). Given the effect COVID has had on the well-being of HCWs, there is a call for research and interventions focused on HCW leaders to support their subordinates' well-being (Obrien et al., 2021). By recognizing that the heavy workload and long hours often prevalent in HCWs can make living a healthy lifestyle difficult, organizations should seek to provide support for their employees' health.

The presence of an integrated health promotion program can help HCWs complete their intentions to participate in healthy behaviors, at least for some employees. One study reviewed showed "work recreation teams" are a facilitator to physical activity, although this was more prevalent in men than in women (25.0% to 5.7%; Blackford et al., 2013). A recent review of studies that utilized simply policy or environmental changes found at least some evidence for the effectiveness specific to positive nutrition and physical activity outcomes (Kahn-Marshall & Gallant, 2012). Much more promising results were found for interventions that had multiple components to them, further emphasizing the importance of organizational and managerial support in creating larger scale, integrated programs that target multiple behaviors and give employees options. A recent review of health intervention in HCWs specifically highlighted a variety of approaches leadership could utilize: those with pre-determined activities, providing employees a wide variety of activity choices, and more participatory strategies that involve employees in planning stages, and overall found that wholistic interventions can improve the health of HCWs (Brand et al., 2017). Some specific interventions are presented in this review, but overall a well-designed, empirically-supported, organizational health initiative can have significant positive effects on employee health, especially when the barriers and facilitators discussed here are considered.

Social and Interpersonal Barriers

Workplace social temptations are a common barrier for those trying to eat healthy, and as previously discussed, vending machines and cafeterias are potential sources of these temptations and poor choices. Moreover, so can workplace gatherings that rely solely on high-calorie, low-nutrient foods (e.g., pizza, donuts) or pressure from co-workers who tend to eat out for meals. Workplace environment and culture were found as barriers to healthy eating and physical activity among recently graduated nurses (Brogan et al., 2021). In a study of barriers among those already participating in workplace obesity intervention, some of the highest factors were "ate a lot of meals away from home," "holidays and special occasions," and "high fat foods are part of my culture" (Stankevitz et al., 2017). Both peer and family influence were cited as barriers in a meta-synthesis of findings on nurses as barriers to healthy eating (Cheong et al., 2021). It can be difficult to turn intentions to act healthy into action when those around you either do not do so themselves, or worse, actively make you feel bad for eating a healthy lunch or taking time to exercise. Interventions can target both improving healthy food choices at work and cultivating a culture where everyone feels safe and respected for their health choices.

Allen and Armstrong found family-work and work-family interference correlated with poor health behaviors of low physical activity and higher fatty food consumption (2006), both of which were also related to overall health in that study. A group of manual workers frequently reported that their food choices are often determined by their spouses (Pridgeon & Whitehead, 2013). These findings again reiterate how organizations cannot ignore family/home life when trying to increase overall employee health behaviors and overall physical health. This ties into the shiftwork concerns discussed earlier, as many HCWs have very little flexibility in their schedules and/or may be on swing/night shifts that make attending family events difficult. Initiatives should target better work-life balance for HCWs, in order to reduce stress and burnout, improve health behaviors, and lower the risk for obesity (e.g., Grzywacz, 2000; Juvanhol et al., 2006).

Similarly, social support can facilitate eating healthy or exercise behavior. "Exercise partners" can be an excellent way to motivate yourself and others, and stay accountable to making sure exercise goals are reached, since social support has been linked to more physical activity completion (Wynd & Ryan-Wagner, 2004). If that partner is a co-worker, it adds an extra element of support, and allows employees to discuss and plan healthy choices at work and feel the culture supports their healthy lifestyle. Nurses that perceived more physical activity by their co-workers were more likely to spend their breaks taking walks and reported burning more work-related calories (Zapka et al., 2009), however the overall norms for healthy behaviors within this sample were perceived as low. Workplace climate for healthy weight management is linked to body mass index, physical health, and health motivation (Sliter, 2013). Interventions that incorporate social support and consider organizational climate can make the behavior change more fun and less likely to return to baseline.

Personal Factors

In a sample of healthcare workers, 83% cited a lack of motivation to getting regular physical activity (Skaal, 2011), as did 45% of military hospital employees (Hearn et al., 2018). Some hospital nurses have reported a general "nonchalance towards unhealthy eating" as a barrier to eating healthier diets (Cheong et al., 2021), and over half of female hospital workers indicated they found physical activity uninteresting (52.7%, Al-Mohannadi et al., 2020). If a person's most prominent belief about a health habit is negative, they are less likely to choose to make those healthy choices (Armitage & Conner, 1999). The TPB posits that our attitudes towards a behavior help to create our intentions towards completing that behavior, so it is important that employers help HCWs understand the importance of healthy behaviors for their long-term physical and mental health, especially among individuals who will end up informing the general public about proper nutrition and exercise behaviors.

Similarly, those who report enjoyment for sedentary behaviors are less likely to partake in physical activity (Salmon et al., 2003). Thus, from the facilitator angle, the enjoyment of healthy behaviors can promote these behaviors, and perhaps healthcare organizations can encourage employees to find the type exercise they actually like by providing a variety of opportunities to try new activities to improve the likelihood of sustained change (Ungar et al., 2016). There is potential that overall enjoyment is higher in some activities than others, with high intensity interval training being one example that is both rated as enjoyable and containing more health benefits (Thum et al., 2017).

Gender could also be a moderating factor in what types of barriers are faced and how/whether health behaviors are completed. Some healthcare positions, such as nurses, are what are considered "pink-collar occupations", meaning the workplace tends to skew disproportionally female (Wood, 2020). For example, 89% of nurses identify as female, while dental hygienists (96%), dental assistants (95%), medical records technicians (93%), and those in home healthcare services (88%) have high proportions as well (Wood, 2020). Further, while the gap has lessened in recent years (Raiber & Verbakel, 2021), females still tend to take on a larger burden in terms of household chores and caregiving (Swinkels et al., 2019). This increased caregiver burden can provide an additional barrier to completing physical activity and eating health meals (e.g., Nomaguchi & Bianchi, 2008; Sisk, 2000).

Another barrier can be the desire for quick results from a lifestyle change, which in reality, rarely occurs when individuals begin a new nutrition or exercise regime. They may believe that a short commitment to these behaviors will result in clear and visible differences, and when this does not happen, they have may get discouraged and stop (Mazzola et al., 2019). This further may affect their future attitude towards healthy behavior change and make it harder to follow healthy programs (Chang et al., 2008). Personal appearance, how their clothes fit, and their ability to be active with their children have been mentioned as motivating factors for low-income mothers to address weight gain (Chang et al., 2008). Thus, these factors that could be harnessed towards getting a person to live a healthier lifestyle, although organizations should both caution employees that quick results are not always possible and beware leading employees towards "toxic diet culture" or extreme measures for achieving a desired physical appearance. Organizations could utilize campaigns that promote not only the physical health benefits of nutritious choices and physical activity, but also the self-esteem, mental health, and overall well-being effects, to increase participation in workplace interventions and healthy behaviors inside and outside of work.

Injuries and illness can also be barriers to healthy behaviors, especially physical activity (Leslie et al., 2013). This connects to the barrier mentioned previously of lacking proper knowledge about proper fitness behaviors and fear of further injury, which can particularly salient for those with injuries or conditions that both need specific direction to exercise safely and may have mental hurdles to work through.

While not technically an "organization barriers," both weather and family responsibilities have come up as barriers to physical activity, both in hospital workers (Al-Mohannadi et al., 2020) and the general population (Mazzola et al., 2017). Specifically, poor weather has been related to a higher probability of sedentary behavior (Salmon et al., 2003). While there is little an organization can do about the weather, creating safe and weather proof opportunities for exercise could help employees complete the exercise intentions.

CONCLUSION

Reducing barriers to healthy nutrition and exercise behaviors in healthcare workers is likely one of the best ways to improve their healthy habits and lower chances of serious illness or injury, and workplace facilitators positively relate to proper diet and physical activity (Mazzola et al., 2017). Organizations and administrators who oversee healthcare workers can take this advocacy a step further by not only eliminating barriers but turning them into facilitators that support healthy behaviors of HCWs and show they value the health and well-being of their employees.

Many potential changes and interventions for HCWs were presented throughout this chapter. Organizations can seek ways to lower workload and stress in their employees, opening up more time availability for planning and completing health behaviors. They can develop interventions that increase healthy food and physical activity options, provide employees with useful and necessary health information, cultivate a healthy workplace culture that provides support for healthy behaviors, and/or incentivize activities that help lower an employee's risk of obesity. The important factor to remember is that any of these efforts are likely to fail if the organization does not recognize and eliminate potential barriers to exercise and nutrition that exist all around HCWs. While much of the research here suggests that these barriers have a profound effect on employee health behaviors (e.g., Mazzola et al., 2017), there is also ample evidence that when organizations commit to employee health, positive outcomes both for the employees and employer are possible (e.g., Jakobsen et al., 2015).

It is also important to consider both the specific nature of the employee sample and their needs when planning health initiatives. Depending on the type of healthcare worker, their demographics and job status, and the setting/organization they work, it might be important to focus on a specific health behavior (e.g., physical activity) over the other (or potentially both). Interestingly, many nurses seem to have at least a moderately healthy diet but do not get enough physical activity (Albert et al., 2014), while another recent article found that 100% of physicians were meeting recommended guidelines for exercise but only 50% were eating the recommended fruits and vegetables servings (Nachnani & Bulchandani, 2019). Thus, this is why it is imperative to do a full needs assessment looking at the specific industry and/or organization before investing resources into a health behavior intervention, if at all possible.

Some researchers have suggested that targeting barriers and facilitators could be one of the best way to target and improve workers' health behaviors in order to lower obesity and increase physical wellness (Goetzel & Ozminkowski, 2008; Mazzola et al., 2019), and this is especially true for HCWs. This chapter has provided a number of barriers to consider in health initiatives and best practices for health promotion among HCWs. Healthcare organizations can and should institute interventions to combat the obesity epidemic because of the profound effect it can have on their own workers health and well-being, but also since these healthcare professionals are well-positioned to affect the general population with their newfound nutrition and exercise knowledge and behaviors. Given the vital role HCWs play in society by keeping the general population safe and well, finding ways to make their work environment healthy is a moral imperative for every healthcare employer.

REFERENCES

Abraham, J. M., Feldman, R., Nyman, J. A., & Barleen, N. (2011). What factors influence participation in an exercise-focused, employer-based wellness program? *INQUIRY: The Journal of Health Care Organization, Provision, and Financing*, *48*(3), 221–241. doi:10.5034/inquiryjrnl_48.03.01 PMID:22235547

Ajzen, I. (1991). The Theory of Planned Behavior. *Organizational Behavior and Human Decision Processes*, *50*(2), 179–211. doi:10.1016/0749-5978(91)90020-T

Al Hazmi, T. M., Alghamdi, A., & Abdulmajeed, I. (2018). Eating habits among healthcare providers during working hours at National Guard Health Affairs-Riyadh, Saudi Arabia. *International Journal of Medical Research & Health Sciences*, *7*(9), 1–14.

Al-Mohannadi, A. S., Albuflasa, A. M., Sayegh, S., Salman, A., & Farooq, A. (2020). A cross-sectional study exploring motivators and barriers to physical activity participation among hospital workers. *Global Journal of Health Science*, *12*(9), 76–85. doi:10.5539/gjhs.v12n9p76

Albert, N. M., Butler, R., & Sorrell, J. (2014). Factors related to healthy diet and physical activity in hospital-based clinical nurses. *OJIN: The Online Journal of Issues in Nursing*, *19*(3).

Albertson, K., Nielsen, M., & Borg, V. (2001). The Danish psychosocial work environment and symptoms of stress, the main, mediating, and moderating role of sense of coherence. *Work and Stress*, *15*(3), 241–253. doi:10.1080/02678370110066562

Aldana, S. G., Anderson, D. R., Adams, T. B., Whitmer, R. W., Merrill, R. M., George, V., & Noyce, J. (2012). A review of the knowledge base on healthy worksite culture. *Journal of Occupational and Environmental Medicine*, *54*(4), 414–419. doi:10.1097/JOM.0b013e31824be25f PMID:22446571

Alexandrova-Karamanova, A., Todorova, I., Montgomery, A., Panagopoulou, E., Costa, P., Baban, A., Davas, A., Milosevic, M., & Mijakoski, D. (2016). Burnout and health behaviors in health professionals from seven European countries. *International Archives of Occupational and Environmental Health, 89*(7), 1059–1075. doi:10.100700420-016-1143-5 PMID:27251338

Allen, T. D., & Armstrong, J. (2006). Further examination of the link between work-faimly conflict and physical health: The role of health-related behaviors. *The American Behavioral Scientist, 49*, 1204–1221. doi:10.1177/0002764206286386

American Nurses Association. (2011). *The ANA Health & Safety Survey: Hazards of the RN work environment.* www.NursingWorld.org

Armitage, C. J., & Conner, M. (1999). Distinguishing perceptions of control from self-efficacy: Predicting consumption of a low-fat diet using the theory of planned behavior. *Journal of Applied Social Psychology, 29*(1), 72–90. doi:10.1111/j.1559-1816.1999.tb01375.x

Atkinson, G., Fullick, S., Grindey, C., & Maclaren, D. (2008). Exercise, energy balance and the shift worker. *Sports Medicine (Auckland, N.Z.), 38*(8), 671–685. doi:10.2165/00007256-200838080-00005 PMID:18620467

Barr-Anderson, D., AuYoung, M., Whitt-Glover, M. C., Glenn, B. A., & Yancey, A. K. (2011). Integration of short bouts of physical activity into organizational routine. *American Journal of Preventive Medicine, 40*(1), 76–93. doi:10.1016/j.amepre.2010.09.033 PMID:21146772

Baumeister, R. F. (2014). Self-regulation, ego depletion, and inhibition. *Neuropsychologia, 65*, 313–319. doi:10.1016/j.neuropsychologia.2014.08.012 PMID:25149821

Blackford, K., Jancey, J., Howat, P., Ledger, M., & Lee, A. H. (2013). Office-Based physical activity and nutrition intervention: Barriers, enablers, and preferred strategies for workplace obesity prevention, Perth, Western Australia, 2012. *Preventing Chronic Disease, 10*(1), 1–11. doi:10.5888/pcd10.130029 PMID:24028834

Bos, C., van der Lans, I. A., van Kleef, E., & van Trijp, H. C. (2018). Promoting healthy choices from vending machines: Effectiveness and consumer evaluations of four types of interventions. *Food Policy, 79*, 247–255. doi:10.1016/j.foodpol.2018.07.001

Brand, S. L., Thompson Coon, J., Fleming, L. E., Carroll, L., Bethel, A., & Wyatt, K. (2017). Whole-system approaches to improving the health and wellbeing of healthcare workers: A systematic review. *PLoS One, 12*(12), 1–26. doi:10.1371/journal.pone.0188418 PMID:29200422

Bredahl, T. V. G., Særvoll, C. A., Kirkelund, L., Sjøgaard, G., & Andersen, L. L. (2015). When intervention meets organisation: A qualitative study of motivation and barriers to physical exercise at the workplace. *TheScientificWorldJournal, 2015*, 1–12. doi:10.1155/2015/518561 PMID:26380361

Brogan, E., Rossiter, C., Duffield, C., & Denney-Wilson, E. (2021). Healthy eating and physical activity among new graduate nurses: A qualitative study of barriers and enablers during their first year of clinical practice. *Collegian (Royal College of Nursing, Australia), 28*(5), 489–497. doi:10.1016/j.colegn.2020.12.008

Burdick, L., Mielke, G. I., Parra, D. C., Gomes, G., Florindo, A., Bracco, M., Lobelo, F., Simoes, E. J., Pratt, M., Ramos, L. R., Moura, L., Brownson, R. C., & Hallal, P. C. (2015). Physicians', nurses' and community health workers' knowledge about physical activity in Brazil: A cross-sectional study. *Preventive Medicine Reports, 2*, 467–472. doi:10.1016/j.pmedr.2015.06.001 PMID:26844104

Chang, M., Nitzke, S., Guilford, E., Adair, C. H., & Hazard, D. L. (2008). Motivators and barriers to healthful eating and physical activity among low-income overweight and obese mothers. *Journal of the American Dietetic Association, 108*(6), 1023–1028. doi:10.1016/j.jada.2008.03.004 PMID:18502238

Chappel, S. E., Verswijveren, S. J. J. M., Aisbett, B., Considine, J., & Ridgers, N. D. (2017). Nurses' occupational physical activity levels: A systematic review. *International Journal of Nursing Studies, 73*, 52–62. doi:10.1016/j.ijnurstu.2017.05.006 PMID:28535398

Chen, D., Jaenicke, E. C., & Volpe, R. J. (2016). Food environments and obesity: Household diet expenditure versus food deserts. *American Journal of Public Health, 106*(5), 881–889. doi:10.2105/AJPH.2016.303048 PMID:26985622

Chen, H.-M., & Hu, H.-M. (2019). Randomized trial of modified stretching exercise program for menstrual low back pain. *Western Journal of Nursing Research, 41*(2), 238–257. doi:10.1177/0193945918763817 PMID:29529975

Cheong, Z. Y., Lopez, V., & Tam, W. S. W. (2021). Barriers to healthy eating among nurses working in hospitals: A meta-synthesis. *Journal of Advanced Nursing*. PMID:34477228

Connor, D. B. O., Jones, F., Conner, M., Mcmillan, B., & Ferguson, E. (2008). Effects of daily hassles and eating style on eating behavior. *Health Psychology, 27*(1), 20–31. doi:10.1037/0278-6133.27.1.S20 PMID:18248102

Cooper, C. L., Dewe, P. J., & O'Driscoll, M. P. (2001). Organizational Stress: A Review and Critique of Theory, Research, and Applications. *Sage (Atlanta, Ga.).*

Dall'Ora, C., Ball, J., Redfern, O., Recio, S. A., Maruotti, A., Meredith, P., & Griffiths, P. (2019). Are long nursing shifts on hospital wards associated with sickness absence? A longitudinal retrospective observational study. *Journal of Nursing Management, 27*(1), 19–26. doi:10.1111/jonm.12643 PMID:29978584

de Moor, M. H. M., Beem, A. L., Stubbe, J. H., Boomsma, D. I., & de Geus, E. J. C. (2006). Regular exercise, anxiety, depression and personality: A population-based study. *Preventive Medicine, 42*(4), 273–279. doi:10.1016/j.ypmed.2005.12.002 PMID:16439008

Donald, I., Taylor, P., Johnson, S., Cooper, C., Cartwright, S., & Robertson, S. (2005). Work environments, stress, and productivity: An examination using ASSET. *International Journal of Stress Management, 12*(4), 409–423. doi:10.1037/1072-5245.12.4.409

Embriaco, N., Papazian, L., Kentish-Barnes, N., Pochard, F., & Azoulay, E. (2007). Burnout syndrome among critical care healthcare workers. *Current Opinion in Critical Care, 13*(5), 482–488. doi:10.1097/MCC.0b013e3282efd28a PMID:17762223

Emmons, K. M., Linnan, L., Shadel, W. G., Marcus, B., & Abrams, D. B. (1999). The Working Healthy Project: A worksite health-promotion trial targeting physical activity, diet, and smoking. *Journal of Occupational and Environmental Medicine*, *41*(7), 545–555. doi:10.1097/00043764-199907000-00003 PMID:10412096

Feeney, S., O'Brien, K., O'Keeffe, N., Iomaire, A. N. C., Kelly, M. E., McCormack, J., McGuire, G., & Evans, D. S. (2016). Practise what you preach: Health behaviours and stress among non-consultant hospital doctors. *Clinical Medicine*, *16*(1), 12–18. doi:10.7861/clinmedicine.16-1-12 PMID:26833509

Fried, Y., Laurence, G. A., Shirom, A., Melamed, S., Toker, S., Berliner, S., & Shapira, I. (2013). The relationship between job enrichment and abdominal obesity: A longitudinal field study of apparently healthy individuals. *Journal of Occupational Health Psychology*, *18*(4), 458–468. doi:10.1037/a0033730 PMID:24001329

Gameiro, M., Chambel, M. J., & Carvalho, V. S. (2020). A person-centered approach to the job demands–control model: A multifunctioning test of additive and buffer hypotheses to explain burnout. *International Journal of Environmental Research and Public Health*, *17*(23), 8871. doi:10.3390/ijerph17238871 PMID:33260306

Geaney, F., Kelly, C., Di Marrazzo, J. S., Harrington, J. M., Fitzgerald, A. P., Greiner, B. A., & Perry, I. J. (2016). The effect of complex workplace dietary interventions on employees' dietary intakes, nutrition knowledge and health status: A cluster controlled trial. *Preventive Medicine*, *89*, 76–83. doi:10.1016/j.ypmed.2016.05.005 PMID:27208667

Geaney, F., Kelly, C., Greiner, B. A., Harrington, J. M., Perry, I. J., & Beirne, P. (2013). The effectiveness of workplace dietary modification interventions: A systematic review. *Preventive Medicine*, *57*(5), 438–447. doi:10.1016/j.ypmed.2013.06.032 PMID:23850518

Goetzel, R. Z., & Ozminkowski, R. J. (2008). The health and cost benefits of work site programs. *Annual Review of Public Health*, *29*(1), 303–323. doi:10.1146/annurev.publhealth.29.020907.090930 PMID:18173386

Grzywacz, J. G. (2000). Work-family spillover and health during midlife: Is managing conflict everything? *American Journal of Health Promotion*, *14*(4), 236–243. doi:10.4278/0890-1171-14.4.236 PMID:10915535

Grzywacz, J. G., Casey, P. R., & Jones, F. A. (2007). The effects of workplace flexibility on health behaviors: A cross-sectional and longitudinal analysis. *Journal of Occupational and Environmental Medicine*, *49*(12), 1302–1309. doi:10.1097/JOM.0b013e31815ae9bc PMID:18231077

Hammerback, K., Hannon, P. A., Harris, J. R., Clegg-Thorp, C., Kohn, M., & Parrish, A. (2015). Perspectives on workplace health promotion among employees in low-wage industries. *American Journal of Health Promotion*, *29*(6), 384–392. doi:10.4278/ajhp.130924-QUAL-495 PMID:25162321

Han, K., Trinkoff, A. M., Storr, C. L., & Geiger-Brown, J. (2011). Job stress and work schedules in relation to nurse obesity. *JONA: The Journal of Nursing Administration, 41*(11), 488-495. https://www.healthypeople.gov/2020/leading-health-indicators/2020-lhi-topics/Nutrition-Physical-Activity-and-Obesity

Hearn, D., Schuh-Renner, A., Canham-Chervak, M., Hodges, E. U., & Evarts, L. (2018). Barriers to physical activity among military hospital employees. The United States Army Medical Department, 1(205), 76.

Heesch, K. C., Brown, D. R., & Blanton, C. J. (2000). Perceived barriers to exercise and stage of exercise adoption in older women of different racial/ethnic groups. *Women & Health*, *30*(4), 61–76. doi:10.1300/J013v30n04_05 PMID:10983610

Howard, K. J., Howard, J. T., & Smyth, A. F. (2012). The problem of absenteeism and presenteeism in the workplace. In R. J. Gatchel & I. Z. Schultz (Eds.), *Handbook of Occupational Health and Wellness* (pp. 151–917). Springer Science + Business Media. https://doi-org.proxy108.nclive.org/10.1007/978-1-4614-4839-6_8

Humpel, N., Owen, N., & Leslie, E. (2002). Environmental factors associated with adults' participation in physical activity: A review. *American Journal of Preventive Medicine*, *22*(3), 188–199. doi:10.1016/S0749-3797(01)00426-3 PMID:11897464

Jakobsen, M. D., Sundstrup, E., Brandt, M., & Andersen, L. L. (2018). Effect of physical exercise on musculoskeletal pain in multiple body regions among healthcare workers: Secondary analysis of a cluster randomized controlled trial. *Musculoskeletal Science & Practice*, *34*, 89–96. doi:10.1016/j.msksp.2018.01.006 PMID:29414757

Jakobsen, M. D., Sundstrup, E., Brandt, M., Jay, K., Aagaard, P., & Andersen, L. L. (2015). Physical exercise at the workplace prevents deterioration of work ability among healthcare workers: Cluster randomized controlled trial. *BMC Public Health*, *15*(1), 1–9. doi:10.118612889-015-2448-0 PMID:26607232

Jeffrey, R. W., French, S. A., Raether, C., & Baxter, J. E. (1994). An environmental intervention to increase fruit and salad purchases in a cafeteria. *Preventive Medicine*, *23*(6), 788–792. doi:10.1006/pmed.1994.1135 PMID:7855111

Juvanhol, L. L., Silva-Costa, A., Rotenberg, L., Moreno, A. B., Melo, E. C. P., Santos, I. S., Nunes, M. A. A., Toivanen, S., Chor, D., & Griep, R. H. (2022). Is work-family conflict a pathway between job strain components and binge eating? A cross-sectional analysis from the ELSA-Brasil study. *Journal of Eating Disorders*, *10*(1), 1–9. doi:10.118640337-022-00540-x PMID:35123594

Kahn-Marshall, J. L., & Gallant, M. P. (2012). Making healthy behaviors the easy choice for employees. *Health Education & Behavior*, *39*(6), 752–776. doi:10.1177/1090198111434153 PMID:22872583

Kakunje, A. (2011). Stress among health care professionals - The need for resiliency. *Online Journal of Health and Allied Sciences: OJHAS*, *10*, 1.

Kitahara, C. M., Flint, A. J., Berrington de Gonzalez, A., Bernstein, L., Brotzman, M., MacInnis, R. J., Moore, S. C., Robien, K., Rosenberg, P. S., Singh, P. N., Weiderpass, E., Adami, H. O., Anton-Culver, H., Ballard-Barbash, R., Buring, J. E., Freedman, D. M., Fraser, G. E., Beane Freeman, L. E., Gapstur, S. M., ... Hartge, P. (2014). Association between Class III obesity (BMI of 40–59 kg/m2) and mortality: A pooled analysis of 20 prospective studies. *PLoS Medicine*, *11*(7), 1–14. doi:10.1371/journal.pmed.1001673 PMID:25003901

Kyle, R. G., Wills, J., Mahoney, C., Hoyle, L., Kelly, M., & Atherton, I. M. (2017). Obesity prevalence among healthcare professionals in England: A cross-sectional study using the Health Survey for England. *BMJ Open*, *7*(12), e018498. doi:10.1136/bmjopen-2017-018498 PMID:29203505

Laschinger, H. K. S., & Leiter, M. P. (2006). The impact of nursing work environments on patient safety outcomes: the mediating role of burnout/engagement. *JONA: The Journal of Nursing Administration, 36*(5), 259–267. https://doi-org.proxy108.nclive.org/10.1097/00005110-200605000-00019

Leslie, J. H., Braun, K. L., Novotny, R., & Mokuau, N. (2013). Factors affecting healthy eating and physical activity behaviors among multiethnic blue-and white-collar workers: A case study of one healthcare institution. *Hawai'i Journal of Medicine & Public Health: a Journal of Asia Pacific Medicine & Public Health*, *72*(9), 300. PMID:24069570

Lima Vilela, B., Benedito Silva, A. A., Barbosa de Lira, C. A., & dos Santos Andrade, M. (2015). Workplace exercise and educational program for improving fitness outcomes related to health in workers. *Journal of Occupational and Environmental Medicine*, *57*(3), 235–240. doi:10.1097/JOM.0000000000000393 PMID:25742529

Malik, S., Blake, H., & Batt, M. (2011). How healthy are our nurses? New and registered nurses compared. *British Journal of Nursing (Mark Allen Publishing)*, *20*(8), 489–496. doi:10.12968/bjon.2011.20.8.489 PMID:21537281

Maslach, C., & Jackson, S. E. (1981). *Maslach Burnout Inventory: MBI*. Consulting Psychologists Press.

Mazzola, J. J., Jackson, A., & Thiele, A. (2019). Obesity in the workplace: Physical, social, and environmental barriers and facilitators to healthy lifestyles. *Occupational Health Science*, *3*, 239–264. doi:10.100741542-019-00046-0

Mazzola, J. J., Moore, J. T., & Alexander, K. A. (2017). Is work preventing us from acting healthy? The relationship between daily workplace barriers and facilitators on nutrition and exercise behaviors. *Stress and Health*, *33*(5), 479–489. doi:10.1002mi.2731 PMID:27891758

McNeill, L. H., Wyrwich, K. W., Brownson, R. C., Clark, E. M., & Kreuter, M. W. (2006). Individual, social environmental, and physical environmental influences on physical activity among black and white adults: A structural equation analysis. *Annals of Behavioral Medicine*, *31*(1), 36–44. doi:10.120715324796abm3101_7 PMID:16472037

Medisauskaite, A., & Kamau, C. (2019). Does occupational distress raise the risk of alcohol use, binge-eating, ill health and sleep problems among medical doctors? A UK cross-sectional study. *BMJ Open*, *9*(5), e027362. doi:10.1136/bmjopen-2018-027362 PMID:31092661

Merrifield, N. (2017). Essex trust switches to 12-hour nursing shifts to alleviate staffing and cost concerns. *Nursing Times*. Retrieved from: https://www.nursingtimes.net/news/hospital/trust-makes-12-hour-shifts-standard-for-most-nursing-staff/7017911.article

Moen, P., Kelly, E. L., Fan, W., Lee, S.-R., Almeida, D., Kossek, E. E., & Buxton, O. M. (2016). Does a flexibility/support organizational initiative improve high-tech employees' well-being? Evidence from the work, family, and health network. *American Sociological Review*, *81*(1), 134–164. doi:10.1177/0003122415622391

Nachnani, E., & Bulchandani, D. (2019). Do doctors practice what they preach regarding nutrition, exercise and sleep. *Endocrine Practice*, *25*, 188–189. doi:10.1016/S1530-891X(20)46747-3

Nahm, E. S., Warren, J., Zhu, S., An, M., & Brown, J. (2012). Nurses' self-care behaviors related to weight and stress. *Nursing Outlook*, *60*(5), e23–e31. doi:10.1016/j.outlook.2012.04.005 PMID:22770679

National Heart, Lung, and Blood Institute. (1998). *Clinical guidelines on the identification, evaluation, and treatment overweight and obesity in adults.* NIH Publication, No. 98-4083.

Nea, F. M., Kearney, J., Livingstone, M. B. E., Pourshahidi, L. K., & Corish, C. A. (2015). Dietary and lifestyle habits and the associated health risks in shift workers. *Nutrition Research Reviews*, *28*(2), 143–166. doi:10.1017/S095442241500013X PMID:26650243

Nepper, M. J., McAtee, J. R., & Chai, W. (2021). Effect of a workplace weight-loss program for overweight and obese healthcare workers. *American Journal of Health Promotion*, *35*(3), 352–361. doi:10.1177/0890117120960393 PMID:32969262

Nicholls, R., Perry, L., Duffield, C., Gallagher, R., & Pierce, H. (2017). Barriers and facilitators to healthy eating for nurses in the workplace: An integrative review. *Journal of Advanced Nursing*, *73*(5), 1051–1065. doi:10.1111/jan.13185 PMID:27732741

Nies, M. A., Vollman, M., & Cook, T. (1996). African American women's experiences with physical activity in their daily lives. *Public Health Nursing (Boston, Mass.)*, *16*(1), 23–31. doi:10.1046/j.1525-1446.1999.00023.x PMID:10074819

Nixon, A. E., Mazzola, J. J., Bauer, J., Krueger, J. R., & Spector, P. E. (2011). Can work make you sick? A meta-analysis of the relationship between job stressors and physical symptoms. *Work and Stress*, *25*(1), 1–22. doi:10.1080/02678373.2011.569175

Nomaguchi, K. M., & Bianchi, S. M. (2004). Exercise time: Gender differences in the effects of marriage, parenthood, and employment. *Journal of Marriage and Family, 66*(2), 413–430. https://doi-org.proxy108.nclive.org/10.1111/j.1741-3737.2004.00029.x

Obrien, N., Flott, K., & Durkin, M. (2021). COVID-19: Leadership on the frontline is what matters when we support healthcare workers. *International Journal for Quality in Health Care*, *33*(1), 1–2. doi:10.1093/intqhc/mzaa153 PMID:33227137

Oenema, A., Brug, J., & Lechner, L. (2001). Web-based tailored nutrition education: Results of a randomized controlled trial. *Health Education Research*, *16*(6), 647–660. doi:10.1093/her/16.6.647 PMID:11780705

Payne, N., Jones, F., & Harris, P. R. (2010). A daily diary investigation of the impact of work stress on exercise intention realisation: Can planning overcome the disruptive influence of work? *Psychology & Health*, *25*(1), 111–129. doi:10.1080/08870440903337622 PMID:20391210

Pelletier, K. R. (2001). A review and analysis of the clinical- and cost-effective studies of comprehensive health promotion and disease management programs at the worksite: 1998-2000 update. *American Journal of Health Promotion*, *16*(2), 107–116. doi:10.4278/0890-1171-16.2.107 PMID:11727590

Perry, L., Gallagher, R., & Duffield, C. (2015). The health and health behaviours of Australian metropolitan nurses: An exploratory study. *BMC Nursing*, *14*(1), 1–11. doi:10.118612912-015-0091-9 PMID:26339200

Persson, M., & Mårtensson, J. (2006). Situations influencing habits in diet and exercise among nurses working night shift. *Journal of Nursing Management*, *14*(5), 414–423. doi:10.1111/j.1365-2934.2006.00601.x PMID:16787477

Phiri, L. P., Draper, C. E., Lambert, E. V., & Kolbe-Alexander, T. L. (2014). Nurses' lifestyle behaviours, health priorities and barriers to living a healthy lifestyle: A qualitative descriptive study. *BMC Nursing*, *13*(1), 1–11. doi:10.118612912-014-0038-6 PMID:25506262

Piko, B. F. (2006). Burnout, role conflict, job satisfaction and psychosocial health among Hungarian health care staff: A questionnaire survey. *International Journal of Nursing Studies*, *43*(3), 311–318. doi:10.1016/j.ijnurstu.2005.05.003 PMID:15964005

Pridgeon, A., & Whitehead, K. (2013). A qualitative study to investigate the drivers and barriers to healthy eating in two public sector workplaces. *Journal of Human Nutrition and Dietetics*, *26*(1), 85–95. doi:10.1111/j.1365-277X.2012.01281.x PMID:22906402

Proper, K. I., & van Oostrom, S. H. (2019). The effectiveness of workplace health promotion interventions on physical and mental health outcomes—A systematic review of reviews. *Scandinavian Journal of Work, Environment & Health*, *45*(6), 546–559. doi:10.5271jweh.3833 PMID:31134284

Raiber, K., & Verbakel, E. (2021). Are the gender gaps in informal caregiving intensity and burden closing due to COVID-19 pandemic? Evidence from the Netherlands. *Gender, Work and Organization*, *28*(5), 1926–1936. doi:10.1111/gwao.12725 PMID:34548767

Salmon, J., Owen, N., Crawford, D., Bauman, A., & Sallis, J. F. (2003). Physical activity and dedentary behavior : A population-based study of barriers, enjoyment, and preference. *Health Psychology*, *22*(2), 178–188. doi:10.1037/0278-6133.22.2.178 PMID:12683738

Shanafelt, T. D., Hasan, O., Dyrbye, L. N., Sinsky, C., Satele, D., Sloan, J., & West, C. P. (2015, December). Changes in burnout and satisfaction with work-life balance in physicians and the general US working population between 2011 and 2014. *Mayo Clinic Proceedings*, *90*(12), 1600–1613. doi:10.1016/j.mayocp.2015.08.023 PMID:26653297

Shang, J., Needleman, J., Liu, J., Larson, E., & Stone, P. W. (2019). Nurse staffing and healthcare associated infection, unit-level analysis. *The Journal of Nursing Administration*, *49*(5), 260–265. doi:10.1097/NNA.0000000000000748 PMID:31008835

Shrestha, A., Pyakurel, P., Shrestha, A., Gautam, R., Manandhar, N., Rhodes, E., Tamrakar, D., Karmacharya, B., Malik, V., Mattie, J., & Spiegelman, D. (2017). Facilitators and barriers to healthy eating in a worksite cafeteria: A qualitative study from Nepal. *Heart Asia*, *9*(2), 1–7. doi:10.1136/heartasia-2017-010956 PMID:29225703

Sisk, R. J. (2000). Caregiver burden and health promotion. *International Journal of Nursing Studies*, *37*(1), 37–43. doi:10.1016/S0020-7489(99)00053-X PMID:10687808

Skaal, L., & Pengpid, S. (2011). Obesity and health problems among South African healthcare workers: Do healthcare workers take care of themselves? *South African Family Practice*, *53*(6), 562. doi:10.1080/20786204.2011.10874153

Sliter, K. A. (2013). Development and validation of a measure of workplace climate for healthy weight maintenance. *Journal of Occupational Health Psychology*, *18*(3), 350–362. doi:10.1037/a0033132 PMID:23834449

Smith, C. S., Folkard, S., Tucker, P., & Evans, M. S. (2003). Work schedules, health, and safey. In J. C. Quick & L. E. Tetrick (Eds.), *Occupational Health Psychology Handbook* (2nd ed.). American Psychological Association.

Sonnentag, S., & Jelden, S. (2009). Job stressors and the pursuit of sport activities: A day-level perspective. *Journal of Occupational Health Psychology*, *14*(2), 165–181. doi:10.1037/a0014953 PMID:19331478

Stankevitz, K., Dement, J., Schoenfisch, A., Joyner, J., Clancy, S. M., Stroo, M., & Østbye, T. (2017). Perceived barriers to healthy eating and physical activity among participants in a workplace obesity intervention. *Journal of Occupational and Environmental Medicine*, *59*(8), 746–751. doi:10.1097/JOM.0000000000001092 PMID:28692017

Swinkels, J., van Tilburg, T., Verbakel, E., & van Groenou, M. B. (2019). Explaining the gender gap in the caregiving burden of partner caregivers. *The Journals of Gerontology. Series B, Psychological Sciences and Social Sciences*, *74*(2), 309–317. PMID:28379560

Tessaro, I., Campbell, M., Benedict, S., Kelsey, K., Heisler-MacKinnon, J., Belton, L., & DeVellis, B. (1998). Developing a worksite health promotion intervention: Health Works for Women. *American Journal of Health Behavior*, *22*(6), 434.

Thum, J. S., Parsons, G., Whittle, T., & Astorino, T. A. (2017). High-Intensity Interval Training Elicits Higher Enjoyment than Moderate Intensity Continuous Exercise. *PLoS One*, *12*(1), 1–11. doi:10.1371/journal.pone.0166299 PMID:28076352

Tryon, K. (2014). Healthy staff increase productivity. *Occupational Health*, *66*(4), 11.

Ungar, N., Sieverding, M., Weidner, G., Ulrich, C. M., & Wiskemann, J. (2016). A self-regulation-based intervention to increase physical activity in cancer patients. *Psychology Health and Medicine*, *21*(2), 163–175. doi:10.1080/13548506.2015.1081255 PMID:26367803

U.S. Census Bureau. (2019). *2019 American Consumer Survey.* Retrieved from https://www.census.gov/programs-surveys/acs/

U.S. Department of Agriculture and U.S. Department of Health and Human Services. (2020). *Dietary Guidelines for Americans, 2020-2025* (9th ed.). DietaryGuidelines.gov.

van Dorssen-Boog, P., de Jong, J., Veld, M., & Van Vuuren, T. (2020). Self-leadership among healthcare workers: A mediator for the effects of job autonomy on work engagement and health. *Frontiers in Psychology*, *11*, 1420. doi:10.3389/fpsyg.2020.01420 PMID:32765341

Vogel, M., Braungardt, T., Meyer, W., & Schneider, W. (2012). The effects of shift work on physical and mental health. *Journal of Neural Transmission (Vienna, Austria)*, *119*(10), 1121–1132. doi:10.100700702-012-0800-4 PMID:22488445

Wang, Y., Beydoun, M. A., Min, J., Xue, H., Kaminsky, L. A., & Cheskin, L. J. (2020). Has the prevalence of overweight, obesity and central obesity levelled off in the United States? Trends, patterns, disparities, and future projections for the obesity epidemic. *International Journal of Epidemiology*, *49*(3), 810–823. doi:10.1093/ije/dyz273 PMID:32016289

Wardle, J., Steptoe, A., Oliver, G., & Lipsey, Z. (2000). Stress, dietary restraint and food intake. *Journal of Psychosomatic Research*, *48*(2), 195–202. doi:10.1016/S0022-3999(00)00076-3 PMID:10719137

Winston, J., Johnson, C., & Wilson, S. (2008). Barriers to healthy eating by National Health Service (NHS) hospital doctors in the hospital setting: Results of a cross-sectional survey. *BMC Research Notes*, *1*(1), 1–7. doi:10.1186/1756-0500-1-69 PMID:18755022

Wong, H., Wong, M. C., Wong, S. Y., & Lee, A. (2010). The association between shift duty and abnormal eating behavior among nurses working in a major hospital: A cross-sectional study. *International Journal of Nursing Studies*, *47*(8), 1021–1027. doi:10.1016/j.ijnurstu.2010.01.001 PMID:20116059

Wood, M. (2020). *How Pink-Collar Jobs Have Changed Since 1940*. Retrieved February 19, 2022. https://internationalwim.org/how-pink-collar-jobs-have-changed-since-1940/

Wright, J. D., Donley, A. M., Gualtieri, M. C., Strickhouser, S. M., & Wright, J. D. (2016). Food deserts: What is the problem? What is the solution? *Social Science and Public Policy*, *53*(2), 171–181. doi:10.100712115-016-9993-8

Wynd, C. A., & Ryan-Wenger, N. A. (2004). Factors predicting health behaviors among army reserve, active duty army, and civilian hospital employees. *Military Medicine*, *169*(12), 942–947. doi:10.7205/MILMED.169.12.942 PMID:15646182

Yates, M., & Samuel, V. (2019). Burnout in oncologists and associated factors: A systematic literature review and meta-analysis. *European Journal of Cancer Care*, *28*(3), 1–19. doi:10.1111/ecc.13094 PMID:31090179

Zapka, J. M., Lemon, S. C., Magner, R. P., & Hale, J. (2009). Lifestyle behaviours and weight among hospital-based nurses. *Journal of Nursing Management*, *17*(7), 853–860. doi:10.1111/j.1365-2834.2008.00923.x PMID:19793242

Zunker, C., Cox, T. L., Wingo, B. C., Knight, B., Jefferson, W. K., & Ard, J. D. (2008). Using formative research to develop a worksite health promotion program for African American women. *Women & Health*, *48*(2), 189–207. doi:10.1080/03630240802313514 PMID:19042216

Section 2
Organizational Issues

Chapter 6
Prioritizing Well-Being for Healthcare Professionals

Melyssa Allen
Mind-Body-Thrive Lifestyle, USA

ABSTRACT

Many rising issues within the healthcare industry were highlighted due to the COVID-19 pandemic. Burnout among healthcare professionals, increasing rates of lifestyle-related chronic illness, and lack of emphasis on professional self-care have contributed to a continued crisis within healthcare organizations. Numerous organizational and systemic issues have been combined with societal norms to create an unsustainable healthcare system operating on mechanisms of disease management versus of health promotion. This chapter aims to address the factors contributing to the overall health of healthcare professionals and proposed solutions to these issues through an integrative resilience model consisting of lifestyle medicine and positive psychology.

INTRODUCTION

Wellness has been defined as the absence of illness and a lifestyle of active prevention from illness, while well-being includes wellness with the addition of positive emotions. The literature has not agreed on an operational definition of these two terms, but Holdsworth (2019) provided the simplified explanation of "wellness has come to mean living well, and wellbeing means living well and enjoying happiness." Many healthcare professionals, those who are supposed to be keeping individuals and communities healthy, struggle to incorporate basic health habits into their own lives to stay well.

Many rising issues within the healthcare industry became highlighted due to the COVID-19 pandemic. Burnout among healthcare professionals, increasing rates of lifestyle related chronic illness, and lack of emphasis on professional self-care and resilience building strategies during training have contributed to a continued crisis within healthcare organizations. Numerous organizational and systemic issues have been combined with societal norms to create an unsustainable healthcare system (Shanafelt & Noseworthy, 2017). Healthcare professionals are left feeling vastly unfulfilled in the work they conduct due to patient readmissions and relapses. Shorter patient visits, constantly evolving insurance reimbursement models,

DOI: 10.4018/978-1-7998-8813-0.ch006

and overly prescribed medications treating lifestyle related diseases have shifted our healthcare systems into disease management instead of health promotion (Rippe, 2020).

Within healthcare systems, the Triple Aim was introduced from the Institute for Healthcare Improvement as a method of optimizing health system performance (Lacagnina, 2019). The Triple Aim was based on measures of enhancing patient experience, improving population health, and reducing costs (Merlo & Rippe, 2021). The pervasiveness of these chronic issues within healthcare systems and the decline of healthcare professional well-being led to the creation of the Quadruple Aim in 2014, which included the addition of improving the work life of healthcare professionals to optimize health systems performance (Parkinson, 2018; Merlo & Rippe, 2020). Considering the patient experience is largely influenced by provider well-being, it is imperative to include improving the lives of providers through resources and organizational systems addressing resilience, burnout, and suicide (Lacagnina, 2019).

The recognition of promoting and prioritizing professional self-care has become even more important amongst the global pandemic of COVID-19, and the residual effects of the pandemic will require continued emphasis for mental and emotional wellness efforts to serve healthcare professionals. Effective solutions at both the individual and organizational levels are needed to protect healthcare professionals' psychological and physical well-being (Wald, 2020; Lianov, 2019). In this chapter we will cover an overview of the current state of health among healthcare professionals, the importance of professional self-care within training programs, and the need for total well-being interventions.

The mental health of healthcare professionals is currently in crisis – with the most common concerns reported as chronic and complex stress, low job satisfaction, burnout, compassion fatigue, secondary and vicarious traumatization (Lianov, 2019). Until recently, healthcare professionals were expected to exude an unrealistic tolerance for traumatic events in the workplace and continue to perform their duties without interruption, and the COVID-19 pandemic highlighted the necessity for proper resiliency training for healthcare professionals (Bozdağ & Ergün, 2020). Without proper training and awareness, healthcare professionals may turn to maladaptive coping strategies like substance use, isolation, and suicidal ideation and may experience depression, burnout, and complex trauma (Adikey et al., 2018).

Burnout is characterized by three domains: emotional exhaustion, depersonalization, and low personal accomplishment. In 2022, the World Health Organization's International Classification of Diseases (ICD) 11 will include "burnout" as an occupational syndrome. Although it will not be a medical disorder, this inclusion of burnout further justifies the need for effective interventions for prevention and treatment efforts. The phenomenon of burnout has reached classification as an epidemic due to the prevalence being near or over 50% of US physicians (Shanafelt & Noseworthy, 2017; Patel et al. 2019). Research has demonstrated burnout leads to increased medical errors, decreased patient quality of care and satisfaction scores, and higher rates of turnover and professionals leaving the healthcare industry due to lack of fulfillment in their careers (Shanafelt & Noseworthy, 2017; Lianov, 2019). While research has emphasized physician burnout, similar prevalence of burnout has been suggested in populations of nurses, nurse practitioners, physician assistants, residents, and fellows (Dyrbye et al. 2017).

Organizational contributions to burnout include the current healthcare systems model, disease management over health promotion, and lack of integrating a culture of well-being within the healthcare organizations (Shanafelt & Noseworthy, 2017). Additionally, there is a disconnect between promoting self-care practices throughout training that result in the absence of a foundation of well-being habits for healthcare professionals to support themselves. While the upfront costs of investing in programs to reduce burnout may not result in immediate monetary return of investment, the long-term gains from this investment outweigh the long-term costs.

The physical health of our healthcare professionals must also be addressed given the rapidly rising rates of lifestyle-related chronic diseases, such as type 2 diabetes, obesity, hypertension, and cardiovascular disease (Parkinson, 2018). In comparison with the general population, healthcare professionals have an increased risk of developing type 2 diabetes, cardiovascular disease, obesity, musculoskeletal injuries, and certain types of cancers (Holtzclaw et al., 2021). Many of these physical health conditions also have mental health comorbidities, indicating a whole health approach to wellness is needed (Merlo & Vela, 2021). Healthcare workplaces pose significant barriers to practicing health promoting behaviors due to inflexible schedules and strenuous shifts which contribute to the development of adverse health effects (Kasila et al., 2018; Holtzclaw et al., 2021).

Promoting the well-being of healthcare professionals not only empowers them to make more positive health choices, but research has also shown more positive work-related indicators, such as decreased absenteeism, increased performance, and lower health care costs (Kottke et al., 2013; Kasila et al., 2018). Adopting healthy lifestyles has been shown to increase the likelihood for healthcare professionals to encourage healthy living among their patients while also serving as role models for desirable client behaviors (Hasson et al., 2018). By encouraging healthcare professionals to optimize their health through adopting healthy lifestyle behaviors, such as increased physical activity, improved nutrition, decreased tobacco use and exposure, decreased alcohol use, practiced positive thinking, stress management, and sleep hygiene, it will not only improve the health and well-being among healthcare professionals, but it will also result in improved patient health promotion practices (Kottke et al., 2013; Holtzclaw et al., 2021).

When it comes to promoting healthy lifestyles for patients, healthcare professionals are quite knowledgeable but may have difficulty translating their knowledge to motivating and encouraging their patients to reduce their behavioral risk factors (Kasila et al., 2018; Hasson et al., 2018). Additionally, many healthcare providers struggle when implementing healthy behavior changes into their lives due to occupational stress, maladaptive coping mechanisms, and lack of motivation. Historically, provider well-being was not incorporated into training programs for healthcare professionals due to the perceived lack of time and importance. More attention has recently been drawn to the impact of provider well-being on patient care and the implications of an "unwell" workforce. Classes on theoretical principles and treatment modalities have taken priority in the academic curricula. The intensely competitive nature of training programs for roles as healthcare professionals fostered a toxic environment that praised individual's "dedication" to their programs where students were encouraged to prioritize their training over everything else, including their own health and well-being. This type of unsustainable lifestyle leads to destructive habits upon entering the workforce and creates healthcare professionals without a foundation of well-being who are expected to help patients create healthier lives.

During professional training, knowledge of the benefits to health promoting behaviors is shared, yet a knowledge-behavior gap exists where students, residents, and fellows are not actively encouraged to prioritize their own well-being through these behaviors. The mental and emotional health of trainees begins to deteriorate as they progress through their programs which, in effect, can adversely impact the quality of patient care. Healthcare professionals that do not practice healthy lifestyle behaviors themselves are less likely to counsel their patients on these behaviors due to the experience of cognitive dissonance (Frates et al., 2019). Cognitive dissonance results in lower rates of counseling patients on healthy lifestyle behaviors, while providers who disclosed their own experiences regarding health behavior changes had patients who reported they were two times more likely to implement the change due to the provider being viewed as more trustworthy and credible (Holtzclaw et al., 2021). While healthcare professionals understand the knowledge to share with their patients to promote healthy lifestyles, the cognitive dissonance resulting from professionals who don't practice elements of healthy living leads to a 50% decrease in their likelihood of counseling their patients on those behaviors (Frates et al., 2019). When healthcare professionals are practicing the elements of a healthy lifestyle, they are more likely to counsel their patients on these positive health behaviors.

Practicing healthy lifestyle behaviors offers a solution to promoting the health of our healthcare professionals and serves as a protective factor against burnout. Lifestyle medicine is the use of evidence-based therapeutic lifestyle interventions to prevent, treat, and often reverse noncommunicable chronic diseases (Frates et al., 2019). It addresses the root cause of lifestyle-related diseases instead of treating the symptoms, which leads to more fulfilled provider-patient interactions. The six pillars of lifestyle medicine include regular physical activity, a plant-predominant eating pattern, practicing mindfulness and stress management, positive social connections, restorative sleep, and avoiding risky substances like tobacco and alcohol (American College of Lifestyle Medicine website, 2021).

Additionally, healthcare professionals who practice positive psychology activities in combination with lifestyle medicine enhance their resilience and well-being (Lianov et al., 2019). In her book, Roots of Positive Change: Optimizing Health Care with Positive Psychology, Dr. Liana Lianov provides a framework for integrating the practices of lifestyle medicine and positive psychology within the health-care system to address the existing challenges regarding healthcare professional burnout and prevalence of chronic disease. In the sections below we will provide a brief overview of the research for lifestyle medicine and positive psychology for healthcare professional well-being, in addition to practical strategies for implementing these health promoting habits.

LIFESTYLE MEDICINE INTERVENTIONS

Sleeping Well

Sleep deprivation has been linked to a multitude of adverse effects on mental, emotional, and physical health (Terre, 2014). Poor quality sleep or inadequate amounts of sleep can lead to an increased risk of conditions like cardiovascular disease, weakened immune functioning, metabolic dysfunction, cognitive impairment, and increased psychiatric symptomology (Kline, 2014; Rossman, 2019). Healthcare professionals face significant challenges when it comes to sleep habits due to long shift hours and overnight shift schedules (Holtzclaw et al., 2021).

Sleep problems are prevalent with between 33-50% of adults reporting regular difficulty falling or staying asleep and about 7-18% meeting criteria for insomnia (Rossman, 2019). Sleep loss significantly impacts job performance and increases the risk of mistakes made by healthcare professionals, jeopardizing patient safety (Bani-Issa et al., 2020). In a Physician Health Survey conducted by MDVIP in 2017, researchers found that 76% of physicians get inadequate sleep (Udell, 2017). The implications for quality of care provided by healthcare professionals impaired by lack of proper sleep demonstrate a need for shift work and current shift schedules to be reevaluated.

Without proper sleep, cognitive functioning becomes significantly impaired. Given the national measure of blood alcohol concentration (BAC) constituting drunk driving is 0.08, driving while drowsy has been shown to cause a similar number of roadway fatalities as driving while drunk. In an Australian study examining the effects of sleep deprivation with driving safety, it was found that being awake for 18 hours was equivalent to a BAC of 0.05 and being awake for 24 hours was equivalent to a BAC of

0.10 in terms of impaired driving ability (Powell et al., 2001). Chattu et al. (2018) found between 50-70 million Americans experience sleep difficulties or disorders, which have been linked to numerous accidents with motor vehicles, medical procedures, and other occupational scenarios (Frates et al., 2019).

Healthy, restorative sleep allows the brain and the body time to repair and replenish energetic resources that result in optimal functioning. Proper amounts of restorative sleep allow for learning and memory consolidation, regulation of hormone levels, and repairing of muscle tissue (Frates et al., 2019). The recommended guidelines for sleep and sleep needs vary across the lifespan and research has strongly suggested adults 17 and older require 7-9 hours of sleep per night (National Sleep Foundation).

Sleep needs to be a priority for healthcare professionals, however, the nature of working within healthcare settings is not the most conducive to supporting healthy sleep habits (Holtzclaw et al., 2021). While shift work and schedules may interfere with health promoting sleep practices, the practices of cognitive-behavioral therapy for insomnia (CBT-I) have been demonstrated as effective interventions for certain types of sleep disturbances. Cognitive-behavioral therapy for insomnia is an evidence-based psychotherapy that helps patients identify unhelpful thoughts and behaviors contributing to poor sleep and replace those unhelpful patterns with more helpful thoughts and behaviors that promote restorative sleep. Below are some of the recommendations from CBT-I protocols shared by Rossman (2019) that can be incorporated into sleep routines:

Practice stimulus control

- Use the bed and bedroom for sleep only, with sexual activity as the only exception.
- Any activities that are incompatible with sleep, such as watching television, being on your phone, worrying, eating, or reading in bed, should be eliminated to reestablish the association for the brain and the body to recognize that the bedroom is for sleep.

Keep the bedroom environment comfortable

- Make an effort to minimize any ambient noise or light sources that could disrupt sleep and set a comfortable temperature. If there are sources of light or noise that you cannot control, such as a neighbor's barking dog, utilizing an eye mask or ear plugs can be helpful. If working overnight, invest in blackout curtains help eliminate the daylight during sleep.

Practice sleep restriction

- Limit the time spent in bed to reduce the amount of time awake in bed. Instead of trying to go to bed earlier or stay in bed later, which often makes the situation worse, staying awake causes the sleep drive to increase and can result in falling asleep faster.

Practice relaxation techniques

- Relaxation techniques can facilitate a faster onset of Stage 1 sleep, the lightest stage of sleep, which better prepares for entering deeper sleep stages. Relaxation practices like deep breathing, guided imagery, body scan, and progressive muscle relaxation can assist in the release of mental and physical tension.

Staying Active

Exercise has been referred to as the most "underutilized antidepressant" due to research findings that demonstrate comparable efficacy of routine exercise to that of antidepressant medications (Frates et al., 2019). There are numerous benefits of regular physical activity including increased energy, improved focus and attention, reduced stress, reduced symptoms of depression and anxiety, improved sleep quality, improved sexual functioning and desire, and improved mood (American College of Sports Medicine [ACSM] Exercise is Medicine ®, 2014). Physical inactivity is one of the top four behavioral risk factors contributing to increased lifestyle-related chronic diseases and mortality rates globally (Blair, 2009; Pratt et al., 2012).

For healthcare professionals, it can be challenging to find adequate time to dedicate to engaging in physical activity. Long shift hours and a lack of time or resources while on breaks during shifts contribute to the barriers faced by healthcare professionals regarding physical activity. With the Exercise is Medicine ® initiative growing worldwide, there is still a lot of work to be done for including physical activity as a vital sign in patient encounters. Regular physical activity promotes total health, but the majority of the global population is not meeting the minimum guidelines for physical activity.

An outline of the physical activity guidelines for healthy adults from the U.S. Department of Health and Human Services Physical Activity Guidelines for Americans – 2nd Edition is below:

- **Moving more, sitting less**: Reducing the amount of sedentary time throughout the day will provide some health benefits
- **Aerobic activity**: At least 150-300 minutes of moderate-intensity activity per week, or at 75-150 minutes of vigorous-intensity physical activity per week. Aerobic activity sessions should be performed throughout the week
- **Resistance training**: At least two days per week of resistance training working the major muscle groups, but making sure to include a rest day between working the same muscle groups
- **Flexibility/Balance training**: Incorporating various active recovery into regular physical activity regimens, especially for older adults who have increased fall risk

Avoiding Substances

Tobacco – Smoking results in significant physical and mental health concerns and remains the leading preventable cause of death in the United States (Frates et al., 2019). While the health risks are widely known and publicized, cigarette smoking remains a public health issue. The addictive quality of nicotine leads to both psychological and physiological dependence, which leads to challenges and complications for individuals who attempt to quit (Ockene & Miller, 1997). Healthcare professionals have a responsibility to patients to inquire about smoking habits but may face barriers to discuss smoking cessation such as lack of knowledge for available resources, jeopardizing the provider-patient relationship, or cognitive dissonance if the healthcare professional is a smoker (van Rossem et al., 2015). There are numerous behavioral counseling and pharmacotherapy treatment programs available for smoking cessation, which can reduce the risk of many chronic diseases and even death. It is important for healthcare professionals to recognize the significant health benefits that result when they quit smoking and to reach out for help to achieve smoking cessation for improved health and well-being.

Caffeine – In moderation and appropriate amounts of consumption, caffeine does not result in significant impairment of functioning. However, caffeine is a stimulant and can lead to adverse health experiences due to the side effects and can impair sleep quality depending on the time of day and amount being consumed (Nawrot et al., 2002). Symptoms such as an increased heart rate and respiration rate may mirror the experience of a panic or anxiety attack, which can then be onset or exacerbated by the consumption of caffeine (Lara, 2010). For healthcare professionals, the accessibility of coffee, energy drinks, and soda within cafeterias and breakrooms tend to lead to overconsumption while on shift. Therefore, it is important for healthcare professionals to be mindful of the time and amount of caffeine consumption related to the potential impacts on their well-being.

Alcohol – In a recently published review from Smirmaul et al. (2021), it is stated that alcohol "represents the leading risk factor for premature mortality and disability among those aged 15-49 years." The adverse health effects of alcohol, outside of the warning label about risks of consuming alcohol while pregnant, are typically not well known or acknowledged unlike the health risks of tobacco. Unfortunately, due to the quarantine period that resulted from efforts to minimize the spread of COVID-19, there is likely to be an increased rate of substance use disorder as many individuals may have turned to alcohol consumption to cope with the stressors caused by the pandemic. In a study published in 2008 by George Kenna & David Lewis they stated, "[g]iven the increasingly stressful environment due to manpower shortages in the healthcare system in general, substance induced impairment among some healthcare professions is anticipated to grow." With the additional stressors and traumas experienced during the COVID-19 pandemic, it is important to recognize the impact of alcohol consumption on both physical and mental well-being for healthcare professionals and providing appropriate treatment, resources, and referrals. While optimal health can be achieved by avoiding alcohol consumption, below are the guidelines for standard drink sizes and the low risk drinking according to the National Institutes of Health "Rethinking Drinking: Alcohol & Your Health" campaign:

Standard drink size

- 12 oz of beer (5% alcohol)
- 5 oz of wine (12% alcohol)
- 1.5 oz of 80-proof distilled spirits (40% alcohol)

Low risk drinking

- For men: no more than 4 standard size drinks on any day and no more than 14 standard size drinks in 7 days
- For women: no more than 3 standard size drinks on any day and no more than 7 standard size drinks in 7 days
- "Binge" drinking is defined as 5 standard size drinks in 2 hours for men and 4 standard size drinks in 2 hours for women

Eating Healthfully

The association of nutrition and physical health has been long supported by research, with lifestyle medicine using a whole food, plant-predominant lifestyle as the "North Star" for nutrition (Frates et al., 2019). Numerous health organizations, such as the American Diabetes Association, American Cancer Society, American Medical Association, American Heart Association, and more all share an aligned message that optimal health is promoted by eating more unrefined plant foods (ACLM, "Many Voices, One Theme," 2020). While nutrition plays a crucial role in health and is often a root cause for many lifestyle-related chronic diseases, little to no education is provided during training for healthcare professionals to coach their patients in adopting healthful nutrition practices (Frates et al., 2019).

Nutrition is a mediating and modifiable factor that can serve as a protective mechanism against mental health conditions like burnout, depression, anxiety, stress, in addition to numerous physical health conditions (Esquivel, 2021). Blanchflower et al. (2013) conducted a large epidemiological study in the UK which found a dose-response relationship with consuming 7-8 servings of fruits and vegetables with increased feelings of happiness, even when confounding factors known to affect emotional well-being were controlled for. Research investigating the gut-brain connection has emerging evidence supporting the notion "food feeds mood," due to findings demonstrating a link between diet quality and mental health (Morton, 2018).

With an abundance of processed, nutrient poor foods that are the most easily accessible and widely available, it is important to move towards eating more whole, nutrient rich foods like vegetables, fruits, nuts, seeds, legumes, and whole grains to promote health (DiMaria-Ghalili et al., 2014; Devries et al., 2017). The American College of Lifestyle Medicine's *Food as Medicine Jumpstart* includes a step-by-step approach to incorporating a more whole food, plant-based lifestyle (WFPB), which encourages the consumption of more fiber-filled, nutrient dense foods to promote overall health.

Managing Stress

The damaging effects of chronic stress on well-being are well documented throughout the research and healthcare professionals are at an increased risk of adverse health conditions due to their occupational demands (Burton et al., 2017). Chronic stress has adverse effects on physical health, such as weakened immune system, sleep deprivation, high blood pressure, and increased risk for cardiovascular disease (Smirmaul et al., 2021). With the COVID-19 pandemic, there were numerous chronic stressors for healthcare professionals serving on the front-line response: the worry of contracting COVID, shortage of personal protective equipment, lockdown and quarantine regulations, financial hardships. Considering healthcare professionals are already at an increased risk for many lifestyle-related chronic diseases, the addition of the chronic stress experienced by the pandemic made matters worse (Babore et al., 2020; Holtzclaw et al., 2021). Below are some evidence-based stress management techniques as shared by Varvogli & Darviri (2011):

- Mindfulness-based stress reduction (MBSR): This 8-week program created by Dr. Jon Kabat-Zinn teaches participants to become more aware of, and relate differently to thoughts, feelings, and body sensations while cultivating a nonjudging awareness moment by moment (Shapiro et al., 2005).
- Cognitive-behavioral therapy (CBT): This approach examines maladaptive thoughts and behaviors and looks to identify reframing them into more adaptive thoughts and behaviors, which can be helpful when working to reframe our appraisal of stressors (McGonigal, 2016).
- Diaphragmatic breathing: Deep breathing can assist with vagal nerve activation, which can trigger the relaxation response and help suppress the stress response.
- Guided imagery: This practice can use an audio track to lead the listener through a visualization to promote relaxation or imagine positive life outcomes.
- Biofeedback: This process helps individuals identify and modify their physiological activity to improve health and performance.

Fostering Positive Social Connections

Humans are social creatures that experience physical, mental, and emotional health benefits from positive social interactions, including micro-moments of connection such as eye contact (Lianov, 2019). The physical benefits experienced by positive social connections include decreased blood pressure, release of oxytocin, improved cancer survival, decreased cardiovascular mortality, maintenance of a healthy body mass index, and better control of blood sugar levels (Martino, Pegg, Frates, 2017). Social engagement leads to mental and emotional health benefits like reduced loneliness, reduced posttraumatic stress disorder symptomology, and increased likelihood of achieve positive health behavior change due to social support and accountability (Walsh, 2011; Martino, Pegg, Frates, 2017).

At a time when social isolation and quarantine was required during the COVID-19 public health crisis, more attention was drawn to the importance of social health for our overall well-being. The loneliness and isolation experienced during the quarantine period resulted in the onset or exacerbation of mental health conditions (Smirmaul et al., 2021). It is important for healthcare professionals to form and strengthen their positive social connections both within and outside of the workplace to support well-being and enhance resilience. Social support networks and resources will be crucial in buffering the effects of the impending mental health crisis among healthcare professionals following the COVID-19 pandemic (Pearman et al., 2020, Stuijfzand et al., 2020).

POSITIVE PSYCHOLOGY INTERVENTIONS

Engagement has been described as the "positive antithesis" of burnout, with vigor, dedication, and absorption in work serving as the contrasting characteristics to the symptoms of burnout (Shanafelt & Noseworth, 2017). Comprehensive efforts to promote engagement, build resilience, and enhance well-being need to be at the forefront of addressing this growing crisis among healthcare professionals (Parkinson, 2018). When healthcare professionals can rediscover and reconnect with meaning and purpose in the work they do, it serves as a protective factor to burnout (Lianov, 2021).

Positive psychology activities have been suggested as effective interventions to facilitate positive health behavior change and improve psychological health (Lianov et al., 2019). Positive psychology is defined as the scientific study of strengths that enable individuals and communities to thrive and lead meaningful and fulfilled lives and can act synergistically with healthy lifestyle habits to promote positive health (Seligman & Csikszentmihalyi, 2014). Positive psychology activities include gratitude practices, mindfulness, savoring, and acts of kindness (Lianov et al., 2020). Additionally, increasing positive emotions through the PERMA model (outlined below) developed by Dr. Martin Seligman has been shown to have physiological benefits, such as increased parasympathetic nervous system functioning, improved vagal tone and greater heart rate variability, increased release of positive neurotransmitters, strengthened immunity, and longer telomeres (Lianov, 2021). The PERMA model can guide individuals and organizations to find activities that increase positive emotions for improving well-being:

- P – Positive emotions: Increasing the experience of positive emotions, such as optimism, gratitude, hope, and more serve to enhance resilience and well-being.
- E – Engagement: Also referred to as a state of "flow," is the experience of an individual being immersed in an activity where they lose track of time.
- R – Relationships: As mentioned in the previous section, positive social interactions create improved physiological and emotional health.
- M – Meaning: Having meaning and purpose in work is associated with improved productivity and success in the workplace, as well as increased quality of life measures.

- A – Accomplishment: A sense of accomplishment improves feelings of satisfaction, self-efficacy, and self-confidence.

CONCLUSION

While a reactive approach to solving these professional crises has been employed, COVID-19 has highlighted the desperate need for proactive solutions to these issues moving forward. Programs focused on promoting well-being and wellness beginning in the early stages of training will provide a foundation for sustainable self-care practices of healthcare professionals to support resiliency and optimize job performance. Organizational changes must also be implemented, but healthcare professionals can adopt individual self-care behaviors necessary to ensure their well-being (Lianov, 2021).

Wald (2020) developed an integrative resilience model to optimize resilience and well-being for healthcare trainees and professionals during the COVID-19 pandemic. His program contained twelve tips with educational and practical strategies targeting the promotion of well-being and resilience to burnout. There are many takeaways from Wald's integrative resilience model that can be applied on an individual and organizational basis utilizing evidence-based strategies that can help develop emotional competencies for occupational demands faced by healthcare professionals.

The literature suggests these well-being programs should be comprised of an integration of evidence-based practices, such as positive psychology and lifestyle medicine (Lianov et al., 2019; Morton, 2018; Frates et al., 2019). Healthy lifestyles and positive emotions have demonstrated a reciprocal, reinforcing link referred to as the *upward spiral theory of lifestyle change* which explains how positive affect can facilitate long-term adherence to positive health behaviors (Lianov, 2021; Van Cappellen et al., 2019). This complementary interaction of health promoting behaviors and positive psychology practices cultivates a framework for sustainable self-care practices that contribute to enhanced resilience, improved well-being, and optimized performance for healthcare professionals.

In addition to the lifestyle medicine and positive psychology interventions, there is an opportunity to teach emotional and mental well-being skills to enhance resilience. Therapeutic skills training incorporating techniques from cognitive-behavioral therapy, acceptance and commitment training, and mindful self-compassion have been suggested as methods to improve the well-being of healthcare professionals (Rogers, 2016; Wald, 2020). While there are many evidence-based approaches that can effectively prevent and treat conditions like burnout, an important aspect shared by Wald (2020) from the integrative resilience model is *self-awareness*.

Normalizing the process of healthcare professionals checking-in with their state of well-being will begin to reinforce a proactive approach to the prevention of mental, emotional, and physical health conditions. At the time this book is being written, we find ourselves at a pivotal moment to create a massive paradigm shift in the way healthcare professionals are trained by their programs and treated by their employers. It is time for organizations to prioritize genuine and thoughtful efforts to help the helpers who have given so much of their lives to caring for their communities and allow our healthcare professionals the chance to achieve their optimal health and happiness.

REFERENCES

Ahmad, W., Taggart, F., Shafique, M. S., Muzafar, Y., Abidi, S., Ghani, N., Malik, Z., Zahid, T., Waqas, A., & Ghaffar, N. (2015). Diet, exercise and mental-wellbeing of healthcare professionals (doctors, dentists and nurses) in Pakistan. *PeerJ*, *3*, e1250. doi:10.7717/peerj.1250 PMID:26401460

Babore, A., Lombardi, L., Viceconti, M. L., Pignataro, S., Marino, V., Crudele, M., Candelori, C., Bramanti, S. M., & Trumello, C. (2020). Psychological effects of the COVID-2019 pandemic: Perceived stress and coping strategies among healthcare professionals. *Psychiatry Research*, *293*, 113366. doi:10.1016/j.psychres.2020.113366 PMID:32798932

Baldisseri, M. R. (2007). Impaired healthcare professional. *Critical Care Medicine*, *35*(2, Suppl), S106–S116. doi:10.1097/01.CCM.0000252918.87746.96 PMID:17242598

Bani-Issa, W., Radwan, H., Al Marzooq, F., Al Awar, S., Al-Shujairi, A. M., Samsudin, A. R., Khasawneh, W., & Albluwi, N. (2020). Salivary cortisol, subjective stress and quality of sleep among female healthcare professionals. *Journal of Multidisciplinary Healthcare*, *13*, 125–140. doi:10.2147/JMDH.S229396 PMID:32103972

Blair, S. N. (2009). Physical inactivity: The biggest public health problem of the 21st century. *British Journal of Sports Medicine*, *43*(1), 1–2. PMID:19136507

Bozdağ, F., & Ergün, N. (2020). Psychological resilience of healthcare professionals during COVID-19 pandemic. *Psychological Reports*. PMID:33050800

Burton, A., Burgess, C., Dean, S., Koutsopoulou, G. Z., & Hugh-Jones, S. (2017). How effective are mindfulness-based interventions for reducing stress among healthcare professionals? A systematic review and meta-analysis. *Stress and Health*, *33*(1), 3–13. doi:10.1002mi.2673 PMID:26916333

Chattu, V. K., Sakhamuri, S. M., Kumar, R., Spence, D. W., BaHammam, A. S., & Pandi-Perumal, S. R. (2018). BaHammam AS, Pandi-Perumal SR. Insufficient Sleep Syndrome: Is it time to classify it as a major noncommunicable disease? *Sleep Science*, *11*(2), 56. doi:10.5935/1984-0063.20180013 PMID:30083291

Devries, S., Agatston, A., Aggarwal, M., Aspry, K. E., Esselstyn, C. B., Kris-Etherton, P., Miller, M., O'Keefe, J. H., Ros, E., Rzeszut, A. K., White, B. A., Williams, K. A., & Freeman, A. M. (2017). A deficiency of nutrition education and practice in cardiology. *The American Journal of Medicine*, *130*(11), 1298–1305. doi:10.1016/j.amjmed.2017.04.043 PMID:28551044

Díaz Ramiro, E. M., Rubio Valdehita, S., López Núñez, M. I., & Aparicio García, M. E. (2020). *Sleep habits as predictors of psychological health in healthcare professionals*. Academic Press.

DiMaria-Ghalili, R. A., Mirtallo, J. M., Tobin, B. W., Hark, L., Van Horn, L., & Palmer, C. A. (2014). Challenges and opportunities for nutrition education and training in the health care professions: Intraprofessional and interprofessional call to action. *The American Journal of Clinical Nutrition*, *99*(5), 1184S–1193S. doi:10.3945/ajcn.113.073536 PMID:24646823

Dyrbye, L. N., Shanafelt, T. D., Sinsky, C. A., Cipriano, P. F., Bhatt, J., Ommaya, A., ... & Meyers, D. (2017). Burnout among health care professionals: A call to explore and address this underrecognized threat to safe, high-quality care. *NAM Perspectives*.

Esquivel, M. K. (2021). Nutrition strategies for reducing risk of burnout among physicians and health care professionals. *American Journal of Lifestyle Medicine*, *15*(2), 126–129. doi:10.1177/1559827620976538 PMID:33790697

Frates, B. (2019). *Lifestyle medicine handbook: An introduction to the power of healthy habits*. Healthy Learning.

Hasson, R., Stark, A. H., Constantini, N., Polak, R., Verbov, G., Edelstein, N., ... Soltz-Aharony, H. (2018). "Practice What You Teach" Public Health Nurses Promoting Healthy Lifestyles (PHeeL-PHiNe): Program Evaluation. *The Journal of Ambulatory Care Management*, *41*(3), 171–180. doi:10.1097/JAC.0000000000000243 PMID:29847404

Holdsworth, M. A. (2019). Health, wellness and wellbeing. *Revue Interventions Économiques. Papers in Political Economy*, (62).

Holtzclaw, L., Arlinghaus, K. R., & Johnston, C. A. (2021). The Health of Health Care Professionals. *American Journal of Lifestyle Medicine*, *15*(2), 130–132. doi:10.1177/1559827620977065 PMID:33790698

Kasila, K., Hallman, M., Kautiainen, H., Vanhala, M., & Kettunen, T. (2018). The gap between behavioral risk status and willingness to change behavior among healthcare professionals. *Perspectives in Public Health*, *138*(6), 311–315. doi:10.1177/1757913917751564 PMID:29356601

Kenna, G. A., & Lewis, D. C. (2008). Risk factors for alcohol and other drug use by healthcare professionals. *Substance Abuse Treatment, Prevention, and Policy*, *3*(1), 1–8. doi:10.1186/1747-597X-3-3 PMID:18230139

Kottke, T., Baechler, C., Canterbury, M., Danner, C., Erickson, K., & Hayes, R. (2013). *ICSI Health Care Guideline: Healthy Lifestyles*. Institute for Clinical Systems Improvement (ICSI).

Lacagnina, S. (2019). The Triple Aim Plus More. *American Journal of Lifestyle Medicine*, *13*(1), 42–43. doi:10.1177/1559827618806183 PMID:30627077

Lara, D. R. (2010). Caffeine, mental health, and psychiatric disorders. *Journal of Alzheimer's Disease*, *20*(s1), S239–S248. doi:10.3233/JAD-2010-1378 PMID:20164571

Lianov, L. (2019). *Roots of Positive Change: Optimizing Health Care with Positive Psychology*. American College of Lifestyle Medicine.

Lianov, L. (2021). A Powerful Antidote to Physician Burnout: Intensive Healthy Lifestyle and Positive Psychology Approaches. *American Journal of Lifestyle Medicine*, *15*(5), 15598276211006626. doi:10.1177/15598276211006626 PMID:34646108

Lianov, L. S., Barron, G. C., Fredrickson, B. L., Hashmi, S., Klemes, A., Krishnaswami, J., Lee, J., Le Pertel, N., Matthews, J. A., Millstein, R. A., Phillips, E. M., Sannidhi, D., Purpur de Vries, P., Wallace, A., & Winter, S. J. (2020). Positive psychology in health care: Defining key stakeholders and their roles. *Translational Behavioral Medicine*, *10*(3), 637–647. doi:10.1093/tbm/ibz150 PMID:32766868

Lianov, L. S., Fredrickson, B. L., Barron, C., Krishnaswami, J., & Wallace, A. (2019). Positive psychology in lifestyle medicine and health care: Strategies for implementation. *American Journal of Lifestyle Medicine*, *13*(5), 480–486. doi:10.1177/1559827619838992 PMID:31523213

Martino, J., Pegg, J., & Frates, E. P. (2017). The connection prescription: Using the power of social interactions and the deep desire for connectedness to empower health and wellness. *American Journal of Lifestyle Medicine*, *11*(6), 466–475. doi:10.1177/1559827615608788 PMID:30202372

McGonigal, K. (2016). *The upside of stress: Why stress is good for you, and how to get good at it*. Penguin.

Merlo, G., & Rippe, J. (2021). Physician burnout: A lifestyle medicine perspective. *American Journal of Lifestyle Medicine*, *15*(2), 148–157.

Merlo, G., & Vela, A. (2021). Mental Health in Lifestyle Medicine: A Call to Action. *American Journal of Lifestyle Medicine*. PMID:35185421

Monti, K., Monti, J. D., & Thomas, D. (2021). Knowledge and Attitudes of Lifestyle Medicine–Based Care in a Military Community. *Military Medicine*, usab279. doi:10.1093/milmed/usab279 PMID:34254645

Nawrot, P., Jordan, S., Eastwood, J., Rotstein, J., Hugenholtz, A., & Feeley, M. (2003). Effects of caffeine on human health. *Food Additives and Contaminants*, *20*(1), 1–30. doi:10.1080/0265203021000007840 PMID:12519715

Nowson, C. (2020). Opportunities for innovation in nutrition education for health professionals. *BMJ Nutrition. Prevention & Health*, *3*(2), 126. PMID:33521520

Owens, J. A. (2007). Sleep loss and fatigue in healthcare professionals. *The Journal of Perinatal & Neonatal Nursing*, *21*(2), 92–100. doi:10.1097/01.JPN.0000270624.64584.9d PMID:17505227

Parry, D. A., Oeppen, R. S., Amin, M. S. A., & Brennan, P. A. (2018). Sleep: Its importance and the effects of deprivation on surgeons and other healthcare professionals. *British Journal of Oral & Maxillofacial Surgery*, *56*(8), 663–666. doi:10.1016/j.bjoms.2018.08.001 PMID:30173962

Patel, R. S., Sekhri, S., Bhimanadham, N. N., Imran, S., & Hossain, S. (2019). A review on strategies to manage physician burnout. *Cureus*, *11*(6). Advance online publication. doi:10.7759/cureus.4805 PMID:31404361

Pearman, A., Hughes, M. L., Smith, E. L., & Neupert, S. D. (2020). Mental health challenges of United States healthcare professionals during COVID-19. *Frontiers in Psychology*, *11*, 2065. doi:10.3389/fpsyg.2020.02065 PMID:32903586

Powell, N. B., Schechtman, K. B., Riley, R. W., Li, K., Troell, R., & Guilleminault, C. (2001). The road to danger: The comparative risks of driving while sleepy. *The Laryngoscope*, *111*(5), 887–893. doi:10.1097/00005537-200105000-00024 PMID:11359171

Pratt, M., Norris, J., Lobelo, F., Roux, L., & Wang, G. (2014). The cost of physical inactivity: Moving into the 21st century. *British Journal of Sports Medicine*, *48*(3), 171–173. doi:10.1136/bjsports-2012-091810 PMID:23134760

Raab, K., Sogge, K., Parker, N., & Flament, M. F. (2015). Mindfulness-based stress reduction and self-compassion among mental healthcare professionals: A pilot study. *Mental Health, Religion & Culture, 18*(6), 503–512. doi:10.1080/13674676.2015.1081588

Rippe, J. M. (2020). Lifestyle Medicine Is Truly the Strong Foundation for Modern Health Care. *American Journal of Lifestyle Medicine, 14*(5), 468–470. doi:10.1177/1559827620912165 PMID:32922230

Rogers, D. (2016). Which educational interventions improve healthcare professionals' resilience? *Medical Teacher, 38*(12), 1236–1241. doi:10.1080/0142159X.2016.1210111 PMID:27573430

Rossman, J. (2019). Cognitive-behavioral therapy for insomnia: An effective and underutilized treatment for insomnia. *American Journal of Lifestyle Medicine, 13*(6), 544–547. doi:10.1177/1559827619867677 PMID:31662718

Sallis, R. (2011). Developing healthcare systems to support exercise: Exercise as the fifth vital sign. *British Journal of Sports Medicine, 45*(6), 473–474. doi:10.1136/bjsm.2010.083469 PMID:21292925

Seligman, M. E., & Csikszentmihalyi, M. (2014). Positive psychology: An introduction. In *Flow and the foundations of positive psychology* (pp. 279–298). Springer.

Shanafelt, T. D., & Noseworthy, J. H. (2017, January). Executive leadership and physician well-being: Nine organizational strategies to promote engagement and reduce burnout. *Mayo Clinic Proceedings, 92*(1), 129–146. doi:10.1016/j.mayocp.2016.10.004 PMID:27871627

Shapiro, S. L., Astin, J. A., Bishop, S. R., & Cordova, M. (2005). Mindfulness-based stress reduction for health care professionals: Results from a randomized trial. *International Journal of Stress Management, 12*(2), 164–176. doi:10.1037/1072-5245.12.2.164

Smirmaul, B. P., Chamon, R. F., de Moraes, F. M., Rozin, G., Moreira, A. S. B., de Almeida, R., & Guimarães, S. T. (2021). Lifestyle medicine during (and after) the COVID-19 pandemic. *American Journal of Lifestyle Medicine, 15*(1), 60–67. doi:10.1177/1559827620950276 PMID:33456421

Stuijfzand, S., Deforges, C., Sandoz, V., Sajin, C. T., Jaques, C., Elmers, J., & Horsch, A. (2020). Psychological impact of an epidemic/pandemic on the mental health of healthcare professionals: A rapid review. *BMC Public Health, 20*(1), 1–18. doi:10.118612889-020-09322-z PMID:32787815

Terre, L. (2014). Clinical implications of impaired sleep. *American Journal of Lifestyle Medicine, 8*(6), 352–370. doi:10.1177/1559827614521955

Van Cappellen, P., Rice, E. L., Catalino, L. I., & Fredrickson, B. L. (2018). Positive affective processes underlie positive health behaviour change. *Psychology & Health, 33*(1), 77–97.

van Rossem, C., Spigt, M. G., Kleijsen, J. R., Hendricx, M., van Schayck, C. P., & Kotz, D. (2015). Smoking cessation in primary care: Exploration of barriers and solutions in current daily practice from the perspective of smokers and healthcare professionals. *The European Journal of General Practice, 21*(2), 1–7. doi:10.3109/13814788.2014.990881 PMID:25649048

Varvogli, L., & Darviri, C. (2011). Stress management techniques: Evidence-based procedures that reduce stress and promote health. *Health Science Journal, 5*(2), 74.

Wald, H. S. (2020). Optimizing resilience and wellbeing for healthcare professions trainees and healthcare professionals during public health crises–Practical tips for an 'integrative resilience' approach. *Medical Teacher*, *42*(7), 744–755. doi:10.1080/0142159X.2020.1768230 PMID:32449867

Walsh, R. (2011). Lifestyle and mental health. *The American Psychologist*, *66*(7), 579–592. doi:10.1037/a0021769 PMID:21244124

Williams, I. M., & Lewis, W. G. (2020). Stress in the workplace for healthcare professionals. *Physiological Reports*, *8*(13). Advance online publication. doi:10.14814/phy2.14496 PMID:32744802

Chapter 7
Conceptual Understanding of Provider Responses to the Complexity of Healthcare Delivery

Tracey C. Arnold
Southern Connecticut State University, USA

E. Carol Polifroni
University of Connecticut, USA

ABSTRACT

This chapter introduces complexity science as a framework for understanding the healthcare delivery system and the inherent challenges it poses for healthcare providers. The Institute for Healthcare Improvement's triple aim, which focuses on the patient experience, population health, and decreased costs, served the health disciplines for a short period of time. It was then recognized that the healthcare provider, the worker at the point of care, was instrumental in the success of the triple aim. This concept, the health and wellbeing of the worker, came to be crystallized as meaning and joy in one's work. The chapter explores this positive affect concept as well as that of compassion satisfaction along with negative affect occupational-based strains occurring for the healthcare provider as they navigate working in the complex healthcare delivery system of the United States.

INTRODUCTION

The healthcare system in the United States (US) is complex. It is difficult to navigate as a patient, and at times it is even more difficult for the healthcare provider. Most healthcare providers, when asked, will state they entered healthcare to help people. They felt a calling and/or recognized behaviors in themselves congruent with helping others. They entered the profession with bright eyes and cheerful smiles knowing they were on the path to fulfillment through assisting others. They envisioned saving lives, bringing

DOI: 10.4018/978-1-7998-8813-0.ch007

comfort, guiding one's health and well-being, and easing the process of death amongst other things. Many find meaning and joy in that work; they are satisfied as their purpose is fulfilled. Others felt the stress of the complexity of the healthcare system and lost that passion and satisfaction. They burned out as the morally distressing situations stayed with them; in turn, they lost their compassion, and they were affected by others' tragedies. In most instances, the quality of care they delivered suffered and, usually, they left the work they deliberately selected to do. The providers lost meaning and joy ad were no longer fulfilled. In the following chapter these topics will be explored in depth to enhance understanding of these healthcare provider responses to the complex system of healthcare delivery.

After completing the chapter, the reader will be able to:

1. Recognize the complex nature of health care delivery.
2. Discern the essence of meaning and joy.
3. Identify the factors contributing to meaning and joy.
4. Address the states of burnout, moral distress, compassion fatigue, and secondary traumatic stress.
5. Propose well-being strategies for themselves to promote meaning and joy.

HEALTHCARE PROVIDERS' RESPONSES TO THE COMPLEXITY OF HEALTHCARE DELIVERY

Complexity of Healthcare Delivery

The US health care delivery system in 2021 is not really a system. It can be characterized as a collection of parts that do not connect with each other unless mandated by payment mechanisms or other regulatory initiatives. Access is difficult unless you have resources, know how to use the resources, speak the language available at the resource, and know how to finance the resource utilization. Cost is an issue that is challenging not driven by typical economic forces of the market, involves the government and individuals, and is institution by institution dependent. Quality, however one defines it, is equally as challenging. Care varies across the nation and quality is often not the measurement or word we would use to characterize care that is delivered. The Institute of Medicine (IOM) in 2002 said quality was safety, timely, efficient, effective, equitable, and patient centered (IOM, 2001). The Covid-19 pandemic experience illustrates that care is not equitable, it is not about the patient per se, it is effective sometimes and rarely efficient, and not safe when misinformation is delivered each night through the media. Yet, there is persistence in calling the sources of health care one receives a health care delivery system. Thus, there must be another lens to examine our health care delivery system and that is the lens of complexity.

Complexity science (Uhl Bien & Russ, 2009) yields to the fact that complex systems are composed of many individual parts which relate to each other in some ways and should relate to each other in many other ways. Complex systems are interactive, and when examined at the fundamental core level, it is noted that each part of a system lies within itself. These individual parts are known as complex adaptive systems and whole systems, e.g., the health care delivery system, are many interactive complex adaptive systems. Complex adaptive systems are characterized as being nonlinear meaning there is not necessarily order or a clear starting and ending point. There is a sense of chasing one's tail which confronts our energy and patience. Order for one is not the order for another because the lens used to judge the order is different. Complex adaptive systems emerge; the emergence is based on need and a commitment to meet that need. The outcome of emergence is often spontaneous because the need is powerful. Complex adaptive systems have the word adaptive in their name. They are adaptive because if they did not, they would cease to exist. There is a bit of Darwinian thought within complex adaptive system i.e., survival of the fittest. Complex adaptive systems also change with feedback; they are in constant motion and thus dynamic. There is also an inherent uncertainty with complex systems and particularly complex adaptive systems; complexity requires one to examine the here and now while constantly looking at what is ahead. Complexity requires attention to the details while appreciating the impact on the whole. Complexity mandates the openness of individuals within the organizations as this openness facilitates the ability to change and to adapt. Such dynamic interactiveness is somewhat antithetical to the health care system which has been described as bureaucratic and immobile. Yet, without an appreciation for the complexity involved, at all levels, the organization, the system, will be replaced by something different.

Experiences within the Covid-19 pandemic in 2021 serve as a perfect illustration of the complex health care delivery system composed of many parts, complex adaptive systems, which has changed the way health care is delivered. Telehealth, discovered in the 1960's, yet rarely used due to payment mechanisms, provider and patient resistance, and lack of the needed technology is now sought after as a prime medium for health care delivery (Robeznieks, 2021). The pandemic made the system adapt as health care remained a need, yet no one wanted to enter into environments other than their own known space; their homes. In intensive care areas (ICUs), we learned patients needed physical assistance to breathe and proning them (putting them on their stomachs instead of their backs) was beneficial; not something routinely done in ICUs prior to 2020 yet now there are proning teams and it is part of care for patients on ventilators with respiratory challenges (Miguel et al., 2021). Technology facilitated interactions with and between providers. The medical record, now electronic in most instances, was visible and accessible regardless of where one was physically located. A national vaccination administration system (https://vams.cdc.gov/vaccineportal/s/login/?language=en_US&startURL=%2Fvaccineportal%2Fs%2F&ec=302) was created quickly to document the covid vaccines being administered and data was accessible on a national and worldwide scale so that the vaccination rates could be tracked and used as datapoints in the evolution of the pandemic's spread. There are many more examples, but complexity as a lens to examine the health care delivery system works when one look at the parts and need to see the whole. As Aristotle said centuries ago, the whole is greater than the sum of its parts.

A component of the whole health care delivery system is human resource. It is perhaps the most precious and fragile resource within the health care delivery system. Protection and promotion of that workforce is crucial for the system to continue to evolve, to be effective and efficient, to deliver quality care and to focus on the patient. Yet, until the Institute for Healthcare Improvement (IHI) introduced its triple aim and subsequently the fourth component of the triple aim, the health care human resource received little attention.

Affective Responses

Healthcare providers' affective responses to the complexity of healthcare delivery are typically positive or negative. These affective responses, known as one's affective wellbeing, involve feelings or emotions and have the potential to influence healthcare providers' future actions and decisions based on whether the responses are positive or negative (Luhmann, 2017). Research has supported a relationship between affective emotions and prosocial behaviors such as helping others (Igou et al., 2020; Xiao et al., 2021), a buffering effect from negative affect emotions after helping others (Spitzmuller et al., 2020), and the act of helping others increasing one's positive affect emotions (Hui et al., 2020).

While these two affective states appear to be on opposite ends of a spectrum, they often overlap with one having both positive and negative affect emotions at the same time affecting how one lives. For instance, a healthcare provider may be happy that a patient survived a traumatic situation but also anxious that they might experience the same type of situation themself.

Positive Affect

Positive affect refers to emotions such as cheerfulness, meaning and joy, and enthusiasm with potential feelings of contentment, engagement, and/or pride (Fortenberry et al., 2017) among others. Those with a propensity for positive affect emotions tend to deal with life's challenges in a positive manner, often affectionally referred to as seeing through rose colored glasses or having a glass half full. They find the silver linings and can find something good in any bad situation.

This chapter will focus on both meaning and joy and compassion satisfaction as the positive affect responses of healthcare providers. Research, definitions, and examples of these concepts will be offered. As well, the authors would like to stress the importance of the positive affect emotions for healthcare providers because research supports that positive affect emotions are required for healthcare providers to stave off burnout, moral distress, compassion fatigue, and secondary traumatic stress (Beauvais et al., 2017). Positive affect emotions and desire to help have a reciprocal relationship in that helping others causes positive affect emotions while positive affect emotions cause a desire to help others (Hui et al., 2020).

Meaning and Joy

In 2008 the IHI created the triple aim for health care which addressed the patient experience, a change to focus on population health instead of individuals, and a commitment to reduce health care costs (Institute for healthcare improvement, n.d.a). It is long recognized that the US health care costs are greater than most other industrialized nations and yet our outcomes are worse in many aspects. Therefore, a focus on reduction of costs is not misplaced. Attention to the patient experience is directly related to cost reduction as it is related to patient centered care. The experience one has with the system, their own or someone close to them, makes a major difference in how, when, where and if care is sought again. The patient experience makes a financial difference for an agency as cost and experience are connected. Slightly less directly connected to the individual experience is the issue of population health; directly connected to cost. Population health involves the attention to causation, disease entities, and the social determinants of health; all subjects for more detailed exploration and examination in other resources. IHI's triple aim became common language for health care providers, economists, and those in the political realm.

In 2014 it was finally appreciated that the experience of the health care provider (the human resource) made a difference in an institution's ability to implement and achieve the triple aim (Bodenheimer & Sinsky, 2014). The worker at the point of care delivery, the provider at a bedside, the administrator in the office, and the director serving on a board for the health care system, all have experience that makes a difference. When the worker, and their numbers are in the millions and millions, does not have meaning and joy in their everyday work they risk delivering less than quality care which impacts the ability of the institution to implement the triple aim (Sikka, et al., 2015).

The literature today is replete with information on and studied about burnout and compassion fatigue. Additionally, newspapers and the lay media ask healthcare providers to share their stories of burnout and intent to leave their respective positions. The authors do not dismiss the reality of burnout and its associated conditions; however, the authors believe that meaning and joy needs to become the catalyst for successful implementation of the IHI's triple aim and the flourishing of the US health care delivery system. In this context, success is defined as the worker returning to work the next day (retention), students seeking to learn how to be health care workers (recruitment), patients receiving the quality care they need (experience), access to care being created through innovative arrangements (population health), and care becoming more efficient and effective (cost). Without meaning and joy for the workforce, success will not happen.

So, what is this catalyst? What is meaning and joy? While meaning and joy is just beginning to be studied in health care, certain things about meaning and joy are known. The IHI states "The most joyful, productive, engaged staff feel both physically and psychologically safe, appreciate the meaning and purpose of their work, have some choice and control over their time, experience camaraderie with others at work, and perceive their work life to be fair and equitable." (Institute for healthcare improvement, n.d.b). In 2013 the National Patient Safety Foundation asserted that workplaces which provided physical, psychological, and emotional safety facilitated the enhancement of meaning and joy. Without safety, meaning and joy could not occur. This is much like Maslow's hierarchy of personal needs for growth & development; safety comes first. Thus, it is relatively easy to see that the concept of burnout may emerge before meaning and joy are discovered if one does not feel safe in their work environment.

Meaning and joy, in nurses across the country, is the sense of purpose, the sense of doing good, and the ability to do what providers what into their respective disciplines and professional practice to do. It is not all that difficult to discern. Meaning and joy is the treatment as a professional person, the respect for one's voice, the treatment with dignity by the other healthcare providers and the patients they are treating, and the ability to pursue what is best for the patient without unexpected barriers of the bureaucracy. Galuska et al. (2018) interviewed 28 nurses across the country in a variety of patient care areas (medical surgical, critical care, emergency departments, perinatal and pediatric, as examples). Each nurse was asked to describe their experiences with meaning and joy as they chose to define it. This latter piece is important; it is not an artificially created definition, but one used by the nurses' themselves. The researchers reported four themes which addressed the experience of meaning and joy. First was a sense of fulfilling a purpose. The nurses believed there was a reason they were doing the work they did, and the reason provided purpose for them. The reason (purpose) differed among the nurses but the inherent and steadfast belief in the larger purpose grounded the nurses and provided them both meaning and joy. It is this very purpose which is being challenged in today's pandemic world as nurses are now caring for people who deliberately chose not to be vaccinated against a powerful virus and yet expect care when they become sick; this morally challenging situation brings the purpose of a nurses' work into question. It makes nurses and other healthcare providers question the meaning and joy that was once found in their positions. The meaning and joy are removed when the systems do not promote the nurses' ability to find the purpose.

Meaningful connections is a second theme found by the research team. The role of interpersonal involvement with healthcare providers, families, and patients enabled the nurses to find meaning and joy. The connectedness between humans was deemed to be powerful. Nurses found meaning and joy when connections were made even for brief moments in time. Again, this need for connectedness became quite clear during the pandemic. Nurses needed to connect with each other and with their patients while their patients needed to connect with their families. Story after story has been heard of nurses and other providers using facetime, iPads, and other mechanisms to enable quarantined patients to connect with loved ones. Additionally, the one-on-one connection between nurse and patient was showcased in the pandemic when nurses were holding the hands and being with the patients as they were dying because their loved ones could not be there. When nurses became overwhelmed with the death, they sought solace with each other…meaningful connections. Health care is a human driven discipline; it is a human science wherein personal growth is achieved when individuals can relate to each other as equals, as one. Meaningful connections contribute to meaning and joy in the workplace.

A few decades ago, when accelerated nursing programs for individuals with degrees in other fields were created to enable quicker preparation for an individual to become a nurse, recruiters often heard from physical scientists who were behind the microscope. They desired a career change to be connected to the people their discoveries were aimed at helping. They wanted the connection, the human-to-human exchange, without the barrier of an instrument as vital as the instrument is to the success of the science. These individuals appreciated the work of discovery and the opportunity to find mechanisms to aid the progress and pursuit of health, but they yearned for the application, the ability to work directly with individuals to implement the discoveries. In other words, the need for human science became their quest rather than the physical science to which they had been committed. Thus, meaning and joy was found when there is a sense of purpose and an ability to develop meaningful connections to fulfill that purpose.

Nurses shared a third theme of impact…the wow factor which described the joy of practice and the joy of their work. The ability to make a difference, large or small, the ability to do good, and the ability to change a trajectory for some equaled an impact with a wow factor. The wow factor was on the individual level for some and the organizational level for others. The breadth or depth of the wow factor was not the significant piece; it was the knowledge that their work had an impact, and the impact created a wow for the provider. The wow housed the joy and meaning for them. Nurses recognized that the wow was not in the everyday necessarily, but when it was known it could stand alone. Meaning and joy happened, were discovered, when the wow factor was present. Organizations facilitated the power of the wow by acknowledging it. Organizations which recognized the worth, the impact and the significant contributions of the nurses made a difference. The acknowledgement that the work of nurses is not something every person wants to do or can do was impactful. Public and private recognition of the work done was important for nurses to appreciate the impact themselves.

The wow factor in health care differs from healthcare provider to healthcare provider and setting to setting. Yet, it is a known contributory factor to meaning and joy. Patients who walked out of a building on their own after being hospitalized for months at a time, provided the wow factor. A peaceful and dignified end of life brought the wow factor to the healthcare providers at the point of care. The recovery from a virus which has crippled the world provided this wow factor and brought joy and meaning to the care team. The ability to decrease an individual's physical or psychological suffering with a back rub, a repositioning experience after hours in the same bed, an opportunity to be outside and see the sky and breathe in the fresh air, and/or the ability to bring joy into a dark experience all provided the wow factor for healthcare providers. In the pandemic situation, the ability of a team to come together from various positions within an organizational structure to do what was needed to meet the ever-changing needs of the individuals with the virus is a wow factor. It is impactful to the people involved, healthcare providers, patients, and families alike.

The fourth theme within the experience of meaning and joy as identified by nurses was the practice environment itself. The world in which they worked provided meaning and joy. It did not matter whether the world was inpatient care delivery or outpatient care delivery, in an operating room, or on a general medical surgical unit, meaning and joy were found within the environment itself. Nurses specifically spoke of three characteristics within the practice environment: the team, the leaders, and the opportunities. The team members make a difference. Everyone can identify people in their work environments who facilitate the work to be done and those who are in the way. These are the people who put up barriers and others who take the barriers down or develop work arounds for the barriers. These are the individuals who are optimistic and those who look at the glass as half empty no matter what and when. The individuals in the Galuska et al. (2018) study spoke about the team members who embraced every experience as one for growth, who accepted the uncertainty of the complex health care delivery system, and who relied on the team members to help shepherd through the experience. Again, another way to speak about the human-to-human connectedness and the importance of relationships.

The current US health care system is hierarchical and, as a result, leaders make a difference. If the leaders embraced autocracy, then there was a lack of meaning and joy. When leaders embraced participation, facilitation of the voice of the provider at the point of care, and provided meaningful opportunities for exchange of ideas with transparent discussions, nurses found meaning in their work. Contemporary leadership theories of transformational leadership, inclusive leadership, and authentic leadership (Northouse, 2022) all contribute to the finding of meaning and joy for the healthcare providers. The words themselves showcase the components which are important to the nurses. The ability to transform environments with multiple complex adaptive systems in play, with limited resources, physical, fiscal and human, and with major societal changes occurring is a hallmark of a leader who facilitates the discovery of meaning and joy by their team members. Authentic and inclusive leadership illustrate the need to be genuine, to truly value the voice of the team and to regard every member as a valuable player are also contributing factors to meaning and joy.

Opportunities for growth is a final subset of the practice environment and it has been addressed throughout the above. Complex adaptive systems are ever changing, and nurses found meaning and joy when they were provided the opportunities to learn how to adapt, to be dynamic and to embrace the change. Gone are the days of change theories which were linear and suggested change was not a daily event. These pinwheel theories of change illustrate that change is all the time and its pace may accelerate or slow down, but its presence is the omnipresent rule of the day.

Meaning and joy is both external and internally driven. Healthcare providers find meaning and joy through the work they do when it is appreciated and valued, when they are treated with respect and dignity, and when there is an esprit de corps. This illustrates the connectedness between the internal and external; the person makes a difference but so does the system in which they work.

Compassion Satisfaction

Compassion satisfaction, another positive concept within the work environment is "the pleasure and satisfying feeling that comes from helping others" (Lightbody-Warner, 2020). Compassion satisfaction is the result of providing care one wants to provide, in systems where the care is valued, and, at the end of their day, healthcare providers are pleased, satisfied, and comforted by the care they delivered. When compassion satisfaction exists, healthcare providers leave their health care environments with a sense of purpose fulfilled and this level of positiveness carries over into their personal life outside the health care environment. Compassion satisfaction facilitates a solid work life balance because there is not a carry-over effect of negativity from one to the other.

Compassion satisfaction proponents suggest that caregivers, of all types and professions, can enhance compassion satisfaction by caring for themselves. They posit that sleep, good diet, exercise, and other strategies are ways to enhance compassion satisfaction by attending to their own personal needs. An example of this is a pocket card developed by Stamm (2010) and later revised, again by Stamm (ProQOL, n.d.) due to the Covid-19 pandemic, entitled Caring for Yourself in the Face of Difficult Work. It focuses on 10 daily self-care items, the healthcare provider's empathy, and switching between work and off-work modes. Figure 1 contains this pocket card.

Figure 1. Helper pocket card
Source: https://proqol.org/helper-pocket-card

CARING FOR YOURSELF IN THE FACE OF DIFFICULT WORK

Our work can be overwhelming. Our challenge is to maintain our resilience so that we can keep doing the work with care, energy, and compassion.

10 things to do each day

1. Get enough sleep.
2. Get enough to eat.
3. Vary the work that you do.
4. Do some light exercise.
5. Do something pleasurable.
6. Focus on what you did well.
7. Learn from your mistakes.
8. Share a private joke.
9. Pray, meditate or relax.
10. Support a colleague.

For More Information see your supervisor or visit www.istss.org, www.proqol.org and www.compassionfatigue.org

FOCUSING YOUR EMPATHY

Your empathy for others helps you do your job. It is important to take good care of your feelings and thoughts by monitoring how you use them. The most resilient workers are those that know how to turn their feelings to work mode when they go on duty, but off-work mode when they go off duty. This is not denial; it is a coping strategy. It is a way they get maximum protection while working (feelings switched to work mode) and maximum support while resting (feelings switched off-work mode).

How to become better at switching between Work and Off-Work Modes

1. Make this a conscious process. Talk to yourself as you switch.
2. Use images that make you feel safe and protected (work-mode) or connected and cared for (non-work mode) to help you switch.
3. Develop rituals that help you switch as you start and stop work.
4. Breathe slowly and deeply to calm yourself when starting a tough job.

Furthermore, a Caregiver's Bill of Rights (Compassion fatigue awareness project, 2013) was created to assist caregivers in understanding, appreciating, and advocating for their own satisfaction. The Bill of Rights states 12 specific rights of healthcare providers in assisting them with this feeling of satisfaction in their work. Figure 2 is a graphic of this bill of rights.

Consistent with the discussion of meaning and joy, compassion satisfaction is internal and external.

Figure 2. Caregiver Bill of Rights
Source: http://compassionfatigue.org/pages/TheBillOfRights.pdf

CFAP
COMPASSION FATIGUE AWARENESS PROJECT®

The Caregiver's Bill Of Rights

As a caregiver I have the right...

. . . to be respected for the work I choose to do.

. . . to take pride in my work and know that I am making a difference.

. . . to garner appreciation and validation for the care I give others.

. . . to receive adequate pay for my job as a professional caregiver.

. . . to discern my personal boundaries and have others respect my choices.

. . . to seek assistance from others, if and when it is necessary.

. . . to take time off to re-energize myself.

. . . to socialize, maintain my interests, and sustain a balanced lifestyle.

. . . to my own feelings, including negative emotions such as anger, sadness, and frustration.

. . . to express my thoughts and feelings to appropriate people at appropriate times.

. . . to convey hope to those in my care.

. . . to believe those in my care will prosper in mind, body and spirit as a result of my caregiving.

In health care, hospitals can be designated as Magnet hospitals® (American Nurses Credentialing Center, n.d.). This is a program sponsored by the American Nurses Association. Hospitals with this designation embrace a model which includes transformational leadership, structural empowerment, exemplary professional practice, and new knowledge & innovation which all lead to quality empirical outcomes. Nurses and other healthcare providers in these designated organizations are hypothesized to have greater meaning and joy in their work because the five components of the model are all addressed in the research findings described. The Baldrige award (National Institute of Standards and Technology, 2021) embraces similar values through system initiatives addressing leaders, customers, the workforce, strategy, operations, and measurement which lead to results. The purpose here is not to endorse either Magnet® or Baldrige but rather to illustrate that organizations can be focused on meaning and joy. When they are, it is hypothesized that there is less burnout and more satisfaction.

Figure 3 is an author drawn concept map that highlights the connection between the components discussed. When there is meaning and joy, there is also compassion satisfaction. This is characterized by personal resiliency and organizational culture which promotes meaning. Compassion satisfaction leads to workforce retention which results in improved quality of care delivered and received. Conversely, burnout and secondary traumatic stress lead to compassion fatigue which creates an intent to leave the workplace ending in moral distress and or moral injury. The latter needs to be prevented through organizational structures and cultures which promote meaning and joy.

Negative Affect

Negative affect refers to emotions such as sadness, disgust, anger, fear, or sadness potentially resulting in lethargy, anxiety, and/or depression (Fortenberry et al., 2017). Those with a propensity for negative affect emotions tend to have an overall negative view the world and generally react to situations and relationships in a negative light. This is often referred to as a bleak outlook or having a glass half empty. These people tend to only find the bad in any situation despite positive circumstances existing within the situation.

Burnout, Moral Distress, Compassion Fatigue, and Secondary Traumatic Stress

Despite the frequent usage of the occupational-based strains of burnout, moral distress, compassion fatigue, and secondary traumatic stress, within the healthcare delivery literature enduring conceptual conflation and lack of conceptual clarity exists. As such, misuse of these terms results in the inability to properly identify, prevent, mitigate, and treat which occupational-based strains the healthcare provider is suffering from. As burnout, moral distress, compassion fatigue, and secondary traumatic stress are negative affect occupational-based strains, it can be surmised they would be damaging to a caregiver's professional quality of life resulting in emotional distress, emotional trauma, and caregiver turnover introducing the potential for negative patient outcomes. As such healthcare provider understanding of these concepts is imperative. Additionally, this understanding and perspective is imperative to help ground the reader in the dynamic and ever-changing environment and appreciate why the healthcare provider reacts as they do, whether it be positively or negatively.

As previously mentioned within this chapter, in 2014 the healthcare workforce (the human resource) described feeling burned out. They felt a lack of compassion for patients. They described occupational stressors and strains that spilled over into their personal and social lives. They asked for help. This led to the IHI developing that fourth aim (though not formally labelled as such) for health care, in which the experience of the healthcare provider was taken into consideration. While the authors recommend positive affect concepts and emotions such as meaning and joy or compassion satisfaction to combat occupational strain, it would be remissive to not adequately describe some of those occupational based strains here especially since the Covid-19 pandemic has had significant negative effects on these problems, bringing them to epidemic proportions.

Figure 3. Joy and meaning concept map
Source: Author drawn

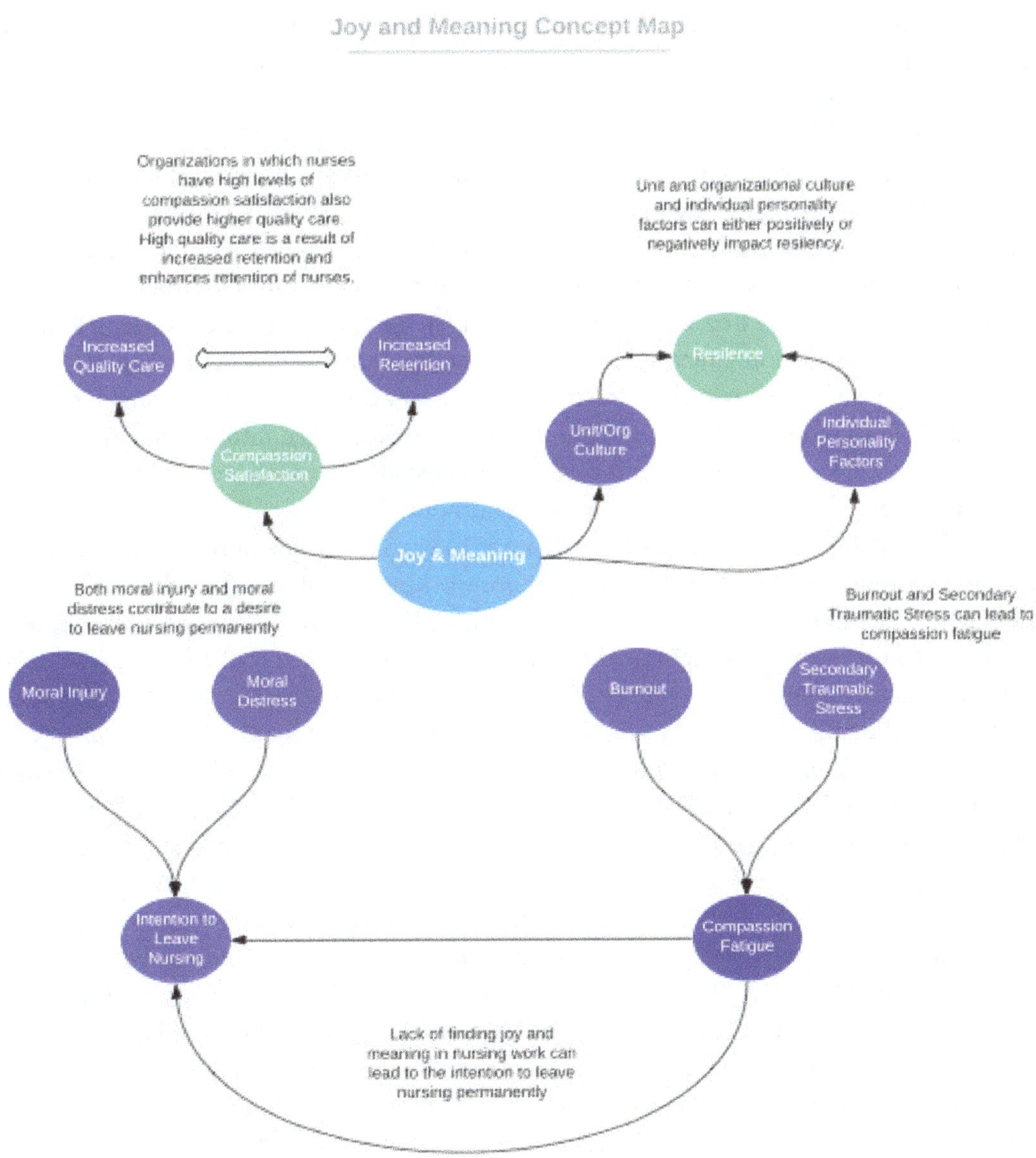

So, what is burnout? Moral distress? Compassion fatigue? Secondary traumatic stress? Answering these questions can help achieve conceptual clarity, identify which occupational based strain the healthcare provider is experiencing, and help the healthcare provider regain their passion for what led them to this career choice to begin.

Burnout has been studied in multiple professions since being introduced into the helping profession literature by Freudenberger in 1974. He noticed the volunteers who helped in drug treatment centers begin to lose their emotional responses and motivation mirroring the destructive results of chronic illicit drug usage seen in their clients. Using an illicit drug use reference, he described these volunteers as burned out. Simultaneously and independently, those loses of emotional response and motivation were being observed by Maslach (1982), an American social psychology researcher, in her work with human service workers. Maslach and colleagues (1996) noted emotional exhaustion, cynicism, professional devaluing, and the questioning of one's ability to perform. Metaphorically, this has been described as one's candle being extinguished (Schaufeli et al., 2009, p. 205). Burnout has global reach and has significantly increased since the Covid-19 pandemic began in 2019. A meta-analysis of 45,539 nurses in 49 countries supports burnout in 11.23% of nurses prior to the pandemic (Woo et al., 2020) while prevalence reported after the pandemic being 51% globally in healthcare professionals (Morgantini et al., 2020).

In other words, the healthcare provider can no longer perform as there is no replenishment of their psychological and/or physical resources. The development of burnout is multifactorial. With both external and internal drivers, burnout is tied to resource availability for the healthcare worker. What then, are these resources? As described in a metasynthesis of burnout in physicians (Sibeoni et al., 2019), stress factors and protective factors seem to be the resources necessary for both the development of and protection from burnout. These stress and protective factors are further divided into organizational, relational, and individual factors. Organizational factors have the highest allostatic load toward the development of burnout and the lowest protective value in preventing burnout (Sibeoni et al., 2019). The organizational factors described by the physicians included such things as workload, lack of time, inability to take time off, organizational structure, work/life balance, and poor working conditions. These factors are supported within the nursing literature on burnout and within general burnout literature across multiple occupations. Relational factors such as professional working relationships with colleagues and relationships with patients and families have a plus/minus effect on burnout depending on whether the professional relationships are collegial or adversary and whether healthcare providers can maintain professional boundaries with patients and families. Individual characteristics have the highest protective ability yet are dependent on the individual. For example, healthcare providers who practice self-care, have high self-confidence, and positive affect personalities have the most protection against developing burnout while healthcare providers with negative affect personalities and emotions such as lack of confidence in their abilities and hopelessness at baseline have the least protection against developing burnout. To clarify, as organizational factors begin to place strain on the healthcare provider, the negative relational factors become more noticeable. Once these relational factors begin to place strain on the healthcare provider, the negative individual factors are highlighted, and the onset of burnout has begun.

Jameton (1984) introduced the concept of moral distress in his book *Nursing Practice: The Ethical Issues*. According to Jameton, he conceived this concept after discussions of problematic situations faced by his students such as death and dying, life support options, and communication difficulties with patients and families. He noted students described the inability to act, typically due to multifactorial constraints, despite knowing what they should do in these situations (Jameton, 2017). It then becomes easy to see that moral distress has impact on the entire healthcare cycle including patients and their family members, nurses, organizational culture, an idea that is supported in Corley's (2002) proposed theory of moral distress.

One might wonder how these ethical dilemmas, which Corley (2002) described as pain and suffering, dehumanization, health policy constraints, staffing and healthcare costs, and brain death, become morally distressing. A methasynthesis of 150 critical care and emergency nurses across 10 qualitative studies of moral distress resulted in the central theme of "the battle within" along with five subthemes (Arnold, 2020, p. 1685). A closer look at these themes may lead to better understanding of how moral distress occurs. For example, nurses described the desire to follow their conscience in delivering care yet having to face a different reality to deliver that care. They had great difficulty eliciting the difference between harming and saving leading to lasting inner conflict. They viewed nursing as their positive yet conflicting identity. They felt a sense of purpose as a nurse, yet also felt as if they had to forgive themselves for things they were required to do; nursing did not turn out to be what they envisioned. This feeling of conflict spilled into their professional relationships as they relished their colleagues who understood their feelings yet were appalled at colleagues who did not seem to care about their patients. They described their care, at times, as futile, a form of torture, and care that was morally questionable.

The Covid-19 pandemic has further exacerbated these morally distressing situations and introduced new ones. Silverman et al. (2021) interviewed 31 nurses caring for Covid-19 patients. Distressing situations such as uncertainty of care of a new illness, the severity of the illness, changes in visitation policies resulting in lack of family presence, the inability of nurses to care for patients as they are used to due to personal protective equipment, and medical resource scarcity were introduced. These new morally distressing situations were also well documented in the media from the perspective of the healthcare provider and the patient/family. For example, heart-wrenching choices were highlighted when Italy announced it did not have enough intensive care beds and ventilators for all their critical Covid-19 patients. How does one decide which patients receive these services and which patients do not? How does this not leave a mark on the soul of the healthcare provider?

Moral distress has a well-documented crescendo effect on the healthcare worker (Epstein & Hamric, 2009). Each mark on the healthcare provider's soul that is not resolved leaves some residue. Over time this residue builds up. Each new situation reminds one of past situations further adding to the residue deposit. What started as individual moral dilemmas now have become a full-on case of moral distress. The healthcare provider then is either morally numb to new situations, elicits a conscious objection to the situation they find themselves in, or becomes burned out (Epstein & Hamric, 2009).

Compassion fatigue was introduced by Joinson (1992) when she noticed a burnout-like condition in emergency nurses. Joinson's initial description of compassion fatigue was quite similar to burnout, but she thought it was a special type of burnout associated with people in the helping professions. Her initial descriptions of stories of compassion fatigue really lend credence to it being the cost of caring as later noted by Figley (1995). Since they care, healthcare providers give so much of themselves by being compassionate and empathetic, by coming in early and staying late, by working extra shifts, and by giving all of themselves despite less-than-ideal working conditions. However, this is not sustainable. Every time the answer is yes, a small intangible payment is made by the healthcare provider. Over time this payment becomes bigger and bigger until it can no longer be paid; the resource bank is empty.

The inability to continue to make this payment has multiple effects not only on the healthcare provider but on their organization and eventually the patient. These effects are due to the emotional and physical exhaustion that leads to the inability to connect with patients and a desensitization to their situations (Mathieu, 2012). A metasynthesis of compassion fatigue in nurses is full of metaphors for what compassion fatigue feels like: "just plain worn out", "walking on a tight rope", "unbearable weight on shoulders", "alone in a crowded room", and "who has my back?" (Nolte et al., 2017). It is easy to see that these nurses have no meaning and no joy in their work anymore. It can be surmised they are no longer entering into the nurse-patient relationship. They no longer feel empathy or compassion for their patients. One can then argue that these nurses are not adequately caring for their patients anymore, a situation known as missed care. Missed care involved care that is only partially done or completely undone and can involve care that is quantified as clinical, emotional, or administrative. When care is missed, multiple nursing metrics are affected including increases in medication errors, falls, pressure injuries, and hospital acquired infections, and an overall decrease in quality of care (Recio-Saucedo et al., 2017). Hence, the importance of recognizing compassion fatigue. A quick literature search of compassion fatigue supports this being a global problem like burnout. Studies of compassion fatigue in healthcare providers (especially nurses) from multiple countries are easy to find. Prevalence appears to be highly variable, yet present across healthcare provider types (Cavanagh et al., 2020) and is both internally and externally driven.

A few years after compassion fatigue was introduced within the literature, another occupational based strain was coming to light. In 1995 traumatologist Charles Figley introduced secondary traumatic stress describing it as the stress a felt after helping someone traumatized or suffering (Figley, 1995). Conceptual conflation between compassion fatigue and secondary traumatic stress ensued when Figley later described compassion fatigue as a "friendlier" (1995, p. 14) term for secondary traumatic stress, stating its preference by nurses and emergency workers. At that time, it was accepted that the two terms were the same and could be used interchangeably although it is not thought that Joinson intended this (Coetzee & Klopper, 2010). Further conceptual conflation ensued when Stamm (2010) described compassion fatigue as a two-part concept made of burnout and secondary traumatic stress.

Since their introduction and usage within the multidisciplinary literature, both compassion fatigue and secondary traumatic stress have undergone evolutionary changes. For example, as introduced, Joinson (1992) described compassion fatigue as a specific type of occupational burnout while later Mathieu (2012) described compassion fatigue as an inability to connect to patients due to the emotional exhaustion from taking care of them. Figley (1995) initially described secondary traumatic stress as the stress from wanting to help someone suffering while later Bride (2011) described secondary traumatic stress as the result from being secondarily traumatized by helping a client or patient. Over time, secondary traumatic stress was noted to have symptoms that parallel the symptoms of post-traumatic stress disorder (PTSD) with hearing about or indirectly finding out about someone's trauma as the source of symptoms for the caregiver (American Psychiatric Association, 2013). These traumatic symptoms parallel previous diagnostic criteria for post-traumatic stress disorder (PTSD) except that the trauma is secondary rather than primary for the secondary traumatic stress sufferer (Figley, 1995).

Occurring in high numbers within the helping professions due to the nature of working with traumatized individuals, secondary traumatic stress is considered an occupational hazard (Bride et al., 2004). Within secondary traumatic stress the sufferer carries the emotional burden of the trauma suffered by their patient, client, or family member. Consistent with the discussion of meaning and joy, secondary traumatic stress is both internally and externally driven.

The conceptual understanding of these negative affect occupational based strain concepts is imperative because although we have noted previously that a focus on meaning and joy or compassion satisfaction is the way to successfully implement the IHI's quadruple aim and the flourishing of the US health care delivery system, there will be times that a healthcare provider's focus will move to the negative affect.

When this happens, helping the healthcare worker by mitigating or treating the condition will only be possible if we are aware of which occupational based strain they are suffering from.

On a global scale, a 2021 metasynthesis of nurses' experience of working with patients with Covid-19 (Zipf, Polifroni & Beck, 2021) found four themes of fear and moral conflict, duty, a calling and a sense of moral obligation, mental & physical side effects ending in exhaustion, and growth and a renewed calling. These four themes summarize the emotional roller coaster presented in this chapter. Healthcare providers, and nurses in particular, have a deep sense of and commitment to their work and yet experience moral distress and mental and physical exhaustion. This occurs at the very same time they are faced with increased complexity in the workplace. For example, prior to Covid-19, proning patients was rare and prone teams did not exist, personal protective equipment was used for very few patients, and negative pressure units were unique and not the norm. Though it all, purpose, meaning and joy reign. Zipf, Polifroni and Beck found that nurses have a renewed commitment to their work when they focus on their duty which is a calling.

SOLUTIONS AND RECOMMENDATIONS

The authors appreciate the public's attention on the negatives and the shock value of focusing on stories of burnout, moral distress, compassion fatigue, and secondary stress. A quick look at the psychology literature gives rise to why the public, and healthcare providers, focus their attention on these negative affect positions. The human brain is just wired that way. This is known as negativity bias. It is also sometimes referred to as negative dominance or simply the negativity effect (Tierney & Baumeister, 2019). One hears a negative comment and perseverates on it for days. One hears a compliment and thinks it cannot be true. Knowing this is the case, one can see why the healthcare provider would tend to focus on the negative affect; think all they are seeing and doing is bad.

Yet, the authors recommend that one focus on meaning and joy instead. The onus for this is multifactorial; on both the healthcare provider and the organization they work for. Simply stating the provider needs to be more resilient is not enough just as stating the organization is at fault is wrong. It is imperative healthcare providers change their way of thinking. They must recognize leaning towards the negative affect is a normal human response, yet they must also change these destructive patterns of thinking. Additionally, it is imperative that organizational leaders create structures wherein nurses and other professionals in health care can do the work they were prepared to do. Structures are largely responsible for the experiences of its employees, and they need to be orchestrated in such a way as to promote well-being and satisfaction with one's ability to do the work at hand.

Patients, consumers, and other providers recognize the complexity of health care. Covid-19 has exacerbated the complexity and the recognition that every unit and actually every team within a unit in a hospital or long-term care setting is a complex adaptive system. Thus, one size does not fit all, and structures need to be flexible enough to recognize the uniqueness of every unit and team. This flexibility will promote individualized approaches to the care delivered and the well-being of the providers. Without the individuality, the one size fits all approach promotes the negative affect and the subsequent burnout rather than the satisfaction which is found when meaning and joy are present.

FUTURE RESEARCH DIRECTIONS

The authors recommendation future research to find answers to these, and other similar questions:

1. What structures promote meaning and joy?
2. Which leadership behaviors and approaches promote compassion satisfaction and decrease burnout?
3. What is the relationship between meaning and joy in the workplace and the presence of moral distress?
4. How does organizational structure contribute to the development of the positive affect?
5. What is the relationship of transformational leadership versus transactional leadership to the optimization of meaning and joy?
6. In states with legislation governing staff to patient ratios, do providers report less burnout and more compassion satisfaction?
7. What is the experience of working in complex adaptive system?
8. How do leaders promote meaning and joy and how do employees optimize it in their practice?
9. What interventions are most beneficial to break the destructive patterns of negative affect emotions in the healthcare provider?

As much as there are recommendations for research, the authors feel need to provide recommendations for caring for yourself. The complexity of healthcare will continue to rise, and the speed at which it does is often externally dictated, such as what happened during the Covid-19 pandemic. No matter the legislation or the legislative efforts, the complexity is inherent in the US health care system. Therefore, learning to care for oneself within it is paramount.

The authors recommend a handful of items, all inextricably interwoven (a characteristic of complexity).

First, each of us needs to know what *our* well-being looks like and feels like. It is different for everyone, and we must become self-aware of where we are in the well-being area. Take the time to do that assessment; know what feels right and what feels not so right. Be conscious of what triggers feeling right and what stimulates one down a track of not feeling right. We are educated to continually assess our patients and this self-assessment is equally if not more important. One cannot do their best if their own well-being is not at its best.

Second, plan for your paid time off. By planning, a few things will be in place. One is the fact that you will use your time. It is known that in the US, too much vacation time is left on the table. This is not healthy in the best of times and it certainly is a problem during a pandemic. This paid time off then serves as a goal, a target for recharging one's batteries and replenishing one's resources. Ask yourself: How far do I need to go? Is there a way to meter out the resources I have so they are not all depleted weeks before the paid time off is scheduled? Do I need an extra day, a boost? Your well-being should contribute to these decisions. For example, schedule your time based on your own well-being determining whether it is in blocks, several days in a row, or single days throughout.

Third, work with your colleagues to create respite areas and signals for need of respite. When your well-being is off kilter, will a few minutes away from the chaos of the unit (chaos is part of complexity) help? Where do you go? To the messy locker room or an area dedicated to replenishment? Can you find an area where you can sit, put your feet up, listen to music, smell a fragrance which brings you calm and healing? Can you talk and share with others if that is your thing, and block out the activity on the unit for a specified time period? There are timers on hot tubs and there can be timers in respite areas.

Fourth, work with leadership to create organizational structure which leads to a change in organizational culture. Find a culture that promotes participating, hearing the voice of the provider at the point of care, and creating a path for implementation of what is possible. Recognition of the voice comes first. Knowing the voice is valued and is not merely complaining but rather being constructive in substantive change is important so that meaning and joy can be maximized and burnout and moral distress minimized if not eliminated.

None of these will work by themselves, but rather they are a package. Activities toward each is a start in the direction of finding the meaning and joy which brough one to the health care career in the first place. Something needs to be done to promote well-being and stop the tide of nurses, in particular, leaving the bedside before they can even become competent in their work. A focus on environments which promote meaning and joy may help turn this crisis around.

CONCLUSION

This chapter presented a view of the complexity of healthcare delivery occurring today in the US. It is a system that is difficult to navigate from the perspectives of both the patient and the healthcare provider. It is wrought with parts that do not make a whole, access difficulties, high costs, and a lack of standardization of both quality of care and care delivery. The Covid-19 pandemic exacerbated this. The lens of complexity science was used to analyze the healthcare delivery system in order set the stage for the identification of the human resource. This human resource is identified as the most precious and fragile component of this entire system. As such, healthcare providers' responses to the complexity of healthcare delivery were described as varied with subsequent feelings and emotions within both the positive and negative affect. Concepts central to these affects (meaning and joy, compassion satisfaction, burnout, moral distress, compassion fatigue, and secondary traumatic stress) were identified and discussed. General recommendations of acknowledgement of negative affect emotions were given with an emphasis on the importance of meaning and joy as a catalyst to remaining satisfied and passionate about one's work within the healthcare profession.

ACKNOWLEDGMENT

The authors acknowledge and appreciate the assistance of Anne Reeder, University of Connecticut School of Nursing PhD student, in the drawing of the concept map.

REFERENCES

American Nurses Credentialing Center. (n.d.). *Magnet recognition program®*. Nursing World. https://www.nursingworld.org/organizational-programs/magnet/

American Psychiatric Association. (2013). *Diagnostic and statistical manual of mental disorders (DSM-5®)*. American Psychiatric Pub.

Arnold, T. C. (2020). Moral distress in emergency and critical care nurses: A metaethnography. *Nursing Ethics*, *27*(8), 1681–1693. doi:10.1177/0969733020935952 PMID:32700649

Beauvais, A., Andreychik, M., & Henkel, L. A. (2017). The role of emotional intelligence and empathy in compassionate nursing care. *Mindfulness & Compassion*, *2*(2), 92–100. doi:10.1016/j.mincom.2017.09.001

Bodenheimer, T., & Sinsky, C. (2014). From triple to quadruple aim: Care of the patient requires care of the provider. *Annals of Family Medicine*, *12*(6), 573–576. doi:10.1370/afm.1713 PMID:25384822

Bride, B. E., & Kintzle, S. (2011). Secondary traumatic stress, job satisfaction, and occupational commitment in substance abuse counselors. *Traumatology*, *17*(1), 22–28. doi:10.1177/1534765610395617

Bride, B. E., Robinson, M. M., Yegidis, B., & Figley, C. R. (2004). Development and validation of the secondary traumatic stress scale. *Research on Social Work Practice*, *14*(1), 27–35. doi:10.1177/1049731503254106

Cavanagh, N., Cockett, G., Heinrich, C., Doig, L., Fiest, K., Guichon, J. R., Page, S., Mitchell, I., & Doig, C. J. (2019). Compassion fatigue in healthcare providers: A systematic review and meta-analysis. *Nursing Ethics*, *27*(3), 639–665. doi:10.1177/0969733019889400 PMID:31829113

Coetzee, S. K., & Klopper, H. C. (2010). Compassion fatigue within nursing practice: A concept analysis. *Nursing & Health Sciences*, *12*(2), 235–243. doi:10.1111/j.1442-2018.2010.00526.x PMID:20602697

Compassion Fatigue Awareness Project. (2013). *The Caregiver's Bill of Rights*. https://compassionfatigue.org/pages/TheBillOfRights.pdf

Corley, M. C. (2002). Nurse moral distress: A proposed theory and research agenda. *Nursing Ethics*, *9*(6), 636–650. doi:10.1191/0969733002ne557oa PMID:12450000

De Hert, S. (2020). Burnout in healthcare workers: Prevalence, impac and preventative strategies. *Local and Regional Anesthesia*, *13*, 171–183. doi:10.2147/LRA.S240564 PMID:33149664

Demerouti, E., Bakker, A. B., Vardakou, I., & Kantas, A. (2003). The convergent validity of two burnout instruments: A multitrait-multimethod analysis. *European Journal of Psychological Assessment*, *19*(1), 12–23. doi:10.1027//1015-5759.19.1.12

Epstein, E. G., & Hamric, A. B. (2009). Moral distress, moral residue, and the crescendo effect. *The Journal of Clinical Ethics*, *20*(4), 330–342. PMID:20120853

Figley, C. R. (Ed.). (1995). *Compassion fatigue: Coping with secondary traumatic stress disorder in those who treat the traumatized*. Brunner/Mazel.

Fortenberry, K. T., Jansen, K. L., & Clark, M. S. (2017). Positive Affectivity. In M. D. Gellman & J. R. Turner (Eds.), *Encyclopedia of behavioral medicine*. Springer. doi:10.1007/978-1-4614-6439-6_977-2

Freudenberger, H. J. (1974). Staff burn-out. *The Journal of Social Issues*, *30*(1), 159–165. doi:10.1111/j.1540-4560.1974.tb00706.x

Galuska, L., Hahn, J., Polifroni, E. C., & Crow, G. (2018). A narrative analysis of nurses' experiences with meaning and joy in nursing practice. *Nursing Administration Quarterly*, *42*(2), 154–163. doi:10.1097/NAQ.0000000000000280 PMID:29494451

Hui, B. P., Ng, J. C., Berzaghi, E., Cunningham-Amos, L. A., & Kogan, A. (2020). Rewards of kindness? A meta-analysis of the link between prosociality and well-being. *Psychological Bulletin, 146*(12), 1084–1116. doi:10.1037/bul0000298 PMID:32881540

Igou, E. R., Blake, A. A., & Bless, H. (2020). Just-world beliefs increase helping intentions via meaning and affect. *Journal of Happiness Studies, 22*(5), 2235–2253. doi:10.100710902-020-00317-6

Institute for healthcare improvement. (n.d.a). *The IHI Triple Aim*. Improving Health and Health Care Worldwide | IHI - Institute for Healthcare Improvement. https://www.ihi.org/Engage/Initiatives/TripleAim/Pages/default.aspx

Institute for healthcare improvement. (n.d.b). *Joy in work*. Improving Health and Health Care Worldwide | IHI - Institute for Healthcare Improvement. https://www.ihi.org/Topics/Joy-In-Work/Pages/default.aspx

Institute Of Medicine Committee on Quality Healthcare in America. (2001). *Crossing the quality chasm*. National Academies Press. What Physicians need to do to optimize telehealth after the pandemic.

Jameton, A. (1984). *Nursing practice: The ethical issues*. Prentice Hall.

Jameton, A. (2017). What moral distress in nursing history could suggest about the future of health care. *AMA Journal of Ethics, 19*(6), 617–628. doi:10.1001/journalofethics.2017.19.6.mhst1-1706 PMID:28644792

Joinson, C. (1992). Coping with compassion fatigue. *Nursing, 22*(4), 116–121. doi:10.1097/00152193-199204000-00035 PMID:1570090

Kristensen, T. S., Borritz, M., Villadsen, E., & Christensen, K. B. (2005). The Copenhagen Burnout Inventory: A new tool for the assessment of burnout. *Work and Stress, 19*(3), 192–207. doi:10.1080/02678370500297720

Lightbody-Warner, M. (2020, December 4). *Compassion satisfaction and compassion fatigue: Helpful tips for our frontline workers*. The Louis A. Faillace, MD, Department of Psychiatry and Behavioral Sciences, McGovern Medical School. https://med.uth.edu/psychiatry/2020/10/29/compassion-satisfaction-and-compassion-fatigue-helpful-tips-for-our-frontline-workers/

Luhmann, M. (2017). The development of subjective well-being. In J. Specht (Ed.), *Personality development across the lifespan* (pp. 197–218). Ruhr University Bochum. doi:10.1016/B978-0-12-804674-6.00013-2

Maslach, C. (1982). *Burnout: The Cost of Caring*. Prentice-Hall.

Maslach, C., Jackson, S. E., & Leiter, M. (1996). Maslach Burnout Inventory. In C. P. Zalaquett & R. J. Wood (Eds.), *Evaluating stress: A book of resources* (3rd ed., pp. 191–218). Scarecrow Education.

Mathieu, F. (2012). *The compassion fatigue workbook: Creative tools for transforming compassion fatigue and vicarious traumatization.* Routledge/Taylor & Francis Group.

Miguel, K., Snyderman, C., Capasso, V., Walsh, M., Murphy, J., & Wang, X. (2021). Development of a prone team and exploration of staff perceptions during COVID-19. *AACN Advanced Critical Care, 32*(2), 159–168. doi:10.4037/aacnacc2021848 PMID:33878151

Morgantini, L. A., Naha, U., Wang, H., Francavilla, S., Acar, Ö., Flores, J. M., Crivellaro, S., Moreira, D., Abern, M., Eklund, M., Vigneswaran, H. T., & Weine, S. M. (2020). Factors contributing to healthcare professional burnout during the COVID-19 pandemic: A rapid turnaround global survey. *PLoS One*, *15*(9), e0238217. doi:10.1371/journal.pone.0238217 PMID:32881887

National Institute of Standards and Technology. (2021). *Malcolm Baldrige national quality award*. NIST. https://www.nist.gov/baldrige/baldrige-award

Nolte, A. G., Downing, C., Temane, A., & Hastings-Tolsma, M. (2017). Compassion fatigue in nurses: A metasynthesis. *Journal of Clinical Nursing*, *26*(23-24), 4364–4378. doi:10.1111/jocn.13766 PMID:28231623

Northouse, P. (2022). *Leadership: Theory & Practice* (9th ed.). Sage.

ProQOL. (n.d.). *Helper pocket card*. https://proqol.org/helper-pocket-card

Recio-Saucedo, A., Dall'Ora, C., Maruotti, A., Ball, J., Briggs, J., Meredith, P., Redfern, O. C., Kovacs, C., Prytherch, D., Smith, G. B., & Griffiths, P. (2017). What impact does nursing care left undone have on patient outcomes? Review of the literature. *Journal of Clinical Nursing*, *27*(11-12), 2248–2259. doi:10.1111/jocn.14058 PMID:28859254

Robeznieks, A. (2021). *What physicians need to do to optimize Telehealth after pandemic*. American Medical Association. https://www.ama-assn.org/practice-management/digital/what-physicians-need-do-optimize-telehealth-after-pandemic?gclid=EAIaIQobChMIvdiajaeZ9AIVw513Ch2BZArpEAAYAiAAEgJzE_D_BwE

Schaufeli, W. B., Bakker, A. B., & Van Rhenen, W. (2009). How changes in job demands and resources predict burnout, work engagement, and sickness absenteeism. *Journal of Organizational Behavior*, *30*(7), 893–917. doi:10.1002/job.595

Sibeoni, J., Bellon-Champel, L., Mousty, A., Manolios, E., Verneuil, L., & Revah-Levy, A. (2019). Physicians' perspectives about burnout: A systematic review and Metasynthesis. *Journal of General Internal Medicine*, *34*(8), 1578–1590. doi:10.100711606-019-05062-y PMID:31147982

Sikka, R., Morath, J. M., & Leape, L. (2015). The quadruple aim: Care, health, cost and meaning in work. *BMJ Quality & Safety*, *24*(10), 608–610. doi:10.1136/bmjqs-2015-004160 PMID:26038586

Silverman, H. J., Kheirbek, R. E., Moscou-Jackson, G., & Day, J. (2021). Moral distress in nurses caring for patients with COVID-19. *Nursing Ethics*, (7-8), 1137–1164. Advance online publication. doi:10.1177/09697330211003217 PMID:33910406

Spitzmuller, M., Park, G., Van Dyne, L., Wagner, D. T., & Maerz, A. (2020). When do you benefit? Differential boundary conditions facilitate positive affect and buffer negative affect after helping others. *European Journal of Work and Organizational Psychology*, *30*(4), 482–494. doi:10.1080/1359432X.2020.1843436

Stamm, B. H. (2010). The Concise ProQOL Manual (2nd ed.). Pocatello, ID: ProQOL.org.

Tierney, J., & Baumeister, R. F. (2019). *The power of bad: How the negativity effect rules us and how we can rule it*. Penguin.

Uhl Bien, M., & Russ, M. (2009). Complexity leadership in bureaucratic forms of organizing: A meso model. *The Leadership Quarterly*, *20*(4), 631–650. doi:10.1016/j.leaqua.2009.04.007

Woo, T., Ho, R., Tang, A., & Tam, W. (2020). Global prevalence of burnout symptoms among nurses: A systematic review and meta-analysis. *Journal of Psychiatric Research*, *123*, 9–20. doi:10.1016/j.jpsychires.2019.12.015 PMID:32007680

Xiao, W., Lin, X., Li, X., Xu, X., Guo, H., Sun, B., & Jiang, H. (2021). The influence of emotion and empathy on decisions to help others. *SAGE Open*, *11*(2). doi:10.1177/21582440211014513

Zipf, A. L., Polifroni, E. C., & Beck, C. T. (2021). The experience of the nurse during the COVID-19 pandemic: A global meta-synthesis in the year of the nurse. *Journal of Nursing Scholarship*. Advance online publication. doi:10.1111/jnu.12706 PMID:34738314

ADDITIONAL READING

Foli, K. J., & Thompson, J. R. (2019). *The influence of psychological trauma in nursing*. Sigma.

McKinney, J. (2020). *Manifesting your heart's desire: How to create a life of abundance, meaning & joy!* FriesenPress.

Nagoski, E., & Nagoski, A. (2019). *Burnout: The Secret to Unlocking the Stress Cycle*. Ballantine Books.

Norris, C. J. (2019). The negativity bias, revisited: Evidence from neuroscience measures and an individual differences approach. *Social Neuroscience*, *16*(1), 68–82. doi:10.1080/17470919.2019.1696225 PMID:31750790

Parks, P. (2018). Naturalizing negativity: How journalism textbooks justify crime, conflict, and "bad" news. *Critical Studies in Media Communication*, *36*(1), 75–91. doi:10.1080/15295036.2018.1533990

Pearson, C. S. (1998). *The hero within: Six archetypes we live by*. Turtleback.

Smith, P. (2009). *To weep for a stranger: Compassion fatigue in caregiving*. CreateSpace.

Smith, P. (2012). *Compassion satisfaction: 50 steps to healthy caregiving*. Createspace Independent Pub.

Trzeciak, S., & Mazzarelli, A. (2019). *Compassionomics (The Revolutionary Scientific Evidence that Caring Makes a Difference)*. Studer Group.

KEY TERMS AND DEFINITIONS

Affective Responses: The emotional responses to a situation.

Burnout: The cynicism and questioning of professional value resulting from unresolved chronic occupational stressors.

Compassion Fatigue: The exhaustion and emotional withdrawal experienced by those in the helping professions that results in the diminishment or loss of compassion towards one's clients or patients.

Compassion Satisfaction: The sense of comfort and achievement one experiences when their work meets their own expectations.

Meaning and Joy: The raison d'être for doing one's work. It is the intangible but powerful reason one chose to enter the career they did, and the search for meaning and joy is what keeps us providing care in the best and the worst of times.

Moral Distress: The knowledge of the right thing to do, yet the inability to act accordingly due to multifactorial systemic constraints.

Organizational Culture: The activities below the surface which permeate the organization. Much like an iceberg, what we see is one thing but what we do not see is quite another. Culture is what we do not see but its presence is powerful.

Organizational Structure: The way an organization is set up from the bottom to the top; is its focus on patients, on hierarchy, on participation? How is the vice of the provider encouraged and heard?

Secondary Traumatic Stress: The indirect stress felt by caregivers resulting from caring for someone undergoing a traumatic situation.

Chapter 8
Mentally Healthy Healthcare:
Main Findings and Lessons Learned From a Needs Assessment Exercise at Multiple Workplace Levels

Davide Giusino
https://orcid.org/0000-0003-0878-1748
Alma Mater Studiorum – University of Bologna, Italy

Marco De Angelis
https://orcid.org/0000-0001-9351-5940
Alma Mater Studiorum – University of Bologna, Italy

Greta Mazzetti
Alma Mater Studiorum – University of Bologna, Italy

Ilaria Rita Faiulo
Azienda Unità Sanitaria Locale di Bologna, Italy

Siw Tone Innstrand
https://orcid.org/0000-0002-8132-962X
Norwegian University of Science and Technology, Norway

Marit Christensen
https://orcid.org/0000-0002-6246-4383
Norwegian University of Science and Technology, Norway

Karina Nielsen
University of Sheffield, UK

ABSTRACT

Interventions addressing healthcare workers' mental health should build upon an exhaustive understanding of the major causes of both work-related stress conditions (i.e., job demands) and positive mental health (i.e., job resources) in the workplace at all the levels they might unfold, namely the individual, the group, the leader, and the organization. The chapter draws upon a multilevel workplace mental health needs assessment exercise performed within three different departments of a large healthcare institution and involving both managers and employees. It aims to illustrate the job demands and resources at multiple levels in the targeted organization, differentiate among healthcare workers' mental models of their working conditions, and discuss the research and practical implications of such findings. Also, it offers practical recommendations on how to effectively conduct such activities by, on the one hand, considering both healthcare workers' mental health risk and protective factors and, on the other hand, encompassing multiple workplace levels of analysis.

DOI: 10.4018/978-1-7998-8813-0.ch008

INTRODUCTION

In the healthcare sector, workers are at risk of suffering from poor mental health due to the characteristics of their jobs. For instance, systematic reviews and meta-analyses (e.g., Membrive-Jiménez et al., 2020) have found adverse working conditions – such as work overload, need to mediate interpersonal conflicts, time pressure, and lack of supervisor support – to contribute to the development of nursing managers' burnout symptoms like emotional exhaustion and depersonalization. Shift work may also negatively impact mental health in healthcare, so that there might be relevant differences between daytime versus night-time healthcare workers' mental health (Brown et al., 2020). Conversely, favorable working conditions – such as work autonomy, opportunities for development at work, and influence over one's work – have been found to negatively correlate with burnout in palliative care nurses (Gómez-Urquiza et al., 2020).

Drawing upon the Job Demands-Resources (JD-R) model (Bakker & Demerouti, 2017, 2018; Schaufeli, 2017), academic literature has highlighted both negative and positive aspects of working in healthcare. The JD-R model conceives the work environment as a potential source of either positive or negative mental health depending on how the work environment is designed, organized, and managed. According to this framework, the work environment can be considered as a constellation of job demands and resources, which differently influence workers' mental health. On the one hand, job demands refer to physical, psychological, social, or organizational aspects of the job that require physical or psychological efforts from the worker. Examples may be emotional demands, team conflict, heavy workload, time pressure. As such, job demands can be understood as risk factors for healthcare workers' mental health. Nevertheless, job demands have recently been differentiated into hindering job demands and challenging job demands (Van den Broeck et al., 2010), where the former hinder the optimal functioning of the individual and the latter stimulate work engagement and individual well-being. On the other hand, job resources correspond to physical, psychological, social, or organizational aspects of the job, that healthcare workers can use to counterbalance the costs implied by job demands in terms of physical, cognitive, and emotional energy. Examples may be personal protective equipment, safety devices, cognitive and behavioral patterns, job autonomy, skill variety, performance feedback, support from colleagues or supervisors, role clarity, job control, adequate pay, job security, career opportunities. In addition, recent studies (e.g., Chen et al., 2018) have integrated job resources with personal resources from the positive psychological tradition – such as, for instance, resilience, adaptability, flexibility, optimism, self-efficacy, hope, psychological capital. Job resources are intrinsically motivating and may help healthcare workers fulfill their basic needs, achieve work-related goals, and positively influence their personal growth and development. Although both job demands and job resources can independently impact individual well-being, job resources may buffer job demands by enabling healthcare workers to cope with job demands. In this framework, distress results from an imbalance between job demands and resources; when job demands exceed resources, poor mental health may show up. Specifically, the JD-R model postulates two distinct processes leading to workers' mental health; through the health impairment process, high job demands are causally linked to burnout over time, while through the motivation process, high job resources result in positive outcomes.

Broetje et al. (2020) performed an integration of previous literature reviews on the topic and identified the key job demands and job resources that nursing staff perceive to be present in their work environment. Healthcare workers' main job demands included work overload, lack of formal rewards, and work-life interference. In contrast, main job resources included supervisor support, fair and authentic management, transformational leadership, positive interpersonal relations, autonomy, and professional resources such as work equipment, access to necessary information, organization of work tasks.

Healthcare workers' mental illness not only constitutes an inherently undesirable human cost – that is, being mentally ill is an unpleasant experience in itself –, but it also translates into worsened quality of care (e.g., Garman et al., 2002; Teoh et al., 2020) and reduced patient safety (e.g., Cheng et al., 2020; Teo et al., 2021). Thus, effective measures should address the working conditions of healthcare workers to positively impact their mental health. On the one hand, interventions should prevent, remove, or reduce factors of healthcare workers' mental illness, namely risk factors or job demands. On the other hand, interventions should promote factors of healthcare workers' positive mental health through protective factors or job resources, thus leveraging what is already going well (e.g., Christensen et al., 2020; Nielsen & Christensen, 2021).

From an ecological perspective, the workplace can be viewed as a system made of different sub-systems, where various patterns of relationships between workers and different working environments occur. Also, workers' mental health can be seen as embedded in such a system. Consequently, mental health interventions should be developed at all systemic levels of the workplace to address potential sources of either good or poor workers' mental health (e.g., Bakker & Demerouti, 2018; Chen et al., 2018; Martin et al., 2016; Teoh et al., 2020). Specifically, sources of mental health and well-being at work can exist at four levels, such as the individual (I), the group or work team (G), the leader (L), and the organization (O). These levels are framed as the IGLO model (Day & Nielsen, 2017; Nielsen & Christensen, 2021; Nielsen et al., 2017). At the individual level, one worker's mental health can derive from work-specific cognitive, affective, and behavioral factors or resources, for instance, work-related self-efficacy and job crafting. At the group level, work-related well-being can be associated with colleagues' support and workgroup climate. The leader level encompasses workers' mental health predictors like line managers' knowledge, skills, abilities, attitudes, behaviors, and support. Finally, at the organizational level, Human Resources Management practices and policies, job design, and occupational health services can play a meaningful role in promoting or hindering workers' psychological well-being. To summarize, the individual level has to do with personal variables, the group level is about team states, processes, and dynamics, the leader level refers to characteristics of and actions implemented by managers, and the organizational level points to how both the work and the working environment are designed, managed, and organized.

When mental health interventions are introduced in organizations, an exhaustive understanding of the work environment is needed (e.g., Di Tecco et al., 2020; Fridrich et al., 2015; Ramos et al., 2020), which can be achieved through a workplace mental health needs assessment exercise. Consistent with JD-R and IGLO, such assessment should encompass, on the one hand, both job demands and job resources and, on the other hand, cover all levels of the workplace system. So, since they can allow the identification of multilevel sources of either good or bad workers' mental health within a given working environment – i.e., barriers to positive mental health at work/major causes of work-related stress and positive aspects of work/major causes of work-related mental health and well-being –, JD-R and IGLO can be deemed as flexible and easy-to-use instruments, not only to perform actual interventions, but also to conduct workplace mental health needs assessment exercises. In this regard, an integration between JD-R and IGLO can be achieved by making the individual, group, leader, and organizational levels serve as a classificatory framework for job demands and job resources. Ultimately, this framework can be deployed as a guide for a workplace mental health needs assessment exercise.

Workplace assessment activities are useful to tailor subsequent interventions according to the specific workers' needs. However, these needs may depend on how workers perceive their work environment. According to Persson et al. (2012), each worker has his/her mental model about his/her work environment. That is, people take cues from the work environment and make sense (e.g., Weick, 1995) and develop a certain understanding of it. This understanding is collectively shared because of common conditions that people may find themselves in together. For instance, one worker's type of perception of a given work environment may depend on the position the worker occupies within the work environment as well as on local working conditions. Similarly, a perceptual distance phenomenon (Gibson et al., 2001, 2009) may occur, whereby managers and employees do not always interpret a given work situation in the same way. This might be the case in healthcare too, where healthcare workers' perceptions of their work environment may differ depending on the hierarchical position they occupy as well as on the belonging department.

To summarize the above, by taking cues from each other at work, people develop shared mental models about their working conditions. So, these appraisals influence what workers see as being a job demand or a job resource. Therefore, it is important to gather workers' mental models of their working environment and to identify which aspects of the work environment they share according to the positions they find themselves in or local conditions. In this vein, workplace mental health needs assessment exercises should be properly contextualized (Nielsen et al., 2014; Vignoli et al., 2017). This means conducting them within the field of homogeneous work environments – e.g., same roles, same physical space, same set of activities, same cultural setting, same working patterns, and so on –, as each work environment is likely to show its own characteristics, peculiarities, and idiosyncrasies, and therefore is not necessarily comparable to others, as much as the knowledge retrieved in one work environment is not necessarily generalizable to another one. In addition, needs assessment activities should adopt a multi-source approach to combine information from different action and acquire a comprehensive picture thanks to the triangulation of perspectives on the targeted assessment issues.

To capture workers' mental models, assessment activities need to involve workers directly (Nielsen et al., 2021). The bottom-up, participatory approach is a guiding principle in this regard. It is one of the most critical success factors of assessment and intervention activities and it consists of the direct participation of relevant employees and stakeholders throughout the whole process. According to Nielsen et al. (2010), the importance of employee participation is because it can (1) help optimize the fit with the local organizational context, (2) be considered an intervention, and (3) facilitate the intervention process. In a bottom-up perspective on workplace mental health promotion, employees should not be seen as passive subjects, but rather as active actors able to change their work environment. Such an approach is able to (1) ensure the use of relevant stakeholders' local knowledge of what the key issues are concerning job demands and job resources, (2) show what changes need to be made and how, and (3) ensure stakeholders feel valued, empowered, and looked after. By using a participatory approach, workers and their managers collectively gain resources, knowledge, and skills to identify workplace problems, develop solutions, and implement changes to improve their working conditions (Nielsen et al., 2014). Thus, employees and managers are to be considered key informants along the assessment activities (Christensen et al., 2019; Tafvelin, 2018).

The present chapter draws upon a multilevel workplace mental health needs assessment exercise performed within a healthcare setting. The overarching aim was to collect suggestions to inform the subsequent design, development, and implementation of multilevel interventions, actions, and initiatives addressing healthcare workers' mental health. The chapter will present the main findings from the needs assessment exercise and discuss a list of key insights and lessons learned from performing the field experience. Particularly, the importance of locally assessing healthcare workers' mental health by means of a contextualized, bottom-up, participatory approach will be argued. Consistently, the focus of the needs assessment was on three hierarchical positions (i.e., senior managers, middle managers, employees) from three departments of the targeted healthcare organization, since (1) the implementation of subsequent interventions, actions and initiatives was planned in each of these departments, (2) this was thought to enable comparisons across both hierarchical positions and departments as well as to (3) clarify whether mental models of job demands and job resources at the different IGLO levels differed across hierarchical positions and/or departments. Thus, along the chapter, study results will be synthesized and organized according to hierarchical roles and departments and framed using JD-R and IGLO analytical categories. Finally, insights into facilitators and barriers to the implementation and effectiveness of workplace mental health needs assessment exercises in healthcare will be provided, thus raising some practical implications, solutions, recommendations, and directions for future research.

THE WORKPLACE MENTAL HEALTH NEEDS ASSESSMENT EXERCISE

The workplace mental health needs assessment exercise, designed to capture job demands and job resources at IGLO levels, was carried out in three departments of a large healthcare institution in Northern Italy. The institution is one of Italy's largest public healthcare organizations in terms of size and care complexity. Its jurisdiction includes 46 municipalities on approximately 3.000 square kilometers, encompassing over 870.000 inhabitants, of which over 23% is over 65 years old, 8% is over 80 years old, and 11% is made of foreign residents. The organization is divided into six territorial districts, extending across the metropolitan area, and is composed of six hospital departments, four territorial department, and five support departments. It has nine district clinics, a growing number of healthcare facilities for older adults, and outpatient clinics spread throughout the whole metropolitan area. It employs over 9.000 professionals, more than 1.300 of which are physicians and 5.100 are care workers.

In the present chapter, the three targeted departments will be named Department A, Department B, and Department C to preserve privacy and anonymity. Each department is different from the others not only in terms of size and discipline, but also because of unique work and organizational cultures. First, Department A counts around 600 employees and most of the clinical activities performed here by healthcare workers are characterized by emergency and urgency. These activities are multidisciplinary and take place in different buildings spread over and beyond the metropolitan area. Second, Department B counts around 600 employees, and it is a multidisciplinary medical institute whose clinical activities – e.g., prevention, diagnosis, and non-surgical treatment of several diseases – are quite routine as compared to Department A. These activites are also spread over the urban territory, such that Department B may include both people working in central hospitals and people working in peripheral hospitals. Third, Department C counts about 300 employees and it consists of a both clinical and research institute, where the medical and the academic mindsets intertwine. Given its monodisciplinary focus and strive for scientific excellence, Department C is considered as more of a specialized hospital. Different from the other two departments, all activities performed by Department C's healthcare workers take place in one building only. Despite the General Director of the main healthcare organization being the same for all three departments, the management style may differ significantly across them, also due to the presence of different senior and middle managers. Also, the three department do not necessarily show the same working patterns, processes, and procedure, as well as they are not necessarily equipped in the same way in terms of technical, financial, and human resources. All these differences between the three departments legitimated the need for differently investigating working conditions and healthcare workers' mental models in each of them.

The workplace mental health needs assessment methodology comprised four main parts, such as (1) a quali-quantitative contextual measurement, aiming to capture the extent to which management was committed to dealing with mental health issues, what sort of policies, practices, and programmes were in place in the healthcare setting and how they were perceived, (2) semi-structured individual interviews with middle and senior managers, aiming to understand middle and senior managers' experiences, ideas and perspectives around the needs for multilevel interventions to improve mental health for their employees, (3) focus groups with employees, aiming to gain mutual knowledge of psychosocial factors affecting mental health at work, and (4) an action plan workshop with a Steering Committee composed of main organizational stakeholders, aiming to identify strategies and interventions needed to improve mental health in the workplace in each department. In the targeted organization, middle managers corresponded to coordinators of work teams within the hospital departments – for instance, they might be head nurses managing other nurses or head physicians managing other physicians. In contrast, senior managers corresponded to directors or heads managing all the employees of the hospital departments.

Contextual Measurement: The Organizational Perspective

Methods

Contextual measurement consisted of a survey to be completed by a small group of employee representatives and investigating three thematic areas, namely (1) description of policies, programs, and practices within the organization, (2) perception of policies, programs, and practices, and (3) management support, commitment and priority, and organizational communication, involvement, and participation. The instrument was composed of 7 open-ended questions for part (1). Eleven Likert-type items were used for part (2) and inspired from the Workplace Integrated Safety and Health (WISH) assessment by Sorensen et al. (2018) and López Gómez et al. (2021). Twelve Liker-type items were used for part (3) and inspired from the Psychosocial Safety Climate (PSC-12) assessment by Hall et al. (2010). The Health and Safety Manager, the Workers Safety Representative, and each Director of the three departments contributed to completing the survey. Qualitative text data went through full NVivo content analysis (Bazeley & Jackson, 2013), while quantitative answers were used to complement the summaries of qualitative findings.

Results

Despite work was not reported to be systematically and preventatively designed, organized, and managed with the explicit aim of promoting healthcare workers' mental health – with the only exception being the organization of work shifts –, some structured practices could be identified. Monthly team meetings were reported to be held whereby employees can discuss both work-related issues and concerns about mental health. These meetings were reported to help conflict management thanks to adopting a mediating leadership style. A "feedback meeting" was mentioned as part of a more extensive performance evaluation system and reported as an occasion for employees to express concerns. A "Counsellors of Confidence" group was reported to be elected by senior management to be voluntarily consulted by employees about psychosocial issues. Psychological support service was reported to be provided to employees by the

Health and Safety Department. The occupational physician was reported to hold a decisive role "as a proxy" in guiding workers to suitable facilities for their needs.

Several initiatives aimed to promote workplace mental health were mentioned such as, for instance, organizational climate assessments and work-related stress surveys. However, participation in such initiatives was described as increasable, lack of impact from these initiatives beyond mere diagnosis was perceived, and some participants appeared more aware than others. Interviewees themselves agreed about internal organizational communication being a need to address for the organization to be able to support workers' mental health. Specific professional categories – e.g., vulnerable workers, workers caring for the elderly, workers with problematic children, workers with work-life balance issues – were reported to be able to take advantage of some mental health-related benefits such as telework, flex time, part-time work, reduced waiting time for healthcare professionals when needing medical diagnostic services, and specially discounted public transport subscriptions.

The COVID-19 pandemic outbreak was reported to have negatively impacted these organizational services, compelling workers to remain at work with limited opportunities for holidays. Nevertheless, extra hours were reported to have been rewarded by regional incentives. Organization-wise, COVID-19 impact on the working environment was reported as a passed test for organizational resilience and adaptability, teaching the organization to implement flexible and agile organizational models instead of old and rigid ones. Breaks, training opportunities, adequate equipment, and financial affordability of basic survival needs – i.e., board and lodging – were reported as organization's strengths. On the other hand, despite a reported increase in managerial sensitivity towards workplace mental health matters, it was reported that senior management commitment to the topic could increase by providing substantial support beyond the formal responsibilities, giving employees' mental health priority above productivity, and being proactive rather than reactive towards initiatives to promote mental health at work.

Semi-Structured Individual Interviews: The Managerial Perspective

Methods

Twenty-one one-hour semi-structured individual interviews with senior and middle managers were conducted. In Department A, two senior managers and three middle managers were interviewed (n = 5). In Department B, four senior managers and six middle managers were interviewed (n = 10). In Department C, two senior managers and four middle managers were interviewed (n = 6). The interviews investigated (1) perceptions, knowledge, and attitudes towards mental health in the workplace, (2) hindering and facilitating aspects for the middle/senior managers' role in promoting and/or preventing mental health issues at work, (3) needs towards creating a mentally healthy workplace, (4) barriers and triggers related to implementing workplace mental health initiatives, and (5) proposals to create and implement workplace mental health initiatives successfully. Interviews were audio-recorded and transcribed qualitative text data went through NVivo deductive content analysis (Bazeley & Jackson, 2013).

Results: Job Demands and Job Resources at IGLO levels in the Healthcare Institution as Reported by Senior Managers

In Department A, healthcare workers' intrinsic motivation to ensure patients' health and well-being was mentioned as an individual-level personal resource. At times, this motivation was reported to drive employees to take initiatives to improve their own well-being. A positive team climate was reported as a group-level resource, as indicated by effective teamwork, cooperation, collaboration, cohesion, open communication, and ability to manage interpersonal conflicts. Especially cooperation among and between senior and middle managers was mentioned, as it was stated, "[...] through working groups, through meetings, which we do periodically, through observation, we try to understand how to strengthen the service and individuals". Nevertheless, mental health problems were reported to be perceived as an individual weakness, which may be due to some degree of stigma – i.e., group-level demand. At the leader level, a compassionate, supportive, and empowering leadership style was self-reported as a crucial resource, especially to pay attention to younger employees and to make employees feel valued; for instance, "I involve interns in our activities and meetings as much as possible. In my opinion, it is an involvement that gives them the feeling of being valued". The middle managers' role was depicted as extremely important, as they hold direct and constant contact with employees – "they are the first contact with the staff, so it is a vital role because they are the ones that absorb a whole series of situations, which are not only organizational but also relational and emotional, at times". At the organizational level, understaffing and high turnover rates were linked to high workload. Continuous and rapid organizational changes, such as departmental restructuring, were linked to employees feeling pressed to adapt to top-down superimposed changes. There was a perception of lacking workplace mental health organizational policies. Limited physical space to properly treat all patients was mentioned. A desire for more open and inclusive organizational communication was expressed. On the other hand, the availability of the Health and Safety Department was perceived as a resource helping to support workers' positive mental health.

In Department B, low employee motivation was mentioned among individual-level job demands. At the group level, the main resource reported was the availability of multidisciplinary teams composed of diverse expertise, skills, and abilities, which were deemed necessary to deal with patients' medical complexity. Team cohesion and open attitudes towards mental health in the workplace were also mentioned. Still, communication between doctors was described as fragmented. At the leader level, leading by example, actively working within the healthcare unit, valuing employee participation and involvement, bottom-up decision-making, and encouraging all professionals to adopt a shared vision supporting departmental identity were self-reported as job resources. For instance, it was stated, "my colleagues have embraced my idea of seeing and thinking of this department as a large operational unit, as a whole". About job demands, a lack of open discussion among all decision-making's stakeholders was mentioned as raising the risk of affecting employees adversely. At the organizational level, senior managers felt their needs supported by the organization as well as workers' psychological well-being ensured by participatory, bottom-up decision-making process. On the other hand, lack of recognition of Department B's value for patients' health, politically determined cuts to beds and personnel, high turnover rates, patient-specific medical complexity, lack of control over tasks and work pace, workload, long shifts, work-life unbalance, lack of professional recognition, and dealing with interpersonally challenging patients and patients' relatives were reported as job demands. For instance, it was stated, "It is a department where the patient is dependent on you, it can be a chronic patient, an elderly patient, a fragile patient as if to say it is a patient who needs commitment and involves a high workload".

In Department C, low work engagement and employee commitment were mentioned as individual-level job demands, especially related to older workers. High work-related emotional loads were linked to medical situations involving children and patients' families. Employees' resistance to change, poor flexibility, and poor openness to learning and development opportunities were cited as to potential obstacles to future interventions' effectiveness. At the group level, interpersonal conflicts, both among peers and different hierarchical roles, were reported as a job demands, whereas no group-level job resources were mentioned. At the leader level, a supportive, empowering, and intellectually stimulating managerial style was self-reported as fostering team cohesion and providing followers' needs with proper listening as much as possible. Several demands were attached to leaders' role, such as coordination of multiple tasks, monitoring collaboration after organizational changes, and poor learning opportunities for leaders. These demands were reported as preventing leaders from always ensuring a positive team climate. At the organizational level, job demands included excessive bureaucracy, top-down management decisions, lack of workers' involvement in decision-making processes, lack of technological support, unequal distribution of technological devices around the hospital, inaccurate evaluation feedback, and poor career opportunities. These demands were perceived as linked to organizational management's unawareness of actual ward issues. On the other hand, equal career and learning opportunities, high task rotation against boredom and monotony, and the psychological support service in the department were reported as job resources.

Table 1 summarizes job demands and job resources at IGLO levels in the healthcare institution as reported by senior managers.

Results: Job Demands and Job Resources at IGLO levels in the Healthcare Institution as Reported by Middle Managers

In Department A, no job resources were mentioned at the individual level. Conversely, high physical, psychological, and emotional demands were referred to, as well as symptoms of psychological distress and physical fatigue. For instance, it was stated, "As soon as you arrive in the morning, you have to take charge a little bit of the whole team, and also manage their specific situations, person by person, so you have to involve everyone at the same time". At the group level, exchange of positive feedback within teams was reported among job resources. Among job demands, interpersonal conflict was linked to unfair career opportunities and lack of recognition from the management. At the leader level, a supportive and participatory leadership style was described as prompting a sense of organizational identification and shared mission and vision. On the other hand, poor learning opportunities for leaders were perceived as job demands. At the organizational level, long shifts affecting healthcare workers' work-life balance and conflicts with patients and/or patients' relatives were listed among job demands. For instance, it was stated, "[…] the typical customer/patient has changed. The user's expectations have changed, everyone comes a bit arrogant, and it is a very, very difficult position the one that you have". No organizational-level job resources were mentioned by middle managers in Department A.

In Department B, no job demands, nor job resources were mentioned at the individual level. A positive team climate was reported as a group-level resource, as indicated by cohesion, support, collaboration, trust, and good group communication. For instance, it was stated, "[…] being able to feel like someone whose point of view is being asked is already a great openness". At the leader level, lack of leadership training was reported as a job demands, whereas informally acquired leadership skills to manage employees' health and well-being were self-reported as job resources. At the organizational level, organizational support towards workplace mental health initiatives was reported as a job resource, even if such support was described as reactive rather than proactive, and although such initiatives were described as discontinuous and little participated. Understaffing, high turnover rates, long shifts, work overload, and work-life unbalance were listed as job demands. Continuous and rapid organizational changes, such as departmental restructuring, were reported as a further job demand, as it was stated, "There were times when people found themselves embedded in a new setting and therefore the references between peers and superiors were not yet clear". Finally, infrequent organizational communication and top-down decision-making were reported to make employees' professional value feel not recognized, as it was stated, "there would be a strong need to share what are the goals that we all have to try to achieve, and not so much between peers but between the different existing hierarchies".

Table 1. Job demands and job resources at IGLO levels as reported by senior managers

	Job Demands	Job Resources
Department A	*Individual* • None. *Group* • Mental health stigma. *Leader* • None. *Organization* • Understaffing. • Turnover. • Workload. • Organizational changes. • Lacking workplace mental health policies. • Limited physical space. • Poor organizational communication.	*Individual* • Intrinsic motivation. *Group* • Positive team climate. *Leader* • Compassionate, supportive, and empowering leadership. *Organization* • Health and Safety Department.
Department B	*Individual* • Low employee motivation. *Group* • Fragmented communication between doctors. *Leader* • Lack of open discussion among decision-making's stakeholders. *Organization* • Lack of recognition. • Cuts to beds and personnel. • Turnover. • Patients' medical complexity. • Lack of job control. • Workload. • Long shifts. • Work-life unbalance. • Organizational changes. • Interpersonally challenging customers.	*Individual* • None. *Group* • Multidisciplinary teams. • Team cohesion. • Open attitudes towards mental health. *Leader* • Leading by example. • Working within healthcare unit. • Valuing employee participation. • Bottom-up decision-making. • Supporting departmental identity. *Organization* • Organizational support.
Department C	*Individual* • Low employee engagement/commitment. • Emotional load. • Resistance to change. *Group* • Interpersonal conflicts. *Leader* • Coordination of multiple tasks. • Managing organizational changes. • Poor learning opportunities for leaders. *Organization* • Bureaucracy. • Top-down management. • Lack of technological support. • Inaccurate feedback. • Poor career opportunities.	*Individual* • None. *Group* • None. *Leader* • Supportive, empowering, and intellectually stimulating leadership. *Organization* • Equal career opportunities. • Equal learning opportunities. • Task rotation. • Psychological support service.

In Department C, poor personal flexibility was mentioned as an individual-level job demand. At the group level, positive team climate was reported as a job resource, as indicated by cohesion, openness to mental health problems, and quality teamwork. For instance, it was stated, "There is a beautiful environment and exchange between specialists, which allows us to grow together". On the other hand, concern was expressed that such a cohesive, established, and long-lasting team may reveal counterproductive over time when faced with needs for change or adaptations. For instance, it was stated, "When I came to run this facility, I felt as if I was dealing with people who were all very rigid and reluctant to change". Lack of communication skills training was also mentioned. At the leader level, a supportive, proactive, democratic, and bottom-up leadership style was described. At the organizational level, a lack of psychological support was linked to poor employee involvement. Work overload and cumbersome bureaucracy were mentioned as additional job demands, along with lack of support when dealing with interpersonally challenging patients' relatives. Low rates of sick leaves were mentioned as an organizational-level resource.

Table 2. Job demands and job resources at IGLO levels as reported by middle managers

	Job Demands	Job Resources
Department A	*Individual* • Psychological distress. • Emotional demands. • Physical fatigue. *Group* • Interpersonal conflicts. *Leader* • Poor learning opportunities for leaders. *Organization* • Unfair career opportunities. • Long shifts. • Work-life unbalance. • Interpersonally challenging customers.	*Individual* • None. *Group* • Mutual positive feedback. *Leader* • Supportive and participatory leadership. *Organization* • None.
Department B	*Individual* • None. *Group* • None. *Leader* • Lack of leadership training. *Organization* • Understaffing. • Turnover. • Long shifts. • Workload. • Work-life unbalance. • Poor organizational communication. • Top-down decision-making.	*Individual* • None. *Group* • Positive team climate. *Leader* • Employee well-being management skills. *Organization* • Support to workplace mental health initiatives.
Department C	*Individual* • Poor flexibility. *Group* • Excessive cohesiveness. • Lack of communication skills training. *Leader* • None. *Organization* • Lack of psychological support. • Workload. • Bureaucracy.	*Individual* • None. *Group* • Positive team climate. *Leader* • Supportive, proactive, democratic, bottom-up leadership. *Organization* • Low rates of sick leaves.

Table 2 summarizes job demands and job resources at IGLO levels in the healthcare institution as reported by middle managers.

Focus Groups and Cognitive Mapping: The Employee Perspective

Methods

Four two-hour focus groups with 27 healthcare professionals were conducted. In Department A, two focus groups took place with a total of three doctors, eight nurses, and four healthcare assistants (n = 15). In Department B, one focus group was conducted with two doctors, three nurses, and one healthcare assistant (n = 6). In Department C, one focus group was conducted with six nurses and two healthcare assistants (n = 8), whereas doctors could not participate. The focus groups investigated (1) perceptions, knowledge, and attitudes towards mental health in the workplace, (2) hindering and facilitating working conditions for mental health issues at work, and (3) needs towards creating a mentally healthy workplace. Focus groups were audio-recorded and transcribed qualitative text data went through NVivo deductive content analysis (Bazeley & Jackson, 2013).

Each focus group included a cognitive mapping exercise to gather healthcare workers' reflections on how job demands and job resources at different IGLO levels interact with each other. To ensure all employees having the same understanding about workplace mental health, the exercise started with an explanatory video of the JD-R model. Then, participants were given five minutes to individually note up to three keywords reflecting the current main issues for their mental health they perceived in their workplace. With this reflection in mind, participants were asked to fill in green post-it notes with at least three job resources and red post-it notes with at least three job demands. This first part of the exercise was carried out without seeing the cognitive map not to bias participants' ideas with predefined categories, but to make them think freely.

Subsequently, the facilitator introduced the actual cognitive map. On the map, some gears illustrated how the IGLO levels interact with each other in the workplace system. There were three smaller gears for the individual (I), the group (G), and the leader (L), placed within a larger gear for the organization (O). Each gear had some example work-related categories attached to its teeth, typical for a (un)healthy workplace, which the facilitator provided some brief explanation about. However, there was also room for additional categories, if needed, which the facilitator could fill in by the unmarked teeth on the gears. Employees were instructed to place their post-it notes on the most suitable category. The facilitator could assist participants by discussing the reported job demand or job resource. Post-it notes that could not be placed clearly could be parked on a "P" area and discussed further later. Finally, participants' statements were discussed collectively in the group. The facilitator sorted participants' statements according to the map categories to check whether some were misplaced and/or pertained to multiple categories. "Parked" statements were discussed to identify the best fit on the map. The facilitator moved the green and red post-it notes around the map and drew relationships, if any, with a marker pen. (S)he summarized the most important discussion points and asked if participants had anything to add before concluding the meeting.

Results: Job Demands and Job Resources at IGLO levels in the Healthcare Institution as Reported by Employees

In Department A, healthcare professionals mostly mentioned intrinsic motivation to ensure patients' health and well-being as an individual-level personal resource. This motivation was described as necessary when facing difficult situations or interpersonally challenging customers. Personal initiative for discussing workplace mental health with colleagues and searching for improvement strategies was cited. Feeling adrenalin from emergency activities was reported as a challenging job demand. For instance, it was stated, "We become emergency-addicted". One the other hand, repetitiveness and boredom from most work activities were reported as hindering job demands. At the group level, teamwork was referred to as a fundamental job resource. For instance, it was stated, "My motivation for this work stays high only because of the group support". Doctors and nurses listed peer mutual support, listening in difficult working conditions, organizational citizenship behaviors, strong sense of community, positive work climate, and team cohesion as crucial group-level job resources. Nevertheless, interpersonal conflicts, blaming attitudes, and disrespectful behaviors could be identified as group-level job demands. At the leader level, the importance of team coordinators' role was underlined, but communication from and to leaders was described as improvable. At the organizational level, lack of scheduled meetings, policies, practices, and trainings on workplace mental health was reported as job demand making employees perceive the organization as distant from their needs. Also, top-down decision-making process about shift management, turnover, and job rotation between central and peripheral hospitals were reported to negatively impact work-life balance. For instance, it was stated, "You are not asked if you want to do the rotation, or if you are available". Among job resources, a specialized team member offering psychological support was reported to be available in one team. Desire for generalizing this service to the whole department was expressed.

Figure 1 and Figure 2 show the cognitive maps from the first and second focus group at Department A. The maps allowed to gather links and interactions among job demands and job resources at different IGLO levels. For instance, an organizational-level job demand such as lack of structured psychological support was linked to an individual-level job demand such as emotional burden. Two organizational-level job demands, such as perceived lack of autonomy and perceived task unclarity, were traced back to a leader-level job demand such as lack of middle managers' communication as well as to an organizational-level job demand such as top-down decision-making. An individual-level job resource such as initiative for discussing workplace mental health was reported to lead to a group-level job resource such as positive relationships with colleagues. Consistent with JD-R theory, some job resources were reported as potentially buffering some job demands. For instance, an individual-level job resource such as further development of stress management skills was mentioned as a possible solution to both emotional burden and conflicts with customers. At the group level, team cohesion was mentioned as a possible resource to increase the sharing of both positive and negative experiences at work.

In Department B, high intrinsic motivation was mentioned as an individual-level personal resource. For instance, it was stated, "[...] let us do not forget, first of all, our passion about patients and medicine". At the group level, team cohesion, effective cooperation, and positive relationships with colleagues were listed as job resources. At the leader level, job demands included inadequate middle managers' behaviors and skills, such as poor communication and neglecting employees' health and well-being needs. At the organizational level, several job demands were reported such as attributing more value to performance rather than to human needs – for instance, it was stated, "they think of us as numbers, not as people"

–, lack of workplace mental health policies, top-down decision-making about holidays and shifts, and personnel understaffing as affecting workload. The latter was described as potentially undermining team cohesion. Organizational demands were described as negatively influencing employee commitment. For instance, it was stated, "a psychologically healthy workplace does not make you want to run away". Additional job demands included work-life balance issues and aggressive customers – healthcare professionals stated patients and their relatives should be made aware of the specific healthcare roles. Answering patterns could be observed per occupational categories. For instance, nurses mentioned consistently higher workload than doctors. Healthcare assistants expressed desire for being included in morning debriefings occurring between doctors and nurses.

Figure 1. Cognitive map from first focus group at Department A. Red boxes = job demands; green boxes = job resources

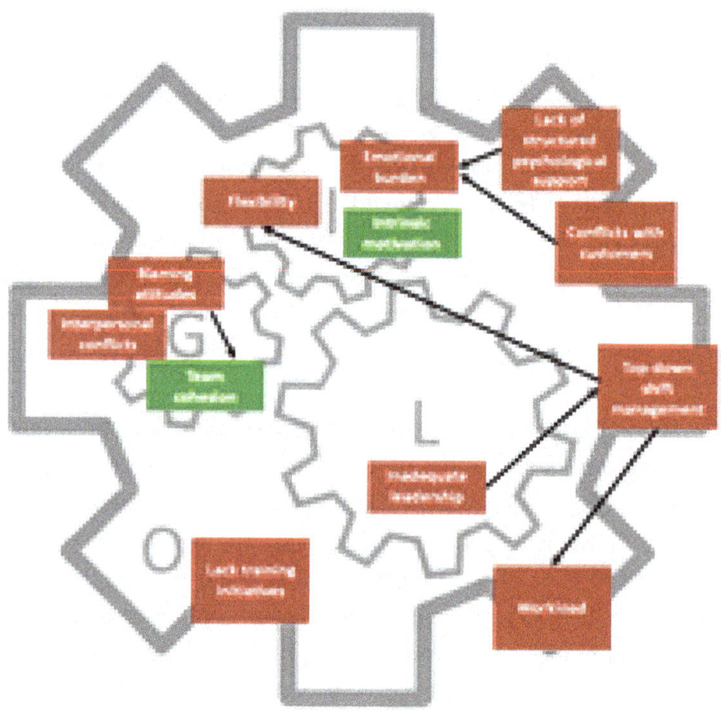

Figure 3 shows the cognitive map from focus group at Department B. Organizational-level job demands such as lack of recognition, lack of workplace mental health policies and practices, top-down decision-making, personnel understaffing, and high workload were linked to individual-level job demands such as low organizational commitment. A vicious cycle was established between the organizational and individual level, whereby organizational-level job demands would decrease organizational commitment which, in turn, would determine personnel understaffing and high workload. The latter was also described as threatening team cohesion and positive relationships with colleagues at the group level. Finally, an individual-level job demand such as frustration was traced back to a leader-level job demand such as managers' poor communication.

Figure 2. Cognitive map from second focus group at Department A. Red boxes = job demands; green boxes = job resources; KSAOs = knowledge, skills, abilities, and other characteristics

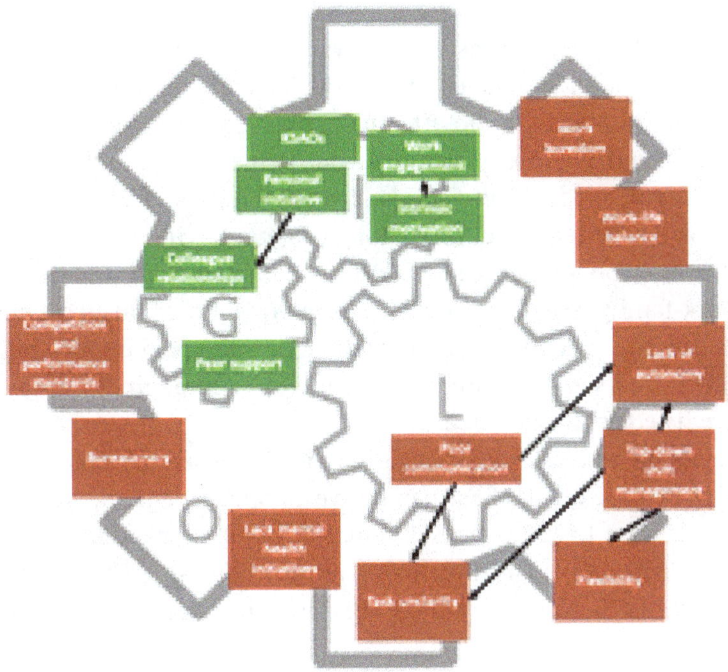

Figure 3. Cognitive map from focus group at Department B. Red boxes = job demands; green boxes = job resources; HR = human resources

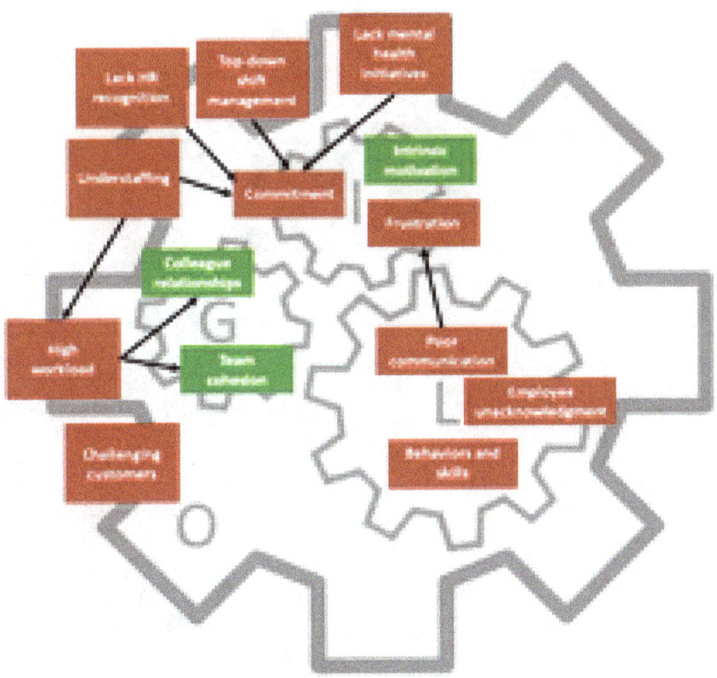

In Department C, intrinsic motivation and healthcare workers' dedication to work were mentioned among individual-level job resources. At the group level, team cohesion, team support, and positive team climate were listed among job resources. On the other hand, ineffective communication processes were also reported as a job demand. For instance, it was stated, "There is a lack of communication on how information is received and how it is given". At the leader level, inadequate leadership was mentioned as a job demand entailing inability to effectively manage communication processes, conflictual interpersonal relationships, and employees' workload due to the need to manage one's own already high workload. For instance, it was stated, "Even if you have no family and you are young, it is still a problem not knowing shifts and schedules and, in the long run, not having stability". At the organizational level, lack of involvement in rota planning and short notice about work schedule were reported as job demands leading to work-family issues, especially among younger employees. On the other hand, positive relationships with patients, recognition, appreciation, development opportunities through intensive job rotation – especially for nurses –, and implementation of – although discontinuous – psychological support initiatives were listed as job resources.

Figure 4 shows the cognitive map from focus group at Department C. Organizational-level job demands such as lack of workplace mental health initiatives, policies, and practices and lack of structured and psychological support were linked to an individual-level job demand such as emotional burden. In turn, emotional burden was perceived as threatening an individual-level job resource such as intrinsic motivation to ensure patients' health and well-being. Organizational issues were also traced back to leadership issues.

Figure 4. Cognitive map from focus group at Department C. Red boxes = job demands; green boxes = job resources; HR = human resources

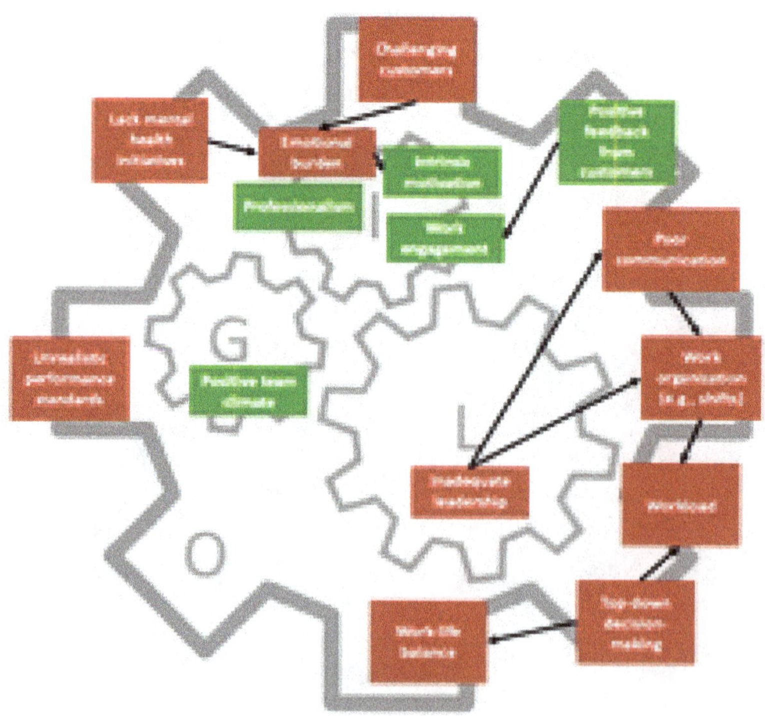

KEY INSIGHTS

The workplace mental health needs' assessment exercise allowed to achieve three main goals, such as (1) gathering job demands and job resources that healthcare workers perceived at different IGLO levels in their workplace, (2) identifying similarities and differences in perceptions – i.e., shared versus diverging mental models – of working conditions across the considered hierarchical positions and departments, and (3) informing a tailored action plan to enhance workplace mental health within the targeted organizational contexts. These goals are delved in the sections below.

Similarities and Differences Among Healthcare Workers' Mental Models

Integration between the JD-R and the IGLO models allowed to identify job demands and job resources that healthcare workers perceived at the individual, group, leader, and organizational levels in the targeted healthcare organization. Also, the contextualizing, bottom-up, participatory approach towards the workplace mental health needs' assessment exercise allowed to gather the extent to which different key stakeholders in different departments agreed or disagreed about major issues related to workplace mental health. That is, it was possible to capture similarities and differences in both the nature and the content of reported workplace mental health issues across hierarchical positions and healthcare departments. Ultimately, such an approach allowed to verify whether workplace mental health needs from senior managers versus middle managers versus employees – both within and between departments –, as well as those from Department A versus Department B versus Department C – both within and between hierarchical positions –, aligned or misaligned. In other words, a picture of shared versus diverging mental models of working conditions within the targeted organizational contexts across the considered hierarchical positions and departments could be taken thanks to collecting a variety of views, perceptions, and needs.

Senior managers tended to agree about low employee motivation and low work engagement as individual-level job demands, although this was not the case for senior managers in Department A. While senior managers from Department B and Department C agreed on employee motivation as an area for improvement, senior managers from Department A mentioned healthcare workers' intrinsic motivation to promote patients' health and well-being. Also, senior managers tended to agree about teamwork – e.g., team cohesion, peer support – as a group-level job resource. However, this was not the case for senior managers in Department C, who consistently reported frequent interpersonal conflicts as a group-level job demand. Senior managers from all three departments agreed about effective leadership as a crucial leader-level job resource, entailing supporting, valuing, and empowering employees as well as listening to their needs. Senior managers from Department A and Department B agreed about high turnover rates as an organizational-level job demand, while senior managers from Department C did not mention it. Senior managers from Department A and Department C agreed about top-down decision-making as an organizational-level job demand, whereas senior managers from Department B even reported bottom-up decision-making as an organizational-level job resource. Finally, senior managers from Department A and Department C agreed about psychological support services as an organizational-level job resource, while senior managers from Department B did not mention it.

Middle managers tended to report few or no issues at the individual level. As an exception, middle managers from Department C – like senior managers – mentioned low employee flexibility as an individual-level job demand. Middle managers from all three departments agreed about teamwork – e.g., team cohesion, peer support, positive social climate – as a group-level job resource. Nonetheless, middle managers from Department C reported concerns about excessive team cohesion in face of needs for change and adaptation. Also, middle managers from Department B mentioned effective team communication as a group-level job resource, whereas middle managers from Department C reported lack of training in communication skills as a group-level job demand. Middle managers from all three departments agreed about supportive and participatory leadership as a crucial leader-level job resource. Nonetheless, middle managers tended to agree about lack of formal training in leadership skills as a leader-level job demand. Middle managers from all three departments agreed about high workload, long shifts, and work-life balance issues as intertwining organizational-level job demands. Middle managers from Department B and Department C agreed about top-down decision-making as an organizational level job demand, whereas middle managers from Department A did not mention it. Also, middle managers from Department B and Department C agreed about limited psychological support services, although middle managers from Department B described workplace mental health initiatives as discontinuous and little participated, whereas middle managers from Department C described workplace mental health initiatives as poor.

Employees from all three departments reported intrinsic motivation to promote patients' health and well-being as an individual-level job resource – and this finding was quite at odds with both senior and middle managers' reports. All employees mentioned positive social climate, team support, and team cohesion as crucial group-level job resources – and this finding was consistent with both senior and middle managers' reports. Nevertheless, employees from Department A and Department C mentioned interpersonal conflicts and ineffective team communication as group-level job demands. Employees from all three departments agreed about ineffective leadership as a leader-level job demand, which was also associated with interpersonal conflicts and poor communication. Finally, all employees agreed about top-down decision-making, lack of professional recognition, and work-life conflicts as organizational-level job demands. Employees from Department B reported conflicts with customers as a job demand, whereas employees from Department C even described positive relationships with patients and patients' relatives as a job resource. Employees from Department A and Department B agreed about lack of workplace mental health policies and practices, whereas employees from Department C mentioned an organizational effort to implement – even if discontinuous – psychological support initiatives.

Overall, shared versus diverging mental models of local working conditions could be gathered across both hierarchical positions and departments. On the one hand, employees mentioned intrinsic motivation as an individual-level job resource more than senior and middle managers did. In fact, senior and middle managers described low employee motivation as an individual-level job demand. On the other hand, senior and middle managers mentioned effective leadership as a leader-level job resource more than employees did. In fact, employees described ineffective leadership as a leader-level job demand. All healthcare workers tended to agree about effective teamwork as a crucial group-level job resource. Also, all healthcare workers tended to agree about organizational-level job demands, such as top-down decision-making, lack of workplace mental health initiatives, and lack of psychological support services. In general, employees seemed to agree on workplace mental health issues more than senior and middle managers. Also, the organizational level seemed to be the most critical one for all healthcare workers.

Ultimately, workplace mental health needs' assessment findings might vary within the same healthcare organization, as well as within the same hierarchical position – depending on healthcare departments – and within the same healthcare department – depending on hierarchical positions. Differences in results from assessment exercises may depend on perceptions of local working conditions. This was the case in the herein described workplace mental health needs' assessment exercise since each department the assessment activities took place in corresponded to a unique work and organizational culture – e.g., workers providing healthcare versus research services, workers in central versus peripheral hospital, and so on. Thus, such differences reflect the organizational complexity of the targeted public healthcare institution, which is to be considered when performing workplace mental health needs' assessment exercises.

Suggestions for Improvement and Action Plan

The needs' assessment exercise allowed to inform a tailored action plan to enhance workplace mental health within the targeted organizational contexts. To ensure fit between the organizational context and subsequently implemented interventions (Peters et al., 2020), and thanks to the participatory approach, healthcare workers themselves offered concrete, practical, and applicable suggestions for improving mental health in their work environments. These suggestions varied according to shared or diverging mental models about local working conditions.

In Department A, middle managers suggested individual-level training programmes for employees to reduce the emotional burden associated with dealing with interpersonally challenging customers, as well as leader-level training programmes for managers to develop stronger delegating skills. Training was recommended to take place during working hours to ensure healthcare workers' participation by preventing prolonging workload after the working day. Suggestions for organizational-level interventions included the provision of better career development opportunities and structured psychological support services. Particularly, debriefing sessions were envisaged whereby healthcare workers could discuss lessons learned from the COVID-19 experience. Also, a structured job rotation plan was suggested to increase individual skills and reduce boredom and resistance to change. Special attention was recommended to newcomers and older workers, since the former may find themselves involved in sudden and unstructured job rotations, whereas the latter's expertise should be exploited in end-of-career plans. Another suggestion entailed the implementation of flexible and innovative management models to overcome heavy bureaucracy; for instance, it was stated, "We have a shift management system that appeared to look innovative, but it is cumbersome".

Employees from Department A suggested scheduled clinical discussions to enhance individual skills and critical thinking about work. Structured psychological support was described as a priority. Particularly, top-down psychological support program was suggested to reduce workplace mental health stigma. For instance, it was stated, "We may need some hours of supervision, in which a psychologist comes to us, and everyone in the group talks about what they want. It could also be useful on an individual level, to talk about work but also other stuff, and this should be openly welcomed".

In Department B, senior managers mainly suggested leader-level interventions, with particular attention to middle managers as they find themselves between managing employees' needs and achieving organizational goals (cfr., Gjerde & Alvesson, 2020). Leveraging upon top managerial support towards workplace mental health initiatives and ensuring constant monitoring of activities were recommended as strategies to promote interventions' long-term sustainability as well as workers' participation and perceptions of usefulness. Also, organizational-level interventions were suggested as solutions to work unpredictability, resource cuts, and patients' medical complexity; these included the refinement of organizational models and the conduction of thematic workshops where healthcare workers could disclose problems and perspectives.

Middle managers from Department B suggested individual-level training programmes for employees to promote communication skills when dealing with healthcare customers. Also, training on technical skills was suggested to facilitate staff rotation in hospital departments suffering from personnel shortages.

Suggestions for group-level interventions included the improvement of interdepartmental communication. Leader-level training programmes for managers were suggested to support open dialogue with employees. Managing technological malfunctioning, providing structured psychological support – particularly to deal with COVID-19's mental health aftermaths –, and raising awareness about workplace mental health issues were listed as organizational-level interventions.

In Department C, middle managers suggested individual-level training programmes for employees to promote coping strategies in face of emotional distress associated with COVID-19 and interpersonally challenging customers. Physical activity group sessions were suggested to promote interprofessional team climate. Suggestions for organizational-level interventions included providing structured psychological support to guide healthcare workers through the COVID-19 experience, establishing periodical job rotation to facilitate a shared vision of organizational needs, enhancing work-life flexibility, valorizing human resources, and scheduling shifts based on individual preferences – e.g., based on where one lives, based on whether one prefers to work at day rather than at night, and so on.

Employees from Department C suggested regular meetings to share objectives, work plans, and updates. Psychological support services were suggested to improve healthcare workers' communication skills and behavioral strategies to manage problematic work situations or challenging customers.

As a final phase of the workplace mental health needs' assessment process, an action plan was developed. Healthcare workers' needs and suggestions were reported to the project's Steering Committee, which was composed of key stakeholders from each targeted hospital department. The aim was to define consistent interventions for each department. Factors to job resources – i.e., elements to preserve – and factors to reduce job demands – i.e., elements to improve – were identified. In Department A, elements to preserve included work engagement and resilience, team cohesion and support, leader-member exchange and support, and internal psychological support services. On the other hand, elements to improve included intra-team and inter-departmental team building, leader-level training courses, and job rotation. In Department B, elements to preserve included shared vision and identity, engagement, intrinsic motivation, team cohesion and support, and internal psychological support services. On the other hand, elements to improve included communication skills – i.e., between healthcare workers and customers, as well as between managers and employees. Finally, in Department C, elements to preserve included intrinsic motivation, intergenerational collaboration, and internal psychological support services. On the other hand, elements to improve included stress management skills, team building, and leadership skills.

LESSONS LEARNED AND RECOMMENDATIONS

Some lessons could be learned from performing the workplace mental health needs assessment exercise. It yielded several insights which may reveal useful to both researchers and occupational mental health practitioners to carry out workplace assessment exercises in the healthcare sector.

First, in line with Nielsen et al. (2013), the constant interaction with an organizational representative acting as a main contact person can be recommended to implement activities as planned. For instance, this may prove particularly relevant about sampling. At the time of conducting the herein described assessment exercise, healthcare personnel's working time in the targeted organization was fully devoted to facing COVID-19's first wave in Italy. Also, work shifts rotation influenced recruitment in focus groups. As a result, this scenario made convenience sampling unavoidable. Then, available healthcare workers were recruited thanks to close collaboration with the Health and Safety Manager, who played a pivotal role in facilitating employee participation and engaging the final interviewed sample.

Similarly, the instalment of a project's Steering Committee can be recommended. In the current case, the Steering Committee was composed of the Health and Safety Manager, the Workers Safety Representative, the Directors of the three targeted departments, and the Nursing Manager. Each stakeholder provided a specific contribution. The Health and Safety Manager and the Workers Safety Representative planned and implemented a structured communication strategy, while the three Directors and the Nursing Manager facilitated employee participation and ensured the project-organization fit. Employee participation was facilitated by encouraging healthcare workers to take part in the upcoming needs assessment activities, while project-organization fit was ensured by making sure that the relevance and usefulness of the upcoming needs assessment activities were correctly perceived in each working environment. In addition, communications from the General Director of the healthcare institution revealed crucial to show the importance of the project and to guarantee healthcare workers' commitment. Ultimately, it is important to involve all the relevant stakeholders of the foreseen activities, otherwise it may be difficult to access the targeted working environments. Nevertheless, due to ongoing organizational changes, the stakeholders' engagement operation was not without obstacles. That is, when relevant stakeholders changed, effort was required to take the new stakeholders on board. For instance, the election of a new General Director called for a need to re-establish a common vision on the running workplace mental health project. Also, the Health and Safety Manager's retirement slowed down the process due to bureaucracy, despite this person not leaving the project itself.

Regarding the quality of gathered data, recruiting healthcare workers from different hierarchical positions and hospital departments may have ensured a sufficient degree of triangulation (Ramos et al., 2020). It also allowed to take the perceptual distance phenomenon into account (Gibson et al., 2001, 2009). However, as a drawback of the deployed recruitment and data collection strategy, ingroup bias might have occurred within focus groups. For instance, doctors, nurses, and healthcare assistants in Department B seemed to express consistent opinions depending on the belonging occupational group. Further, a positive image of leadership was likely to stem from the semi-structured individual interviews. Leaders may tend to overestimate themselves and their contribution (Stone et al., 2002) to creating a mentally healthy workplace. Therefore, the role of the interviewer in clarifying expectations related to the needs assessment is crucial; (s)he should encourage participants' willingness to reveal their sincere viewpoints by creating a climate of psychological safety within a comfortable and convivial meeting environment.

Another challenge in interviews and focus groups related to ethics. In the herein described assessment exercise healthcare workers were reassured that their privacy would be protected. Accordingly, each worker was asked to self-generate a code to preserve their anonymity when data would have been stored while allowing researchers to link them to the participants. Before participation, all workers were allowed to read an informed consent form detailing the participation procedure, the contents of the project, the purpose of the data collection, the modalities of future dissemination of data, the participants' rights, and the contact points for any inquiry. It was underlined that participation in the assessment activities was voluntary and that it could be withdrawn at any time without any consequence. Trust-based measures were taken by focus groups' facilitators by clearly explaining the importance of every participant's compliance with the ethical requirements of anonymity, privacy, and confidentiality. Each worker was advised to respect the confidentiality of what was shared by others during the focus group as well as to respect the others' words and viewpoints without judging or attacking anyone. Also, facilitators committed to a strict code of ethical scientific and professional conduct whereby they should not disclose any sensitive information they might be aware of regarding the interviewed persons.

Finally, the development of an actional plan as a final phase of the workplace mental health needs' assessment process can be recommended. The action plan signals that the assessment exercise is not an end, but rather a means to the design and development of effective interventions to reduce job demands and promote job resources at multiple workplace levels. As such, this phase may help to strengthen the partnership between the assessors and the organizational stakeholders. Involving organizational representatives within the action plan phase allows them to have their say about future initiatives based on the results from the needs assessment, which can maximize the feasibility and monitorability of implemented actions.

CONCLUSION

Interventions addressing healthcare workers' mental health should build upon an exhaustive understanding of causes of stress and factors of positive mental health in the workplace. Also, interventions should reduce job demands and promote job resources at all workplace levels, such as the individual, the group, the leader, and the organization. As a mean to the design and development of tailored interventions, workplace mental health needs assessment exercises should follow the same logic. Particularly, participatory, bottom-up assessment activities are required to directly ask healthcare workers what they feel about their working environment, as this cannot be known a priori.

The present chapter drawn upon a workplace mental health needs assessment exercise involving senior managers, middle managers, and employees from three departments of a large healthcare institution in Northern Italy. Healthcare workers' perceptions of local working conditions could be gathered at different IGLO levels via semi-structured individual interviews and focus groups. By integrating the JD-R and IGLO models into one analytical framework, two separate research strands were linked, and such an integrated framework can be used in future healthcare workers' mental health studies. Also, in line with Nielsen et al. (2013), Nielsen et al. (2014), and Abildgaard et al. (2018), cognitive mapping revealed effective in mapping job demands and job resources at different IGLO levels, how they interact and, thus, what interventions can be developed. Furthermore, similarities and differences in mental models across hierarchical positions and hospital departments could be analyzed.

Practical recommendations on how to effectively conduct assessment activities could be developed. Therefore, the present chapter contributes to informing some core design and implementation principles of workplace mental health needs' assessment activities in healthcare settings. These includes, among others, encompassing both job demands and job resources at individual, group, leader, and organizational levels; constantly interacting with relevant organizational representatives and stakeholders; installing a devoted Steering Committee; clarifying expectations towards the needs assessment exercise; ensuring psychological safety while conducting the assessment activities; and including an action plan phase at the end of the needs' assessment process. Moreover, throughout the workplace mental health needs assessment exercise, healthcare workers themselves, both managers and employees, provided some practical suggestions for improvement of mental health in their workplaces, to inform an action plan and choose interventions to enhance workplace mental health. Main foreseen solutions included, among others, training programs on both hard – e.g., job-related techniques – and soft skills – e.g., emotional distress and interpersonal conflict management, leadership, and communication –; creating better career development opportunities; refining job rotation plans; renewing the organizational management models; introducing both work-oriented and people-oriented workshops; scheduling physical activity group sessions; and providing structured psychological support services.

Researchers and occupational mental health practitioners are hereby provided with a usable assessment methodology to gather job demands and job resources that healthcare workers might experience at different workplace levels. The methodology considers the local conditions healthcare workers may find themselves working in or their hierarchical positions within their peculiar work environment. In general, the described procedure might inform the design and implementation of workplace mental health needs' assessment activities in healthcare settings, but also the development of interventions based on suggestions for improvement from participants – as long as some critical issues are taken care of, such as, for instance, the engagement of all relevant stakeholder, the recruitment and sampling of participants, the potential methodological bias which may threaten the quality of collected data, and ethical challenges.

One limitation of the presented work relates to the concept of shift work and the negative effects that shift work has been found to cause to healthcare workers (Brown et al., 2020). Relevant differences might exist in the mental health of daytime versus nighttime healthcare workers. However, in the described study, information about whether the involved healthcare workers were shift workers, daytime workers or nighttime workers was not systematically collected, as it was out of the scope of the research and intervention project that the chapter was based on. It may have happened to come across this type of information during the interviews and focus groups that have been run with the healthcare workers, but this would not be enough to perform a proper analysis or state a precise distinction between such categories of workers. Thus, it is not exactly clear if all healthcare workers that participated in the study were daytime workers or whether any nighttime workers were tested. This could impact the generalizability of the retrieved results. Nighttime workers may have provided different responses and may have different managers, which could influence the results.

Recommendations for effective implementation of workplace mental health needs' assessment activities in healthcare should be considered considering the constraints that may be imposed by the highly dynamic contingencies that healthcare settings may find themselves in. The organizational impact of COVID-19 could be one example. Contingencies may prevent the involvement of key actors, delay the process as compared to what was initially planned, and determine deviations from or adjustments to the original project. Therefore, flexibility and adaptivity of deployed instruments, tools, procedures, techniques, and methodologies may reveal critical factors for those willing to perform workplace mental health assessments in the healthcare sector.

ACKNOWLEDGMENT

This research has received funding from the European Union's Horizon 2020 research and innovation programme under the project H-WORK – Multilevel Interventions to Promote Mental Health in SMEs and Public Workplaces (grant agreement No 847386).

REFERENCES

Abildgaard, J. S., Nielsen, K., & Sverke, M. (2018). Can job insecurity be managed? Evaluating an organizational-level intervention addressing the negative effects of restructuring. *Work and Stress*, *32*(2), 105–123. doi:10.1080/02678373.2017.1367735

Bakker, A. B., & Demerouti, E. (2017). Job demands-resources theory: Taking stock and looking forward. *Journal of Occupational Health Psychology*, *22*(3), 273–285. doi:10.1037/ocp0000056 PMID:27732008

Bakker, A. B., & Demerouti, E. (2018). Multiple levels in job demands-resources theory: Implications for employee well-being and performance. In E. Diener, S. Oishi, & L. Tay (Eds.), *Handbook of Well-Being* (pp. 1–13). DEF Publishers. https://nobascholar.com

Bazeley, P., & Jackson, K. (2013). *Qualitative Data Analysis with NVivo* (2nd ed.). SAGE Publications Ltd.

Broetje, S., Jenny, G. J., & Bauer, G. F. (2020). The key job demands and resources of nursing staff: An integrative review of reviews. *Frontiers in Psychology*, *11*, 84. doi:10.3389/fpsyg.2020.00084 PMID:32082226

Brown, J. P., Martin, D., Nagaria, Z., Verceles, A. C., Jobe, S. L., & Wickwire, E. M. (2020). Mental health consequences of shift work: An updated review. *Current Psychiatry Reports*, *22*(7), 1–7. doi:10.100711920-020-1131-z PMID:31955278

Chen, S.-L., Shih, C.-T., & Chi, N.-W. (2018). A multilevel job demands-resources model of work engagement: Antecedents, consequences, and boundary conditions. *Human Performance*, *31*(5), 282–304. doi:10.1080/08959285.2018.1531867

Cheng, H., Yang, H., Ding, Y., & Wang, B. (2020). Nurses' mental health and patient safety: An extension of the job demands-resources model. *Journal of Nursing Management*, *28*(3), 653–663. doi:10.1111/jonm.12971 PMID:32052511

Christensen, M., Innstrand, S. T., & Saksvik, P. Ø. (2020). Healthy workplaces: Designing and implementing health-promoting organizational interventions in healthcare. In L. Tevik Løsveth & A. de Lange (Eds.), *Integrating the Organization of Health Services, Worker Wellbeing and Quality of Care* (pp. 1–15). Springer. doi:10.1007/978-3-030-59467-1_14

Christensen, M., Innstrand, S. T., Saksvik, P. Ø., & Nielsen, K. (2019). The line manager's role in implementing successful organizational interventions. *The Spanish Journal of Psychology*, *22*(e5), 1–11. doi:10.1017jp.2019.4 PMID:30819272

Day, A., & Nielsen, K. (2017). What does our organization do to help our well-being? Creating healthy workplaces and workers. In N. Chmiel, F. Fraccaroli, & M. Sverke (Eds.), *An Introduction to Work and Organizational Psychology: An International Perspective* (pp. 295–314). Wiley-Blackwell. doi:10.1002/9781119168058.ch16

Di Tecco, C., Nielsen, K., Ghelli, M., Ronchetti, M., Marzocchi, I., Persechino, B., & Iavicoli, S. (2020). Improving working conditions and job satisfaction in healthcare: A study concept design on a participatory organizational level intervention in psychosocial risks management. *International Journal of Environmental Research and Public Health*, *17*(10), 3677. doi:10.3390/ijerph17103677 PMID:32456147

Fridrich, A., Jenny, G. J., & Bauer, G. F. (2015). The context, process, and outcome evaluation model for organisational health interventions. *BioMed Research International, 414832*, 1–12. doi:10.1155/2015/414832 PMID:26557665

Garman, A. N., Corrigan, P. W., & Morris, S. (2002). Staff burnout and patient satisfaction: Evidence of relationships at the care unit level. *Journal of Occupational Health Psychology*, *7*(3), 235–241. doi:10.1037/1076-8998.7.3.235 PMID:12148955

Gibson, C. B., Conger, J. A., & Cooper, C. (2001). Perceptual distance: The impact of differences in team leader and member perceptions across cultures. In J. Osland, M. E. Mendenhall, R. S. Reiche, & B. Szkudlarek (Eds.), *Advances in Global Leadership* (Vol. 2, pp. 245–276). Emerald Group Publishing Limited. doi:10.1016/S1535-1203(01)02122-0

Gibson, C. B., Cooper, C. D., & Conger, J. A. (2009). Do you see what we see? The complex effects of perceptual distance between leaders and teams. *The Journal of Applied Psychology*, *94*(1), 62–76. doi:10.1037/a0013073 PMID:19186896

Gjerde, S., & Alvesson, M. (2020). Sandwiched: Exploring role and identity of middle managers in the genuine middle. *Human Relations*, *73*(1), 124–151. doi:10.1177/0018726718823243

Gómez-Urquiza, J. L., Albendín-García, L., Velando-Soriano, A., Ortega-Campos, E., Ramírez-Baena, L., Membrive-Jiménez, M. J., & Suleiman-Martos, N. (2020). Burnout in palliative care nurses, prevalence and risk factors: A systematic review and meta-analysis. *International Journal of Environmental Research and Public Health*, *17*(20), 7672. doi:10.3390/ijerph17207672 PMID:33096682

Hall, G. B., Dollard, M. F., & Coward, J. (2010). Psychosocial safety climate: Development of the PSC-12. *International Journal of Stress Management*, *17*(4), 353–383. doi:10.1037/a0021320

Lavrakas, P. (2008). *Encyclopedia of Survey Research Methods*. SAGE Publications. doi:10.4135/9781412963947

López Gómez, M. A., Gundersen, D. A., Boden, L. I., Sorensen, G., Katz, J. N., Collins, J. E., Wagner, G., Vriniotis, M. G., & Williams, J. A. R. (2021). Validation of the Workplace Integrated Safety and Health (WISH) assessment in a sample of nursing homes using Item Response Theory (IRT) methods. *BMJ Open*, *11*(6), e045656. doi:10.1136/bmjopen-2020-045656 PMID:34145013

Martin, A., Karanika-Murray, M., Biron, C., & Sanderson, K. (2016). The psychosocial work environment, employee mental health and organizational interventions: Improving research and practice by taking a multilevel approach. *Stress and Health*, *32*(3), 201–215. doi:10.1002mi.2593 PMID:25044861

Membrive-Jiménez, M. J., Pradas-Hernández, L., Suleiman-Martos, N., Vargas-Román, K., Cañadas-De la Fuente, G., Gomez-Urquiza, J. L., & De la Fuente-Solana, E. I. (2020). Burnout in nursing managers: A systematic review and meta-analysis of related factors, levels and prevalence. *International Journal of Environmental Research and Public Health*, *17*(11), 3983. doi:10.3390/ijerph17113983 PMID:32512738

Nielsen, K., Abildgaard, J. S., & Daniels, K. (2014). Putting context into organizational intervention design: Using tailored questionnaires to measure initiatives for worker well-being. *Human Relations*, *67*(12), 1537–1560. doi:10.1177/0018726714525974

Nielsen, K., Antino, M., Rodríguez-Muñoz, A., & Sanz-Vergel, A. (2021). Is it me or us? The impact of individual and collective participation on work engagement and burnout in a cluster-randomized organisational intervention. *Work and Stress*, *35*(4), 374–397. Advance online publication. doi:10.1080/02678373.2021.1889072

Nielsen, K., & Christensen, M. (2021). Positive participatory organizational interventions: A multilevel approach for creating healthy workplaces. *Frontiers in Psychology*, *12*, 696245. doi:10.3389/fpsyg.2021.696245 PMID:34262513

Nielsen, K., Nielsen, M. B., Ogbonnaya, C., Känsälä, M., Saari, E., & Isaksson, K. (2017). Workplace resources to improve both employee well-being and performance: A systematic review and meta-analysis. *Work and Stress*, *31*(2), 101–120. doi:10.1080/02678373.2017.1304463

Nielsen, K., Randall, R., Holten, A.-L., & González, E. R. (2010). Conducting organizational-level occupational health interventions: What works? *Work and Stress*, *24*(3), 234–259. doi:10.1080/02678373.2010.515393

Nielsen, K., Stage, M., Abildgaard, J. S., & Brauer, C. V. (2013). Participatory intervention from an organizational perspective: Employees as active agents in creating a healthy work environment. In G. Bauer & G. Jenny (Eds.), *Salutogenic Organizations and Change* (pp. 327–350). Springer. doi:10.1007/978-94-007-6470-5_18

Persson, R., Hansen, Å. M., Garde, A. H., Kristiansen, J., Nordander, C., Balogh, I., Ohlsson, K., Östergren, P.-O., & Ørbæk, P. (2012). Can the job content questionnaire be used to assess structural and organizational properties of the work environment? *International Archives of Occupational and Environmental Health*, *85*(1), 45–55. doi:10.100700420-011-0647-2 PMID:21573960

Peters, S. E., Nielsen, K. M., Nagler, E. M., Revette, A. C., Madden, J., & Sorensen, G. (2020). Ensuring organization-intervention fit for a participatory organizational intervention to improve food service workers' health and wellbeing: Workplace organizational health study. *Journal of Occupational and Environmental Medicine*, *62*(2), e33–e45. doi:10.1097/JOM.0000000000001792 PMID:31815814

Ramos, S., Costa, P., Passos, A. M., Silva, S. A., & Sacadura-Leite, E. (2020). Intervening on burnout in complex organizations – The incomplete process of an action research in the hospital. *Frontiers in Psychology*, *11*, 2203. doi:10.3389/fpsyg.2020.02203 PMID:33071844

Schaufeli, W. B. (2017). Applying the Job Demands-Resources model: A "how to" guide to measuring and tackling work engagement and burnout. *Organizational Dynamics*, *46*(2), 120–132. doi:10.1016/j.orgdyn.2017.04.008

Sim, J., & Waterfield, J. (2019). Focus group methodology: Some ethical challenges. *Quality & Quantity*, *53*(6), 3003–3022. doi:10.100711135-019-00914-5

Sorensen, G., Sparer, E., Williams, J. A. R., Gundersen, D., Boden, L. I., Dennerlein, J. T., Hashimoto, D., Katz, J. N., McLellan, D. L., Okechukwu, C. A., Pronk, N. P., Revette, A., & Wagner, G. R. (2018). Measuring best practices for workplace safety, health and wellbeing: The Workplace Integrated Safety and Health Assessment. *Journal of Occupational and Environmental Medicine*, *60*(5), 430–439. doi:10.1097/JOM.0000000000001286 PMID:29389812

Stone, A. A., Turkkan, J. S., Bachrach, C. A., Jobe, J. B., Kurtzman, H. S., & Cain, V. S. (2002). *The Science of Self-Report: Implications for Research and Practice*. Lawrence Erlbaum Associates.

Tafvelin, S., von Thiele Schwarz, U., Nielsen, K., & Hasson, H. (2018). Employees' and line managers' active involvement in participatory organizational interventions: Examining direct, reversed, and reciprocal effects on well-being. *Stress and Health*, *35*(1), 69–80. doi:10.1002mi.2841 PMID:30303299

Teo, S. T. T., Nguyen, D., Trevelyan, F., Lamm, F., & Boocock, M. (2021). Workplace bullying, psychological hardiness, and accidents and injuries in nursing: A moderated mediation model. *PLoS One*, *16*(1), e0244426. doi:10.1371/journal.pone.0244426 PMID:33417612

Teoh, K. R. H., Hassard, J., & Cox, T. (2020). Individual and psychosocial predictors of hospital doctors' work-related: A multilevel and moderation perspective. *Health Care Management Review*, *45*(2), 162–172. doi:10.1097/HMR.0000000000000207 PMID:29957704

Van den Broeck, A., De Cuyper, N., De Witte, H., & Vansteenkiste, M. (2010). Not all job demands are equal: Differentiating job hindrances and job challenges in the Job Demands-Resources model. *European Journal of Work and Organizational Psychology*, *19*(6), 735–759. doi:10.1080/13594320903223839

Vignoli, M., Nielsen, K., Guglielmi, D., Tabanelli, M. C., & Violante, F. S. (2017). The importance of context in screening in occupational health interventions in organizations: A mixed methods study. *Frontiers in Psychology*, *8*, 1347. doi:10.3389/fpsyg.2017.01347 PMID:28848468

Weick, K. E. (1995). *Sensemaking in Organizations*. Sage Publications, Inc.

ADDITIONAL READING

de Lange, A. H., Løvseth, L. T., Teoh, K. R.-H., & Christensen, M. (2020). Editorial: Healthy healthcare: Empirical occupational health research and evidence-based practice. *Frontiers in Psychology*, *11*, 2236. doi:10.3389/fpsyg.2020.02236 PMID:33178057

Demerouti, E., Bakker, A. B., Nachreiner, F., & Schaufeli, W. B. (2001). The job demands-resources model of burnout. *The Journal of Applied Psychology*, *86*(3), 499–512. doi:10.1037/0021-9010.86.3.499 PMID:11419809

Hsieh, H.-F., & Shannon, S. E. (2005). Three approaches to qualitative content analysis. *Qualitative Health Research*, *15*(9), 1277–1288. doi:10.1177/1049732305276687 PMID:16204405

International Labour Organisation. (2020). *Workplace Well-Being*. Retrieved from: https://www.ilo.org/safework/areasofwork/workplace-health-promotion-and-well-being/WCMS_118396/lang--en/index.htm

Juniper, B. (2011). Defining employee wellbeing. *Occupational Health*, *63*(10), 25.

LaMontagne, A. D., Martin, A., Page, K. M., Reavley, N. J., Noblet, A. J., Milner, A. J., Keegel, T., & Smith, P. M. (2014). Workplace mental health: Developing an integrated intervention approach. *BMC Psychiatry*, *14*(1), 131. doi:10.1186/1471-244X-14-131 PMID:24884425

Maassen, S. M., van Oostveen, C., Vermeulen, H., & Weggelar, M. (2021). Defining a positive work environment for hospital healthcare professionals: A Delphi study. *PLoS One*, *16*(2), e0247530. doi:10.1371/journal.pone.0247530 PMID:33630923

Salanova, M., Llorens, S., Cifre, E., & Martínez, I. M. (2012). We need a HERO! Toward a validation of the Healthy and Resilient Organization (HERO) model. *Group & Organization Management*, *37*(6), 785–822. doi:10.1177/1059601112470405

Søvold, L. E., Naslund, J. A., Kousoulis, A. A., Saxena, S., Qoronfleh, M. W., Grobler, C., & Münter, L. (2021). Prioritizing the mental health and well-being of healthcare workers: An urgent global public health priority. *Frontiers in Public Health*, *9*, 679397. doi:10.3389/fpubh.2021.679397 PMID:34026720

Taris, T. W., & Schaufeli, W. B. (2016). The Job Demands-Resources model. In S. Clarke, T. M. Probst, F. Guldenmund, & J. Passmore (Eds.), *The Wiley Blackwell Handbook of the Psychology of Occupational Safety and Workplace Health* (pp. 157–180). John Wiley.

World Health Organization. (2018). *Mental Health: Strengthening Our Response*. Retrieved from: https://www.who.int/news-room/fact-sheets/detail/mental-health-strengthening-our-response

KEY TERMS AND DEFINITIONS

Bottom-Up Decision-Making: A type of organizational decision-making process whereby employees are seen as key informants about working conditions as well as active actors able to change their workplace environment. As such, employees are directly involved and called to participate in, contribute to, and influence the decision-making process itself.

IGLO: Ecological model of mental health in the workplace. The model posits that sources of mental health and well-being at work exist at five different levels, namely the individual (I), the group or work team (G), the leader (L), and the organization (O).

Job Demands: The physical, social, or organizational job aspects requiring sustained physical or psychological effort and costs, which have a detrimental effect on employees' well-being and job performance.

Job Resources: The physical, psychological, social, and organizational aspects of a job that can help employees achieve work goals, which can boost employees' well-being and job performance and buffer the detrimental effect of job demands.

Mental Health: A state of well-being in which an individual realizes his/her own abilities, can cope with the everyday stresses of life, can work productively, and can contribute to his/her community. Mental health is an integral and essential component of health, which is a state of complete physical, mental, and social well-being and not merely the absence of disease or infirmity. Mental health is more than just the absence of mental disorders or disabilities.

Needs Assessment: Data collection process aimed to identify organizational needs in terms of work-related mental health, and to select tailored interventions addressing the satisfaction of those needs subsequently.

Personal Resources: The physical or psychological aspect of an individual that can help achieve work goals, well-being, and performance.

Top-Down Decision-Making: A type of organizational decision-making process whereby employees are seen as passive subjects of the workplace environment and, therefore, unable to change their workplace environment. As such, employees are not involved in the process and decisions are made by the managers only.

Workplace Well-Being: All aspects of working life, from the quality and safety of physical environment, to how workers feel about their work, their working environment, the climate at work and work organization, which is perceived to be primarily determined by work, and that can be influenced by workplace interventions.

Chapter 9
Health-Oriented Leadership in Healthcare:
The Role of Supervisor Attitude, Cognition, and Behavior

Claire E. Burnett
Georgia Institute of Technology, USA

Cooper Drose
Georgia Institute of Technology, USA

Keaton A. Fletcher
Georgia Institute of Technology, USA

ABSTRACT

The purpose of this chapter is to explore a model of health-oriented leadership in which healthcare leaders' attitudes and cognitions precipitate their health-oriented leadership behaviors and ultimately impact frontline healthcare workers' health and well-being. To better understand these relationships, this chapter will explore this model at different levels of specificity of leadership including general (e.g., transformational), specific (e.g., health-oriented), and targeted (e.g., sleep). The authors separately examine the ways in which healthcare leaders' health-oriented attitudes, cognitions, and behaviors can impact followers' health and well-being. In doing so, they highlight that internal antecedents (e.g., attitudes and cognitions) are necessary precursors for effective health-oriented leadership behaviors. Then they provide recommendations for research and practice based on the model and the current state of the literature in order to better their understanding of health-oriented leadership while simultaneously improving the health and wellness of frontline healthcare workers.

DOI: 10.4018/978-1-7998-8813-0.ch009

INTRODUCTION

Workplace leadership has a clear and strong impact on followers' work-related attitudes, cognitions, behaviors, and outcomes (e.g., Judge et al., 2004). Although less frequently explored, there is ample evidence to suggest that leadership is also a key antecedent to follower health behaviors and outcomes (Aronsson & Lindh, 2004; Nyberg et al., 2005). For example, within healthcare organizations, destructive leadership has been negatively associated with employee well-being (Schyns & Schilling, 2013), while fair leadership behavior and leadership support have been linked to better employee mental health (Finne et al., 2014). Although many studies have explored the impact of general leadership constructs (e.g., transformational leadership, destructive leadership, leadership support) on follower health and wellness, there has been a recent increase in the empirical examinations of health-oriented leadership and similar specific leadership approaches that explicitly focus on the health and well-being of followers (Rudolph et al., 2020).

Health-oriented leadership is defined as a leader's attitudes toward, and awareness of, followers' health, and behaviors such as effective health-related communication and the design of health promoting working conditions (Franke & Felfe, 2011). Within this specific leadership approach, there are several health-oriented leader cognitions and attitudes that express themselves through domain-specific, health-oriented leader behaviors. Health-oriented leadership is particularly promising for the healthcare industry given the wide range of negative health outcomes that healthcare workers tend to face (Khamisa et al., 2013). Further, the expertise of healthcare employees and leaders ought to make health-oriented leadership particularly effective in healthcare organizations. Although this area of leadership is nascent and few direct studies of health-oriented leadership within healthcare organizations are currently published, we seek to draw upon empirically supported findings from similarly challenging occupations (e.g., military settings) to outline a roadmap for practitioners and researchers alike to better understand and explore the potential mechanisms and outcomes of health-oriented leadership within healthcare organizations.

Specifically, the purpose of this chapter is to explore a model of health-oriented leadership in which healthcare leaders' attitudes and cognitions precipitate their health-oriented leadership behaviors and ultimately impact frontline healthcare workers' health and well-being (see Table 1 for an overview). We separately examine the ways in which healthcare leaders' health-oriented attitudes, cognitions, and behaviors can impact followers' health and well-being. In doing so we highlight that internal antecedents (e.g., attitudes and cognitions) are necessary precursors for effective health-oriented leadership behaviors. Then we provide recommendations for research and practice based on our model and the current state of the literature in order to better our understanding of health-oriented leadership while simultaneously improving the health and wellness of frontline healthcare workers.

LEADERS' HEALTH-ORIENTED COGNITIONS

Cognition is comprised of knowledge (i.e., *what* people know, also referred to as declarative knowledge; Campbell, 1990), the manner in which that knowledge is organized and recalled, and the ability to use that knowledge (Gagne, 1984; Kraiger et al., 1993). Together these aspects of cognition capture not only what an individual knows, but how that knowledge is manipulated and put to use. In the context of leadership, leaders' cognitions ultimately impact followers, the organization, and other stakeholders (Mumford, Watts, & Partlow, 2015). Similarly, although the theory of planned behavior (Ajzen, 1991)

Table 1. Summary Table of Major Topics

	Cognitions	Attitudes	Behaviors
Organization-oriented	Knowledge of organizational policies • Family/medical leave • Employee assistance programs	Attitudes toward organizational policies and change • Champion current health policies • Value diversity • Open to new health policies	Self-directed health behaviors • Set example about self-care • Emotion regulation
Follower-oriented	Knowledge of followers' health needs • Mental health needs • Discrimination based issues	Attitudes toward work and health • Value employee health • Normalize mental health	Follower-directed health behaviors • Provide support to followers • Reduce workplace stressors • Target specific health behaviors

points toward cognitive processes such as cognitive self-regulation as key predictors of individuals' behaviors, it also suggests that one's understanding of norms, resources, and one's own own cognition ultimately impact what behaviors they engage in. In other words, leaders are charged with making sense of the environment, deciding what knowledge is relevant, creating a vision for moving forward (Partlow et al., 2015), and also determining which aspects of that process to share with followers (e.g., Arain et al., 2020).

Asking leaders to actively value, protect, and improve follower health and wellbeing requires a shift in focus and significant effort. Employers have traditionally viewed protecting employee health as a legal requirement (Miller & Haslam, 2009) or a means to improve profit (Pfeffer et al., 2020). Resolving the discrepancy between this perspective and an active interest in employee health may require significant cognitive effort on the part of leaders. Even with regard to one's own health behaviors, change requires significant cognitive effort (Schwarzer, 2001). However, a comprehensive report by the National Health Services (NHS) succinctly captures the importance of leaders' health-related cognitions in their recommendation "that all NHS leaders and managers are developed and equipped to recognise the link between staff health and well-being and organizational performance and that their actions are judged in terms of whether they contribute to or undermine staff health and well-being" (p. 9, Boorman, 2009). The report goes on to recommend that healthcare leaders are explicitly trained in the health and well-being of healthcare employees. Similarly, Dellve and Eriksson (2017) center their model of health-promoting managerial work around leader's "evidence-based knowledge of health-promoting psychosocial work conditions as well as their capability to apply, adapt, and craft sustained managerial work practices" (p. 3). These recommendations highlighting the importance of leaders' health-oriented knowledge echo the broader findings that when multiple paths exist, or problems are novel, ambiguous, or complex, leaders' cognitions are particularly important in predicting outcomes (Mumford et al., 2007; Judge et al., 2004).

Certainly, healthcare professionals already possess a strong foundation of declarative knowledge regarding health, health behaviors, and health outcomes. However, healthcare leaders need to know not only about health behaviors (e.g., smoking, exercise) and their outcomes, but also their organizations' health-related policies (e.g., employee assistance programs, sick leave, family supportive policies; McCarthy et al., 2010). Further, these leaders need to have knowledge of each of their individual subordinates' needs since one of the primary reasons supportive policies go unused is lack of supervisor support (French & Shockley, 2020). Lastly, healthcare leaders need to know about the unique health challenges that healthcare workers are facing (e.g., burnout, abuse, discrimination, etc.; DiBenedetto, 1995; Mohanty et al., 2019). Below we outline these three specific considerations and methods healthcare leaders may use to elicit and learn this information.

Knowledge of Organizational Policies

Within the context of healthcare organizations, health-related knowledge may be readily available, but difficult to apply in the workplace. Ryan and Kossek (2008) developed a model to explain the role supervisors play in work-life policy use, but this model translates to policy use regarding other employee benefits such as employee assistance programs, worker's compensation, or flexible scheduling. Specifically, the model highlights the need for supervisor support of policy use, high quality communication between the leader and subordinates in order to ensure effective policy use, and universal implementation of policies for all employees coupled with an ability to negotiate policy use for employees' specific needs. Unfortunately, many workplace leaders are unfamiliar with employee benefits policies. For example, Laharnar and colleagues (2013) found that roughly 35% of supervisors had not been trained on the Family Medical Leave Act or effective implementation of this policy. Further, roughly 35% did not feel confident in their ability to guide employees through use of the Family Medical Leave Act. Boorman and colleagues (2009) identified lack of supervisor knowledge of employee health services as a target for intervention to improve healthcare worker health, recommending that healthcare leadership should "be fully aware of the role of health and well-being services, including occupational health, as a core service to support and help staff" (p. 12). Similarly, Casper and colleagues (2004) found that supervisors' average self-rated awareness of family-friendly workplace policies was only "to a slight extent", and that this knowledge in turn predicted how frequently leaders referred employees to employer-sponsored work-family programs. With regard to other organizational policies that have direct impacts on employee health, Shanafelt and Noseworthy (2017) point toward flexible scheduling policies and vacation policies as two organizational levers managers can capitalize on to reduce healthcare worker burnout. But leaders need to have knowledge of these policies and how to effectively use them without causing harm to their followers' careers.

Clearly, even if healthcare organizations take steps to promote employee health through provision of flexible work arrangement policies, employee assistance programs, or other related policies, leaders' lack of knowledge of these programs/policies is a limiting factor in their effectiveness. Therefore, to ultimately enhance employee health, healthcare organizations should ensure their workplace leaders and managers are trained in all of the employee health related benefits the company offers. This may be too much information to remember, so providing easy-to-use cognitive aids such as handouts or mobile apps to help offload this cognition (Fletcher & Bedwell, 2017) may further encourage leadership support of these policies.

Knowledge of Followers' Health Needs

Healthcare workers face unique physical hazards (abuse and violence), chemical and infectious hazards, as well as psychological hazards such as stress and burnout (Moore & Kaczmarek, 1990; Gorman et al., 2013). Zuckerman highlights shiftwork and long hours as a potentially underrecognized threat to healthcare employee health and safety which leaders need to be educated about (2013). Healthcare leaders need to be aware of these hazards, the appropriate methods of prevention, and the appropriate methods of mitigating harm once they have occurred. One barrier to gaining this knowledge is the well-documented underreporting of incidents of injury or harm. For example, less than one third of healthcare workers report their experiences of workplace violence (Phillips, 2016). This underreporting may lead to distortions in the cognitions of healthcare leaders, resulting in their underestimation of these hazards and their own ability to prevent them. Simple awareness of the range and severity of hazards, as well as their frequency, is a necessary cognitive foundation for leaders working to protect and improve the health of their followers.

However, employee health needs and goals are likely to not all be the same, suggesting that there will rarely be a one-size-fits-all implementation of any health-oriented policy or practice. One of the key requirements of leaders is individualized consideration (Bass, 1985) in which leaders learn the unique needs and motivators of each follower. Some have even argued that healthy leadership is "a specific manifestation of the broader leadership style of individualized consideration, which involves leaders showing an awareness of and concern for their followers' health and wellbeing" (p. 18, Rudolph et al., 2020). Fundamentally, this component of leadership is rooted in changes in leader cognition. An example of individualized consideration is the creation and enactment of idiosyncratic deals (i-deals; Liao et al., 2016). By working with individual subordinates to understand what their specific needs and motivations are, leaders are able to establish i-deals which allow for customization of the work environment and tasks. These i-deals are not made in isolation, instead being formed in the context of the work unit and thus interacting with one another (e.g., Vidyarthi et al., 2016). Thus, it is important to gain an understanding of what each followers' specific needs are and how they fit together before enacting i-deals. Depending on the number of subordinates a healthcare leader has, this can be a daunting task. Again, we suggest using external cognitive aids to help organize, distribute, and manipulate this information. Similarly, when seeking information about what i-deals would be beneficial to employees, it is important to offer this opportunity to all followers and ask about the same potential needs (e.g., flexible scheduling, more frequent breaks) with all employees.

When considering individual subordinates' unique needs, it is also worth considering their unique exposure to stressors. Equality of policy enforcement would remove manager discretion and ensure that all employees have equal access to, and use of policies. However, not all healthcare workers face the same stressors, and thus equitable distribution and enforcement of policies based on need may be more appropriate, which places a greater burden and responsibility on the healthcare leader. For example, female physicians and male nurses face gender-based discrimination (Hu et al., 2019; Kronsberg et al., 2017), and healthcare workers who are racial minorities also face discrimination from both patients as well as their colleagues (Nunez-Smith et al., 2007). Among surgical residents that over 30% had experienced gender-based discrimination, nearly 17% had experienced racial discrimination and 30% had experienced some form of abuse (verbal and/or physical; Hu et al., 2019). This discrimination came from both patients and their families; further, attending surgeons themselves were responsible for large portions of the sexual harassment and abuse experiences. Discrimination can lead to burnout and suicidal ideation (Hu et al., 2019) as well as physical symptoms and long-term health conditions (Mays et al., 2007). Leaders have a responsibility to acknowledge that members of minority groups face unique stressors that may require additional support and resources to protect their health. Therefore, it is critical for healthcare leaders to take active steps to learn about the unique experiences and stressors that healthcare workers face based on their perceived group membership. In doing so, leaders will create a cognitive foundation upon which they can alter their own behaviors (e.g., reducing supervisor perpetrated abuse and harassment) but also establish equitable distribution of resources to ensure that particularly vulnerable workers are receiving the access to policies and resources they need.

Lastly, one of the biggest, and potentially underreported, challenges facing healthcare workers, in particular, is mental health struggles. Healthcare workers face burnout, depression, trauma, and high rates of suicidal ideation (e.g., Coughlan et al., 2017; West et al., 2018). Workplace-related post-traumatic stress disorder (PTSD) has been linked to a range of somatic symptoms (Milligan-Saville et al., 2017). Strikingly, one study found that one in three participating healthcare providers screened positive for PTSD, but only 55% of healthcare providers had received education on PTSD (Luftman et al., 2017). Burnout and mental health challenges, like PTSD, among healthcare workers have been associated with alcohol use disorders, neck and back pain, sleep disturbances, and memory challenges (Peterson et al., 2008). To effectively support workers' health and wellbeing, healthcare leaders need to understand the prevalence of mental health challenges, as well as methods of preventing or mitigating them. Further, before leaders can change their behavior to address worker wellbeing, including sharing information about the realities of mental health challenges, they need to understand their own role in this process. One study suggests that supervisor behavior can have a direct impact on employee psychological wellbeing above and beyond social support, work and life stressors, age, and health practices (Gilbreath & Benson, 2004). This knowledge alone should help increase leaders' ability to impact followers' wellbeing as improved expertise and familiarity with a problem is linked to improved behavioral changes (Mumford et al., 2015). However, knowledge alone is not enough to change leaders' behaviors and impact followers' health.

LEADERS' HEALTH-ORIENTED ATTITUDES

Operating in concert with cognitions, individuals' attitudes are among the most proximal predictors of their behaviors (Armitage & Christian, 2003). As such, it is imperative to better understand how leaders' attitudes regarding health can influence their own behavior, and ultimately, the health of their subordinates. One model introduced by Fazio (1986) mapped the attitude-behavior relationship. This model states that "motivation and opportunity act as determinants of spontaneous versus deliberate attitude-to-behavior processes" (Fazio, 1995 p.257). In other words, given the opportunity and motivation, one's attitudes ought to directly influence their behaviors. This is echoed in the Theory of Planned Behavior, which suggests that if individuals are sufficiently motivated and have the cognitive availability to act on their attitudes, those attitudes are a significant driver for their behaviors (Ajzen, 1991).

Attitudes are a learned association between an object and an emotional outcome, and the strength of this attitude is equal to the strength of the relationship between the object and its subsequent emotional link (Fazio, 1990). If an attitude towards an object is strong, the likelihood that someone acts on that behavior is much more likely, and less consciously driven. Further, the amount of effort necessary to engage in a behavior aligned with one's attitudes is lower than engaging in behavior that contradicts one's attitudes (Ajzen, 1991). For example, if a leader has learned to strongly associate smoking cigarettes with feelings of disgust or shame, they have a negative attitude towards smoking and are much more likely to speak up when they see someone smoking than someone who has positive emotional reactions to, and attitudes toward, cigarette smoking. When someone has a strong attitude towards an object or action, their behavioral response tends to be more automatic or non-conscious. However, to engage in a manner that is contrary to one's attitudes one must make a conscious and effortful decision. Shifting leader attitudes within the healthcare industry towards health promotion is therefore critical as organizations will see greater action from leaders in the promotion of positive health practices in their followers.

Additionally, leaders' attitudes are not only important as antecedents to their own behavior, but as direct influences on the attitudes of their followers. The theory of emotional contagion states that through subconscious mimicry, individuals will emulate the cues of others, causing them to adopt opinions that may not have originally been their own (Dasborough et al. 2009). Along these lines, Barsade (2002) found that not only are behaviors spread between individuals, but that attitudes are as well. Further, social learning theory would place strong emphasis on the attitudes of leaders as it suggests that individuals imitate others, particularly those in a position of power (Bandura, 1977, 1986). In this sense, leader attitudes themselves can be seen as both predictors and/or creators of employee attitudes and subsequent behaviors (Weierter, 1997). Thus, is it is critical to explore leaders' attitudes toward organizational interventions to promote employee health, as well as their attitudes toward the role of work on employee health in general, including mental health.

Attitudes Toward Organizational Policies and Change

Many organizations (42% overall, 62% of hospitals; CDC, 2017) already have workplace health programs designed to protect or promote the health of employees. Further, one study of 26 manufacturing workplaces participating in a health-oriented program found that a sizeable majority of managers believe that workplace health promotion programs are important (75%), improve employee health (80%), and reduce health care costs while boosting employee morale (Linnan et al., 2007). However, as noted above, supervisors can be a potential limiting factor with regard to the enactment of these policies if they do not possess these positive attitudes. Assuming leaders are aware of workplace health-oriented policies and programs, it is also critical that they have positive attitudes towards the policies or programs and value their implementation. For example, Hurtado and colleagues (2015) found that supervisors' support for nurses taking their meal breaks led to greater use of full meal breaks, which was associated with lower psychological distress. In other words, although all nurses had officially recognized meal breaks as part of company policy, supervisors' support for these policies resulted in their use and ultimately positive health outcomes. Similarly, a qualitative study of a paid parental leave policy found that "departmental characteristics and supervisor attitudes ultimately set the tone for the level of support offered to and experienced by leave-taking employees" (p. 121, Richardson et al., 2019).

One specific issue organizations are trying to tackle that has clear implications for employee health and wellbeing is workplace diversity. Many organizations have policies regarding diversity and inclusion, and it is critical for healthcare leaders to commit and buy into these policies. For example, Hammer and colleagues (2020) found that leaders' positive attitudes towards military veteran employees improved the impact of a supervisor training designed to improve sleep and wellbeing among workers. Further, the leaders' attitudes themselves improved following the training. On the other hand, one study found that women were more likely to experience gender harassment if their supervisors had a negative bias toward women (Piotrkowski, 1998), particularly if the leader was male. Similarly, Marchiondo et al. (2021) found that leaders' attitudes toward diversity were associated with male followers' perceptions of gender-based bias in the workplace and support for diversity initiatives. This suggests a leaders' attitudes may themselves be a risk factor for the experience of unique workplace stressors and health threats. Clearly, leaders' attitudes towards subgroups within the workforce are important predictors of the impact work can have on employee health, and these attitudes are malleable. It is necessary, then, for leaders to maintain (or generate) positive attitudes towards particularly vulnerable populations of employees within their workforce in a way that aligns with organizational policies and values to ensure the health and wellbeing of all employees.

That being said, many initiatives to promote health and wellbeing within the workplace require significant organizational change (Nielsen et al., 2010). Thus, interventions are frequently met with resistance from front-line workers (e.g., Nielsen et al., 2010). Workplace leaders may serve as champions for this change (Rafferty et al., 2013), smoothing the transition into the intervention and garnering buy-in from employees; however, they themselves must first have positive attitudes towards the change.

One of the most important jobs of a leader is to effectively facilitate and implement change (Kanter et al., 1992). In order to effectively implement organizational change, there are different models which can be used (Kanter et al., 1992; Kotter, 1996; Luecke, 2003). Though each model is applied differently, the vital role of leadership is expressed throughout. Within the organizational change literature, much of the focus is on employee resistance. The goal of this research is to better understand how to lead individuals through change when they are already satisfied with existing norms. Yet, what influence is a leader able to have on their followers when not only their employees are resistant to change, but they are as well? In order to understand this influence, Rubin and colleagues (2009) measured leadership and organizational cynicism, and the subsequent outcomes this had on their followers. They found that leaders who were cynical about organizational change resulted in reduced follower commitment and increased follower cynicism regarding organizational change. These leaders were also more likely to manage employees who shared this cynicism, leading to overall increased cynicism within the organization and greater difficulty implementing effective change. (Rubin et al., 2009). Similarly, gaining manager buy-in for health interventions was reported by one participant in a qualitative study as the most notable hurdle in making organizational changes (Whysall et al. 2006). Results of this study suggest leaders' attitudes towards the implementation of new organizational health initiatives determined whether or not health interventions would be successful. It is important that even if interventions are met with hesitancy, leaders maintain a positive attitude toward health and safety initiatives, as they are beneficial for both their employees and their organization as a whole. Whysall et al. (2006) also found that leaders' attitudes surrounding health and safety interventions directly influenced their employees when committing to new health-oriented behaviors. Specifically, *managerial enthusiasm and support* were seen as the greatest facilitators for successful health and safety interventions (Whysall et al. 2006).

Overall, ensuring leaders' have positive attitudes toward organizational health interventions and change is critically important for healthcare organizations if they hope to improve the health of their employees. However, if leaders do not have the proper attitude with regard to their follower's health, many of these planned improvements will not be as successful as intended. Thus, for leaders within the healthcare industry to truly influence the health of their followers, they must have buy-in and change their attitudes in order to see health initiatives as an important use of both their own and their employees' time and effort.

Attitudes Toward Work and Health

Beyond holding positive attitudes toward organizational policies and changes regarding employee health, healthcare leaders must hold positive attitudes towards the value of employee health and wellbeing in the workplace. These beliefs move beyond attitudes toward organizational policies by shifting perspective toward health and safety behaviors themselves. Leaders' attitudes toward health establish and perpetuate cultures of health, and are particularly important regarding potentially stigmatized health outcomes and behaviors such as those surrounding mental health.

Leaders' beliefs regarding health and wellbeing and the role of work in employees' lives can help promote a health culture. For example, Bronkhorst and colleagues (2018) found that leaders' attitudes towards safety were significant predictors of followers' perceptions of a safety climate as well as their safety behaviors. Similarly, Frear and Colleagues (2018) found that leaders who believed provision of support was valued by the organization provided support to their followers, whereas those that believed support necessitated reciprocity actually made their followers work harder in response to receiving support themselves. Additionally, O'Neill et al. (2009) found that top managements' own negative experiences with work-family conflict impacted lower level managements' perceived work-family climate, suggesting that across multiple levels of the organization, leaders' experiences and attitudes towards the interface between work and wellbeing can have impacts on perceived climate. Clearly, leaders' attitudes are critical for establishing or perpetuating a culture from the top down. By establishing health-oriented cultures, healthcare organizations will increase their employee health outcomes and decrease levels of burnout and job stress (Kuoppala et al.,2008; Skakon et al., 2010). It is critical, then, for leaders to understand the weight their own attitudes have for creating these social environments.

Another major component of health culture is the acceptance and normalization of discussing and protecting the mental health of employees. Previous studies found roughly 10% of healthcare workers had possibly clinical levels of depression and 25% had possibly clinical levels of anxiety (Lindwall et al., 2014) and these rates, particularly those of depression, may have increased during the COVID-19 pandemic (Pappa et al., 2020). Due to the stressful, fast-paced nature of the healthcare industry, it is crucial that organizations are aware of these statistics and monitoring leaders' attitudes towards mental healthcare seeking. Negrini and colleagues found supervisors' attitudes towards followers' mental health recovery and return to work were significant predictors of the successful return to work (2018). Similarly, Hoge and colleagues (2004) found that concerns about stigma from coworkers and leaders was a barrier to mental health treatment seeking among soldiers returning from deployment, particularly those who met screening criteria for a mental health disorder. Ultimately, it is critical that researchers find ways to help eliminate the stigma of help seeking for mental illness, and for healthcare leaders themselves to have positive attitudes regarding the normalization and promotion of self-care regarding mental health.

Overall, leaders' attitudes likely play a key role in influencing follower health outcomes. Healthcare organizations must do their best to implement strategies in order to first change and/or secure leaders' positive attitudes about the importance of follower health outcomes, and in doing so, they will be able to change organizational structure to promote a healthier workplace. By having greater leader support, the implementation of different interventions and healthy practices will have a greater chance of success, leading to happier, healthier employees.

LEADERS' HEALTH-ORIENTED BEHAVIORS

As the theory of planned behavior (Ajzen, 1991) suggests, attitudes and cognitions combine to influence individuals' behavior which is what directly impacts those around them. Leader behavior, therefore, is critical to understand as it has an impact on direct followers, and potentially further down the hierarchy or across teams. By understanding and altering leaders' health-oriented behaviors, researchers and practitioners can help create far-reaching, beneficial impacts on healthcare workers' wellbeing.

Leaders' interactions with followers can be impactful for followers both inside and outside of the workplace. We argue that it is through their behavior that leaders convert their internal attitudes and cognitions into meaningful change in employees' health. Existing research in leadership and follower health link supportive leader behavior to improved follower health and decreased levels of burnout (Kuoppala, et al., 2008). Despite these established associations, less work has been done with regard to health-specific leadership behaviors (Franke et al., 2014). Recent research has begun to ask what leaders can specifically do to positively impact follower health, and with it comes important implications for the influential nature of leadership both inside and outside of the workplace.

Health-oriented leadership centers around the idea that leaders' behaviors can impact follower health in multiple ways, including directly, through planned behavior, and indirectly, through role modeling of behavior (Franke & Felfe, 2011; Franke, Felfe & Pundt, 2014). In highlighting the importance of employee health and actively promoting it, leaders impact their followers' health. Further, health-oriented leadership serves as a resource that improves working conditions to reduce stressors. Gurt et al. (2011) extends this argument, stating that leaders' impact follower health by altering their followers' experience of the organization (e.g., role ambiguity, health climate). Specifically, Franke and colleagues (2014) identify two different types of health-oriented leadership behaviors that serve equally important, yet distinct purposes: self-directed behaviors and follower-directed behaviors.

Self-Directed Health Behaviors

Self-directed, health-oriented leadership behaviors, what Franke and colleagues (2014) coin "SelfCare," are behaviors that leaders themselves take in order to improve or maintain their health (e.g., engaging in healthy eating habits). The authors argue that these self-directed leader behaviors form the basis from which healthy leaders are then able to promote health for their followers via follower-directed behaviors. This study found that employees' ratings of their supervisor's health behaviors were positively correlated with their own self-reported measure of self-care. In a similar study looking at police officers, Santa Maria and colleagues (2019) found that leader health behaviors were significantly correlated to follower health behaviors. To that end, it is important that leaders in the healthcare industry not only promote healthy behaviors such as stress mitigation and a nutritious diet, but demonstrate them for followers. Leaders are, after all, creators of group social identity, workplace climate, and designers of work systems (Wegge et al., 2014). Specifically, role modeling is a self-management strategy of health-oriented leadership behaviors (Franke et al., 2014). To the extent that followers see their leader as a role model of their own health behaviors, leader health behaviors can shape follower health behaviors (Wegge et al., 2014). In other words, a leader that embraces and models health behaviors for followers is also one that positively shapes follower health behaviors.

Beyond serving as a role model, leaders may need to actively engage in self-management strategies such as emotional regulation. Glasø and Eianersen (2008) investigated connections between emotional regulation during follower-leader interactions and found that the suppression of emotions such as disappointment and annoyance, and faking of emotion such as enthusiasm and calmness, were both positively linked to follower and leader health complaints. This is an important takeaway for followers and leaders alike, as the suppression of the instinct to fake emotion is a skill that ought to be mastered in order to facilitate transparent and authentic communication. Actionable items for leaders in the healthcare field might include controlled expression of true emotions during interactions with employees and modelling healthy lifestyle behaviors such as discussing a personal prioritization of sleep on nights before shifts with employees.

Follower-Directed Health Behaviors

A general behavior in which healthcare leaders can engage that will have implications for follower health is providing support. House (1981) constructed a theoretical framework for supervisory support at work, with four dimensions of leader support behaviors: emotional, appraisal, instrumental, and informational. Emotional support helps the target cope with the negative emotions of a stressor, appraisal support helps the target think about the stressor differently (e.g., as a challenge rather than a threat or hindrance), instrumental support is actively aiding the target in overcoming the stressor, and informational support is the provision of information that can be used to overcome the stressor. These behaviors are in turn associated with improved follower health. In a longitudinal study, Dormann and Zapf (1999) investigated the effects of social support by supervisors on both social stressors at work and depressive symptoms, and they found that under conditions of high social stressors at work, those receiving high levels of supervisor social support saw reduced depressive symptoms. This study illuminates the far-reaching effects of leader behavior on followers and the mitigating effects of positive leader behaviors on follower workplace stress. In a study investigating the relationships between supervisor support and job stress, Yang et al. (2015) found a significant, direct negative effect of supervisor support on job stress. Provision of support by supervisors is impactful in reducing followers' job stress and improving their health.

Leaders in the healthcare field can also improve follower health by reducing work-related pressures. This reduction constitutes the creation of health-promoting, psychosocial work conditions for followers (Rudolph et al., 2020). There are multiple ways in which healthcare leaders might reduce work-related pressure that still allow for an efficient, productive work environment. Eberz and Antoni (2016; 2018) explore salutogenic leadership, in which leaders can mitigate pressures by building trust and managing incidents. Practice of salutogenic leadership better accounted for employees' health sense of work coherence than general measures of leadership behaviors. In another study of leadership reducing work pressure for followers, Adler and colleagues (2014) explored leader promotion of stress management for deployed US soldiers; these strategies improved follower mental health and attitudes toward seeking mental health treatment. Boehm et al. (2016) suggested taking both a person- and task-oriented approach in health-focused leadership behaviors such that these approaches might complement successful, general leadership styles. Behaviors that reduce work-pressures by building trust, promoting stress management, and managing incidents are critically important to enact in the healthcare field due to its already-high pressure nature and the high-cost of error.

Lastly, Frank and colleagues (2014) also highlight follower-directed, health-oriented leadership behaviors, what they coin "StaffCare," as behaviors that target positive health outcomes for followers, such as actively providing healthy working conditions (e.g., assembling/leading a healthy workplace workshop). For example, within the healthcare industry, sleep is critically important for job performance, and often suffers due to shift work demands (Ferri et al., 2016). Longstanding poor sleep quality and quantity can eventually lead to negative long-term health outcomes including memory loss, obesity, and hypertension (Ganster, Crain, & Brossoit, 2017). Despite these linkages, the CDC reports that the average American adult does not get the seven to eight hours of sleep recommended by American Academy of Sleep Medicine and the Sleep Research Society (Liu et al., 2016; Watson, et al., 2015). Sleep leadership behaviors are those that aid followers in getting more sleep and express concern for follower sleep outcomes (Gunia et al., 2015). These behaviors might involve encouraging followers to get a good night's rest before an important work day or generally inquiring into their sleep habits. Though this domain specific, health-oriented leadership behavior may sound arbitrary, Gunia and colleagues (2015) studied the effects of sleep leadership in the military setting and found that sleep-specific leadership behaviors extend beyond the influence of general, positive leader behaviors in decreasing sleep problems in followers. Further supporting these findings, Sianoja et al. (2020) found a link between increased sleep leadership practices and reduced sleep disturbance and sleep impairment among military service members. These findings are transferable to high-risk, high-pressure healthcare occupations and involve very limited effort on behalf of leaders. Further, in addition to sleep outcomes, leaders hoping to impact follower health may note problem areas in other target outcome areas, such as smoking habits, dietary habits, or physical activity of followers.

IMPROVING LEADERS' HEALTH COGNITIONS, ATTITUDES, AND BEHAVIORS

Previously, we outlined cognitions, attitudes, and behaviors that healthcare leaders need to improve in order to be more effective at promoting and protecting their subordinates' health and wellbeing. Below we outline intentional steps healthcare leaders can take to gain the improve their knowledge, attitudes, and behaviors they need as well as methods of synthesizing this information into actionable plans. See Table 2 for a specific practical recommendations.

Table 2. Practical Takeaways

Practical Takeaways for Leaders in Healthcare		
Cognitions	**Attitudes**	**Behaviors**
Provide training to leaders on all employee health-related benefits.	Generate positive attitudes towards existing health-oriented policies and programs.	Promote healthy behaviors and role model them for followers.
Provide training to leaders on occupational hazards, prevention, and mitigation.	Generate positive attitudes toward new health-oriented policies and programs.	Regulate emotional displays and discuss personal prioritization of health with followers.
Provide training on employee mental health challenges, prevention, and mitigation.	Normalize and promote self-care regarding mental health.	Provide support in at least one (or more) of the four dimensions: emotional, appraisal, instrumental, and informational.
Establish formal and informal mechanisms to learn about followers' wellbeing needs and goals.	Establish a health-oriented culture through valuing employee health.	Reduce work-related stressors for followers.
Establish formal and informal mechanisms to learn about effects of discrimination and group-based stressors faced by followers.	Generate or maintain positive attitudes towards particularly vulnerable employees.	Encourage specific health behaviors through conversation and daily interactions.

Formal and Informal Learning

Multiple studies suggest that formal training programs are associated with improved leader knowledge, attitudes, and behaviors regarding subordinate health. Meta-analytic evidence as well as systematic reviews suggest that training managers in mental health of employees improves leaders' knowledge of, attitudes toward, and behaviors regarding followers' mental health problems (Gayed et al., 2018; Tsutsumi, 2011), ultimately improving follower wellbeing. For example, Mohr and colleagues (2021) completed a randomized control trial with supervisors in the experimental group receiving supportive supervisor training. Results suggest veteran followers had improved wellbeing. Brady and colleagues (2021) also showed this intervention could improve veteran followers' relationships with their families, particularly when they are under stress. Similarly, Kawakami et al. (2005) found that a web-based training designed to improve leader support for followers' mental health resulted in maintenance of levels of support, whereas supervisors who received a control training were perceived as having provided less support over time. This suggests that some trainings may serve as "booster shots", reminding leaders of the importance of knowledge and attitudes they already have, rather than letting them decay over time as other pressures take precedent. Within healthcare, one study found that a training designed to encourage supervisors within long-term health care organizations to be safety-specific transformational leaders improved leaders' attitudes regarding safety, self-efficacy and intentions to promote safety, and ultimately follower perceptions of leaders' safety-specific transformational leadership as well as safety climate (Mullen & Kelloway, 2009).

On the other hand, Dellve and Eriksson (2017) suggest that formal training mechanisms may not be the best method for conveying health-promoting knowledge to leaders, but rather that leaders can engage in informal learning through conversations and reflections with peers, subordinates, and supervisors. This echoes sentiments by Telford and colleagues (2017) that much non-technical learning in the healthcare field occurs informally. However, a risk associated with informal learning is that the knowledge gained is incomplete, incorrect, or unorganized (Dale & Bell, 1999). With regard to learning about the importance of work in the healthcare workers' health and wellbeing, the workplace conditions may not immediately be conducive to adequate informal learning. Specifically, a lack of time and social/organizational support, a lack of preparedness or willingness by leaders to learn these lessons, and a lack of clear or immediate feedback mechanisms are all barriers to adequate informal learning (Dale & Bell, 1999). That said, these barriers can be overcome.

One method healthcare leaders can take to facilitate better outcomes for themselves and followers is to be intentional about their informal learning experiences. Perhaps healthcare leaders can set up journal clubs (e.g., Lachance, 2014) or debriefs (Telford et al., 2017) focused on employee health and wellbeing. Or, leaders can set an intention for themselves of learning about a specific employee health concern per month, and actively engage their subordinates in conversations about their experiences with that concern.

Action Planning

Ultimately, the theory of planned behavior (Ajzen, 1991) points toward the intention to engage in a behavior as the direct cognitive antecedent to behavior. It is through the intentional creation of specific and clear action plans, then, that leaders can convert their knowledge and attitudes into behaviors that impact employee health and wellbeing. Marks and colleagues (2001) suggest that planning is "the formulation and transmission of a principal course of action for mission accomplishment" (p. 365). Plans ought to include information about the time frame, the necessary resources, and the sequencing and timing of events. These plans ought to focus on causes of employee health that can be manipulated, that influence multiple health outcomes, and will have large effects if changed (Marcy & Mumford, 2010). In the context of healthcare workers' wellbeing, action plans will focus on the process of information gathering and its ultimate use. Leaders should plan out and engage in the formal and informal routes they will use to learn about their organizations' health-related policies, the health needs and goals of their followers, and potential threats to these needs. Leaders should then plan on what they, themselves, will do with this information. How will they share it with followers? How will they change their own behavior if it is itself a threat to follower wellbeing?

Not only do leaders need to create action plans for themselves, but they need to be able to share these with their units, often in the form of visions. Partlow and colleagues (2015) suggest that simplification of ideas and preempting future negative affect are key to effective vision creation. Therefore, as leaders create their action plans and work to distill them down to a shareable vision with followers, they ought to focus on key points and changes and ensure that possible negative reactions are accounted for. With regard to focusing on health and wellbeing, this is challenging due to the broad and sensitive nature of the topic at hand. For example, subordinates may not be comfortable discussing their health behaviors or mental health needs with their supervisor or colleagues. Leaders need to plan for alternative ways to ensure employees have access to the resources and protections they need even if they are not willing to share their personal needs. Lastly, leaders need to plan on *when* will be the most opportune times to implement their new action plans (Mumford et al., 2007). Ultimately, as Mumford and colleagues (2007) point out, declarative knowledge, situational monitoring, plan formation, and range of other internal cognitions come together to change the leaders' behaviors and, thus, followers' outcomes.

CONCLUSION

In the wake of the COVID-19 pandemic, healthcare workers are at higher risk than ever for burnout, anxiety, and depression (García-Fernández et al., 2020). A more recent study conducted by Klebe, Felfe, and Klug (2021) investigated the specific effects of health leadership on follower health during times of crisis and found that in times of crisis, the positive relationship between healthy leadership and follower health was stronger than before a time of crisis. Leaders in the healthcare field are charged with the enormous responsibility of ensuring taskwork is completed while also paying heed to the needs of their followers. The idea of a health-oriented leader is a newer concept in leadership literature, but no less important than more commonly discussed general leadership theories. The healthcare industry is subject to many unique challenges, including high-stakes tasks, shift work, dynamic multiteam systems, and high team interdependence, therefore the fulfillment of follower needs must also be approached in a specific, unique way. Domain-specific, health-oriented leadership presents a feasible avenue for leaders to promote mental, social, and physical wellbeing. Though the field still has room for growth, health-oriented leadership has demonstrated promise in improving follower wellbeing and workplace outcomes. As presented in this chapter, a successful health-oriented leader in healthcare organizations is one who is able to (1) cultivate general knowledge of employee health and emphasize its importance in order to (2) direct positive attitudes and energy towards health and health promotion and (3) exhibit health-oriented leadership behaviors to maximize positive impact on followers.

We suggest that healthcare organizations ought to take steps to improve their leaders' attitudes toward follower health and wellbeing, increase their knowledge of workplace health policies and follower health goals and status, and ultimately improve their health-oriented behavior. In doing so, we argue that healthcare organizations will be capitalizing upon one of their greatest levers with regard to employee health. From a theoretical perspective, there remains much work to be done with regard to health-oriented leadership, particularly within healthcare organizations. A better understanding of leaders' health-oriented attitudes and cognitions and how these predict leaders' health-oriented behaviors is necessary. We also need to better understand the incremental validity of targeted and specific health-oriented leadership behaviors above and beyond general leadership behaviors when predicting follower health and wellness. Further, any attempts to alter leaders' health-oriented attitudes, cognitions, or behaviors should be met with a critical eye toward timing. Specifically, researchers and practitioners need a much better understanding of how long the effects of trainings or other interventions take to emerge and how long they last. See Table 3 for suggested future research directions.

Table 3. Future Research Directions

Future Research Directions	
Overall Directions	How do leaders' health-oriented cognitions, attitudes, and behaviors differ in the hospital setting versus the family care setting?
	How do health-oriented leadership cognitions, attitudes, and behaviors differ across health professions?
	How can changes in health-oriented cognition and attitudes be better translated to health-oriented leadership behaviors?
Cognitions	How might healthcare organizations aid in offloading cognition of health policies and benefits for leaders in a way that makes them accessible yet memorable?
	How do mental models of follower health differ between novice and experienced leaders? Effective and ineffective leaders?
	What are cognitive or attitudinal barriers to gaining knowledge about diversity-based challenges to health?
Attitudes	What methods might be used to encourage positive leader attitudes toward health-oriented policies and programs?
	How might workplace leaders champion change and create buy in for health-oriented interventions from followers?
	What tactics are most effective in creating a culture centered around wellbeing?
Behaviors	What health-specific leader behaviors are most effective in creating change and positive impact on follower health?
	What mechanisms translate leaders' own health behaviors to followers' health behaviors?
	How do the dimensions of leader support interact with specific health needs to impact follower wellbeing?
	What drives/mitigates resistance to leaders' targeted health-oriented behaviors?

This chapter makes several important contributions to literature. First, it clarifies the differences between general leadership, more specific health-oriented leadership, and targeted health-oriented leadership cognitions, attitudes, and behaviors. Then, it proposes a model in which health-oriented leadership cognitions and attitudes lead to health-oriented leadership behavior, which ultimately impact follower cognitions, attitudes, behaviors, and ultimately outcomes. Finally, this chapter raises further questions into the future directions of leadership by identifying the state of extant literature on health-oriented leadership in the healthcare field as well as key areas in need of exploration, including the ultimate impact of leader behavior on follower health outcomes.

REFERENCES

Adler, A. B., Saboe, K. N., Anderson, J., Sipos, M. L., & Thomas, J. L. (2014). Behavioral Health Leadership: New Directions in Occupational Mental Health. *Current Psychiatry Reports*, *16*(10), 1–7. doi:10.100711920-014-0484-6 PMID:25160794

Ajzen, I. (1991). The theory of planned behavior. *Organizational Behavior and Human Decision Processes*, *50*(2), 179–211. doi:10.1016/0749-5978(91)90020-T

Arain, G. A., Bhatti, Z. A., Ashraf, N., & Fang, Y. H. (2020). Top-down knowledge hiding in organizations: An empirical study of the consequences of supervisor knowledge hiding among local and foreign workers in the Middle East. *Journal of Business Ethics*, *164*(3), 611–625. doi:10.100710551-018-4056-2

Armitage, C. J., & Christian, J. (2003). From attitudes to behaviour: Basic and applied research on the theory of planned behaviour. *Current Psychology (New Brunswick, N.J.)*, *22*(3), 187–195. doi:10.100712144-003-1015-5

Aronsson, G., & Lindh, T. (2004). *Långtidsfriskas arbetsvillkor: En populationsstudie. Arbete och Hälsa, 10*. Arbetslivsinstitutet.

Bandura, A. (1977). Self-efficacy: Toward a unifying theory of behavioral change. *Psychological Review*, *84*(2), 191–215. doi:10.1037/0033-295X.84.2.191 PMID:847061

Bandura, A. (1986). The explanatory and predictive scope of self-efficacy theory. *Journal of Social and Clinical Psychology*, *4*(3), 359–373. doi:10.1521/jscp.1986.4.3.359

Barsade, S. G. (2002). The ripple effect: Emotional contagion and its influence on group behavior. *Administrative Science Quarterly*, *47*(4), 644–675. doi:10.2307/3094912

Bass, B. M. (1985). *Leadership and performance beyond expectations*. Free Press.

Boehm, S. A., Baumgärtner, M. K., & Kreissner, L. M. (2016). The relationship between leadership and health: A comparison of general and health-focused leadership approaches. In M. Wiencke, M. Cacace, & S. Fischer (Eds.), *Healthy at Work*. Springer. doi:10.1007/978-3-319-32331-2_7

Boorman, S. (2010). Health and well-being of the NHS workforce. *Journal of Public Mental Health, 9*(1), 4-7.

Brady, J. M., Hammer, L. B., Mohr, C. D., & Bodner, T. E. (2021). Supportive supervisor training improves family relationships among employee and spouse dyads. *Journal of Occupational Health Psychology*, *26*(1), 31–48. doi:10.1037/ocp0000264 PMID:33119332

Bronkhorst, B., Tummers, L., & Steijn, B. (2018). Improving safety climate and behavior through a multifaceted intervention: Results from a field experiment. *Safety Science*, *103*, 293–304. doi:10.1016/j.ssci.2017.12.009

Campbell, J. P. (1990). Modeling the performance prediction problem in industrial and organizational psychology. In M. D. Dunnette & L. M. Hough (Eds.), *Handbook of industrial and organizational psychology* (pp. 687–732). Consulting Psychologists Press.

Casper, W. J., Fox, K. E., Sitzmann, T. M., & Landy, A. L. (2004). Supervisor referrals to work-family programs. *Journal of Occupational Health Psychology*, *9*(2), 136–151. doi:10.1037/1076-8998.9.2.136 PMID:15053713

Centers for Disease Control and Prevention. (2018). *Workplace Health in America 2017.* Centers for Disease Control and Prevention, U.S. Department of Health and Human Services.

Coughlan, B., Powell, D., & Higgins, M. F. (2017). The second victim: A review. *European Journal of Obstetrics, Gynecology, and Reproductive Biology*, *213*, 11–16. doi:10.1016/j.ejogrb.2017.04.002 PMID:28526169

Dale, M., & Bell, J. (1999). *Informal learning in the workplace, Research Brief, Number 134.* Department for Education and Employment. www.dfes.gov.uk/research/data/uploadfiles/RB134.doc

Dasborough, M. T., Ashkanasy, N. M., Tee, E. Y., & Herman, H. M. (2009). What goes around comes around: How meso-level negative emotional contagion can ultimately determine organizational attitudes toward leaders. *The Leadership Quarterly*, *20*(4), 571–585. doi:10.1016/j.leaqua.2009.04.009

Dellve, L., & Eriksson, A. (2017). Health-promoting managerial work: A theoretical framework for a leadership program that supports knowledge and capability to craft sustainable work practices in daily practice and during organizational change. *Societies (Basel, Switzerland)*, *7*(2), 12. doi:10.3390oc7020012

DiBenedetto, D. V. (1995). Occupational hazards of the health care industry: Protecting health care workers. *AAOHN Journal*, *43*(3), 131–137. doi:10.1177/216507999504300303 PMID:7702679

Dormann, C., & Zapf, D. (1999). Social support, social stressors at work, and depressive symptoms: Testing for main and moderating effects with structural equations in a three-wave longitudinal study. *The Journal of Applied Psychology*, *84*(6), 874–884. doi:10.1037/0021-9010.84.6.874 PMID:10639907

Eberz, S., & Antoni, C. H. (2016). The Systemic Salutogenic Interaction Modell (SSIM) - A holistic approach for explanation and development of health-promoting interactions between leaders and employees. Gruppe. Interaktion. Organisation. *Zeitschrift für Angewandte Organisationspsychologie*, *47*(3), 265–273. doi:10.1007/11612.1862-2615

Eberz, S., & Antoni, C. H. (2018). The TIMP-inventory – a contribution to the identification of core-factors of salutogenic leadership. *Zeitschrift für angewandte Organisationspsychologie, 1,* 69-80. doi:10.1007/s11612-017-0384-4

Fazio, R. H. (1986). How do attitudes guide behavior? In R. M. Sorrentino & E. T. Higgins (Eds.), *Handbook of motivation and cognition: Foundations of social behavior* (pp. 204–243). Guilford Press.

Fazio, R. H. (1990). Multiple processes by which attitudes guide behavior: The MODE model as an integrative framework. In Advances in experimental social psychology (Vol. 23, pp. 75–109). Academic Press. doi:10.1016/S0065-2601(08)60318-4

Fazio, R. H. (1995). Attitudes as object-evaluation associations: Determinants, consequences, and correlates of attitude accessibility. *Attitude strength: Antecedents and consequences, 4*, 247-282.

Ferri, P., Guadi, M., Marcheselli, L., Balduzzi, S., Magnani, D., & Di Lorenzo, R. (2016). The impact of shift work on the psychological and physical health of nurses in a general hospital: A comparison between rotating night shifts and day shifts. *Risk Management and Healthcare Policy*, *9*, 203–211. doi:10.2147/RMHP.S115326 PMID:27695372

Finne, L. B., Christensen, J. O., & Knardahl, S. (2014). Psychological and social work factors as predictors of mental distress: A prospective study. *PLoS One*, *9*(7), e102514. doi:10.1371/journal.pone.0102514 PMID:25048033

Fletcher, K. A., & Bedwell, W. L. (2017). Cognitive Aids in Emergency Medical Services. In J. R. Keebler, E. H. Lazzara, & P. Misasi (Eds.), *Human Factors and Ergonomics of Prehospital Emergency Care* (pp. 123–140). CRC Press. doi:10.1201/9781315280172-9

Franke, F., & Felfe, J. (2011). Diagnose gesundheitsförderlicher führung - Das instrument "health-oriented leadership". In B. Badura, A. Ducki, H. Schröder, J. Klose, & K. Macco (Eds.), *Fehlzeiten-Report 2011* (pp. 3–13). Springer. doi:10.1007/978-3-642-21655-8_1

Franke, F., Felfe, J., & Pundt, A. (2014). The impact of health-oriented leadership on follower health: Development and test of a new instrument measuring health-promoting leadership. *German Journal of Human Resource Management*, *28*(1–2), 139–161. doi:10.1177/239700221402800108

Frear, K. A., Donsbach, J., Theilgard, N., & Shanock, L. R. (2018). Supported supervisors are more supportive, but why? A multilevel study of mechanisms and outcomes. *Journal of Business and Psychology*, *33*(1), 55–69. doi:10.100710869-016-9485-2

French, K. A., & Shockley, K. M. (2020). Formal and informal supports for managing work and family. *Current Directions in Psychological Science*, *29*(2), 207–216. doi:10.1177/0963721420906218

Gagne, R. M. (1984). Learning outcomes and their effects: Useful categories of human performance. *The American Psychologist*, *39*(4), 377. doi:10.1037/0003-066X.39.4.377

Ganster, D. C., Crain, T. L., & Brossoit, R. M. (2018). Physiological Measurement in the Organizational Sciences: A Review and Recommendations for Future Use. *Annual Review of Organizational Psychology and Organizational Behavior*, *5*(1), 267–293. doi:10.1146/annurev-orgpsych-032117-104613

García-Fernández, L., Romero-Ferreiro, V., López-Roldán, P., Padilla, S., Calero-Sierra, I., Monzó-García, M., Perez-Martin, J., & Rodriguez-Jimenez, R. (2020). Mental health impact of COVID-19 pandemic on Spanish healthcare workers. *Psychological Medicine*, *51*, 1–3. doi:10.1017/S0033291720002019 PMID:32456735

Gayed, A., Milligan-Saville, J. S., Nicholas, J., Bryan, B. T., LaMontagne, A. D., Milner, A., Madan, I., Calvo, R. A., Christensen, H., Mykletun, A., Glozier, N., & Harvey, S. B. (2018). Effectiveness of training workplace managers to understand and support the mental health needs of employees: A systematic review and meta-analysis. *Occupational and Environmental Medicine*, *75*(6), 462–470. doi:10.1136/oemed-2017-104789 PMID:29563195

Gilbreath, B., & Benson, P. G. (2004). The contribution of supervisor behaviour to employee psychological well-being. *Work and Stress*, *18*(3), 255–266. doi:10.1080/02678370412331317499

Glasø, L., & Einarsen, S. (2008). Emotion regulation in leader-follower relationships. *European Journal of Work and Organizational Psychology*, *17*(4), 482–500. doi:10.1080/13594320801994960

Gunia, B. C., Sipos, M. L., LoPresti, M., & Adler, A. B. (2015). Sleep leadership in high-risk occupations: An investigation of soldiers on peacekeeping and combat missions. *Military Psychology*, *27*(4), 197–211. doi:10.1037/mil0000078

Gurt, J., Schwennen, C., & Elke, G. (2011). Health-specific leadership: Is there an association between leader consideration for the health of employees and their strain and well-being? *Work and Stress*, *25*(2), 108–127. doi:10.1080/02678373.2011.595947

Hammer, L., Brady, J. M., & Perry, M. (2020). Training supervisors to support veterans at work: Effects on supervisor attitudes and employee sleep and stress. *Journal of Occupational and Organizational Psychology*, *93*(2), 273–301. doi:10.1111/joop.12299

Hoge, C. W., Castro, C. A., Messer, S. C., McGurk, D., Cotting, D. I., & Koffman, R. L. (2004). Combat Duty in Iraq and Afghanistan, Mental Health Problems, and Barriers to Care. *The New England Journal of Medicine*, *351*(1), 13–22. doi:10.1056/NEJMoa040603 PMID:15229303

House, J. S. (1981). *Work stress and social support*. Addison-Wesley Series on Occupational Stress.

Hu, Y.-Y., Ellis, R. J., Hewitt, D. B., Yang, A. D., Cheung, E. O., Moskowitz, J. T., Potts, J. R. III, Buyske, J., Hoyt, D. B., Nasca, T. J., & Bilimoria, K. Y. (2019). Discrimination, Abuse, Harassment, and Burnout in Surgical Residency Training. *The New England Journal of Medicine*, *381*(18), 1741–1752. doi:10.1056/NEJMsa1903759 PMID:31657887

Hurtado, D. A., Nelson, C. C., Hashimoto, D., & Sorensen, G. (2015). Supervisors' Support for Nurses' Meal Breaks and Mental Health. *Workplace Health & Safety*, *63*(3), 107–115. doi:10.1177/2165079915571354 PMID:25994975

Judge, T. A., Piccolo, R. F., & Ilies, R. (2004). The forgotten ones? The validity of consideration and initiating structure in leadership research. *The Journal of Applied Psychology*, *89*(1), 36–51. doi:10.1037/0021-9010.89.1.36 PMID:14769119

Kanter, R. M., Stein, B. A., & Jick, T. D. (1992). *The Challenge of Organisational Change*. The Free Press.

Kawakami, N., Kobayashi, Y., Takao, S., & Tsutsumi, A. (2005). Effects of web-based supervisor training on supervisor support and psychological distress among workers: A randomized controlled trial. *Preventive Medicine*, *41*(2), 471–478. doi:10.1016/j.ypmed.2005.01.001 PMID:15917043

Khamisa, N., Peltzer, K., & Oldenburg, B. (2013). Burnout in relation to specific contributing factors and health outcomes among nurses: A systematic review. *International Journal of Environmental Research and Public Health*, *10*(6), 2214–2240. doi:10.3390/ijerph10062214 PMID:23727902

Klebe, L., Felfe, J., & Klug, K. (2021). Healthy Leadership in Turbulent Times: The Effectiveness of Health-Oriented Leadership in Crisis. *British Journal of Management*, *32*(4), 1203–1218. Advance online publication. doi:10.1111/1467-8551.12498

Kotter, J. P. (1996). Why transformation efforts fail. *Harvard Business Review*.

Kraiger, K., Ford, J. K., & Salas, E. (1993). Application of cognitive, skill-based, and affective theories of learning outcomes to new methods of training evaluation. *The Journal of Applied Psychology*, *78*(2), 311–328. doi:10.1037/0021-9010.78.2.311

Kronsberg, S., Bouret, J., & Brett, A. (2017). Lived experiences of male nurses: Dire consequences for the nursing profession. *Journal of Nursing Education and Practice*, *8*(46), 46. doi:10.5430/jnep.v8n1p46

Kuoppala, J., Lamminpää, A., Liira, J., & Vainio, H. (2008). Leadership, job well-being, and health effects—A systematic review and a meta-analysis. *Journal of Occupational and Environmental Medicine*, *50*(8), 904–915. doi:10.1097/JOM.0b013e31817e918d PMID:18695449

Lachance, C. (2014). Nursing journal clubs: A literature review on the effective teaching strategy for continuing education and evidence-based practice. *Journal of Continuing Education in Nursing*, *45*(12), 559–565. doi:10.3928/00220124-20141120-01 PMID:25401339

Laharnar, N., Glass, N., Perrin, N., Hanson, G., & Anger, W. K. (2013). A training intervention for supervisors to support a work-life policy implementation. *Safety and Health at Work*, *4*(3), 166–176. doi:10.1016/j.shaw.2013.07.001 PMID:24106648

Liao, C., Wayne, S. J., & Rousseau, D. M. (2016). Idiosyncratic deals in contemporary organizations: A qualitative and meta-analytical review. *Journal of Organizational Behavior*, *37*, S9–S29. doi:10.1002/job.1959

Lindwall, M., Gerber, M., Jonsdottir, I. H., Börjesson, M., & Ahlborg, G. Jr. (2014). The relationships of change in physical activity with change in depression, anxiety, and burnout: A longitudinal study of Swedish healthcare workers. *Health Psychology*, *33*(11), 1309–1339. doi:10.1037/a0034402 PMID:24245832

Linnan, L., Weiner, B., Graham, A., & Emmons, K. (2007). Manager Beliefs regarding Worksite Health Promotion: Findings from the Working Healthy Project 2. *American Journal of Health Promotion*, *21*(6), 521–528. doi:10.4278/0890-1171-21.6.521 PMID:17674640

Liu, Y., Wheaton, A. G., Chapman, D. P., Cunningham, T. J., Lu, H., & Croft, J. B. (2016). Prevalence of Healthy Sleep Duration among Adults— United States, 2014. *Morbidity and Mortality; Weekly Report*, *65*(6), 137–141. doi:10.15585/mmwr.mm6506a1 PMID:26890214

Luecke, R. (2003). *Managing change and transition* (Vol. 3). Harvard Business Press.

Luftman, K., Aydelotte, J., Rix, K., Ali, S., Houck, K., Coopwood, T. B., Teixeira, P., Eastman, A., Eastridge, B., Brown, C. V. R., & Davis, M. (2017). PTSD in those who care for the injured. *Injury*, *48*(2), 293–296. doi:10.1016/j.injury.2016.11.001 PMID:27871770

Marchiondo, L. A., Verney, S. P., & Venner, K. L. (2021). Academic leaders' diversity attitudes: Their role in predicting faculty support for institutional diversity. *Journal of Diversity in Higher Education*. Advance online publication. doi:10.1037/dhe0000333

Marcy, R. T., & Mumford, M. D. (2010). Leader cognition: Improving leader performance through causal analysis. *The Leadership Quarterly*, *21*(1), 1–19. doi:10.1016/j.leaqua.2009.10.001

Marks, M., Mathieu, J., & Zaccaro, S. (2001). A temporally based framework and taxonomy of team processes. *Academy of Management Review*, *26*(3), 356–376. doi:10.5465/amr.2001.4845785

Mays, V. M., Cochran, S. D., & Barnes, N. W. (2007). Race, race-based discrimination, and health outcomes among African Americans. *Annual Review of Psychology*, *5*(1), 201–225. doi:10.1146/annurev.psych.57.102904.190212 PMID:16953796

McCarthy, A., Darcy, C., & Grady, G. (2010). Work-life balance policy and practice: Understanding line manager attitudes and behaviors. *Human Resource Management Review*, *20*(2), 158–167. doi:10.1016/j.hrmr.2009.12.001

Miller, P., & Haslam, C. (2009). Why employers spend money on employee health: Interviews with occupational health and safety professionals from British Industry. *Safety Science*, *47*(2), 163–169. doi:10.1016/j.ssci.2008.04.001

Milligan-Saville, J. S., Paterson, H. M., Harkness, E. L., Marsh, A. M., Dobson, M., Kemp, R. I., Bryant, R. A., & Harvey, S. B. (2017). The amplification of common somatic symptoms by posttraumatic stress disorder in firefighters. *Journal of Traumatic Stress*, *30*(2), 142–148. doi:10.1002/jts.22166 PMID:28273379

Mohanty, A., Kabi, A., & Mohanty, A. P. (2019). Health problems in healthcare workers: A review. *Journal of Family Medicine and Primary Care*, *8*(8), 2568–2572. doi:10.4103/jfmpc.jfmpc_431_19 PMID:31548933

Mohr, C. D., Hammer, L. B., Brady, J. M., Perry, M. L., & Bodner, T. (2021). Can supervisor support improve daily employee well-being? Evidence of supervisor training effectiveness in a study of veteran employee emotions. *Journal of Occupational and Organizational Psychology*, *94*(2), 400–426. doi:10.1111/joop.12342

Moore, R. M. Jr, & Kaczmarek, R. G. (1990). Occupational hazards to health care workers: Diverse, ill-defined, and not fully appreciated. *American Journal of Infection Control*, *18*(5), 316–327. doi:10.1016/0196-6553(90)90231-G PMID:2174654

Mullen, J. E., & Kelloway, E. K. (2009). Safety leadership: A longitudinal study of the effects of transformational leadership on safety outcomes. *Journal of Occupational and Organizational Psychology*, *82*(2), 253–272. doi:10.1348/096317908X325313

Mumford, M. D., Friedrich, T. L., Caughron, J. J., & Byrne, C. L. (2007). Leader cognition in real-world settings: How do leaders think about crises? *The Leadership Quarterly*, *18*(6), 515–543. doi:10.1016/j.leaqua.2007.09.002

Negrini, A., Corbiere, M., Lecomte, T., Coutu, M. F., Nieuwenhuijsen, K., St-Arnaud, L., Durand, M.-J., Gragnano, A., & Berbiche, D. (2018). How can supervisors contribute to the return to work of employees who have experienced depression? *Journal of Occupational Rehabilitation*, *28*(2), 279–288. doi:10.100710926-017-9715-0 PMID:28660364

Nielsen, K., Randall, R., Holten, A., & González, E. R. (2010). Conducting organizational-level occupational health interventions: What works? *Work and Stress*, *24*(3), 234–259. doi:10.1080/02678373.2010.515393

Nunez-Smith, M., Curry, L. A., Bigby, J., Berg, D., Krumholz, H. M., & Bradley, E. H. (2007). Impact of race on the professional lives of physicians of African descent. *Annals of Internal Medicine*, *146*(1), 45–51. doi:10.7326/0003-4819-146-1-200701020-00008 PMID:17200221

Nyberg, A., Bernin, P., & Theorell, T. (2005). *The impact of leadership on the health of subordinates.* Report No 1, National Institute for Working Life.

O'Neill, J. W., Harrison, M. M., Cleveland, J., Almeida, D., Stawski, R., & Crouter, A. C. (2009). Work–family climate, organizational commitment, and turnover: Multilevel contagion effects of leaders. *Journal of Vocational Behavior*, *74*(1), 18–29. doi:10.1016/j.jvb.2008.10.004 PMID:19412351

Pappa, S., Ntella, V., Giannakas, T., Giannakoulis, V. G., Papoutsi, E., & Katsaounou, P. (2020). Prevalence of depression, anxiety, and insomnia among healthcare workers during the COVID-19 pandemic: A systematic review and meta-analysis. *Brain, Behavior, and Immunity*, *88*, 901–907. doi:10.1016/j.bbi.2020.05.026 PMID:32437915

Partlow, P., Medeiros, K., & Mumford, M. (2015). Leader cognition in vision formation: Simplicity and negativity. *The Leadership Quarterly*, *26*(3), 448–469. Advance online publication. doi:10.1016/j.leaqua.2015.02.009

Peterson, U., Demerouti, E., Bergström, G., Samuelsson, M., Åsberg, M., & Nygren, Å. (2008). Burnout and physical and mental health among Swedish healthcare workers. *Journal of Advanced Nursing*, *62*(1), 84–95. doi:10.1111/j.1365-2648.2007.04580.x PMID:18352967

Pfeffer, J., Vilendrer, S., Joseph, G., Kim, J., & Singer, S. J. (2020). Employers' Role in Employee Health: Why They Do What They Do. *Journal of Occupational and Environmental Medicine*, *62*(11), e601–e610. doi:10.1097/JOM.0000000000001967 PMID:32769791

Phillips, J. P. (2016). Workplace violence against health care workers in the United States. *The New England Journal of Medicine*, *374*(17), 1661–1669. doi:10.1056/NEJMra1501998 PMID:27119238

Piotrkowski, C. S. (1998). Gender harassment, job satisfaction, and distress among employed white and minority women. *Journal of Occupational Health Psychology*, *3*(1), 33–43. doi:10.1037/1076-8998.3.1.33 PMID:9552270

Rafferty, A. E., Jimmieson, N. L., & Restubog, S. L. D. (2013). When leadership meets organizational change: The influence of the top management team and supervisory leaders on change appraisals, change attitudes, and adjustment to change. The psychology of organizational change: Viewing change from the employee's perspective, 145-172.

Richardson, D. M., Steeves-Reece, A., Martin, A., Hurtado, D. A., Dumet, L. M., & Goodman, J. M. (2019). Employee experiences with a newly adopted paid parental leave policy: Equity considerations for policy implementation. *Health Equity*, *3*(1), 117–123. doi:10.1089/heq.2019.0007 PMID:30989153

Rubin, R. S., Dierdorff, E. C., Bommer, W. H., & Baldwin, T. T. (2009). Do leaders reap what they sow? Leader and employee outcomes of leader organizational cynicism about change. *The Leadership Quarterly*, *20*(5), 680–688. doi:10.1016/j.leaqua.2009.06.002

Rudolph, C. W., Murphy, L. D., & Zacher, H. (2020). A systematic review and critique of research on "healthy leadership". *The Leadership Quarterly, 31*(1), 101335. doi:10.1016/j.leaqua.2019.101335

Ryan, A.M. & Kossek, E.E. (2008), Work-life policy implementation: Breaking down or creating barriers to inclusiveness? *Human Resource Management, 47*(2), 295-310. doi:10.1002/hrm.20213

Santa Maria, A., Wolter, C., Gusy, B., Kleiber, D., & Renneberg, B. (2019). The Impact of Health-Oriented Leadership on Police Officers' Physical Health, Burnout, Depression and Well-Being. *Policing. Journal of Policy Practice, 13*(2), 186–200. doi:10.1093/police/pay067

Schwarzer, R. (2001). Social-cognitive factors in changing health-related behaviors. *Current Directions in Psychological Science, 10*(2), 47–51. doi:10.1111/1467-8721.00112

Schyns, B., & Schilling, J. (2013). How bad are the effects of bad leaders? A meta-analysis of destructive leadership and its outcomes. *The Leadership Quarterly, 24*(1), 138–158. doi:10.1016/j.leaqua.2012.09.001

Shanafelt, T. D., & Noseworthy, J. H. (2017). Executive Leadership and Physician Well-being: Nine Organizational Strategies to Promote Engagement and Reduce Burnout. *Mayo Clinic Proceedings, 92*(1), 129–146. doi:10.1016/j.mayocp.2016.10.004 PMID:27871627

Sianoja, M., Crain, T. L., Hammer, L. B., Bodner, T., Brockwood, K. J., LoPresti, M., & Shea, S. A. (2020). The relationship between leadership support and employee sleep. *Journal of Occupational Health Psychology, 25*(3), 187–202. doi:10.1037/ocp0000173 PMID:31789546

Skakon, J., Nielsen, K., Vilhelm Borg, V., & Guzman, J. (2010). Are leaders' well-being, behaviours and style associated with the affective well-being of their employees? A systematic review of three decades of research. *Work and Stress, 24*(2), 107–139. doi:10.1080/02678373.2010.495262

Telford, B., Fletcher, K., & Bedwell, W. (2017). Informal Learning in the Healthcare Industry. In J. E. Ellingson & R. A. Noe (Eds.), *Autonomous learning in the workplace* (pp. 219–236). Routledge. doi:10.4324/9781315674131-12

Tsutsumi, A. (2011). Development of an evidence-based guideline for supervisor training in promoting mental health: Literature review. *Journal of Occupational Health, 53*(1), 1–9. doi:10.1539/joh.R10002 PMID:21079372

Vidyarthi, P. R., Singh, S., Erdogan, B., Chaudhry, A., Posthuma, R., & Anand, S. (2016). Individual deals within teams: Investigating the role of relative i-deals for employee performance. *The Journal of Applied Psychology, 101*(11), 1536–1552. doi:10.1037/apl0000145 PMID:27513681

Wegge, J., Shemla, M., & Haslam, S. A. (2014). Leader behavior as a determinant of health at aork: Specification and evidence of five key pathways. *German Journal of Human Resource Management, 28*(1–2), 6–23. doi:10.1177/239700221402800102

Weierter, S. J. (1997). Who wants to play "follow the leader?" A theory of charismatic relationships based on routinized charisma and follower characteristics. *The Leadership Quarterly, 8*(2), 171-193.

West, C. P., Dyrbye, L. N., & Shanafelt, T. D. (2018). Physician burnout: Contributors, consequences and solutions. *Journal of Internal Medicine, 283*(6), 516–529. doi:10.1111/joim.12752 PMID:29505159

Whysall, Z., Haslam, C., & Haslam, R. (2006). Implementing health and safety interventions in the workplace: An exploratory study. *International Journal of Industrial Ergonomics*, *36*(9), 809–818. doi:10.1016/j.ergon.2006.06.007

Yang, T., Shen, Y.-M., Zhu, M., Liu, Y., Deng, J., Chen, Q., & See, L.-C. (2015). Effects of Co-Worker and Supervisor Support on Job Stress and Presenteeism in an Aging Workforce: A Structural Equation Modelling Approach. *International Journal of Environmental Research and Public Health*, *13*(1), 72. doi:10.3390/ijerph13010072 PMID:26703705

Zuckerman, N. (2014). Shift work, stress, and violence: Shift work. In T. Gorman (Ed.), *Controlling health hazards to hospital workers: A reference guide* (pp. 126–129). Baywood Publishing Co., Inc. doi:10.2190/NS.23.Suppl

Chapter 10
COVID-19 and Healthcare Staff Wellbeing:
Is Burnout Really a Systemic Issue of Morality?

Lorna French
University of Surrey, UK

Paul Hanna
University of Surrey, UK

Catherine Huckle
University of Surrey, UK

ABSTRACT

This conceptual chapter offers a critical review of contemporary theory and research in relation to 'burnout' and 'moral injury' to consider how understandings of burnout and moral injury can be usefully applied to healthcare workers during the COVID-19 pandemic. The authors find that whilst there are significant overlaps in the conceptualisation of 'burnout' and 'moral injury', there is also significant potential in drawing on systemic understandings of moral injury originating in military literature to understand and support healthcare workers. A focus on the systemic and organisational support needed to work with moral injury in healthcare staff would reduce staff burnout, time-off, and turnover improving patient outcomes and offering economic advantages to healthcare organisations. Whilst much research has been undertaken in relation to healthcare staff burnout, this chapter offers an original contribution to knowledge by offering a conceptual account of the usefulness of systemic understandings of moral injury in healthcare settings during the COVID-19 pandemic.

DOI: 10.4018/978-1-7998-8813-0.ch010

INTRODUCTION

The COVID-19 pandemic has put unprecedented pressure on the healthcare staff throughout the world. Staff have been asked to return from retirement, intermittently self-isolate or take sick leave, cover for staff that may be shielding, be redeployed into unfamiliar areas and work in overrun and under-resourced services (Vindrola-Padros et al., 2020; Willan, King, Jeffery, & Bienz, 2020). Not only are healthcare staff at higher risk of severe illness or death from coronavirus, but they are likely to be impacted by fear of infection, long hours, and delays in the provision of personal protective equipment and adequate COVID-19 testing resources (Heilbron, 2020). Indeed 44% of a sample of UK doctors surveyed in April, at the height of the initial pandemic 'peak', reported suffering from depression, anxiety, stress, burnout, and other mental health issues related to or made worse by their work, with 25% reporting this was directly due to the impact of COVID-19 (BMA, 2020).

In the United States of America and United Kingdom, through the framing of political leaders, the COVID-19 virus has come to represent an invisible enemy, with hospitals and Intensive Care Units as the frontline trenches, and healthcare staff as our 'wartime heroes' (Benziman, 2020). This gives the impression of necessary sacrifice, with rewards for those showing bravery, and implies the following of overarching 'orders' from higher up in the organisational system. Mirroring this wartime narrative is the potential of healthcare staff to suffer 'moral injury' during the pandemic (Borges, Barnes, Farnsworth, Bahraini, & Brenner, 2020; Greenberg, Docherty, Gnanapragasam, & Wessely, 2020; Williams, Brundage, & Williams, 2020; Williamson, Murphy, & Greenberg, 2020). A term traditionally associated with veterans, moral injury is commonly characterised by significant distress resulting from actions (either of an individual or their trusted authority), or lack of action, which violate one's moral or ethical code (Litz et al., 2009; Richardson et al., 2020). More specifically, Shay defined moral injury as "A betrayal of what's right, by someone who holds legitimate authority (e.g., in the military – a leader), in a high stakes situation" (Shay, 2014, p. 183). It has been suggested that the demand placed on healthcare staff during the COVID-19 pandemic, and lack of essential resources such as ventilators, could lead to healthcare workers being unable to provide the treatment that they consider to be ethical and morally 'right', putting them in danger of moral injury (Williamson et al., 2020).

Explorations into moral injury highlight themes of guilt, shame, anger and depression (Richardson et al., 2020). Alienation from colleagues and systems has also been identified as an outcome of moral injury in healthcare professionals (Gibbons, Shafer, Hickling, & Ramsey, 2013; Haight, Sugrue, & Calhoun, 2017). Commonalities can be observed between moral injury and the key features understood to characterise burnout (emotional exhaustion, depersonalisation, and diminished personal accomplishment) (Iliffe & Manthorpe, 2019). The loss of trust in the moral authority associated with moral injury may appear similar to the depersonalised 'cynicism' and emotional exhaustion experienced by healthcare staff (Hall, Johnson, Watt, Tsipa, & O'Connor, 2016). Understanding this potential crossover is essential, as the foundation of distress may change the associated intervention most likely to support the wellbeing of healthcare staff. 'Burnout' has long been used as a catchall term to describe workplace-related emotional distress (Kopacz, Ames, & Koenig, 2019; Orton & Gray, 2015), and understanding what burnout really means for healthcare staff is vital during an emotionally challenging time likely to impact their collective wellbeing for years to come.

While the issue of moral injury has been raised by authors in the context of the pandemic, many have highlighted the likelihood of its occurrence and importance of considering it a target for support (Borges et al., 2020; Greenberg et al., 2020; Williams et al., 2020; Williamson et al., 2020), rather than an extension of a pre-existing issue. Even where authors have considered the context of high burnout (Dean, Jacobs, & Manfredi, 2020), further theoretical exploration is required to understand how burnout and morality are likely to coincide during the COVID-19 pandemic. This chapter therefore aims to: i) understand burnout in healthcare and assess whether it can be indicative of injuries to morality, ii) understand the individual and systemic origins of these phenomena, and iii) explore how this relates to the experiences of healthcare staff during COVID-19.

DEFINING BURNOUT

Since its introduction to the psychological vocabulary in the 1970s (Freudenberger, 1974), the term 'burnout' has been widely used to describe any experience of psychological distress in the workplace (Kopacz et al., 2019; Orton & Gray, 2015). In healthcare literature, burnout is defined by experiences of emotional exhaustion, depersonalisation and low efficacy in the workplace (Brotheridge & Grandey, 2002). These domains are often the focus of assessing the presence of burnout through the Maslach Burnout Inventory (MBI, Maslach, Jackson, Leiter, Schaufeli, & Schwab, 1986).

Emotional exhaustion is the chronic depletion of physical and emotional resources resulting from excessive job demands and continuous 'hassles'(Zohar, 1997), and is considered burnout's most fundamental component (Maslach, Schaufeli, & Leiter, 2001; W. Schaufeli & Enzmann, 1998). The experience of emotional exhaustion has been closely linked to high rates of turnover (Cropanzano, Rupp, & Byrne, 2003; Wright & Cropanzano, 1998) and quality and safety of patient care (Salyers et al., 2017). Alongside emotional exhaustion, depersonalisation has also been investigated within healthcare personnel. Depersonalisation, the experience of feeling detached from the world and others within it, manifests as a 'lack of empathy' and negative attitudes towards patients (Maslach et al., 1986). A large cross-sectional study assessing burnout in doctors found high levels of burnout and depersonalisation (Orton, Orton, & Pereira Gray, 2012), and an online discussion between medical students and practicing physicians highlighted the development and progression of cynicism over the course of medical training as a coping mechanism (Peng, Clarkin, & Doja, 2018). Higher levels of emotional exhaustion and depersonalisation alone have been found to be vital components of burnout, with higher levels of emotional exhaustion causing higher levels of depersonalisation (W. B. Schaufeli, Bakker, Hoogduin, Schaap, & Kladler, 2001; Zhang, Mu, He, Cai, & Li, 2020). The third domain of burnout, reduced personal accomplishment, the experience of failed performance at work and/or the negative evaluation of ones work, appears to be a consequence of burnout rather than a contributing factor (Peiró, González-Romá, Tordera, & Mañas, 2001).

Burnout significantly correlates with high scores on the Symptom Check List, which includes items related to depression, anxiety, and other areas of psychological distress (Bauer et al., 2006). There appears to be a conceptual similarity between burnout, depression and anxiety (Ahola & Hakanen, 2007) all correlating with helpless thinking (Ohue, Moriyama, & Nakaya, 2011). However, the defining feature of burnout versus depression has been considered to be context; "burnout is specific to the work context, in contrast to depression, which tends to pervade every domain of a person's life" (Maslach et al., 2001, p. 404). Although research has demonstrated that individuals with high incidence of burnout symptoms can meet diagnostic criteria for depression (Ahola, Hakanen, Perhoniemi, & Mutanen, 2014; Bianchi, Schonfeld, & Laurent, 2014; Schonfeld & Bianchi, 2016), a recent meta-analysis found no conclusive overlap between burnout and depression or anxiety (Koutsimani, Montgomery, & Georganta, 2019).

Burnout as an Individual Problem vs Systemic Issue

Although burnout is a problem situated within the workplace, it is usually measured by prevalence of individual symptoms and perceptions rather than by workplace experiences. Currently, healthcare staff presenting with 'burnout' tend to be signposted to stress reduction programmes and encouraged to build resilience against stress (Kumar, 2016; Tregoning, Remington, & Agius, 2014). This strategy highlights the individualist approach often taken with burnout, in which the problem is situated within individual staff members and interventions are delivered in light of that. However, in contrast to understanding burnout as an individual pathology, an alternative approach conceptualises burnout as something associated with inadequate staffing, excessive workload, poor leadership, lack of support, and lack of opportunity for development (Bressi et al., 2009; Graber et al., 2008; Pinikahana & Happell, 2004; Willard-Grace et al., 2014). Indeed, in a recent survey, healthcare staff working under pressure, with time constraints and on an understaffed 'frontline' were the most exhausted, stressed and compassion fatigued (McKinley et al., 2020).

Similarly, levels of resilience have been assessed in conjunction with burnout, which is of particular importance as personal resilience is often considered helpful for mitigating burnout (Rushton, Batcheller, Schroeder, & Donohue, 2015) with recent research identifying higher levels of resilience in UK doctors than in the general population, despite even higher levels of secondary traumatic stress (72%) and low compassion satisfaction (24%) (McCain, McKinley, Dempster, Campbell, & Kirk, 2018). While low resilience was positively associated with burnout, non-clinical issues were the main factor perceived to cause low resilience (e.g. career transition, complaints and litigation, professional relationships and senior level support), suggesting that systemic factors are likely to impact individual coping. Research into burnout and psychiatric morbidity in doctors identified both personal and organisational factors, such as low job satisfaction, overload, increased hours worked and neuroticism (Imo, 2017). Therefore, even in cases where personal factors are identified as important for burnout, it seems that organisational factors directly impact these or interact with them.

Although skills-based stress reduction programmes may go some way to supporting resilience and alleviating burnout in healthcare staff, it seems likely that acknowledging and alleviating organisational factors is necessary for improving wellbeing, something rarely done in healthcare organisations (Wilkinson, 2015). This results in an environment where positive change is understood and advised, but not undertaken, and the pressure is placed on individuals to bear greater stress rather than organisations to relieve it (Squiers, Lobdell, Fann, & DiMaio, 2017). Further, a recent report from Health Education England advised three levels of intervention for improving staff mental wellbeing; primary, secondary and tertiary (HEE, 2019). Primary level interventions would seek to remove sources of distress, whereas secondary and tertiary interventions focus more on individual coping and recovery from mental health difficulties. Although the report highlights the benefits of primary interventions, the authors acknowledge the difficulties with this level of organisational adjustment; *"this can be both costly and time consuming, requiring considerable commitment from managers, colleagues and those responsible for the design of organisational systems"* (HEE, 2019, p. 78). This demonstrates the crucial difficulties with healthcare systems; it is not that the benefits of systemic and organisational change are not known, rather ongoing resource constraints, overworked staff and a culture of 'carrying on regardless' mean that guidelines cannot be followed, resulting in secondary and tertiary interventions become the first point of call.

There are aspects to working within a healthcare environment that are known to cause high levels of pressure and stress, and many of these will not be changeable (e.g. high stakes situations, being around death, emotional environment). In addition, as highlighted in the introduction, healthcare settings often embody a culture of the 'hero ideal' which serves to reinforce notions of 'carrying on regardless' and creates additional stress and pressure to deliver services at 'superhuman' levels, another facet which is difficult to change as it is linked to broader cultural narratives concerning healthcare staff. However, there may be specific elements that are contributing to the chronic exhaustion seen across healthcare organisations, particularly those that underfunded and overstretched (Appleby, 2018). For example, experience of 'futile or potentially inappropriate care' seems to correlate with burnout (Lambden et al., 2019). To explore this further, it is important to understand the complex moral and emotional processes underlying exhaustion and depersonalisation, and how these might be important when considering systemic and organisational change.

Compassion, Morality and Moral Distress

Compassion, the 'sensitivity to suffering in self and others with a commitment to try to alleviate and prevent it' (Gilbert et al., 2017, p. 1), is the cornerstone of an effective healthcare system. Compassion, empathy, dignity and respect are fundamental nursing principles (Flynn & Mercer, 2013). In addition to the benefits for recovery and patient outcomes, compassionate care is important for the wellbeing of healthcare staff (Gilbert, 2010). For example, there is evidence that doctors with high empathy scores have more job satisfaction and less burnout (Larson & Yao, 2005; Thomas et al., 2007), and that clinicians who feel compassionately treated by their organisation and team are more robust, creative and open (Cole-King & Gilbert, 2011). Compassion and burnout are therefore inherently linked in a cyclical fashion; lower compassion is linked with higher burnout, and when clinicians are more burned out, they are less able to be compassionate. Likewise, a more compassionate workplace protects against burnout.

Compassion fatigue, a precursor to the depersonalisation and emotional exhaustion seen in burnout, can occur due to long-term emotional investment in patients, having to have difficult and complex conversations at work, and a lack of time to decompress (Mendes, 2014). However, there may also be elements of guilt in being unable to deliver the best care within their time- and resource-limited environment (Mendes, 2014), suggesting a moral component to burnout that may be compounded by under resourced healthcare organisations. For example, healthcare staff in experienced distress as a result of feeling unable to deliver the high standards of care they wanted as a result of understaffing and organisational pressures (Wilkinson, 2015).

When staff cannot carry out what they believe to be ethically appropriate actions, especially if this is repeated over time, 'moral distress' can occur (Lamiani, Borghi, & Argentero, 2017). Moral distress can be triggered by many organisational factors known to be present in healthcare settings, such as lack of resources and time, workload, lack of autonomy and ethical climate of the workplace (Monrouxe, Rees, Dennis, & Wells, 2015), and can be felt not only by doctors and nurses, but anybody who works close to or directly with patients, including porters, ward clerks, and managers (Oliver, 2018). While often discussed as two distinct constructs, moral distress and burnout have been found to be associated (Ann B. Hamric & Blackhall, 2007; Ann Baile Hamric, Borchers, & Epstein, 2012; Meltzer & Huckabay, 2004; Piers et al., 2012). For example, Rushton et al (Rushton et al., 2015) found that nurses in high intensity settings reporting moral distress also scored highly for the three domains of burnout, arguing moral distress causes empathetic over-arousal, leading to emotional exhaustion. Similarly, Morley (Morley, Ives, & Bradbury-Jones, 2019) postulated that the 'dulling' of one's emotions as a result of ongoing moral distress would inevitably lead to compassion fatigue.

The existence of moral distress in the health service is well documented in the United States. Surveys across staff in medical settings have found moral distress to be present in all professional groups, with higher impact on those involved in direct patient care (Whitehead, Herbertson, Hamric, Epstein, & Fisher, 2015). Moral distress can lead to anxiety, depression, job dissatisfaction, burnout, and staff turnover (Allen et al., 2013). There is evidence that moral distress is not only an individual issue (with impact from isolated incidents), but a systemic issue. Moral distress has been negatively associated with ethical workplace climate, with the highest-ranked source being 'watching patient care suffer due to lack of continuity' (Whitehead et al., 2015).

A systematic review identified both organisational factors (perceived poor ethical climate, poor collaboration across medical professionals, lack of support from colleagues, working in acute care, not having enough time available for patients, and experiencing instrumental leadership) and psychological characteristics (low structural empowerment, poor access to resources, poor psychological empowerment, and low levels of autonomy) were associated with moral distress (Lamiani et al., 2017). The authors recommend management investment in organisational change (such as positive ethical climate, team collaboration and support), and educational and supportive interventions such as enhancing empowerment, autonomy and ethical knowledge. Thus, it appears that when healthcare organisations or professional groups have a culture of 'just deal with it', rather than acknowledging and mitigating the risk of moral distress, this can impact psychological health of the workforce and risk subsequent burnout (Houston et al., 2013).

In the UK, Young, Froggatt and Brearley (Young, Froggatt, & Brearley, 2017) identified that moral distress can occur when caring is restricted by organisational processes, resources or the provision of futile care, highlighting the systemic issues that can influence moral distress. Further, a recent survey with intensive care staff also identified situations where care was felt to be futile as engendering the highest levels of moral distress (Colville, Dawson, Rabinthiran, Chaudry-Daley, & Perkins-Porras, 2019). In addition, links have been drawn between moral distress and austerity, with differences between unavoidable and avoidable moral challenges. For example, Morley, Ives and Bradbury-Jones (Morley et al., 2019) argue unavoidable ethical challenges present in healthcare (patient suffering and end-of-life decision making) may require individual resilience support for staff, whereas avoidable ethical challenges related to austerity (withdrawal of treatments, staff reductions, time rationing) require additional organisational responses. These responses could focus on improving the ethical climate of healthcare environments and improving communication at the team level to build more trusting relationships (Morley, 2016). Focusing solely on individual approaches absolves the institution of responsibility (Traynor, 2017, 2018), rather than placing accountability with organisations and the political system (Morley et al., 2019).

Burnout and Moral Distress in Light of COVID-19: The Case of the UK National Health Service

If burnout is not tackled, the NHS will fail – Suzy Jordache, Senior Medical Educator at the UK's Medical Protection Society (Moberly, 2017).

Prior to 2020, the NHS workforce was already struggling with high rates of burnout in combination with moral distress, low funding and resource availability, and reduced staffing levels (Abbasi, 2019). NHS staff were being negatively impacted by a workforce that was overstretched and supplemented by temporary staff (Sizmur & Raleigh, 2018), and the institution was tending towards individualistic interventions for stress, with resource restrictions making systemic change difficult to implement (HEE, 2019).

In March 2020, the UK went into lockdown to slow the spread of the new coronavirus sweeping the globe. The arrival of this virus was in the context of an NHS already on its knees, with lower numbers of intensive care beds (Rhodes et al., 2012) and low staffing levels (Lee & Stoye, 2018). Hospitalisations of those with confirmed COVID-19 diagnoses peaked at a daily rate of 3,564 in April (DHSC, 2020), and the NHS was overwhelmed not only with patients but with new infection control guidelines that vastly altered clinicians' day-to-day working (e.g. personal protective equipment, reduced patient contact, ban on hospital visitors). Prior to November 2020, 600 health and social care workers had caught COVID-19 and died across England, Scotland and Wales (BBC, 2020). Many NHS workers have moved out of their homes due to concerns that personal protective equipment is not adequate to protect them and their loved ones (Jones-Berry, 2020), highlighting the complex moral environment in which NHS staff have been placed.

With the increased demand on services and staff redeployment, many have discussed the potential for staff to suffer 'moral injury' during this time (Borges et al., 2020; Dean et al., 2020; Greenberg et al., 2020; Williams et al., 2020; Williamson et al., 2020). Moral injury is considered a distinct term from moral distress, although moral distress may lead to moral injury (APA, 2020); moral injury can occur from a single, traumatic event, whereas moral distress can occur from less traumatic events that arise repeatedly over a period of time. Potentially Morally Injurious Events (PMIEs) occur in high-stakes environments and violate one's moral code or values, either through one's own actions (doing something you felt you should not have done), or other people's actions or inactions (feeling betrayed by other people's actions or inactions) (Borges et al., 2020). The nature of the pandemic is likely to force the hand of healthcare professionals in situations where resources are restricted, or where they are unable to provide a 'good death' (Selman et al., 2020).

Although prevalence data for moral injury during COVID-19 is somewhat limited at this early stage, initial investigations in US healthcare have identified moral injury scores similar to military service members exposed to 7-month war zone deployments (Hines, Chin, Levine, & Wickwire, 2020). Burnout, however, has been more extensively demonstrated internationally. In Spain, levels of compassion fatigue and burnout have been found to be moderate/high in physicians and nurses (Ruiz-Fernández et al., 2020), 53% of surveyed healthcare workers in Iran reported high levels of pandemic-related burnout (Khasne, Dhakulkar, & Mahajan, 2020), and over 40% of nurses in Japan met criteria for burnout (Matsuo et al., 2020). Further, systemic reviews have identified the increased risk of mental health impact of COVID-19 on care providers, including stress, anxiety, depression, insomnia and distress (Shaukat, Ali, & Razzak, 2020; Vizheh et al., 2020).

Although many theoretical papers are recommending an emphasis on moral injury when considering burnout and staff wellbeing (APA, 2020; Borges et al., 2020; Dean et al., 2020; Greenberg et al., 2020; Williams et al., 2020; Williamson et al., 2020), this is rarely in the context of widespread, pre-existing moral distress. While research has shown increased burnout during COVID-19 (Hines et al., 2020), in the UK this is a heavy impact on an already burned out workforce under moral pressure. Further, despite aftercare for COVID-19 being advised to encourage reflection on experience and replacement of traumatic narratives (Greenberg et al., 2020), there is little suggestion of the limitations of this intervention in the context of the current National Health Service, or the value of this intervention prior to the pandemic.

The difficulties experienced by healthcare staff during this time can be understood as an extension of pre-existing problems within the healthcare service. Individuals already on the edge of burnout experienced a significant increase in work-related stress factors such as high patient mortality and low control, while simultaneously not having access to external coping strategies such as social support or hobbies. Similarly, individuals with underlying moral distress following work in a resource restricted healthcare institution are perhaps more likely to experience moral injury in response to PMIEs during COVID-19. Rather than seeing these issues as distinct, it is important to consider whether burnout in National Health Service staff is indicative of moral distress and injury that has led to emotional overwhelm and exhaustion. This might alter the proposed course of individual intervention from resilience training to access to ethical consultation, palliative care consultation, allowing time off (APA, 2020).

National Health Service trusts in the UK have responded to the COVID-19 pandemic by introducing support measures for their staff, such as reflective spaces for teams to support the development of a meaningful narrative around morally distressing circumstances, or access to a free wellbeing support helpline (Greenberg et al., 2020; NHS, 2020). Many services did not previously have regular access to reflective spaces, and so had reached crisis point in response to the pandemic in order to access this support. In addition, these interventions are indicative of the individualist focus of burnout and moral injury support, placing emphasis on personal resilience and wellbeing rather than practical, organisational change. Given the nature of moral injury, systemic issues (such as lack of access to personal protective equipment) are likely to be central factors in staff experience of burnout and moral injury, as they will reduce likelihood of being able to act in a manner they consider ethical.

The culture of the National Health Service is another factor exacerbated by the pandemic. A pervasive narrative of healthcare staff as 'heroes' on the frontline has dominated the media and political communications, provoking the ideas of individuals doing their best in a 'war' with the country behind them. This places even higher pressure on individuals to 'come through' for their patients, to work against the odds in difficult and traumatic conditions to provide the best care. As being unable to 'do the right thing' and avoid a 'bad death' can cause powerlessness and moral distress in more usual times (Young et al., 2017), encouraging narratives of being 'heroes' always doing the right thing can create an impossible ideal that healthcare staff cannot live up to. Feeling unable to provide ideal and heroic care could contribute to the negative cognitions and guilt, shame and anger associated with burnout and moral injury. This link has been previously drawn in male combat veterans, with those identifying more strongly with the soldier-hero figure being potentially more at risk of moral injury (Farnsworth, 2014).

It is easy to hide behind COVID-19 as the cause for significant distress, burnout and moral injury in the healthcare service. However, research has shown that these issues were already present prior to the pandemic and it is important to acknowledge the role of organisational culture and systemic issues. While individual stress management and support may be helpful for staff during this time, management and policy makers must be held accountable for the working environment that exists across the National Health Service, and a culture change must be implemented within an economic environment that makes this possible. In the current environment, healthcare staff are being placed under extraordinary moral pressure, have been removed from their families and their colleagues, and are under conditions that are aggravating years of underfunding. While individual stress and trauma management is vital and necessary, cultural and systemic change is needed to support staff not just to recover from the impact of the pandemic, but for the workplace to recover from the last ten years of restrictions.

CONCLUSION

Burnout in healthcare staff is widespread to the point of being commonplace and is often co-occurring with symptoms of moral distress. This chapter has highlighted research suggesting the current reality of the healthcare service requires many employees to work in a way that does not measure up to their ethical standards, which leads to emotional exhaustion and burnout. Instead of considering this solely an individual issue, we argue that burnout should be addressed at a systemic level. Individual stress-management and mindfulness strategies may help reduce the personal impact of moral distress and promote resilience, but there cannot be a hope of a well-functioning and healthy healthcare system without practical and cultural changes. Whilst many of these issues have been in existence for a number of years, we suggest that the COVID-19 pandemic has highlighted and exacerbated existing problems, pushing healthcare staff off the metaphorical cliff on which the healthcare system was balanced. It has brought unparalleled moral pressure, isolation and exhaustion to a workforce already impacted by burnout and moral distress.

Therefore, further cross-cultural research is needed to provide evidence on the extent to which healthcare workers have experienced systemic moral injury in order to examine the differences between national healthcare systems and provide examples of how to mitigate such issues. Further, given the variety of employment roles in healthcare systems, coupled with pre-existing forms of marginalisation experienced by different groups working within healthcare systems, we suggest further research is needed to examine the distribution of forms of individual and systemic moral injury between healthcare workers in different employment roles, levels of seniority, employment status (e.g. FT/PT/bank staff) and comparing across individuals from different social groups (e.g. people from marginalised backgrounds). In addition, as this chapter has highlighted, the conceptualisations of burnout, moral injury and morality are often overlapping, therefore we suggest a need for qualitative research to explore the ways in which healthcare workers experience their work in relation to individual and organisational forms of morality and moral injury, whilst also offering a deeper exploration into the three additional principles of nursing, namely empathy, dignity, and respect.

Healthcare organisations typically places emphasis on individualist interventions for staff wellbeing, and this trend continues into the pandemic. We suggest that without acknowledging the contribution of systemic factors, the workforce will continue to experience high turnover, high staff sickness, and low rates of satisfaction and morale. Further, staff members will continue to experience the guilt, shame and anger associated with working in an environment that does not protect them from ethical challenges and thus future research is needed to evidence where, how and why such environments exist and offer a more substantive evidence base to challenge the status-quo. Further, here we also call for research exploring the impact of the cultures within healthcare systems on burnout and moral injury, examining how such cultures have potentially been exacerbated by the COVID-19 pandemic in relation to fear, blame, and hero narratives, providing an understanding of how such culture interacts with morality to create moral emotions like guilt/shame and anger.

It is important to remember that exploring morality and burnout is not for the purpose of creating diagnostic criteria or exact definitions, but to ensure change to the pertinent systemic issues that are increasingly prevalent and damaging to our healthcare staff. It is common for literature on burnout and moral distress to recommend intervention for moral distress due to the associated improvement in patient care, rather than simply the improvement of wellbeing in the workforce. Change is required, not just because it would be better economically and for patient care, by reducing staff turnover and sickness, but because it is time to prioritise healthcare staff. Therefore, as literature highlights some potential systemic solutions and areas of workplace environment that worsen burnout and moral injury, we call for future research seeking to explore what the barriers have been in implementing these systemic solutions to this point.

REFERENCES

Abbasi, K. (2019). A workforce crisis in the NHS. *Journal of the Royal Society of Medicine*, *112*(9), 363–363. doi:10.1177/0141076819875444 PMID:31496348

Ahola, K., & Hakanen, J. (2007). Job strain, burnout, and depressive symptoms: A prospective study among dentists. *Journal of Affective Disorders*, *104*(1-3), 103–110. doi:10.1016/j.jad.2007.03.004 PMID:17448543

Ahola, K., Hakanen, J., Perhoniemi, R., & Mutanen, P. (2014). Relationship between burnout and depressive symptoms: A study using the person-centred approach. *Burnout Research*, *1*(1), 29–37. doi:10.1016/j.burn.2014.03.003

Allen, R., Judkins-Cohn, T., deVelasco, R., Forges, E., Lee, R., Clark, L., & Procunier, M. (2013). Moral Distress Among Healthcare Professionals at a Health System. *JONA'S Healthcare Law, Ethics and Regulation*, *15*(3), 111–118. doi:10.1097/NHL.0b013e3182a1bf33 PMID:23963112

APA. (2020). *COVID-19 pandemic guidance document: moral injury during the COVID-19 pandemic*. Retrieved from American Psychiatric Association: https://www.psychiatry.org/File%20Library/Psychiatrists/APA-Guidance-COVID-19-Moral-Injury.pdf

Appleby, J. (2018). *70 years of NHS spending*. Nuffield Trust. Retrieved from https://ww.nuffieldtrust.org.uk/news-item/70-year-of-nhs-spending

Bauer, J., Stamm, A., Virnich, K., Wissing, K., Müller, U., Wirsching, M., & Schaarschmidt, U. (2006). Correlation between burnout syndrome and psychological and psychosomatic symptoms among teachers. *International Archives of Occupational and Environmental Health*, *79*(3), 199–204. doi:10.100700420-005-0050-y PMID:16258752

BBC. (2020). *Coronavirus: NHS workers who died in the pandemic*. Retrieved from https://www.bbc.co.uk/news/av/uk-53914546

Benziman, Y. (2020). "Winning" the "battle" and "beating" the COVID-19 "enemy": Leaders' use of war frames to define the pandemic. *Peace and Conflict*, *26*(3), 247–256. doi:10.1037/pac0000494

Bianchi, R., Schonfeld, I. S., & Laurent, E. (2014). Is burnout a depressive disorder? A reexamination with special focus on atypical depression. *International Journal of Stress Management*, *21*(4), 307–324. doi:10.1037/a0037906

BMA. (2020). *Almost half of UK doctors suffering from burnout, depression or anxiety, BMA survey reveals*. Retrieved from https://www.bma.org.uk/bma-media-centre/almost-half-of-uk-doctors-suffering-from-burnout-depression-or-anxiety-bma-survey-reveals

Borges, L. M., Barnes, S. M., Farnsworth, J. K., Bahraini, N. H., & Brenner, L. A. (2020). A commentary on moral injury among health care providers during the COVID-19 pandemic. *Psychological Trauma: Theory, Research, Practice, and Policy*, *12*(S1), S138–S140. doi:10.1037/tra0000698 PMID:32496101

Bressi, C., Porcellana, M., Gambini, O., Madia, L., Muffatti, R., Peirone, A., Zanini, S., Erlicher, A., Scarone, S., & Altamura, A. C. (2009). Burnout Among Psychiatrists in Milan: A Multicenter Survey. *Psychiatric Services (Washington, D.C.)*, *60*(7), 985–988. doi:10.1176/ps.2009.60.7.985 PMID:19564233

Brotheridge, C. M., & Grandey, A. A. (2002). Emotional Labor and Burnout: Comparing Two Perspectives of "People Work". *Journal of Vocational Behavior*, *60*(1), 17–39. doi:10.1006/jvbe.2001.1815

Cole-King, A., & Gilbert, P. (2011). Compassionate care: The theory and the reality. *Journal of Holistic Healthcare*, *8*(3).

Colville, G., Dawson, D., Rabinthiran, S., Chaudry-Daley, Z., & Perkins-Porras, L. (2019). A survey of moral distress in staff working in intensive care in the UK. *The Journal of the Intensive Care Society*, *20*(3), 196–203. doi:10.1177/1751143718787753 PMID:31447911

Cropanzano, R., Rupp, D. E., & Byrne, Z. S. (2003). The relationship of emotional exhaustion to work attitudes, job performance, and organizational citizenship behaviors. *The Journal of Applied Psychology*, *88*(1), 160–169. doi:10.1037/0021-9010.88.1.160 PMID:12675403

Dean, W., Jacobs, B., & Manfredi, R. A. (2020). Moral Injury: The Invisible Epidemic in COVID Health Care Workers. *Annals of Emergency Medicine*, *76*(4), 385–386. doi:10.1016/j.annemergmed.2020.05.023 PMID:32586634

DHSC. (2020). *Patients admitted to hospital*. Retrieved from https://coronavirus.data.gov.uk/details/healthcare

Farnsworth, J. K. (2014). Dialogical tensions in heroic military and military-related moral injury. *International Journal for Dialogical Science*, *8*(1), 13–37.

Flynn, M., & Mercer, D. (2013). Is compassion possible in a market-led NHS? *Nursing Times*, *109*(7), 12–14. PMID:23513933

Freudenberger, H. J. (1974). Staff Burn-Out. *The Journal of Social Issues*, *30*(1), 159–165. doi:10.1111/j.1540-4560.1974.tb00706.x

Gibbons, S. W., Shafer, M., Hickling, E. J., & Ramsey, G. (2013). How Do Deployed Health Care Providers Experience Moral Injury? *Narrative Inquiry in Bioethics*, *3*(3), 247–259. doi:10.1353/nib.2013.0055 PMID:24407133

Gilbert, P. (2010). Compassion Focused Therapy: Distinctive Features. Routledge.

Gilbert, P., Catarino, F., Duarte, C., Matos, M., Kolts, R., Stubbs, J., Ceresatto, L., Duarte, J., Pinto-Gouveia, J., & Basran, J. (2017). The development of compassionate engagement and action scales for self and others. *Journal of Compassionate Health Care*, *4*(1), 4. doi:10.118640639-017-0033-3

Graber, J. E., Huang, E. S., Drum, M. L., Chin, M. H., Walters, A. E., Heuer, L., Tang, H., Schaefer, C. T., & Quinn, M. T. (2008). Predicting Changes in Staff Morale and Burnout at Community Health Centers Participating in the Health Disparities Collaboratives: Staff Morale and Burnout at Community Health Centers. *Health Services Research*, *43*(4), 1403–1423. doi:10.1111/j.1475-6773.2007.00828.x PMID:18248402

Greenberg, N., Docherty, M., Gnanapragasam, S., & Wessely, S. (2020). Managing mental health challenges faced by healthcare workers during covid-19 pandemic. *BMJ (Clinical Research Ed.)*, *m1211*, m1211. doi:10.1136/bmj.m1211 PMID:32217624

Haight, W., Sugrue, E. P., & Calhoun, M. (2017). Moral injury among Child Protection Professionals: Implications for the ethical treatment and retention of workers. *Children and Youth Services Review*, *82*, 27–41. doi:10.1016/j.childyouth.2017.08.030

Hall, L. H., Johnson, J., Watt, I., Tsipa, A., & O'Connor, D. B. (2016). Healthcare Staff Wellbeing, Burnout, and Patient Safety: A Systematic Review. *PLoS One*, *11*(7), e0159015. doi:10.1371/journal.pone.0159015 PMID:27391946

Hamric, A. B., & Blackhall, L. J. (2007). Nurse-physician perspectives on the care of dying patients in intensive care units: Collaboration, moral distress, and ethical climate*. *Critical Care Medicine*, *35*(2), 422–429. doi:10.1097/01.CCM.0000254722.50608.2D PMID:17205001

Hamric, A. B., Borchers, C. T., & Epstein, E. G. (2012). Development and Testing of an Instrument to Measure Moral Distress in Healthcare Professionals. *AJOB Primary Research*, *3*(2), 1–9. doi:10.1080/21507716.2011.652337

HEE. (2019). *NHS Staff and Learners' Mental Wellbeing Commission*. Retrieved from https://www.hee.nhs.uk/sites/default/files/documents/NHS%20%28HEE%29%20-%20Mental%20Wellbeing%20Commission%20Report.pdf

Hines, S. E., Chin, K. H., Levine, A. R., & Wickwire, E. M. (2020). Initiation of a survey of healthcare worker distress and moral injury at the onset of the COVID-19 surge. *American Journal of Industrial Medicine*, *63*(9), 830–833. doi:10.1002/ajim.23157

Houston, S., Casanova, M. A., Leveille, M., Schmidt, K. L., Barnes, S. A., Trungale, K. R., & Fine, R. L. (2013). The intensity and frequency of moral distress among different healthcare disciplines. *The Journal of Clinical Ethics*, *24*(2), 98–112.

Iliffe, S., & Manthorpe, J. (2019). Job dissatisfaction, 'burnout' and alienation of labour: Undercurrents in England's NHS. *Journal of the Royal Society of Medicine*, *112*(9), 370–377. doi:10.1177/0141076819855956

Imo, U. O. (2017). Burnout and psychiatric morbidity among doctors in the UK: A systematic literature review of prevalence and associated factors. *BJPsych Bulletin*, *41*(4), 197–204. doi:10.1192/pb.bp.116.054247

Jones-Berry, S. (2020). COVID-19: nurses offered alternative housing to safeguard loved ones. Nursing Standard. *Nursing Standard*. Retrieved from https://rcni.com/nursing-standard/newsroom/news/covid-19-nurses-offered-alternative-housing-to-safeguard-loved-ones-159156

Khasne, R. W., Dhakulkar, B. S., & Mahajan, H. C. (2020). Burnout among Healthcare Workers during COVID-19 Pandemic in India: Results of a Questionnaire-based Survey. *Indian Journal of Critical Care Medicine*, *24*(8), 664–671. doi:10.5005/jp-journals-10071-23518

Kopacz, M. S., Ames, D., & Koenig, H. G. (2019). It's time to talk about physician burnout and moral injury. *The Lancet. Psychiatry*, *6*(11), e28. doi:10.1016/S2215-0366(19)30385-2

Koutsimani, P., Montgomery, A., & Georganta, K. (2019). The Relationship Between Burnout, Depression, and Anxiety: A Systematic Review and Meta-Analysis. *Frontiers in Psychology*, *10*, 284. doi:10.3389/fpsyg.2019.00284

Kumar, S. (2016). Burnout and Doctors: Prevalence, Prevention and Intervention. *Health Care*, *4*(3), 37. doi:10.3390/healthcare4030037

Lambden, J. P., Chamberlin, P., Kozlov, E., Lief, L., Berlin, D. A., Pelissier, L. A., ... Prigerson, H. G. (2019). Association of Perceived Futile or Potentially Inappropriate Care With Burnout and Thoughts of Quitting Among Health-Care Providers. *The American Journal of Hospice & Palliative Care*, *36*(3), 200–206. doi:10.1177/1049909118792517

Lamiani, G., Borghi, L., & Argentero, P. (2017). When healthcare professionals cannot do the right thing: A systematic review of moral distress and its correlates. *Journal of Health Psychology*, *22*(1), 51–67. doi:10.1177/1359105315595120

Larson, E. B., & Yao, X. (2005). Clinical empathy as emotional labor in the patient-physician relationship. *Journal of the American Medical Association*, *293*(9), 1100–1106.

Lee, T., & Stoye, G. (2018). What does the NHS spend its money on? In A. Charlesworth & P. Johnson (Eds.), *Securing the Future: Funding Health and Social Care to the 2030s*. Institute for Fiscal Studies.

Litz, B. T., Stein, N., Delaney, E., Lebowitz, L., Nash, W. P., Silva, C., & Maguen, S. (2009). Moral injury and moral repair in war veterans: A preliminary model and intervention strategy. *Clinical Psychology Review*, *29*(8), 695–706. doi:10.1016/j.cpr.2009.07.003

Maslach, C., Jackson, S. E., Leiter, M. P., Schaufeli, W. B., & Schwab, R. L. (1986). Maslach burnout inventory (Vol. 21). Consulting Psychologists Press.

Maslach, C., Schaufeli, W. B., & Leiter, M. P. (2001). Job Burnout. *Annual Review of Psychology*, *52*(1), 397–422. doi:10.1146/annurev.psych.52.1.397

Matsuo, T., Kobayashi, D., Taki, F., Sakamoto, F., Uehara, Y., Mori, N., & Fukui, T. (2020). Prevalence of Health Care Worker Burnout During the Coronavirus Disease 2019 (COVID-19) Pandemic in Japan. *JAMA Network Open*, *3*(8), e2017271. doi:10.1001/jamanetworkopen.2020.17271

McCain, R. S., McKinley, N., Dempster, M., Campbell, W. J., & Kirk, S. J. (2018). A study of the relationship between resilience, burnout and coping strategies in doctors. *Postgraduate Medical Journal*, *94*(1107), 43–47.

McKinley, N., McCain, R. S., Convie, L., Clarke, M., Dempster, M., Campbell, W. J., & Kirk, S. J. (2020). Resilience, burnout and coping mechanisms in UK doctors: A cross-sectional study. *BMJ Open*, *10*(1), e031765. doi:10.1136/bmjopen-2019-031765

Meltzer, L. S., & Huckabay, L. M. (2004). Critical Care Nurses' Perceptions of Futile Care and Its Effect on Burnout. *American Journal of Critical Care*, *13*(3), 202–208. doi:10.4037/ajcc2004.13.3.202

Mendes, A. (2014). Recognising and combating compassion fatigue in nursing. *British Journal of Nursing (Mark Allen Publishing)*, *23*(21), 1146–1146. doi:10.12968/bjon.2014.23.21.1146

Moberly, T. (2017). Five minutes with . . . Suzy Jordache. *BMJ (Clinical Research Ed.)*, *j2371*. doi:10.1136/bmj.j2371

Monrouxe, L. V., Rees, C. E., Dennis, I., & Wells, S. E. (2015). Professionalism dilemmas, moral distress and the healthcare student: Insights from two online UK-wide questionnaire studies. *BMJ Open*, *5*(5), e007518–e007518. doi:10.1136/bmjopen-2014-007518

Morley, G. (2016). Efficacy of the nurse ethicist in reducing moral distress: What can the NHS learn from the USA? Part 2. *British Journal of Nursing (Mark Allen Publishing)*, *25*(3), 156–161. doi:10.12968/bjon.2016.25.3.156

Morley, G., Ives, J., & Bradbury-Jones, C. (2019). Moral Distress and Austerity: An Avoidable Ethical Challenge in Healthcare. *Health Care Analysis*, *27*(3), 185–201. doi:10.100710728-019-00376-8

NHS. (2020). *Our NHS people: wellbeing support*. Retrieved from NHS Employers: https://www.nhsemployers.org/-/media/Employers/Documents/Retain-and-improve/Health-and-wellbeing/NHSSupportingOurPeople12.pdf?la=en&hash=D49FAA8660A94E578AC08B10553D61DEFC297EEE

Ohue, T., Moriyama, M., & Nakaya, T. (2011). Examination of a cognitive model of stress, burnout, and intention to resign for Japanese nurses: Cognitive model of burnout for nurses. *Japan Journal of Nursing Science*, *8*(1), 76–86. doi:10.1111/j.1742-7924.2010.00161.x

Oliver, D. (2018). David Oliver: Moral distress in hospital doctors. *BMJ (Clinical Research Ed.)*, *k1333*. doi:10.1136/bmj.k1333

Orton, P., & Gray, D. P. (2015). Burnout in NHS staff. *Lancet*, *385*(9980), 1831. doi:10.1016/S0140-6736(15)60921-7

Orton, P., Orton, C., & Pereira Gray, D. (2012). Depersonalised doctors: A cross-sectional study of 564 doctors, 760 consultations and 1876 patient reports in UK general practice. *BMJ Open*, *2*(1), e000274. doi:10.1136/bmjopen-2011-000274

Peiró, J. M., González-Romá, V., Tordera, N., & Mañas, M. A. (2001). Does role stress predict burnout over time among health care professionals? *Psychology & Health*, *16*(5), 511–525. doi:10.1080/08870440108405524

Peng, J., Clarkin, C., & Doja, A. (2018). Uncovering cynicism in medical training: A qualitative analysis of medical online discussion forums. *BMJ Open*, *8*(10), e022883. doi:10.1136/bmjopen-2018-022883

Piers, R. D., Van den Eynde, M., Steeman, E., Vlerick, P., Benoit, D. D., & Van Den Noortgate, N. J. (2012). End-of-Life Care of the Geriatric Patient and Nurses' Moral Distress. *Journal of the American Medical Directors Association*, *13*(1), 80.e87–80.e13. doi:10.1016/j.jamda.2010.12.014

Pinikahana, J., & Happell, B. (2004). Stress, burnout and job satisfaction in rural psychiatric nurses: A Victorian study. *The Australian Journal of Rural Health, 12*(3), 120–125. doi:10.1111/j.1440-1854.2004.00572.x

Rhodes, A., Ferdinande, P., Flaatten, H., Guidet, B., Metnitz, P. G., & Moreno, R. P. (2012). The variability of critical care bed numbers in Europe. *Intensive Care Medicine, 38*(10), 1647–1653. doi:10.100700134-012-2627-8

Richardson, N. M., Lamson, A. L., Smith, M., Eagan, S. M., Zvonkovic, A. M., & Jensen, J. (2020). Defining Moral Injury Among Military Populations: A Systematic Review. *Journal of Traumatic Stress, 33*(4), 575–586. doi:10.1002/jts.22553

Ruiz-Fernández, M. D., Ramos-Pichardo, J. D., Ibáñez-Masero, O., Cabrera-Troya, J., Carmona-Rega, M. I., & Ortega-Galán, Á. M. (2020). Compassion fatigue, burnout, compassion satisfaction and perceived stress in healthcare professionals during the COVID-19 health crisis in Spain. *Journal of Clinical Nursing, 29*(21-22), 4321–4330. doi:10.1111/jocn.15469

Rushton, C. H., Batcheller, J., Schroeder, K., & Donohue, P. (2015). Burnout and Resilience Among Nurses Practicing in High-Intensity Settings. *American Journal of Critical Care, 24*(5), 412–420. doi:10.4037/ajcc2015291

Salyers, M. P., Bonfils, K. A., Luther, L., Firmin, R. L., White, D. A., Adams, E. L., & Rollins, A. L. (2017). The Relationship Between Professional Burnout and Quality and Safety in Healthcare: A Meta-Analysis. *Journal of General Internal Medicine, 32*(4), 475–482. doi:10.100711606-016-3886-9

Schaufeli, W., & Enzmann, D. (1998). *The burnout companion to study and practice: A critical analysis*. CRC Press.

Schaufeli, W. B., Bakker, A. B., Hoogduin, K., Schaap, C., & Kladler, A. (2001). on the clinical validity of the maslach burnout inventory and the burnout measure. *Psychology & Health, 16*(5), 565–582. doi:10.1080/08870440108405527

Schonfeld, I. S., & Bianchi, R. (2016). Burnout and Depression: Two Entities or One?: Burnout and Depression. *Journal of Clinical Psychology, 72*(1), 22–37. doi:10.1002/jclp.22229

Selman, L. E., Chao, D., Sowden, R., Marshall, S., Chamberlain, C., & Koffman, J. (2020). Bereavement Support on the Frontline of COVID-19: Recommendations for Hospital Clinicians. *Journal of Pain and Symptom Management, 60*(2), e81–e86. doi:10.1016/j.jpainsymman.2020.04.024

Shaukat, N., Ali, D. M., & Razzak, J. (2020). Physical and mental health impacts of COVID-19 on healthcare workers: A scoping review. *International Journal of Emergency Medicine, 13*(1), 40. doi:10.118612245-020-00299-5

Shay, J. (2014). Moral injury. *Psychoanalytic Psychology, 31*(2), 182.

Sizmur, S., & Raleigh, V. (2018). *The risks to care quality and staff wellbeing of an NHS system under pressure*. Retrieved from https://www.picker.org/wp-content/uploads/2014/12/Risks-to-care-quality-and-staff-wellbeing-VR-SS-v8-Final.pdf

Squiers, J. J., Lobdell, K. W., Fann, J. I., & DiMaio, J. M. (2017). Physician Burnout: Are We Treating the Symptoms Instead of the Disease? *The Annals of Thoracic Surgery*, *104*(4), 1117–1122. doi:10.1016/j.athoracsur.2017.08.009

Thomas, M. R., Dyrbye, L. N., Huntington, J. L., Lawson, K. L., Novotny, P. J., Sloan, J. A., & Shanafelt, T. D. (2007). How Do Distress and Well-being Relate to Medical Student Empathy? A Multicenter Study. *Journal of General Internal Medicine*, *22*(2), 177–183. doi:10.100711606-006-0039-6

Traynor, M. (2017). Critical Resilience for Nurses: An Evidence-based Guide to Survival and Change in the Modern NHS. Routledge.

Traynor, M. (2018). Guest editorial: What's wrong with resilience. *Journal of Research in Nursing*, *23*(1), 5–8. doi:10.1177/1744987117751458

Tregoning, C., Remington, S., & Agius, S. (2014). Facing change: Developing resilience for staff, associate specialist, and specialty doctors. *BMJ (Clinical Research Ed.)*, *g251*. doi:10.1136/bmj.g251

Vindrola-Padros, C., Andrews, L., Dowrick, A., Djellouli, N., Fillmore, H., Bautista Gonzalez, E., ... Johnson, G. (2020). Perceptions and experiences of healthcare workers during the COVID-19 pandemic in the UK. *BMJ Open*, *10*(11), e040503. doi:10.1136/bmjopen-2020-040503

Vizheh, M., Qorbani, M., Arzaghi, S. M., Muhidin, S., Javanmard, Z., & Esmaeili, M. (2020). The mental health of healthcare workers in the COVID-19 pandemic: A systematic review. *Journal of Diabetes and Metabolic Disorders*, *19*(2), 1967–1978. doi:10.100740200-020-00643-9

Whitehead, P. B., Herbertson, R. K., Hamric, A. B., Epstein, E. G., & Fisher, J. M. (2015). Moral Distress Among Healthcare Professionals: Report of an Institution-Wide Survey: Moral Distress. *Journal of Nursing Scholarship*, *47*(2), 117–125. doi:10.1111/jnu.12115

Wilkinson, E. (2015). UK NHS staff: Stressed, exhausted, burnt out. *Lancet*, *385*(9971), 841–842. doi:10.1016/S0140-6736(15)60470-6

Willan, J., King, A. J., Jeffery, K., & Bienz, N. (2020). Challenges for NHS hospitals during covid-19 epidemic. *BMJ (Clinical Research Ed.)*, *m1117*. doi:10.1136/bmj.m1117

Willard-Grace, R., Hessler, D., Rogers, E., Dube, K., Bodenheimer, T., & Grumbach, K. (2014). Team Structure and Culture Are Associated With Lower Burnout in Primary Care. *Journal of the American Board of Family Medicine*, *27*(2), 229–238. doi:10.3122/jabfm.2014.02.130215

Williams, R. D., Brundage, J. A., & Williams, E. B. (2020). Moral Injury in Times of COVID-19. *Journal of Health Service Psychology*, *46*(2), 65–69. doi:10.100742843-020-00011-4

Williamson, V., Murphy, D., & Greenberg, N. (2020). COVID-19 and experiences of moral injury in front-line key workers. *Occupational Medicine*, *70*(5), 317–319. doi:10.1093/occmed/kqaa052

Wright, T. A., & Cropanzano, R. (1998). Emotional exhaustion as a predictor of job performance and voluntary turnover. *The Journal of Applied Psychology*, *83*(3), 486–493. doi:10.1037/0021-9010.83.3.486

Young, A., Froggatt, K., & Brearley, S. G. (2017). 'Powerlessness' or 'doing the right thing' – Moral distress among nursing home staff caring for residents at the end of life: An interpretive descriptive study. *Palliative Medicine*, *31*(9), 853–860. doi:10.1177/0269216316682894

Zhang, Q., Mu, M.-c., He, Y., Cai, Z.-l., & Li, Z.-c. (2020). Burnout in emergency medicine physicians: A meta-analysis and systematic review. *Medicine*, *99*(32), e21462. doi:10.1097/MD.0000000000021462

Zohar, D. (1997). Predicting burnout with a hassle-based measure of role demands. *Journal of Organizational Behavior: The International Journal of Industrial, Occupational and Organizational Psychology and Behavior*, *18*(2), 101–115.

Chapter 11
How the Prevalence of Work Stress Influences the Quality of Life and Performance of Hospital Employees

Navneesh Tyagi
https://orcid.org/0000-0002-1475-0617
Noida Institute of Engineering and Technology, India

Preeti Tyagi
ICRI, India

ABSTRACT

Recently the COVID-19 pandemic has very clearly revealed the enormous challenges and risks our healthcare workers are facing globally while working in difficult situations. They are more prone to make mistakes which can lead to harmful effects on them and their patients leading to work stress which has become a part of their daily lives. A dearth of studies has examined this concept in an organizational context as it affects an individual's life and work. This study is examining the influence of work stress on employee performance and quality of life of healthcare workers. Data collected from employees of selected hospitals with the help of a structured questionnaire were analyzed using SPSS version 23. Findings of correlation and regression analysis revealed a significant positive influence of the work stress on employee performance and quality of life.

INTRODUCTION

Since medical personnel have to retort to the needs of patients and families very fast, medical practice is stressful. When compared to other occupations, health care professionals experience very high levels of stress. Numerous organisational and behavioural studies have been conducted to ascertain the unique pressures experienced by health care professionals (Jacobsen et al., 2014; Nübling et al., 2010). The

DOI: 10.4018/978-1-7998-8813-0.ch011

primary contributors of occupational stress are workload, leadership style, professional conflict, emotional cost of caring, as well as a lack of incentive and shift work (McVicar, 2003). Bridger et al. (2013) demonstrated high levels of stress and burnout among nurses causing absenteeism or nursing turnover and finally resulting in staff shortages and increased workload intensity. Physicians attribute occupational stress mostly to high quantitative demands (the amount and pace of work), perceived greater obligation toward patients, role uncertainty, personal costs, their relationships with colleagues and employees, and medical bureaucracy (Bernburg et al., 2016; Pedrazza et al., 2016). Radical changes prompted by the need to remain profitable and meet future demographic needs, as well as digitalization, are putting further burden on the healthcare sector and its workforce (Abramovitz and Zelnick, 2010; Farquharson et al., 2013). As health expectancy increases, 11.6 percent of the world's population is projected to be over 65 years old in 2022, leading in an increase in global health care demand (Deloitte, 2018). Additionally, decreases in hospital services, an increased emphasis on outpatient treatment, and staff shortages are structural sources of high expectations that act as additional chronic psychosocial risk factors for remaining personnel (Aiken et al., 2002). Any medical errors or omissions can be costly, detrimental to a patient's life, and occasionally irrevocable. In medical professions, night shifts and extended working hours are also very common. Currently, healthcare system is operating under the most difficult conditions of COVID 19 epidemic which has disturbed the whole world and lead to demises. The psychological health of healthcare workers is facing an intense social work load that is disrupting their critical thinking performance. This decrease in critical thinking ability may give rise to a decline in the efficiency of the services provided to ease the living conditions and to secure the health of individuals.

Working face-to-face with patients can give rise to serious issues such as feeling of isolation, fear of life, and annoyance among healthcare professionals, and stress may be the reaction to these concerns in them (Xiang et al., 2020; Zhang et al., 2020). Cai et al. (2020) revealed that healthcare professionals possess tremendously high stress levels during the COVID-19 epidemic. According to new studies, occupational stress accounts for 50-60% of all non-working days (Golubic et al., 2009). Work-related stress has been shown to be harmful when there is a mismatch between job needs, worker skills, available resources, and required resources (Tyagi, Moses, and Rana, 2017). Work-related stress has been shown to be harmfull when there is a mismatch between job requirements, capabilities of workers, resource availability etc. (Mursali et al., 2009). The majority of studies agree that professional stress can occur from variety of dangers (Clegg, 2001). These dangers are separated into two categories: physical and psychosocial. Workplace exposure to physical dangers has been linked to anxiety, which leads to work-related stress. Psychosocial risks include variables such as organization, job design and administration, over and above the social structure of the workplace, all of which can have a negative effect on individual's quality of life (Cox and Rial-Gonzalez, 2002). Organizational as well as Individual issues such as mental, behavioral, and physical outcomes, work life quality, organizational commitment, and performance are frequently influenced by occupational stress (Beheshtifar et al., 2011). It can escort to injury and bad health. When workforce is stressed, they are more likely to be less motivated, unhealthy, unproductive and insecure at work (Tyagi, 2021). In a competitive market, their businesses are not very successful. Stress can occur as a result of pressures at home and at work. Employers cannot protect their employees from stress that arises outside of the workplace, but they can protect them from stress that arises as a result of their jobs. Workplace stress can cause issues for an organizational performance and its workers quality of life. Proper management and good work environment of organization can prevent stress of employees (Tyagi and Moses, 2020). Poor level of quality of life is linked to high level of work stress related to job discontent that ultimately result in a higher likelihood of leaving the company (Fairbrother and Warn, 2003). This might be viewed as a general impression of the job or as a collection of attitudes towards specific aspects of the profession (Lu et al., 2009). There is increasing evidence that existing employment trends are having a damaging influence on job fulfillment and deteriorating employee health (physical as well as mental) (Faragher et al., 2010), consequently quality of life. The two components (occupational stress and quality of life) can have adverse effect on a workforce performance that consequently increases corporate expense. The necessity for enhancing work quality, productivity, health and safety in the workplace, has been discovered by a review of the current circumstances across the world (Liaudanskiene et al., 2010).

Thus, the present research is directed with the objective of estimating the effect of stress of healthcare professionals on their employee performance and quality of life.

Given the above explanation, in light of the fact that there has been little research combining specifically these three constructs of work stress, performance, and quality of life among healthcare employees, the existing study was directed to evaluate the effect of workplace stress on healthcare employee performance and quality of life.

CONCEPTUAL BACKGROUND

High levels of occupational stress and its detrimental effects on health are well-documented in those who work in the healthcare field. However, little is known regarding its impact on work life quality and performance in healthcare settings (Bischoff et al., 2019). Job stress can happen at any time and at any location (Barzideh et al., 2014) with instant or delayed reactions. The study of relevant literature presented that healthcare employees are stressed by unfavorable psychological factors such as insufficient support, lack of teamwork, and a shortage of personnel (Allisey et al., 2014). Some causes of stress in healthcare include contradictory expectations of patients, colleagues, and organization. Stress causes job dissatisfaction, which leads to poor job performance and the likelihood of turnover. In that case, Job rotation and reinforcement of employees' faith in their individual competencies and skills may increase job satisfaction in stressful work conditions (Ruyter et al., 2001).

Work stress in healthcare may also arise due to role ambiguity, workload pressure, homework interface, performance pressure, interpersonal relationships, role conflicts, and job performance, and even personal motivation. Stressors have a negative impact on job performance (Rana and Munir, 2011; Ahmed and Ramzan, 2013).

This stress is developed if an employee's abilities may not match with the job requirements (Yang et al., 2015). It may further increase under inappropriate working circumstances (Barzideh, Choobineh, and Tabatabaee, 2014) that can have negative health implications. Employees that are able to overcome employment stress and advance their careers are said to have captured "challenge stress" while the employee's workplace stress which cannot be overcome (for instance, tension produced by politics within the organization) is termed as hindrance stress (Yang et al., 2017). The Job stress can lead to a decrease in job dedication and performance of employees (Reilly, Dhingra, & Boduszek, 2014; Abuhashesh et al., 2019). It has an impact on the company as well as employees in terms of emotional, behavioral, and physical consequences such as dedication, work satisfaction, and performance (Hoboubi et al., 2017). Healthcare employees with children have got greater anxiety level (Hacimusalar et al. 2020) in the current epidemic situation where schools were closed and kids were forced to reside at home. For health workers, the circumstances created a slew of issues, including child care and education. They were unable to obtain authorization from their employers to work from home and faced problems in finding somebody to look after their children. Therefore one of them had abandoned their career (Maria et al., 2020; Hazarika and Das, 2020) to manage their family. Thus' anxiety levels have been raised as a result of such stressful life situations. Job performance literature stated that it is a result of the interaction of three factors: skill, effort, and the character of the work environment. Employee skills comprise their knowledge, abilities, and competencies; effort refers to an employee's level of motivation on the job; and the nature of work conditions refers to the degree to which the environment accommodates the employee's performance (Masa'deh, Obeidat, and Tarhini, 2016). Every organisation aspires for improved employee performance regardless of external events and conditions. Stress has a substantial impact on employee performance, which may have an adverse effect on employees' mental and physical health. Numerous research undertaken in western countries have demonstrated that stressors, notably Occupational Stress Inducers (OSI), are negatively connected with employees' quality of life and wellbeing (Raja et al., 2020).

Ha1: There is a significant influence of Job stress on employee performance.

The negative and pricey repercussions of stress highlight the call for solutions to control stress within the workplace. Employees may start searching for opportunities outside their organizations. In healthcare organizations long hour overwork and work intensification are very common that lead to significant and occasional distressing effect. This stress disturbs mental as well as physical health. Employees who are under extreme pressure at work due to uncooperative colleagues and employer, are undervalued, and pushed to work harder and harder. Ozyurek et al. (2021) conducted his study to evaluate quality of life, stress, anxiety sensitivity, and satisfaction with life. They demonstrated that surgical clinic nurses had a lower quality of life and were more stressed. Kowalska and Szwamel (2021) observed that stress also effects well-being and quality of life and finally lead to emotional or psychological problems in life and quality of patient care delivered by these healthcare workers (Shaban et al., 2012). Financial difficulties, sleep problems, and a lack of leisure activities are all significantly correlated with sadness, anxiety, and stress (Cheung et al., 2016). Long practice hours, peer relationships, a lack of recreational opportunities, poor eating habits, a lack of regular exercise, and continual pressure in the healthcare atmosphere may All of these factors have an effect on employees' quality of life (Moura et al., 2016). As a result of the preceding analysis of the literature, it is obvious that few studies have evaluated these characteristics in comparison to other industries, particularly between high-tech and conventional industries, but rarely in the healthcare industry. This study seeks to close this gap by examining the effect of job stress on employee quality of life and performance among healthcare professionals. The proposed Model of this study is as under:

Therefore the following hypothesis is postulated:

Ha2: There is a significant influence of Job stress on Quality of Life.

Figure 1. Conceptual Model of Influence of Work Stress on Employee Performance and Quality of Life

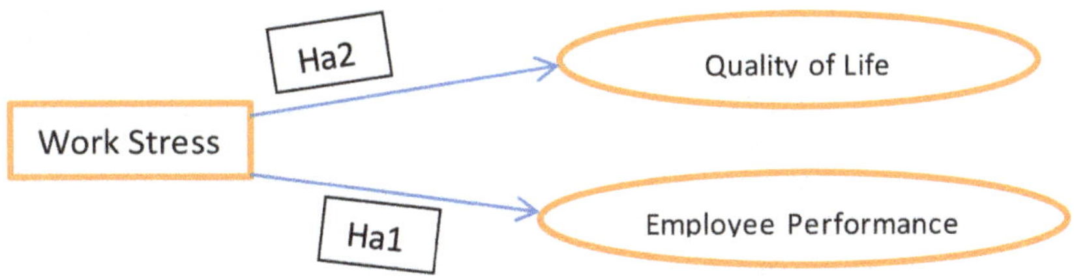

OBJECTIVES OF STUDY

To analyze the influence of Work Stress on Employee Performance and Quality of Life.

METHODOLOGY

Research Design

Correlational research was used in this study. A Likert scale questionnaire was used to obtain data from 150 staff of selected hospitals in Delhi. Explanatory or causal research designs were preferred to assess the effect of stress on employee performance and quality of life. The explanatory study method was chosen because it focuses on the causal effect of stress (an independent variable) on employee performance and quality of life (dependent variables). Second, explanatory research places a premium on empirical research. The study sought empirical evidence of the variables' relationships using statistical analysis.

Data Collection

Research data was collected in two phases, firstly; the secondary sources viz. several journals, Internet, books, magazines, articles etc. were referred for the purpose of literature review. Proceedings of many researchers concerning stress, Employee performance, and Quality of Life were referred. Then a questionnaire was created to collect information from the participants about the impact of these stress variables on employee performance and quality of life. The respondents were polled for the primary data. The organization's approval has to be obtained. The questionnaire was distributed to the employees who were asked to complete it. Participants were asked to inquire anything regarding the questionnaire or the study.

Perceived Stress Scale

Cohen et al. (1983) designed a 14-item scale that was employed in this study. On a 5-point Likert-type scale (Never = 0 to Very often = 4), respondents were asked to rate the items. The scores of seven items with affirmative statements have been reversed. A high score shows the person's extreme perceived stress. The total score goes from 0 to 56.

Table 1. Reliability Statistics

Variable	Cronbach Alpha	No. of Items
Employee Stress	0.766	14
Quality of life	0.858	28
Employee Performance	0.793	10

Employee Performance Questionnaire

It consists of self-structured, Likert five-point scale extending from strongly disagree [1] to strongly agree [5]). The scale has been developed with the help of extensive literature review. The scale consists of 10 items.

Quality of Life Scale

It was created by Menekay and Celmece (2017) to find out how employees felt about their quality of life. Working life, social life, burnout, and satisfaction are the four components of the measure, which has 28 items.

Data Analysis and Discussion

This section deals with the data collected that include all the demographics factors of the respondents and techniques used in this research. After obtaining the data the data was put in SPSS 23 software and different test of reliability, correlation, and regression results were analyzed and result findings and conclusions were discussed.

Reliability was estimated to check the correctness of the questionnaire. The reliability is tested on the response of There were 150 replies. A descriptive cross-sectional study was undertaken in certified hospitals in the Delhi NCT region of India. The study population consisted of hospital staff. The sampling frame includes all physicians, nurses, and paramedical employees in the hospitals' various departments and sections. The sample was drawn via quota sampling from these three occupational groups: physicians, nurses, and paramedical employees. After selecting participants, the researcher described the study's main objective to them. If volunteers consented to participate, the questionnaire was distributed to 250 individuals who were asked to complete and return it. Only 150 valid replics were collected, resulting in a 68 percent response rate for the poll. The sample was selected based on their willingness to participate in the study and at least one year of job experience directly associated with patients. These respondents were requested to complete a 52-question questionnaire in which 14 questions were related to stress, 10 questions related to employee performance, and 28 questions were related to Quality of life. As shown in tables below, the construct reliability (Cronbach α) scores of all the constructs were found to exceed the threshold value of 0.70 (Nunnally, 1978), therefore the scale can reliably be used in the present study.

The data cleaning and data screening was conducted by deleting those responses which were inaccurate.

Table 2. Correlation Analysis (N= 150)

	WS	QWL	EP
WS	1	-.695**	-.473**
QWL	-.695**	1	.436**
EP	-.473**	.436**	1

** Correlation is significant at the P value= 0.0 1

Hypothesis Testing

To justify the objective of the research study, hypotheses were tested using Karl Pearson's correlation and regression analysis. The analysis was done by applying SPSS 23 version.

Correlation coefficients among the variables under investigation were estimated. This table shows that the results are significant. Correlation of work stress is moderately negative (-.473) with employee performance. Significant value should be less than .05 levels and the value calculated is found to be significant at 0.01 levels. Therefore alternative hypothesis (Ha1) is failed to be rejected. Here a moderately negative correlation between work stress and the employee performance is observed. Work stress is found to be highly negatively correlated (-.695) with quality of life. Significant value should be less than .05 and the value calculated is found to be significant at p= 0.000. Therefore alternative hypothesis (Ha2) is also failed to be rejected. There is a moderately positive correlation (.436) between quality of life and the employee performance.

Table 3. Regression Analysis

Model	R	R Square	Adjusted R Square	Std. Error of the Estimate
1 (WS-QWL)	-.695a	.483	.480	4.79612
2 (WS-EP)	-.473b	.224	.219	5.30662

a. Dependent Variable: QWL, EP
b. Predictors: (Constant), WS 1

In the above value, the R square value shows that .224 percent of employee performance is influenced by work stress. It means that 22.4% of changes in employee's performance as a dependent variable is explained by work stress. Work Stress is moderately and positively related to employee performance. It satisfies the hypothesis (Ha1) which succeeds in predicting the significant effect of work stress on employee performance.

Work Stress is significantly and positive correlated to quality of life. In the above value, the R square value showing .483 percent of job satisfaction influencing work stress. It shows that 48.3% of changes in quality of life as a dependent variable is explained by work stress. It satisfies the hypothesis (Ha2) which succeeds in showing the significant effect of work stress on quality of life.

The above table shows the linear relationship between dependent variable and independent variable. Linear analysis is used in view of the study objective and hypothesis. The significant value should be less

Table 4. Coefficients

Model		Standardized coefficients B	Std. Error	Unstandardized Coefficients (Beta)	T	F	Sig
1	(Constant)	4.849	1.569		3.090	138.323	.000
	WS	-.770	.065	-.695	11.761		.025
	a. Dependent Variable: QWL						
2	(Constant)	11.999	1.826 6		.572	42.756	.000
	WS	.498	.076	.473	6.539		.000
	b. Dependent Variable: EP						

than .05 and the calculated result of significant value is found to be .025 which shows there is a weak impact of work stress on quality of life. Stress has a significantly negative influence on quality of life.

The above table shows the linear relationship between the dependent variables (employee performance and quality of life) and independent variable (work stress). Linear analysis is used in view of the study objective and hypothesis. The significant value should be less than .05 and the result of significant value is (p= 0.000) which shows the statistically significantly impact of independent variable on dependent variables. There is a significantly positive impact of work stress on employee performance.

The magnitude of F value also confirms that there is significant relationship between work stress and quality of life. The value of F must be greater than 5. In this study, the value of F is 138.3 that is greater than 5. The results are justified. The output of ANOVA analysis also depicts a statistically significant difference between the means of variables (work stress and quality of life). The significance value is (p= 0.000), which is below 0.05 that confirms a significant relationship between work stress and employee performance. In this study, the value of F is 42.756 that is greater than 5 and therefore statistically significant difference in the means of variable (stress and employee performance) is proved. These findings are consistent with previous studies like Yang et al. (2017), Mittal and Bhasker (2018) etc.

CONCLUSION

Health care professionals require assistance in building their resilience to inevitable occupational stress. The purpose of this systematic review was to determine the effect of work stress on employee performance and quality of life. Nonetheless, this study emphasises the vacuum in prior research in this area and summarises previously published information on this subject, including the following: (a). Employees in the healthcare sector have unusually high levels of occupational stress; (b). Stress among health care workers is connected with a variety of chronic diseases, risky behaviours, staff turnover, and medical blunders; and (c). Physical activity is being discussed for its potential to alleviate or regulate stress.

The gap this paper tried to fill are: (a). Limited evidence is available on this topic and no systematic study specifically combining the influence of Work Stress on Employee Performance and Quality of Life is published yet and (b). This paper identifies work stress studies aimed at improving the Employee Performance and Quality of Life of employees of the healthcare sector.

There is a moderate correlation between different construct under study. R square value shows 22.4% percent of stress that influence employee's performance. Overload, role ambiguity, role conflict, personal responsibility, engagement, a lack of feedback, and rapid technological development all contribute to high levels of stress among health care personnel. The aforementioned constructs are positively connected and exert a bigger influence on employee performance and quality of life (Mittal and Bhasker, 2018; Yang et al., 2017). To alleviate stress, employers should take proactive measures such as optimizing workloads, effectively managing customer expectations, minimizing relationship and role conflict, implementing an adequate reward system, and providing adequate training and counselling to employees in order to improve their job performance and quality of life. Workload had a greater impact on job performance than the other primary characteristics studied in the study. The majority of employees across all age groups agree that job stress has an impact on their performance. An organization must attempt to ease and sort out measures to assist employees in overcoming workplace stress. It basically assesses their potential as a valuable asset to the hospital. It is the supreme responsibility of the management to generate a conducive climate to work stress-free on a day-to-day basis to maintain high morale and productivity among healthcare staff. For this purpose, job stress moderation, counseling, meditation programs, and more incentives can be provided to progress the quality of life and performance of the staff.

This study can help decision-makers make the best business decisions possible through their HR systems, resulting in increased employee satisfaction and work performance. Healthcare organization may organize meditation or sports classes, can offer paid time off to its employees, encourage employees to take breaks, may provide benefits for mental and physical health, may reduce the workload of employees, and management can take pains to delegate the work efficiently. Employees can be owed alternate shift timings that may lead to a healthy work life balance. A job stress audit can be originated at periodic basis in order to establish the job stress area and moderate the same. Seminars and workshops for stress reduction can be organized by the organizations.

LIMITATIONS AND FUTURE IMPLICATIONS

The main limitation of this research was its sample size that was relatively medium compared to other past studies. Furthermore, the questionnaire formed might be more profound. The time to obtain some of the feedbacks of the survey was long due to Covid 19 pandemic that interrupt the motivation of wanting to accomplish a better sample size. Due to busy schedule the respondents may interpret the questions incorrectly. Some of the respondents did not like to share their views. It is also suggested that future researchers could further explore the research on a widespread data and determine other variables that effects employee performance and quality of life. It would allow providing a better analytical result.

REFERENCES

Abramovitz, M., Zelnick, J. (2010). Double jeopardy: the impact of neoliberalism on care workers in the United States and South Africa. *International Journal of Health Services: Planning, Administration, Evaluation, 40*(1), 97–117. . doi:10.2190/HS.40.1.f

Abuhashesh, M., Al-Khasawneh, M., Al-Dmour, R., & Masa'deh, R. (2019). The impact of Facebook on Jordanian consum-ers' decision process in the hotel selection. *IBIMA Business Review,* 1-16.

Ahmed, A., & Ramzan, M. (2013). Effects of job stress on employees job performance: A study on banking sector of Pakistan. *IOSR Journal of Business and Management*, *11*(6), 61–68. doi:10.9790/487X-1166168

Aiken, L. H., Clarke, S. P., Sloane, D. M., Sochalski, J., & Silber, J. H. (2002). Hospital nurse staffing and patient mortality, nurse burnout, and job dissatisfaction. *Journal of the American Medical Association*, *288*(16), 1987–1993. doi:10.1001/jama.288.16.1987 PMID:12387650

Allisey, A. F., Noblet, A. J., Lamontagne, A. D., & Houdmont, J. (2014). Testing a model of officer intentions to quit: The mediating effects of job stress and job satisfaction. *Criminal Justice and Behavior*, *41*(6), 751–771. doi:10.1177/0093854813509987

Barzideh, M., Choobineh, A. R., & Tabatabaee, H. R. (2014). Job stress dimensions and their relationship to musculoskeletal disorders in Iranian nurses. *Work (Reading, Mass.)*, *47*(4), 423–429. doi:10.3233/WOR-121585 PMID:23324727

Beheshtifar, M., Hoseinifar, H., & Moghadam, M. (2011). Effect procrastination on work-related stress. *European JOurnal of Economics Finance Administration Science*, 38-59.

Bernburg, M., Vitzthum, K., Groneberg, D. A., & Mache, S. (2016). Physicians' occupational stress, depressive symptoms and work ability in relation to their working environment: A cross-sectional study of differences among medical residents with various specialties working in German hospitals. *BMJ Open*, *6*(6), e011369. doi:10.1136/bmjopen-2016-011369 PMID:27311909

Bischoff, L. L., Otto, A. K., Hold, C., & Wollesen, B. (2019). The effect of physical activity interventions on occupational stress for health personnel – a systematic review. *International Journal of Nursing Studies*. doi:10.1016/j.ijnurstu.2019.06.002

Bridger, R. S., Day, A. J., & Morton, K. (2013). Occupational stress and employee turnover. *Ergonomics*, *56*(11), 1629–1639. doi:10.1080/00140139.2013.836251 PMID:24047248

Cai, B., Tu, J., Ma, L., Chen, L., Fu, Y., & Jiang, Q. (2020). Psychological impact and coping strategies of frontline medical staff in Hunan between January and March 2020 during the outbreak of coronavirus disease 2019 (COVID19) in Hubei. *China Med. Sci. Monit.*, *26*, e924171. PMID:32291383

Cheung, T., Wong, S. Y., Wong, K. Y., Law, L. Y., Ng, K., Tong, M. T., Wong, K. Y., Ng, M. Y., & Yip, P. S. (2016). Depression, anxiety and symptoms of stress among baccalaureate nursing students in Hong Kong: A cross-sectional study. *International Journal of Environmental Research and Public Health*, *13*(8), 779. doi:10.3390/ijerph13080779 PMID:27527192

Clegg, A. (2001). Occupational stress in nursing: A review of the literature. *Journal of Nursing Management*, *9*(2), 101–106. doi:10.1046/j.1365-2834.2001.00216.x PMID:11879452

Cohen, S., Kamarck, T., & Mermelstein, R. (1983). A global measure of perceived stress. *Journal of Health and Social Behavior*, *24*(4), 385–396. doi:10.2307/2136404 PMID:6668417

Cox, T., & Rial-Gonzalez, E. (2002). Work-related stress: the European picture. *Magazine of the European Agency for Safety and Health at Work*, *5*, 4-6. https://osha.europa.eu/en/publications/magazine/5

Deloitte. (2018). *2019 Global health care outlook: The evolution of smart health care*. Deloitte Touche Thomtsu Limited.

Fairbrother, K., & Warn, J. (2003). Workplace dimensions, stress and job satisfaction. *Journal of Managerial Psychology, 18*(1), 8–21. doi:10.1108/02683940310459565

Faragher, E. B., Cass, M., & Cooper, C. L. (2005). The relationship between job satisfaction and health: A meta-analysis. *Occupational and Environmental Medicine, 62*(2), 105–112. doi:10.1136/oem.2002.006734 PMID:15657192

Farquharson, B., Bell, C., Johnston, D., Jones, M., Schofield, P., Allan, J., Ricketts, I., Morrison, K., & Johnston, M. (2013). Nursing stress and patient care: real-time investigation of the effect of nursing tasks and demands on psychological stress, physiological stress, and job performance: study protocol. *Journal of Advanced Nursing, 69*(10), 2327–2335. doi:10.1111/jan.12090 PMID:23387943

Golubic, R., Milosevic, M., Knezevic, B., & Mustajbegovic, J. (2009). Work-related stress, education and work ability among hospital nurses. *Journal of Advanced Nursing, 65*(10), 2056–2066. doi:10.1111/j.1365-2648.2009.05057.x PMID:19627386

Hacimusalar, Y., Kahve, A. C., Yasar, A. B., & Aydin, M. S. (2020). Effects of coronavirus disease 2019 (COVID-19) pandemic on anxiety and hopelessness levels: A cross-sectional study in healthcare workers and community sample in Turkey. *Journal of Psychiatric Research, 129*, 181–188. doi:10.1016/j.jpsychires.2020.07.024 PMID:32758711

Hazarika, O. B., & Das, S. (2021). Paid and unpaid work during the Covid-19 pandemic: A study of the gendered division of domestic responsibilities during lockdown. *Journal of Gender Studies, 30*(4), 429–439. doi:10.1080/09589236.2020.1863202

Hoboubi, N., Choobineh, A., Ghanavati, F. K., Keshavarzi, S., & Hosseini, A. A. (2017). The impact of job stress and job satisfaction on workforce productivity in an Iranian petrochemical industry. *Safety and Health at Work, 8*(1), 67–71. doi:10.1016/j.shaw.2016.07.002 PMID:28344843

Jacobsen, H. B., Reme, S. E., Sembajwe, G., Hopcia, K., Stiles, T. C., Sorensen, G., Porter, J. H., Marino, M., & Buxton, O. M. (2014). Work stress, sleep deficiency, and predicted 10-year cardiometabolic risk in a female patient care worker population. *American Journal of Industrial Medicine, 57*(8), 940–949. doi:10.1002/ajim.22340 PMID:24809311

Kowalska, W., & Szwamel, K. (2021). Stress management strategies and quality of life in undergraduate nursing and midwifery students in Poland: A pilot study. *Nursing Open*. Advance online publication. doi:10.1002/nop2.982 PMID:34227744

Liaudanskiene, R., Varnas, N., & Ustinovichius, L. (2010). Modelling the application of workplace safety and health act in Lithuanian construction sector. *Technological and Economic Development, 16*(2), 233–253. doi:10.3846/tede.2010.15

Lu, H., While, A. E., & Barriball, K. L. (2005). Job satisfaction among nurses: A literature review. *International Journal of Nursing Studies, 42*(2), 211–227. doi:10.1016/j.ijnurstu.2004.09.003 PMID:15680619

Maria, S., Francesca, L., Massimiliano, P., & Mirco, F. (2020). Parents' Stress and Children's Psychological Problems in Families Facing the COVID-19 Outbreak in Italy. *Frontiers in Psychology*, 11. https://www.frontiersin.org/article/10.3389/fpsyg.2020.01713

Masa'deh, R., Obeidat, B. Y., & Tarhini, A. (2016). A Jordanian empirical study of the associations among transformational leadership, transactional leadership, knowledge sharing, job performance, and firm performance: A structural equation modelling approach. *Journal of Management Development*, *35*(5), 681–705. doi:10.1108/JMD-09-2015-0134

McVicar, A. (2003). Workplace stress in nursing: A literature review. *Journal of Advanced Nursing*, *44*(6), 633–642. doi:10.1046/j.0309-2402.2003.02853.x PMID:14651686

Menekay, M., & Celmece, N. (2017). Investigation of the quality of life scale improvement. *J. Econ. Manag. Perspect.*, *11*, 327–336.

Mittal, M., & Bhakar, S. S. (2018). Examining the impact of role overload on job stress, job satisfaction and job performance: A study among married workingwomen in banking sector. *International Journal of Management Study*, *7*(1), 2231–2528. doi:10.18843/ijms/v5i2(7)/01

Moura, I. H., Nobre, R., Cortez, R. M., Campelo, V., Macedo, S. F., & Silva, A. R. (2016). Quality of life of undergraduate nursing students. Qualidade de vida de estudantes de graduacao em enfermagem. *Revista Gaúcha de Enfermagem*, *37*(2), e55291. doi:10.1590/1983-1447.2016.02.55291 PMID:27253594

Mursali, A., Basuki, E., & Dharmono, S. (2009). Relationship between noise and job stress at private thread spinning company. *University Medicine*, *28*, 8.

Nübling, M., Vomstein, M., Schmidt, S. G., Gregersen, S., Dulon, M., & Nienhaus, A. (2010). Psycho-social work load and stress in the geriatric care. *BMC Public Health*, *10*(1), 428. doi:10.1186/1471-2458-10-428 PMID:20663137

Nunnally, J. C. (1978). *Psychometric theory* (2nd ed.). McGraw-Hill.

Ozyurek, P., Cevik, C., Kılıc, I., & Aslan, A. (2021). Effects of Day and Night Shifts on Stress, Anxiety, Quality of Life, and Oxidative Stress Parameters in Nurses. *Florence Nightingale Journal of Nursing*, *29*(1), 81–92. doi:10.5152/FNJN.2021.19141 PMID:34263226

Pedrazza, M., Berlanda, S., Trifiletti, E., & Bressan, F. (2016). Exploring Physicians' Dissatisfaction and Work-Related Stress: Development of the PhyDis Scale. *Frontiers in Psychology*, *7*, 187. doi:10.3389/fpsyg.2016.01238 PMID:27588013

Raja, M., Azeem, M. U., Haq, I. U., & Naseer, S. (2020). Perceived threat of terrorism and employee outcomes: The moderating role of negative affectivity and psychological capital. *Journal of Business Research*, *110*, 316–326. doi:10.1016/j.jbusres.2020.01.026

Rana, B. U. I., & Munir, K. (2011). *Impact of stressors on the performance of employees.* Munich Personal RePEc Archive.

Reilly, E., Dhingra, K., & Boduszek, D. (2014). Teachers' self-efficacy beliefs, self-esteem, and job stress as determinants of job satisfaction. *International Journal of Educational Management*, *28*(4), 365–378. doi:10.1108/IJEM-04-2013-0053

Ruyter, K., Wetzels, M., & Feinberg, R. (2001). Role stress in call centers: Its effects on employee performance and satisfaction. *Journal of Interactive Marketing*, *15*(2), 23-35. doi:10.1002/dir.1008

Shaban, I. A., Khater, W. A., & Akhu-Zaheya, L. M. (2012). Undergraduate nursing students' stress sources and coping behaviors during their initial period of clinical training: A Jordanian perspective. *Nurse Education in Practice*, *12*(4), 204–209. doi:10.1016/j.nepr.2012.01.005 PMID:22281123

Tyagi, N. (2021). Aligning organizational culture to enhance managerial effectiveness of academic leaders: An interface for employee engagement and retention. *International Journal of Educational Management*, *35*(7), 1387–1404. Advance online publication. doi:10.1108/IJEM-10-2020-0447

Tyagi, N., & Moses, D. B. (2020). Developing and validating the antecedents of managerial effectiveness: Factorial constitution in institutions of higher learning. *International Journal of Leadership in Education*, *0*(0), 1–21. doi:10.1080/13603124.2020.1762003

Tyagi, N., Moses, D. B., & Rana, S. (2017). Influence of Organizational Justice on Managerial Effectiveness in Institutions of Higher Learning. *Productivity*, *58*(3), 286–299.

Xiang, Y. T., Yang, Y., Li, W., Zhang, L., Zhang, Q., Cheung, T., & Ng, C. H. (2020). Timely mental health care for the 2019 novel corona virus outbreak is urgently needed. *The Lancet. Psychiatry*, *7*(3), 228–229. doi:10.1016/S2215-0366(20)30046-8 PMID:32032543

Yang, T., Guo, Y., Ma, M., Li, Y., Tian, H., & Deng, J. (2017). Job stress and presenteeism among Chinese healthcare workers: The mediating effects of affective commitment. *International Journal of Environmental Research and Public Health*, *14*(9), 978. doi:10.3390/ijerph14090978 PMID:28850081

Yang, T., Shen, Y. M., Zhu, M., Liu, Y., Deng, J., Chen, Q., & See, L. C. (2015). Effects of co-worker and supervisor support on job stress and presenteeism in an aging workforce: A structural equation modelling approach. *International Journal of Environmental Research and Public Health*, *13*(1), 72. doi:10.3390/ijerph13010072 PMID:26703705

Zhang, J., Wu, W., Zhao, X., & Zhang, W. (2020). Recommended psychological crisis intervention response to the 2019 novel corona virus pneumonia outbreak in China: A model of West China Hospital. *Precision Clinical Medicine*, *3*(1), 3–8. doi:10.1093/pcmedi/pbaa006

Section 3

Prevention and Treatment Issues

Chapter 12
A Creative Intervention for Supporting the Mental Wellness of Nurses:
The Ameliorative Promise of Graphic Testimonials

J. Blake Scott
University Central Florida, USA

Nathan Holic
University of Central Florida, USA

Christa L Cook
University of Central Florida, USA

University of Central Florida
University of Central Florida, USA

Aislinn Woody
https://orcid.org/0000-0002-1503-5922
University of Central Florida, USA

ABSTRACT

Mental health challenges are prevalent among nurses who have been on the front lines of the COVID-19 pandemic, with dangerous and demoralizing working conditions, mental health stigma, and limited mental health support contributing to such challenges. A wide range of interventions have been developed to support nurses' mental wellness therapeutically, through organizational and broader advocacy, and by educating communities and publics about nurses' experiences. Nurses have produced various forms of artistic expressions, including comics or "graphic testimonials," to document, process, and share their experiences. Yet such forms, as examples of "graphic medicine," remain a relatively untapped and unique resource for supporting the mental health of nurses and advocating for and educating others about their lived experiences, needs, and vulnerabilities. As a unique medium, graphic testimonials have much to offer mental health interventions for nurses, especially through destigmatizing, integrated, and capacity building approaches that empower nurses to decide how best to use them.

DOI: 10.4018/978-1-7998-8813-0.ch012

INTRODUCTION

Even not accounting for the impact of the ongoing pandemic, the United States has a well-established nursing shortage (Haddad, Annamaraju, &Toney-Butler, 2020). In addition to recruiting more people into the nursing profession, retaining practicing nurses is crucial. COVID-19 has heightened the challenge of recruitment and retention, exacerbating difficulties of acute care that threaten the mental wellness of nurses. The prevalence of mental distress among nurses and other healthcare workers constitutes a continuing exigency in need of urgent and inventive interventions; rather than a chronic condition that can be managed and stabilized, such mental distress has manifested as the accumulation of acute distress over time. The issue of nurses' mental health challenges might be conceptualized as a "wicked problem"--that is, a complex, multicausal, variously defined, and at least somewhat intractable problem (Conklin, 2005)--demanding a similarly complex, multipronged solution.

Drawing on emergent research, this chapter's Background section overviews the mental health challenges for nurses, focusing on the context of the COVID-19 pandemic, and addressing institutional and societal contributors to such challenges, including the stigmatization that prevents many nurses from seeking or obtaining help. Here the authors discuss forms of trauma and moral injury that nurses experience, and the sense of duty and sacrifice that is reinforced by public representations and perceptions of nurses. The Background section also highlights and explains stigma's roles in nurses' mental health challenges.

The chapter's second major section examines a range of evidence-based and experimental efforts, some recently initiated, for addressing nurses' and other healthcare workers' mental health challenges and supporting their well-being. Here the authors discuss the potential benefits and the limitations of existing efforts in the U.S. and beyond, including those initiated by individual nurses and those sponsored by networks or groups of nurses, hospitals and other institutions, and professional organizations. The chapter's authors argue that individualizing approaches to self-care, particularly those that depend on a narrow notion of resilience, are insufficient and unfairly put the burden of mental wellness on nurses. Referencing creative, artistic efforts to support nurses' mental wellness in particular, the authors then turn to the under-explored promise of graphic medicine for ameliorating nurses' mental health challenges and for supporting their therapeutic, advocacy, and educational needs. Graphic medicine is an emergent interdisciplinary field described by Williams (2007) as at the "intersection between the medium of comics and the discourse of healthcare" (n.p.).

The chapter's Solutions and Recommendations section reviews and proposes relevant applications of narrative-based, autobiographical comics--what some have called "graphic pathographies" (Green & Myers, 2010, with pathographies being narratives about experiences with illness or care), and what the authors of this chapter call "graphic testimonials." The authors consider ongoing and potential responses to the mental health stigmatization and related challenges of nurses that involve, or could involve, creative applications of graphic testimonials and their unique qualities and functions. The authors argue for collective, integrated, capacity-building, and de-stigmatizing approaches to developing and deploying nurses' graphic testimonials for mental health support, as such approaches have more potential to improve organizational, socio-cultural, and other structural conditions in ways that address nurses' most pressing needs.

The chapter's Future Research Directions section points to gaps in several related bodies of research, including how nurses are experiencing mental health stigma and distress in the U.S. context, the efficacy of different types of interventions to destigmatize and support nurses' mental wellness (particularly in the context of an ongoing pandemic), and the implementation and evaluation of graphic testimonials in therapeutic, educational, and advocacy responses. Finally, the chapter concludes by returning to the promise of graphic medicine for creating better awareness of and enriching multi-pronged responses to the mental health challenges of nurses and other providers.

This chapter's overarching goal is to lay the groundwork for the use and evaluation of graphic testimonials or comics as mechanisms by which nurses experiencing mental health challenges can make meaning from their experiences in a therapeutic manner, advocate for better support, and educate others about their experiences and vulnerabilities in de-stigmatizing ways. The chapter's fuller set of objectives are to:

1. Overview the mental health challenges for nurses in the context of the COVID-19 pandemic through several related frameworks, and outline three types of ameliorative support needed by nurses;
2. Critically examine a range of interventions--from individualizing efforts grounded in resilience to advocacy efforts aimed at structural and policy change--to support nurses' mental wellness in the face of ongoing challenges;
3. Introduce the field of graphic medicine, and explain how graphic testimonials have been created and used in response to the pandemic;
4. Make a case for the unique potential of graphic testimonials to contribute to integrated and multi-pronged initiatives to support nurses' mental wellness, particularly through collective and capacity-building approaches;
5. Recommend lines of inquiry for future research related to understanding the problem and to developing and evaluating responses.

BACKGROUND: MENTAL HEALTH CHALLENGES FOR NURSES DURING THE COVID-19 PANDEMIC

A recent systematic review and meta-analysis of 70 studies (with over 100,000 participants) of healthcare workers in practice during COVID-19 indicated common experiences with anxiety (30%), depression (31.1%), sleep problems (44%), acute stress (56.5%) and post-traumatic stress (20.2%) (Marvaldi et al., 2021). Healthcare workers responding to a recent survey by Mental Health America (2021) indicated factors contributing to their distress as including not only work stress and exhaustion but also worry about exposing loved ones, struggling with parenting, not getting adequate emotional support, and being stigmatized in their communities. The results of national survey of ICU nurses in the Netherlands after the first COVID-19 surge there indicated higher rates of reported anxiety, depression, and posttraumatic stress disorder (PTSD); such rates were higher for nurses working with staffing shortages and lower for those who took time off for holiday, pointing to the necessity of recovery time (Heesakkers, Zegers, van Mol, & van de Boogaard, 2021). Female identity and work experience greater than ten years--characteristics of a large portion of the nursing workforce responding to COVID-19--have been found to be positively associated with poor trauma resilience (Vagni, Maiorano, Giostra, & Pajardi, 2020). Although fewer studies have been conducted about the mental health of nursing students during the COVID-19 pandemic, there is emerging evidence that they, too, experience such mental health problems as PTSD, depression, anxiety, stress, and insomnia (Gao, Wang, Guo, & Hu, 2021).

The working conditions of nurses and other healthcare workers constitute an important set of factors contributing to mental distress and trauma; these conditions include lack of training for those working outside of their areas of expertise (particularly as they are redeployed to critical care settings), changing clinical guidelines, limited and inadequate equipment and supplies (including personal protective equipment, or PPE), long hours due to staff illness, and dealing with death and dying, sometimes as proxies for patients' loved ones (see Maben & Bridges, 2020; Owens, 2020; De Kock et al., 2021). In one international study of the mental health of healthcare workers, survey respondents who reported not being provided appropriate PPE were more than twice as likely to also report depression (Khajuria et al., 2021). In addition to PPE shortages, many staff nurses who have continued to work long hours under risky circumstances have not been offered retention or crisis pay, even as they have watched hospitals hire travel nurses at salaries several times higher than their own. When previously trusted institutions act in a way that is harmful to those who rely on them, members of the team can experience institutional betrayal.

One framework for understanding the challenges of nursing is moral injury (see, for example, Dean, Talbot, & Dean, 2029), or the trauma or distress experienced by individuals who feel compelled to engage in action or inaction that violates a moral or ethical code, manifesting in feelings of guilt, shame, and/or, regret, as well as a loss of meaning and professional identity. Moral injury was first identified in combat settings where service members were forced to confront the necessity of action or inaction that violated their deeply held values (Litz et al., 2009). Subsequent research has identified this experience in other high-stakes situations, too. In the context of nursing during the COVID-19 pandemic, moral injury, like trauma, has been acute but continuous, and has occurred through such changes as triage protocols, the uneven allocation of scant resources to patients, the delivery of sub-standard care due to an overwhelming workload, and working without the guidance of best practices in a novel historical context (Williamson et al., 2021). Although the experience of occupational moral injury in and of itself does not constitute mental illness, it accounted for significant variance in the occurrence of PTSD, depression, suicidality, and anxiety in one systematic review and meta-analysis (Williamson, Stevelink, & Greenberg, 2018). Further, because professional identity is thought to influence nurses' stress levels and quality of care (Sun et al., 2016), the questioning of this identity prompted by moral injury can compound such injury's harmful effects. The framework of moral injury can help expand the target of mitigation from self-care and coping mechanisms to more structural changes in institutional patterns (Doheny, 2021). It can also lead to the recognition that nursing ethics might necessary become more utilitarian in times of crisis, and that "feeling morally compromised in a crisis situation is not a sign of weakness, but rather a clear demonstration of the strength of…moral integrity" (Altman, 2020).

Alongside moral injury, we can understand nurses' mental health challenges through the notion of vicarious trauma. Vicarious trauma, sometimes referred to as secondary traumatic stress, countertransference, compassion fatigue, and shared trauma, is a complex phenomenon experienced by clinicians who bear witness to the suffering of others (Branson, 2019). Even the death of a single patient or the perception of dissatisfaction by patients' families can contribute to poor mental health outcomes in nurses (Andolhe et al., 2015). Elevated death exposures can lead to increased emotional exhaustion and burnout (Kelly, Gee, & Butler, 2021). What is unique about the COVID pandemic, when contrasted against other large scale traumatic experiences, is that this increased exposure has been continuous. More than a year and a half into the public health response, the daily U.S. COVID-19 over a seven-day average climbed to over 2,000 (Rattner & Towey, 2021). Despite the need for recovery, frontline nurses lack the literal and metaphorical distance to process, manage, and seek help with their responses to vicarious trauma.

A related, and similarly shared form of trauma that can be a useful framework for understanding nurses' mental health challenges is community trauma. Community trauma affects a "geographical area and/or social group and fundamentally disrupts the structures of, and bonds within, communities" (Bender et al., 2021). The framework of community trauma can help foreground the ways nurses experience unique occupational distress alongside other kinds individual and collective distress as members of families, communities, and societies (see Blackburn, McAuliffe, & Johns, 2020). Nurses' self-concepts and professional identities are influenced by their workplace values and environments, public perception, and social and cultural values (Hoeve, Jansen, & Roodbol, 2013) related to their familial, religious, political, community, and other roles. Further, aspects of nurses' identities can sometimes be in conflict, as when nurses worry about infecting family members with COVID-19 because of their unsafe work conditions, or when nurses must negotiate competing community views about protection measures such as vaccination. The blurring and compounding of professional and personal challenges caused by the pandemic can exacerbate tensions that could otherwise be compartmentalized in more manageable ways. For example, a nurse may have to decide between avoiding a conflict with a spouse or parent and acquiescing to the demands of a job in which one feels devalued.

One common aspect of nurses' identities that is shaped by both professional values and public perception is a strong sense of duty and sacrifice. A systematic review of nurses' experiences working in acute care hospital settings concluded that their sense of duty and personal sacrifice increased during respiratory pandemics (Fernandez et al., 2020). Dealing with collective and sometimes conflicting trauma requires emotional connectedness, which healthcare workers described in one study as "as having empathy and value, help and support, presence, and vulnerability" (Bender et al., 2021). Yet nurses and other healthcare providers are commonly conceptualized as angels or heroes, superhumans without the same vulnerabilities as other community members. Take, for example, Marvel Comics' *The Vitals: True Nurse Stories* (Ryan, 2020), which "tells tales of some real heroes, the nurses, as they work in high-risk environments in order to care for those in need" (n.p.). Such conceptions can disempower and silence nurses who are struggling with trauma and disconnectedness (Stokes-Parish et al., 2020).

Another identity-based and culturally shaped mental health challenge that nurses can experience in the context of the pandemic--both as healthcare workers and as people experiencing mental distress and trauma--is stigmatization. Stigma can be defined as expressed negative beliefs, assumptions, and attitudes about people, which can involve them being separated and treated differently, and in ways that convey shame, blame, judgment, and disapproval. Goffman (1963) described stigma as a "discrediting" attribute (p. 10), and Hinshaw (2006) described the stigma surrounding mental illness, more specifically, as a "mark of shame" shaped by stereotypes, fear, and rejection.

Pointing to the multidimensional nature of stigma, Goffman (1963) argued that we need "a language of relations, not attributes" to describe it (p. 3). Indeed, stigma has been conceptualized as including multiple mutually influencing domains or types, such as systemic stigma conveyed through institutional policies and structures, community stigma driven by cultural values and attitudes, enacted stigma manifested through language-used, embodied actions, and other means, self-stigma that internalizes other sources, and anticipated or expected stigma. In their conceptual model of HIV stigma, for example, Turan et al. (2017) drew distinctions and connections among the levels of structural, intersectional, and individual stigma, as well as the types of enacted, anticipated, community, and internalized stigma (see, in Turan et al., Figure 1: "Conceptual Framework for HIV-Related Stigma, Engagement in Care, and Health Outcomes"). In a model with even more dimensions, Stangl et al. (2019) included stigma's drivers of fear, stereotypes, blame, and authoritarianism, and its multi-scalar facilitators of broader sociocultural norms, institutional structures and organizational policies, and interpersonal interactions (see, in Stangl et al., Figure 1: "Health Stigma and Discrimination Framework"); they also identified the "marking" of health-related stigma as intersecting with occupation, race, gender, and other aspects of identity. In other words, stigma is often expressed and experienced intersectionally. Knaak, Mantler, & Szeto (2017) specified the following examples of stigma's scales in the healthcare sector: "structural (eg, investment of resources, quality of care standards, organizational culture), interpersonal (eg, patient–provider interactions, discriminatory behaviours, negative attitudes), and intraindividual (eg self-stigma, patient reluctance to seek care, provider reluctance to disclose a mental illness and/or seek care)" (p. 111).

While social psychologists and other professionals have developed models of stigma that capture its various dimensions, rhetoricians of health and medicine have theorized its enactments through and impacts on discursive interactions, in particular. Based on her studies of mental health stigma, Molloy (2019) observed that such stigmatization can create for patients a "rhetorical disability," or discrediting effect on the patient's credibility or character that alters what is possible in their dialogues with providers and others (see p. 44). Johnson (2010) similarly argued that stigma can create a "kakoethos" or anti-ethos that can override other attributes and encompass various "permutations of badness," such as shame, humiliation, and worthlessness, anxiety, fear, and sadness (p. 465).

Nurses and other healthcare providers can be enactors of stigma, of course. As the pandemic has progressed, for instance, many nurses are facing their own stigmatizing attitudes towards patients or co-workers who have refused vaccination, attitudes that can conflict with ethical obligations of beneficence, justice, and respect for persons in the care of patients. As the WHO has recognized, healthcare workers have also been subject to stigma and discrimination because of their roles in the COVID-19 pandemic, including "avoidance by their family or community owing to stigma or fear" (see Bagcchi, 2020). In some cases, the stigmatization of nurses, as the front-line representatives of an overburdened healthcare system during the pandemic, has led to violence. About 20% of the more than 15,000 respondents to a National Nurses United (2020) survey reported facing increased on-the-job violence linked to such pandemic-related changes as staffing shortages and visitor restrictions. A cross-sectional, global study concluded that, even after adjusting for compounding factors, healthcare workers "are significantly more likely to experience COVID-19-related stigma and bullying" in both workplace and community settings (Dye et al., 2020). As explained by nurse-advocates Cipriano, Boston-Leary, Mcmillan, & Peterson (2021), "While nurses were being heralded as heroes, they suffered from involuntary social isolation and abuse from landlords, retail businesses, community members and, in some cases, families. Nurses were falsely viewed as virus spreaders even as evidence showed that nurses had lower infection rates compared to the general public" (n.p.).

Nurses who have been exposed to and become ill from COVID-19 have reported internalized stigma. A systematic review of stigmatization from work-related COVID-19 exposure pointed to common findings of increased self-stigma among healthcare workers (Schubert et al., 2021). The public perception and expectation for nurses to be resolute, sacrificial heroes can compound the self-stigmatization of those who are experiencing mental distress and cause nurses to avoid seeking support and advocating for their needs. Additionally, moral injury can exacerbate self-stigmatization by prompting nurses to question their professional identities and enacted ethics of care.

Like other, often intersecting forms of stigma, mental health stigma has been identified as a barrier to care and linked to poor health outcomes, a pattern that holds for healthcare providers. Citing several studies, Knaak, Mantler, & Szeto (2017) note that mental illness-related stigma has been found to be a "problem of culture, where staff are often discouraged to talk openly or seek help for psychological problems" (p. 112). They go on to explain that has such stigma "has inward-facing impacts for health professionals' own willingness to seek help or disclose a mental health problem, which can result in an over-reliance on self-treatment, low peer support—including ostracization and judgment from co-workers if disclosure does occur—and increased risk of suicide" (p. 112).

The mental health challenges faced by nurses--and magnified by the COVID-19 pandemic--are multifaceted, and therefore forms of ameliorative intervention and support should be multifaceted as well. Take stigma, for example. Since stigma manifests at multiple levels in the healthcare system, interventions to address it should include but also move beyond the individual and address the complex social challenges while engaging populations most impacted (Nyblade et al., 2019; Logie & Turan, 2020). Those addressing mental health stigma and its intersections with other forms of stigma during the COVID-19 pandemic might consider adapting HIV stigma-reduction interventions, including collecting data that depicts people's stories about stigmatization (Logie, 2020).

The following section discusses the following three ways to respond to nurses' mental health needs, offering examples (including artistic responses) of each: 1. therapeutic support, including but moving well beyond self-care; 2. forms of collective workplace and occupational advocacy, and; 3. storytelling that educates and mobilizes more meaningful support from publics and communities. As part of this discussion, the authors note the limitations of responses that focus primarily on self-care, putting the burden of addressing it on individual nurses.

THERAPEUTIC, ADVOCACY, AND EDUCATIONAL RESPONSES

Therapeutic Interventions and Support

One type of response needed to support the mental health of nurses, especially in the context of the COVID-19 pandemic, is therapeutic, here defined broadly to include a range of supportive mechanisms for identifying those who are experiencing mental illness and connecting them to various types of treatment, care, and healing or restoration. Nurses need individual and collective mental health support as professionals and as community members. Among other interventions, such support can include mechanisms for becoming more aware of, making meaning from, and connecting with peers about mental health difficulties; networks of co-workers helping to identify nurses experiencing distress and to connect them with needed mental health resources; expanded organization-sponsored therapeutic support involving mental health specialists; and a workplace culture that incentivizes rather than stigmatizes seeking help and support. It is important to note that this set of needs will persist after the COVID-19 pandemic ends. A systemic review of PTSD symptoms in healthcare workers pointed to increased prevalence of symptoms after the SARS 2003 outbreak and MERS 2012 outbreak, as well as during the COVID-19 pandemic (Carmassi et al., 2020). In addition to supporting nurses who are experiencing mental health problems during and after the pandemic, therapeutic responses can help prevent such problems and prepare nurses and nurses-in-training for coping with them and their contributors, such as dealing with increased levels of death and dying. This is particularly important given that nurses-in-training have been prematurely deployed to become part of the healthcare workforce (Galvin, Richards, & Smith, 2020).

A range of therapeutic responses to mental health challenges of healthcare workers have been implemented across the U.S. and world. Cole-King and Dykes (2020) advocated a multilayered system support based on delivery and level of need, visualizing these with a multilevel pyramid. At the bottom level is self-help or self-care, which is applicable to all workers. The middle levels involve employer-sponsored and workplace-integrated forms of support that include non-medicalized peer support such as buddy systems and supportive listening that can involve colleagues but also link to external specialists (e.g., via hotlines); these levels are for workers who are experiencing anxiety and other symptoms but not severely.

At the top of the pyramid are skilled support and specialized mental health support that an employer would provide but also outsource, depending on worker preferences; these more intense levels are for workers who are struggling with severe distress (p. 1).

In their review of evidence-based psychological support for nurses during COVID-19 and previous outbreaks, Maben and Bridges (2020) pointed to a number of self-care mechanisms, including meditation/mindfulness breaks and calming strategies such as the FACE mnemonic (focus what is in your control, acknowledge thoughts and feelings, come back into your body, engage in what you're doing) (see, in Maben & Bridges, Figure 1: "Strategies and interventions to support nurses' psychological well-being during Covid-19 crisis"). Other forms of support focusing on self-care mentioned in the literature--some provided by employers and involving external resources--include the following: de-stress exercises led by a physical therapist (Gonzalez et al., 2020); digital learning and support materials (e.g., about signs of mental health distress and strategies for coping) (Blake et al., 2020; Zace et al., 2021); apps for self-screening and tracking mental health symptoms (DePierro et al., 2020); resilience-based computer-assisted training (Zace et al., 2020); and tele-education programs focused on mindfulness and stress management (Sockalingam et al., 2020).

More collective or team-based and middle-level types of therapeutic support mechanisms for healthcare workers--most at Cole-King and Dykes' (2020) middle levels of support--have also been developed and implemented. In their review of evidence-based interventions, Maben and Bridges (2020) included peer conversations that show understanding and validate concerns, staff huddles or handovers, shift-based buddy systems, end-of-shift check-ins, and weekly problem-solving review meetings. Other articles mentioned group activities to relieve stress (Chen et al., 2020), peer detection of mental health anxiety or distress (Greenberg & Tracy, 2020); peer-led group workshops on coping strategies (Waterman et al., 2018; Albott et al., 2020), peer counseling and support teams (Zace et al., 2021; Donnelly et al., 2020; Cheng et al., 2020), and group support video calls for healthcare workers at home (Schulte et al., 2020). Owens (2020) cautioned that peer-based debriefing sessions should not take the place of trained critical incident debriefing (CISD) teams, which "should be a part of a network of services such as preevent education, follow-up services, and referral to professional care and postincident education programs" (n.p.). Healthcare systems in Canada and Norway have begun to implement mental health peer support programs for healthcare workers in clinical settings, though better integration of such programs is needed (Mulvale et al., 2019).

More specialized forms of advanced therapeutic support, often outsourced by employers, mentioned in the literature include psychological intervention by medical teams that provide online courses about coping (Chen et al., 2020), cognitive behavior therapy (Geoffrey et al., 2020), teletherapy hotlines (Lefevre et al., 2020; Chen et al., 2020; Hong et al., 2020; Rolling et al., 2021), mental health liaison teams (Shamia et al., 2015), and standardized scenario-based simulation training materials (Cheung et al., 2020).

Some professional and government organizations have developed fuller suites of multi-level resources to support nurses and other healthcare workers during the COVID-19 pandemic. For example, the American Nurses Association (ANA) Enterprise created the Well-Being Initiative, which includes a range of digital resources such as apps and podcasts about self-care and restoration, various downloadable guides and fact sheets, webinars about coping and self-recovery, tools for exploring gratitude practices for nurses, a "Happy App" for calling and connecting to compassionate listeners, videos about dealing with grief, and prompts for an expressive writing journal. Another notable initiative, sponsored by the Mental Health Commission of Canada and co-developed by healthcare workers, is The Working Mind Healthcare, a comprehensive suite of online educational and support resources that includes the standard topics of recognizing the signs of mental distress, improving resilience, and supporting colleagues in distress, but also the less common topic of reducing mental health stigma in healthcare settings.

A less common but still promising type of therapeutic response is art-based interventions. In their systematic review of such interventions for care professionals during and after a healthcare crisis, Havsteen-Franklin et al. (2020) identified common intervention elements and mental health benefits, the former including the development of psychosocial competencies for peer support, emotional processing, "naming the impact of the crisis," and "using an integrative creative approach" (p. 1). They pointed out that art-based therapy has long been used in mental health services, including during crisis situations alongside other treatments, and they documented such art-based approaches as psychodramatic methods for debriefing training, expressive arts that integrate body, mind, and spirit, and art as therapy or self-regulation (see also Shapiro et al., 2021 for an institutional model of integrated support that includes creative arts as part of the psychological and spiritual dimensions). In a notable narrative-based example, U.S.-based example, the University of Colorado Anschutz Medical Campus (2020) offers a program for writing expressive narratives about COVID-19, as a modified form of written exposure therapy, to healthcare providers who are experiencing mental health distress. The ANA Enterprise Well-Being Initiative includes a narrative writing program designed in part for therapeutic self-expression. Beyond institutionally sponsored art-based therapy, a number of healthcare providers have created art individually or in community groups as a way to cope with the challenges of COVID-19, as illustrated in a *Los Angeles Times* piece (Easter, 2020) featuring painting, drawing, photography, mixed-media collage, dance, sewing, food art, and poetry.

In their rapid systematic review, Muller et al. (2020) found that studies about mental health interventions "mainly focused on individual approaches, most often requiring healthcare workers to initiate contact" (n.p.). They also concluded that such approaches are not always well matched to what healthcare workers say they need and the services accessible to them (given their work conditions, workloads, workplace and community cultures of stigmatization, etc.). Another limitation of many mental health support mechanisms designed for individual healthcare workers is their grounding in a narrow notion of resilience, understood and measured as one's ability to cope with distress through a sense of self-efficacy and forms of self-care. There is some evidence that "resilience (measured by self-efficacy or resilience scales) can be protective against poor mental health outcomes" (De Kock et al., 2021), and organizationally sponsored support can build on a foundation of self-care (Cole-King & Dykes, 2020). At the same time, the authors of this chapter are also leery of approaches that over-rely on individual-based notions of and resilience and care, in part because such approaches are insufficient, and in part because nurses may prefer different, non-workplace-based forms of support. One study of nurses' coping strategies during the COVID-19 pandemic (LoGiudice & Bartos, 2021) noted that their participants' most common forms self-care activities were "spending time with those in the same household or arranging virtual visits with friends (social); prayer or meditation (spiritual); exercise, walking, and yoga (physical); arts/crafts/creative endeavors, reading, and writing/journaling (intellectual); and listening to music (emotional)" (p. 18). In his editorial critiquing resilience, Traynor (2018) explained that those researching nurses tend to "understand resilience in purely individual–individualistic–terms," as a personal characteristic, rather than a broader understanding of unit-level or organizational resilience (p. 6). He goes on to point out problems with this understanding, including making assumptions about what nurses need, absolving organizations and institutions of responsibility, and placing the responsibility of coping on nurses whose trauma is caused by organizational conditions and failures. As stated by De Kock et al. (2021) in their rapid review, "Whilst psychological interventions aimed at enhancing resilience in the individual may be of benefit, it is evident that to build a resilient workforce, occupational and environmental factors must be addressed" (n.p.).

Workplace and Occupational Advocacy

In addition to mechanisms for helping nurses prepare for, cope with, and connect to peer-based and specialist support for mental health challenges, nurses need mechanisms to collectively advocate for better working conditions and policies, additional occupational needs and incentives, and increased funding to make better support possible. The rapid systematic review by Muller et al. (2020) noted that healthcare workers "are more interested in occupational protection, rest, and social support than in professional psychological help" (n.p.). It stands to reason that some of the most important and effective ways to ameliorate the mental health challenges of nurses is to mitigate contributing workplace and occupational factors. In addition to mental health support and among other necessities, nurses need adequate PPE and standardized protection processes, clear clinical guidelines, manageable shifts and hours, more rest breaks, more time off, adequate training for working outside of their areas of expertise, fewer redeployments in critical care settings if not trained for such settings, crisis pay, and prioritization of family members for testing, vaccination, and treatment (Adams & Walls, 2020).

Within their workplaces, nurses need additional mechanisms for communicating their challenges, vulnerabilities, and difficulties, and for advocating for their concerns and needs to supervisors and organizational administrators. Freely expressing vulnerabilities without the threat of negative repercussions can be a powerful means of emotional connectedness and mental well-being (Bender et al., 2021). In their editorial on supporting healthcare workers during COVID-19, Adams and Walls (2020) argued that "Frequent information and feedback sessions with local managers and the broader facility community, complemented by clear, concise, and measured communication, will help teams stay focused on care and secure in their roles" (p. 1439). Of course, such channels for feedback should result in work conditions, protocols and other policies, and support mechanisms that match the expressed needs and preferences of nurses. In their review of evidence-based interventions lead by managers and other leaders in organizations, Maben and Bridges (2020) similarly noted the need to invite feedback about and systematically monitor and respond to staff mental health and safety needs, also mentioning the priorities of recognizing symptoms of deteriorating mental health and reducing stigma around help-seeking (see, in Maben & Bridges, Figure 1: "Strategies and interventions to support nurses' psychological well-being during Covid-19 crisis").

Some of the most powerful advocacy efforts have been sponsored by professional organizations. The ANA has been a prominent advocate for expanded mental health help, better working conditions, family support, and other forms of organizational or institutional support. For example, the ANA sponsored the #GetMePPE social media lobbying campaign, partnered with the American Hospital Association to lobby Congress for supplemental emergency funding, and launched the Coronavirus Response Fund to provide "financial assistance, mental health and well-being support, the latest science-based guidance for protection and patient care, and national advocacy for nurses and patients" (Cipriano, Boston-Leary, Mcmillan, & Peterson, 2020, p. 442). Both the ANA Enterprise's Well-Being Initiative and the Mental Health Commission of Canada's Working Mind Healthcare program have substantial advocacy components. The former includes a site for nurses to submit their stories, including using pictures and videos, to be part of the Year of the Nurse and other advocacy campaigns; the latter, Canadian program includes advocacy briefs and reports for organizations and policymakers about how to better support the mental health and de-stigmatization of nurses and other healthcare staff. Similarly, the U.K. COVID Trauma Response Working Group (2020) has issued rapid guidance for planners and organizations for such issues as "responding to stress experienced by hospital staff associated with COVID" and for "moral injury in healthcare workers associated with COVID-19," both of which offer a number of specific actions that can be taken by healthcare policymakers, planners, managers, and other leaders. They have also developed clinical guidelines for such issues as screening and monitoring for PTSD and delivering bereavement and grief support. Yet another example of an organizationally sponsored, nurse-led advocacy effort is the Frontline Nurses WikiWisdom Forum (Brown & Rushton, n.d.), which asks nurses about and reports on what they have "learned from the frontlines of fighting the coronavirus" that they "most want policy makers, health care administrators and your bosses to know" (n.p.). These types of advocacy efforts are crucial for the more structural responses they can advance through policymaking and institution-level support and organizational change.

Public and Community Education Through Storytelling

Somewhat overlapping with advocacy efforts, nurses need mechanisms to document and educate their communities and larger publics about their lived experiences during and beyond the COVID-19 pandemic. Such mechanisms can help nurses provide more realistic pictures of their experiences that combat both superhuman expectations and stigmatization, enlist publics in efforts to lobby governments for funding, and potentially persuade community members to adopt behaviors that better protect nurses and other frontline workers. As with forms of self-therapy, nurses have turned on their own accord to art and writing to document their experiences and better educate others about their lived realities. *Nature Medicine* featured a digital gallery of self-sponsored art produced by healthcare and medical professionals and students for these purposes (Stower & Guennot, 2021). Yet efforts to support nurses in narrating and disseminating their stories have not been as prevalent in healthcare responses as therapeutic and other kinds of efforts, even though the former can also have therapeutic effects.

A few healthcare initiatives have included mechanisms for gathering and sharing nurses' stories—through writing but also other media--in order to educate stakeholders and publics, though the public reach of such efforts is unclear. For example, the Well-Being Initiative provides a narrative writing program, drawing on the established practice of narrative medicine, that collects and disseminates nurses' stories for both advocacy and educational purposes. The American Hospital Association's (n.d.) "Stories from the Front Lines" initiative includes a public-facing website with stories of hospitals workers told in writing, video interviews, and photographs; some of these are about individual workers, and some are about the efforts of groups, programs, hospitals, and larger healthcare systems. The emphasis of this initiative is on "Positive Stories," however, which runs the risk of reinforcing assumptions about providers' resilience and ability to cope and adapt. "They are real people overcoming extraordinary challenges and saving lives," reads the introduction to the website. An AARP-sponsored Web article (Crouch, 2021) takes could be considered a more measured approach to conveying "What Nurses Want You to Know about the Past Year," sharing nurses' perspectives on resilience but also grief, exhaustion, and admonition. The final sections of this piece include nurses' pleas to the public to wear masks and get vaccinated as the best ways to support them.

Healthcare researchers also have helped nurses document their experiences during the COVID-19 pandemic through community-based participatory studies involving Photovoice. This approach can be especially generative because it positions the participants as the authorities and authors of their stories.

In one example, Badanta, Acevedo-Augilera, Lucchetti, & Diego-Cordero (2021) conducted a qualitative descriptive study in which the health professional participants shared photographs about their experiences working during the pandemic and answered questions about the photographs. Two needs communicated by participants were more effective management of institutional resources and stronger community support. Another study (Providence, 2021) asked nurses to submit photographs, writing, and artwork that depicted or symbolized their experiences. The researchers of the study, who plan to synthesize and share the stories they gathered in a series of reports, noted the nurses' expressions of anxiety, frustration, and loneliness

Along with stories of nurses' heroic actions and resilience, national and local media have increasingly reported and shared through various media stories of nurses' challenging and difficult lived experiences. A particularly vivid example--"offering a firsthand perspective of the brutality of the pandemic inside a COVID-19 I.C.U."--is the short film "Death, Through a Nurse's Eyes" published in the Opinion section of the *New York Times* (Stockton & King, 2021). The *New York Times* also created the "Voices from the Pandemic's Front Lines" initiative, in which "scores of Times staff members worked to present the stories of doctors, nurses and other health care professionals who are risking everything to care for Covid-19 patients" (Palmer, 2020, n.p.). This initiative generated the regularly updated digital gallery of photographs and reflective narratives titled "In Harm's Way," organized in the sections "Fighting the Summer Surge" (in the U.S.) and "Around the World." An *Atlantic* article (Yong, 2020) that was part of a collection of work that won the Pulitzer Prize draws its title of "No One is Listening to Us" from the frustrated words of a nurse in Iowa. Through the stories and words of several healthcare workers, this piece captures the exasperation of working in overwhelming conditions while being ignored, distrusted, and threatened by members of their communities and in some cases families. One interviewee expressed his weariness of "walking out of an ICU where COVID-19 has killed another patient, and walking into a grocery store where he hears people saying it doesn't exist" (n.p.).

Through creating fuller and better understandings of the lived experiences and contextualized, firsthand reflections of nurses and other healthcare workers, the abovementioned efforts and stories they amplify have the potential to problematize the public perception of providers as stoic or sacrificial heroes, to counter stigmatizing assumptions about their roles and difficulties in responding to the pandemic, and to mobilize readers to support them through lobbying, educating others in their lifeworlds, and taking personal responsibility to protect themselves and others through various measures, including vaccination. Such functions may become even more important as communities and publics become habituated to the conditions and even conflicts of an ongoing pandemic.

Building on exiting efforts to convey the mental health challenges of nurses' experiences through varied media and for multiple purposes, the following section discusses and endorses a novel, growing, and still-underutilized artistic medium for responding to the mental health challenges of nurses: comics or graphic testimonials. In addition to overviewing the history of graphic medicine as a field and spotlighting the proliferation of graphic testimonials by and about healthcare workers during the COVID-19 pandemic, the next section argues that graphic testimonials by nurses can be used to help advance therapeutic, advocacy, and public educational goals in ways that prioritize nurses' perspectives, problematize stereotypes, and combat stigma.

SOLUTIONS AND RECOMMENDATIONS: THE PROMISE OF GRAPHIC TESTIMONIALS

Memoir and autobiographic narrative have long been used as tools for conveying and educating others about individual and collective experiences, including about health and medicine, and also for self-directed reflection, meaning-making, and therapeutic release. The well-established field of narrative medicine recognized that "the effective practice of medicine requires narrative competence, that is, the ability to acknowledge, absorb, interpret, and act on the stories and plights of others" (including other healthcare workers) and oneself (Charon, 2001, p. 1897). As part of a growing movement and health humanities field known as graphic medicine (Czerwiec et al., 2015), autobiographical comics and graphic memoirs have followed in the narrative medicine tradition, with many authors--including nurses--using such forms to tell their stories and make sense of attempt to heal from illness, pain, stigma, and trauma (see Green & Myers, 2010). Too some, the medium of comics--sometimes culturally (mis)understood as nonserious, trivial, and disposable--might seem ill-suited to such subjects. But health and medical stakeholders (e.g., patients, providers, caregivers, advocates, family members) have increasingly recognized and valued comics' unique potential to convey information or tell a story in a multilayered, approachable, and provoking manner. Comics' interplay of words and images, representational and symbolic renderings, sequential but fragmentary structure, and active engagement of the reader can enable distinct interpretive and affective experiences. Williams (2012) explained that "Comics, like poetry, seem to allow more leeway in terms of meaning and, like film, offer the possibility of words juxtaposed with a contradictory image," adding that

Ambiguity and metaphor can be layered, bestowing properties that see to lend comics to the portrayal of complex or taboo narrative. Where language is lacking to describe bodily sensations or complex emotional states, metaphor can play a vital role...Comics' language is always characterized by a plurality of messages; difficult, ambivalent, chaotic, or incomprehensible impressions, narratives or visions can be articulated (p. 25).

A groundbreaking example of a graphic memoir embodying such qualities and authored by a nurse is M. K. Czerwiec's memoir *Taking Turns* (2017), which focuses on her experiences working in a hospital AIDS unit, depicting her and her patients' challenges in a de-stigmatizing manner. Other notable graphic memoirs have similarly examined the trauma of illness and caregiving as a form of "auto-therapy" (Williams, 2011); these include Brian Fies' *Mom's Cancer* (2006) about how his mother's diagnosis of and treatment for lung cancer affected him and the family, David B.'s *Epileptic* (2006) about the family trauma resulting from a child's misunderstood illness, and Roz Chast's *Can't We Talk About Something More Pleasant?* (2014) about the difficulty of discussing end-of-life plans with one's reluctant parents. Graphic memoirs have also been used to explore community trauma, as with the collection of comics *Love is Love* (Andreyko et al., 2017) about the Pulse shooting, Will Dennis's *Where We Live* (2018) edited anthology about the Las Vegas shootings, and Fies' *A Fire Story* (2019) about fleeing the California wildfires.[1]

Graphic testimonials have also been used by healthcare educators to educate patients about illness and treatment and to help providers-in-training prepare for the challenges of patient care (see George & Green, 2015; Yu, 2018). Graphic testimonials have been found to promote empathetic, patient-centered care in medical students (Tsao & Yu, 2016) and postgraduate medical learners (Sutherland, Choi, & Yu, 2021), and to foster connection and collective bonds of empathy, as with memoirs about illness and death co-created by patients and their loved ones (Czerwiec & Huang, 2017). More recently, medical educators have begun to use comics to educate students about structural racism and ways to address racial disparities in healthcare (Obuobi, Vela, & Callender, 2021).

Finally, graphic testimonials or comics have been used in research practices. In their overview of "comics-based research," Kuttner, Sousanis, and Weaver-Hightower (2018) discussed how comics can be useful to present research, with examples ranging from comics sketches for anthropological fieldwork, to visualized oral histories, to graphic memoir (see also Weaver-Hightower, 2013). Comics, they argued, "provide a frame through which to think, and think differently, about the objects or findings of research" (p. 398). Beyond presenting research, they also considered how comics could be used in data collection, imagining comics as a tool for capturing interviews ("complete with body language and facial expressions") (p. 411), as well as a tool for visualizing field notes and ideas. Comics, they suggested, could be "co-created with participants as a form of participatory meaning-making" (p. 411). The co-authors of this chapter have enacted this latter used of comics as participatory data collection tools in a project aimed at combating HIV stigma. In the data collection phase of this project, the authors of this chapter asked participants to "fill in" minimal comic storyboards depicting their experiences with and reactions to provider-enacted stigma, an approach not unlike the use of Photovoice in community-based participatory research about nurses' experiences during the COVID-19 pandemic (Badanta, Acevedo-Augilera, Lucchetti, & Diego-Cordero, 2021).

Graphic Testimonials in Response to COVID-19

In the more specific context of the COVID-19 pandemic, graphic testimonials and other types of comics have been used for a range of functions in health and medicine, somewhat aligned with the different categories of "COVID-19 Comics" (Jaggers, 2020) on the Graphic Medicine website: "By/About Caregivers," "By Patients" (e.g., "When COVID-19 Stole My Sense of Smell & Taste"), "Educational" (e.g., "Meet the New Strains), "Ethics/Social Justice" (e.g., "In/Vulnerable: Inequity in the Time of Pandemic"), "Coping and Humor" (e.g., "Coping with Pandemic Numbness"), and "Historic" (e.g., "America Isn't Ready for a Pandemic"). The comics in each category were created by cartoonists and/or people working in health and medicine. Gathered from various mainstream media and personal social media sources, the comics by and about caregivers including graphic testimonials that vividly--and in some cases symbolically, metaphorically, and/or humorously--depict the challenges of and reflections about working and living during the pandemic (see Figure 1).

In their analysis of this curated collection, Saji, Venkatesan, and Callender (2021) identified the comics' varied functions as sharing information and persuading laypeople to follow public health precautions and safety measures, exposing and correcting misinformation, raising ethical concerns such as the politicalization of the disease and public health response, sharing the anxieties and vulnerabilities of first-hand experiences, and offering "lessons learnt from past virulent disease outbreaks, particularly the influenza pandemic of 1918 through a comparison-and-contrast approach" (p. 142). Another source that curates a range of "web exclusive" COVID-19-related comics, including many autobiographical testimonials of healthcare providers, is the "Annals Graphic Medicine" website (American College, 2021), searchable by author or publication date. Two other notable collections of COVID-19 comics are *Covid Chronicles* (Sacks, Talajic, & Kim, 2020), including "Vol. 1: A nurse's anguish in the ICU" and *Covid Chronicles: A Comics Anthology* (Boileau & Johnson, 2021). The latter anthology brings together the work of various artists who document and offer cultural commentaries on the emotion-laden reactions of individuals, families, communities, institutions, and societies--many related to healthcare. The former *Covid Chronicles* (2020) more specifically chronicles "ten personal [and nonfictional] accounts of life and death" by healthcare workers on the frontlines, gathered by a journalist, drawn by a comic artist, and distributed online by *NBC News*.

Graphic testimonials that document the lived experiences by nurses and other healthcare workers have both reinforced the problematic hero narrative of healthcare workers (as in Marvel Comics' *The Vitals: True Nurse Stories*, Ryan, 2020) and documented such workers' vulnerability, fear, moral injury, questioning, and trauma, as in many of the comics curated in the Graphic Medicine and Annals Graphic Medicine sites. For example, the latter includes physician Carla Canepa's (2020) "COVID Blues," which depicts various emotions when caring for patients, sadness and emptiness when alone, and a "vitriolic rage" about public health unpreparedness simmering just below the surface. Another example from this site is provider Alice Bellchambers' (2020) "One of My Demons: Crying (or a Lack of)," which depicts her cathartic, coping experience of crying with a housemate after a shift in which a patient dies.

Figure 1. Partial screen shot of Graphic Medicine Web page "COVID-19 Comics: By/About Caregivers" (taken from https://www.graphicmedicine.org/covid-19-comics-by-about-caregivers/)

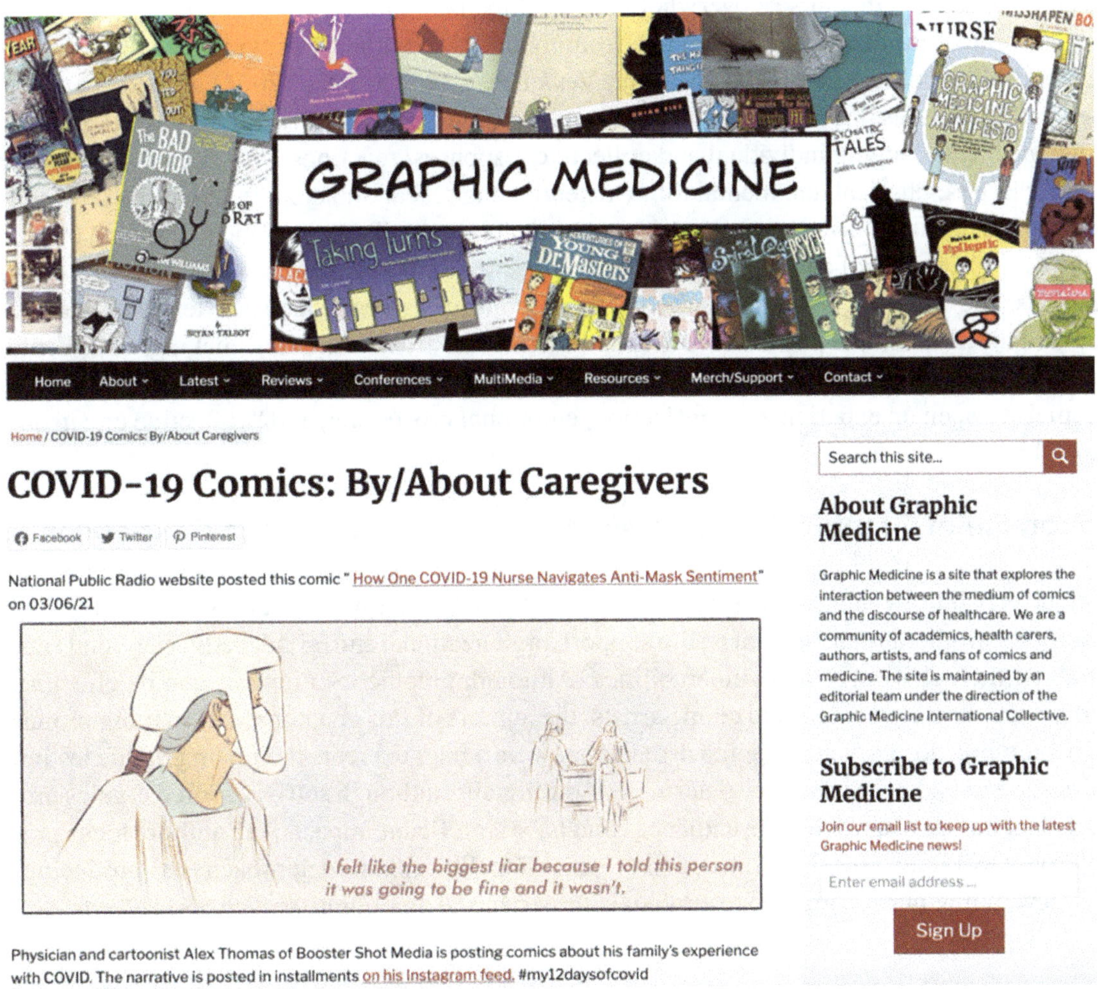

As with other artistic responses to COVID-19 by healthcare providers, many of these autobiographical comics are self-sponsored expressions that we could call auto-therapy, following Williams (2011). Williams suggested that "comics as art therapy" has not become more widespread simply because drawing (like other forms of art) can be intimidating to those without specialized training (p. 356); but in co-launching the graphic medicine movement, Williams and others have developed how-to manuals and pedagogies for training everyday people to produce comics, as with Lynda Barry's widely acclaimed exercises and workshop method (see her book *Syllabus*, 2014) which have been used by such diverse non-artist groups as prison inmates, postal workers, and hairdressers. In addition to teaching people to create their own comics, the field of graphic medicine has linked comic artists with patients and others who need their stories told through this medium. McNicol and Leamy (2020) reported on a pilot project in which people with mild-to-moderate dementia worked collaboratively with artists "to communicate their experiences and express their opinions" about stigma and other issues through graphic narratives (p. 267). In response to the ongoing COVID-19 pandemic, the Graphic Medicine International Collective, in collaboration with the Penn State College of Medicine, recently launched a project that matches frontline healthcare workers with artists who create comics portraying the workers' experiences, offering funding to both (Noe, 2021). As part of this project, one of this chapter's co-authors, a comic artist and teacher, is collaborating with a nurse administrator (see Figure 2 for an example of a thumbnail sketch they created to capture the nurse's overwhelming workload).

In addition to auto-therapies, the graphic testimonials by healthcare providers cited in this section can be conceptualized as expressing what Saji, Venkatesan, & Callender (2021) termed "covidity"--"a neologism that captures philosophical, material, and emotional responses to the COVID-19 pandemic… and embraces wide-ranging individual and collective responses/ reactions, including an intense experience of paradoxes, physical and mental toll, existential angst, fear and anxiety about the return of such pandemics, the need to reinvent oneself in the context of constant disruption, and the trauma of everyday life" (p. 142). The notion of covidity captures the connections across individual and co-authored graphic testimonials, the range of changing and sometimes conflicting reactions such testimonials typically convey, and the need for and power of transformation through artistic meaning-making. Saji, Venkatsen, & Callender focused their analysis of covidity on the interpretive functions of metaphors in graphic testimonials to open up experiences to reflection, emotional processing, and "collective understanding" (pp. 144, 152).

The Promise of Graphic Testimonials for Nurses' Therapeutic Responses

The unique capabilities and already established uses of graphic testimonials are well-suited to the needs of nurses for auto-therapy and mental health support, organizational and broader advocacy, and educating others about their challenges and vulnerabilities. Although graphic testimonials can be effectively co-created by healthcare providers and comic artists, the authors of this chapter see even more promise in a capacity building, do-it-yourself approach that empowers nurses to create their own graphic testimonials for purposes and audiences that they determine. Additionally, although self-sponsored comics produced by individual nurses can reach wide audiences and have significant impacts, the authors focus primarily on the promise of collective, integrated, and organizationally supported approaches to producing, sharing, and leveraging nurses' graphic testimonials for structural ameliorative changes.

Figure 2. Thumbnail sketch of comic depicting overwhelming nature of nurse administrator's workload, by Nathan Holic

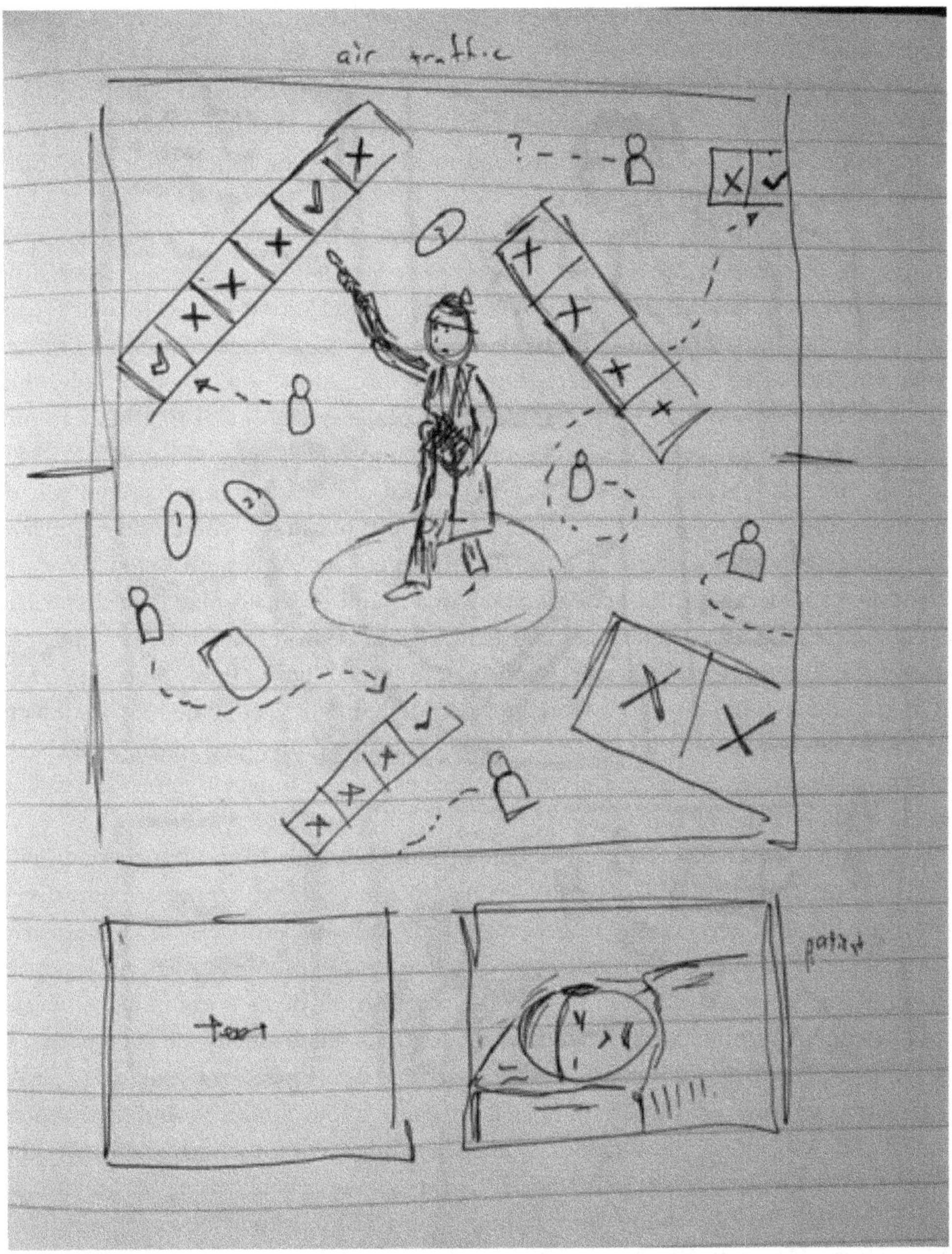

Given that graphic testimonials are already being produced and used by nurses and other healthcare providers to express, interpret and reflect on, and begin to heal from individual and collective trauma, moral injury, anxiety, depression, and other mental health challenges, it stands to reason that such comics could be integrated into a range of therapeutic interventions for nurses, including but also beyond those focused on self-help and individual resilience.

Nurses may be more willing to acknowledge their mental health challenges and be open to self-help materials (e.g., about coping, de-stressing, focusing strategies) if they were communicated through engaging graphic testimonials created by other nurses and depicting familiar experiences and reactions. A similar approach has been used successfully to help medical students and their teachers reflect on the stress and anxiety of their training through reading comics created by students (George & Green, 2015). The successful integration of graphic medicine in medical education suggests that that they could also be used for preparing nursing students, interns, and residents for the moral injury and other types of mental health challenges they will likely face.

Nurses' creation of graphic testimonials could also be integrated into programs that help them create written narratives as a means of therapeutic self-expression, either as an alternative or supplement to such written narratives. Graphic alternatives might make such narratives easier to share (especially via social media) with other nurses and, possibly, other coworkers (e.g., supervisors) and those in nurses' personal lifeworlds. Because therapeutic narrative writing programs (e.g., sponsored by the ANA and the University of Colorado Medical Campus) already include pedagogical materials to aid nurses in crafting their narratives, these could be supplemented with materials around Barry's (2014) workshop approach; ideally, the hospital or other organization would enlist a comic artist/educator or group to offer synchronous workshops (online or in-person) for groups of nurses who could, in turn, teach other nurses. In the authors' region of Central Florida, for example, The Sequential Artists Workshop (SAW) offers various types and levels of online workshops that could be customized for a specific group or population. The Graphic Medicine International Collective also hosts regular "drawing together" and other workshops, and a number of libraries sponsor graphic medicine book club kits. Depending on the uses of the graphic testimonials, such workshops could help nurses decide how to depict aspects of actual experiences and reactions without compromising confidentiality, and they could also help nurses experiment with various representational strategies, such as using animals to depict the characters in the testimonials to enable broader identification.

Graphic testimonials could also be used as part of more advanced forms of therapy led by mental health specialists. The University of Colorado uses healthcare workers' expressive narratives as a form of written exposure therapy, and graphic testimonials could be used similarly if not more effectively, as their medium enables more varied and multilayered depictions of complex affective responses. Graphic testimonials could also be used either to inform the creation of, or as a component of, standardized scenario-based simulation training (e.g., Cheung et al., 2020) in which nurses select depictions of familiar experiences and learn new ways of reacting and coping. The developers of simulations could use comics as data collection or story elicitation tools to learn more about nurses' contextualized experiences (e.g., with trauma, moral injury, stigmatization) and their impacts on mental health, and then develop composite stories to be used in the simulations. These types of interventions using graphic testimonials are especially promising for addressing trauma, including PTSD. In their book *Looking at Trauma: A Tool Kit for Clinicians*, Hershler, Hughes, Nguyen, & Walls (2021) uses comics to present twelve trauma treatment models to help clinicians explain in relatable ways the impacts and management of trauma to patients. A similar resource could be created by and for nurses who have experienced trauma, but focused more on fostering recognition of and empathy for their own and others' traumatic experiences, as more advanced treatments would need to be delivered by specialists.

Regarding peer-based therapeutic interventions, peer-led workshops could involve the drawing and sharing of graphic testimonials about challenges, coping mechanisms, and needs. The quick sketching of comics or filling in of comic storyboards (e.g., with blank thought clouds and speech bubbles) could even be used as a form of shift debriefing that enables nurses to simultaneously engage in internal reflection. Some practitioners of graphic medicine have begun to experiment with new forms of distributing comics, such as a deck of large playing cards. Sharable and short but informative comics about signs of mental health problems and referral information could be used by peer support teams as easy-to-use tools for reminding nurses how to identify peers who are in distress and how to connect them to mental health support and care.

The Promise of Graphic Testimonials in Advocacy and Educational Efforts

Some of the same approaches to helping nurses create graphic testimonials can also be used in advocacy and public education efforts that feature nurses' stories. Comics' approachability and potential to convey serious messages through humor or "serious play" (Williams & Czerweic, 2015) can make them a disarming tool for countering a workplace culture that silences and stigmatizes mental illness; in addition to being part of digital learning materials, graphic testimonials could be made into posters, digital images, and other forms that could be displayed or used in the workplace. Given the multifaceted nature of mental health stigma, for example, graphic testimonials could identify and convey connections across the drivers and facilitators of stigma in their environments. In addition to the authors' own ongoing research on developing graphic testimonials about the experiences of people living with HIV (PLWH) to combat provider-enacted stigma, Teti, Epping, Myroniuk, & Evans-Agnew (2021) explored how PLWH used visual metaphors in creative photography to depict and make sense of stigma. Such studies show the power of visual artistic forms as stigma-addressing mechanisms. Nurses' graphic testimonials, particularly about their fears, vulnerabilities, and stigmatization, could also be shared with family and friends, remembering that healthcare providers have expressed a preference in some studies for home- and community-based care activities (LoGiudice & Bartos, 2021).

Within their organizations, groups of nurses could create graphic testimonials to convey the mental health impacts of moral injury and otherwise demoralizing and unsafe working conditions as potentially more impactful ways to convey and lobby for their workplace needs. Although organizations and institutions might co-sponsor and create opportunities for creating and sharing graphic testimonials, nurses themselves should collectively determine and prioritize workplace advocacy actions using their comic-based stories. Several groups--including the Green Mountain Support Services, the Women in Comics Collective, and the Graphic Advocacy Project--have developed resources for and approaches to the do-it-yourself collective creation and use of comics for advocacy purposes (e.g., accessibility advocacy, community organizing, legal advocacy). Nurses could look to such groups for models of how to advocate for themselves in their workplaces and local communities.

Just as written and PhotoVoice testimonials by providers have been collected and used by ANA and other nursing and healthcare organizations to mobilize stakeholders and publics in broader policymaking advocacy, such organizations could also incorporate graphic testimonials as compelling stories through which to educate and persuade policymakers and their constituents, particularly about such issues as funding for and policies around PPE and workplace safety, pay and benefits, vaccination, and mental health support. The medium of comics is especially well suited for a range of communication channels, from social media memes to political ads to policy briefs. Because such graphic testimonials can be short but still impactful, organizations could include a wide range of stories when using them.

Nurses and other providers have already been expressing and documenting their experiences working and living during the COVID-19 pandemic through various artistic means, including through comics that they create and distribute on their own, through collectives, and/or with the help of others such as the Graphic Medicine Frontlines project or media outlets like *NBC News*. The authors of this chapter believe that graphic testimonials designed in part to educate should involve this full range of efforts in order to reach interpersonal networks, local communities, and broader publics--all of the spheres in which nurses need more robust and meaningful support. With this type of educational response, too, organizations and groups with expertise in graphic medicine and comics might coordinate with local groups of nurses and larger nursing organizations to train nurses in comic creation through a capacity building approach. Empowering nurses with the ability to create and share graphic testimonials about their experiences gives them another mechanism for reclaiming their rhetorical credibility and agency that stigma and other factors can disable.

Continued efforts to educate others about the lived experiences and indispensability of nurses should be wary of explicitly or implicitly reinforcing a (super)hero narrative that can dehumanize nurses by ignoring their vulnerabilities and play into the occupation-based stigma against mental illness in healthcare workers. Such efforts should also go beyond expressing appreciation through "pizza and coffee mugs," as Owens (2020) puts it. Accolades of nurses' sacrifice might be edifying, but they can "camouflage" nurses' vital needs for "ongoing support" (Blackburn, McAuliffe, & Johns, 2020). Finally, educational efforts, like therapeutic and advocacy ones, should remind healthcare stakeholders, communities, and publics that nurses need organizational, institutional, policymaking, sociocultural, and other types of systemic support for mental wellness, and that even graphic testimonials by and about individual nurses reveal broader, wicked problems that cannot be solved by simply asking nurses to become more resilient or victim-blaming them when they struggle to do so. The authors recognize that the range of interventions reviewed, proposed, and advocated for in this chapter require more funding, time, energy and other resources than are currently available to many nurses, their supervisors and other decision-makers, and the institutions in which they work. But supporting the mental health of nurses and other healthcare providers on the front lines is something our society cannot afford *not* to invest in, and this is why lobbying for increased funding is a central component of advocacy.

FUTURE RESEARCH DIRECTIONS

Putting the promise of graphic testimonials aside for a moment, future research is needed to better understand the range of mental health challenges experienced by nurses and the various factors contributing to them. Most of the research about these topics as related to the COVID-19 pandemic has focused on nurses and other healthcare workers in China and, to a lesser extent, Europe, Canada, and other places outside of the United States. In addition, most of this research has focused on workers (including critical care nurses) in hospitals and hospital systems, leaving a research gap about nursing in other healthcare contexts. Although some studies of healthcare providers' mental health during the COVID-19 pandemic have taken a cross-sectional approach to identify demographic factors (e.g., age, gender, years in profession) and workplace factors (e.g., redeployment to critical care, lack of adequate PPE) associated with symptoms of mental illness (see, for example, Khajuria et al., 2021), more research sensitive to these factors is needed, along with qualitative research that could explore some of the possible reasons for these associations and the health disparities they indicate. Future qualitative research about nurses' mental health challenges and contributing factors might utilize comics (or more minimal comic storyboards, as the authors have done in their research) as tools for collecting data from and about nurses.

Regarding nurses' experiences with the stigmatization of mental health, in particular, future research is needed to further explore the relationship between nurses as targets and enactors of stigma, and to better understand the intersectional nature and cross-cutting drivers and facilitators of nurses' mental health stigma (the latter perhaps using Stangl et al.'s "Health Stigma and Discrimination Framework," 2019).

A second major direction for future research is the continued and expanded evaluation of the various interventions that have been implemented to support nurses' and other healthcare workers' mental wellness during and beyond the pandemic. Evaluating the efficacy of mental health support should entail such criteria as mental health outcomes, job satisfaction, and likelihood to stay in the profession, as well as more difficult-to-measure criteria such as the level of workplace stigmatization around mental health. Some research has begun such evaluation, which is why several of the articles cited in this chapter make claims about "evidence-based" interventions, but even most the systematic reviews can only make tentative claims about efficacy, in part because many of the interventions they describe have been implemented fairly recently (and some, like the effects of interventions on PTSD, are not yet fully knowable in an ongoing pandemic). As Mulvale et al. (2019) argue in their review of peer-based mental health support, many such efforts are in need of further integration--a topic that future research could address. Because some interventions to support nurses' mental health are somewhat localized, future research should also examine how such efforts could be further expanded, adapted, and scaled, along with the barriers to doing so.

Third, future research should continue to evaluate the already existing uses of graphic medicine by and for healthcare providers. As Noe & Levin (2020) observe, graphic medicine initiatives aimed at healthcare providers and providers-in-training have only just begun to be evaluated systematically, and therefore more research is needed. Initiatives to evaluate include the Graphic Medicine Frontlines project and the use of graphic testimonials to train providers about stigma.

A final direction of future research pertains to what the authors proposed in the previous section: developing ways to integrate nurses' creation of graphic testimonials into various therapeutic, advocacy, and educational mechanisms for supporting mental health, and then evaluating these. Although the uses of graphic testimonials proposed by the chapter's authors were informed by similar, already-implemented applications, most of these proposals are still somewhat conjectural and therefore need to be developed, implemented, and evaluated. Any such efforts will need to consider how to avoid simply giving nurses and their supervisors more work that they do not have time to do, how to enlist the co-sponsorship of organizational administrators and other decision-makers, how to help nurses become confident creators of their own graphic testimonials, whether and to what extent to enlist comic artists beyond initial training, how to avoid inadvertently reinforcing idealized and stigmatized portrayals of nurses, how to ensure that the uses of graphic testimonials do not replace more advanced mental health support by specialists, and, most of all, how to ensure that efforts are grounded in and responsive to what *nurses* say they want and need. For their part, the chapter's interdisciplinary team of authors (including a public health nurse with a background in mental health, a nurse specializing in trauma-informed care, a teacher and author of graphic narratives, a health communication specialist, and a pre-med student) plans to collaborate with others to integrate the creation and use of nurses' graphic testimonials into an existing peer-based mental health monitoring and intervention program for healthcare workers. Partnering with an organization of comic artists, we will co-design workshops for helping nurses create graphic testimonials to aid in identifying struggling co-workers and connect them to needed mental health support, to de-stigmatize mental distress and illness, and to communicate and advocate for nurses' workplace and broader needs.

CONCLUSION

As mentioned in this chapter's introduction, the stakes of not addressing nurses' and other healthcare providers' mental health distress and trauma have never been higher, not only for their individual well-being but also for the nursing profession and delivery of healthcare. Nurses are a critical component of our healthcare system, and the demand for qualified nurses continues to grow due to our aging population, aging workforce, burnout, family obligations, and violence in the healthcare setting (Haddad, Annamaraju, & Toney-Butler, 2020). This critical component is threatened by mental health challenges that can demoralize and debilitate nurses and that have been linked to lower job satisfaction and burnout. Of the 6,000 acute and critical care nurses responding to a recent survey about the impact of the previous 18 months, 66% reported that their experiences have made them consider leaving the profession (AACN, 2021). Although research has indicated that a "bedside care workforce with a greater proportion of professional nurses is associated with better outcomes for patients and nurses" (Aiken et al., 2016), the increased demand for nurses due to the pandemic has reduced optimal or even adequate staffing. Without an adequate supply of nurses, patient care and health outcomes will be adversely impacted. Complications of an inadequate nursing supply include greater likelihood of hospital readmissions, increased mortality and morbidity, longer length of stay, and decreased overall quality of care (American Association of Colleges of Nursing, 2020). Addressing mental health challenges arising from the pandemic may help us prevent further attrition of the nursing workforce.

In addition to mechanisms for supporting their individual and collective mental wellness, nurses need mechanisms for collective advocacy and for educating others about their lived experiences, vulnerabilities, and needs during and beyond the COVID-19 pandemic. A range of interventions and other responses have begun to address these varied needs, some involving written, visual, and other art forms created by nurses and other healthcare workers. At the same time, the field of graphic medicine has developed a range of uses for comics in health provider education, patient care, auto-therapy, advocacy, and de-stigmatizing educational storytelling about people's experiences with illness, care, and caregiving. More recently, graphic testimonials have been used to document, make sense of, and convey arguments about the experiences of nurses and other healthcare workers during the COVID-19 pandemic, and such uses can be expanded and integrated into other mechanisms of mental wellness support for nurses. The introduction of the *Graphic Medicine Manifesto* (Williams & Czerweic, 2015) asserts that, "Graphic medicine seeks to disrupt…power imbalance! We believe those best positioned to represent illness and care-giving are those living with it" (p. 20). This same ethic applies to graphic testimonials about nurses and their vulnerabilities and needs. Graphic testimonials afford nurses a unique and novel medium for disrupting power imbalances that have demanded their acquiescent "resilience" and silenced their vulnerabilities, difficulties, and needs. Although nurses must be empowered to authoritatively express their mental health needs, it is up to all of us who depend on them to lobby for more responsive forms of support.

REFERENCES

AACN. (2021, September 21). Hear us out campaign reports nurses' COVID-19 reality. *American Association of Critical Care Nurses*. https://www.aacn.org/newsroom/hear-us-out-campaign-reports-nurses-covid-19-reality

Adams, J. G., & Walls, R. M. (2020). Supporting the health care workforce during the COVID- 19 global epidemic. *Journal of the American Medical Association, 323*(15), 1439. doi:10.1001/jama.2020.3972 PMID:32163102

Aiken, L. H., Sloane, D., Griffiths, P., Rafferty, A. M., Bruyneel, L., McHugh, M., Maier, C. B., Moreno-Casbas, T., Ball, J. E., Ausserhofer, D., & Sermeus, W. (2017). Nursing skill mix in European hospitals: Cross-sectional study of the association with mortality, patient ratings, and quality of care. *BMJ Quality & Safety, 26*(7), 559–568. doi:10.1136/bmjqs-2016-005567 PMID:28626086

Albott, C. S., Wozniak, J. R., McGlinch, B. P., Wall, M. H., Gold, B. S., & Vinogradov, S. (2020). Battle Buddies: Rapid deployment of a psychological resilience intervention for health care workers during the COVID-19 pandemic. *Anesthesia and Analgesia, 131*(1), 43–54. doi:10.1213/ANE.0000000000004912 PMID:32345861

Altman, M. (2020, April 10). Shifting ethic in a crisis: Responding to COVID-19. *American Association of Critical Care Nurses*. https://www.aacn.org/blog/shifting-ethics-in-a-crisis-responding-to-covid-19

American Association of Colleges of Nursing. (n.d.). *Nursing Fact Sheet*. https://www.aacnnursing.org/News-Information/Fact-Sheets/Nursing-Fact-Sheet

American College of Physicians. (2021). *Annals graphic medicine*. https://www.acpjournals.org/topic/web-exclusives/annals-graphic-medicine

American Hospital Association. (n.d.). *Stories from the front lines*. https://www.aha.org/issue-landing-page/2020-06-02-stories-front-lines

American Nurses Association. (2021, October 14). Well-being inititative. *Nursing World*. https://www.nursingworld.org/practice-policy/work-environment/health-safety/disaster-preparedness/coronavirus/what-you-need-to-know/the-well-being-initiative/

Andolhe, R., Barbosa, R. L., de Oliveira, E. M., Costa, A. L. S., & Padilha, K. G. (2015). Estresse, coping e burnout da Equipe de Enfermagem de Unidades de Terapia Intensiva: Fatores associados. *Revista Da Escola de Enfermagem Da USP, 49*(spe), 58–64. doi:10.1590/S0080-623420150000700009

Andreyko, M., Gaydos, S., & Rich, J. (Eds.). (2017). *Love is love: A comic book anthology to benefit the survivors of the Orlando Pulse shooting*. IDW Publishing.

B., D. (2006). *Epileptic*. Pantheon.

Badanta, B., Acevedo-Aguilera, R., Lucchetti, G., & de Diego-Cordero, R. (2021). "A picture is worth a thousand words": A photovoice study exploring health professionals' experiences during the COVID-19 pandemic. *Journal of Clinical Nursing, 30*(10.1111), 1-13. doi:10.1111/jocn.15887

Bagcchi, S. (2020). Stigma during the COVID-19 pandemic. *The Lancet. Infectious Diseases, 20*(7), 782. doi:10.1016/S1473-3099(20)30498-9 PMID:32592670

Barry, L. (2014). *Syllabus: Notes from an accidental professor*. Drawn and Quarterly.

Bellchambers, A. S. (2020). One of my demons: Crying (or a lack of). *Annals Graphic Medicine*. https://www.acpjournals.org/doi/10.7326/G19-0054

Bender, A. E., Berg, K. A., Miller, E. K., Evans, K. E., & Holmes, M. R. (2021). "Making sure we are all okay": Healthcare workers' strategies for emotional connectedness during the COVID-19 pandemic. *Clinical Social Work Journal, 49*(4), 445–455. Advance online publication. doi:10.100710615-020-00781-w PMID:33456094

Blackburn, P., McAuliffe, D., & Johns, L. (2020, May 18). Health-care workers share our trauma during the coronavirus pandemic-on top of their own. *The Conversation.* https://theconversation.com/health-care-workers-share-our-trauma-during-the-coronavirus-pandemic-on-top-of-their-own-137887

Blake, H., Bermingham, F., Johnson, G., & Tabner, A. (2020). Mitigating the psychological impact of COVID-19 on healthcare workers: A digital learning package. *International Journal of Environmental Research and Public Health, 17*(9), E2997. doi:10.3390/ijerph17092997 PMID:32357424

Bolieau, K., & Johnson, R. (Eds.). (2021). *COVID chronicles: A comics anthology.* Graphic Mundi. doi:10.1515/9780271091723

Branson, D. C. (2019). Vicarious trauma, themes in research, and terminology: A review of literature. *Traumatology, 25*(1), 2–10. doi:10.1037/trm0000161

Brown, T., & Rushton, C. (n.d.). *Frontline Nurses WikiWisdom Forum.* https://nurses.wikiwisdomforum.com/

Canepa, C. M. (2020). COVID Blues. *Annals graphic medicine.* https://www.acpjournals.org/doi/10.7326/G20-0053

Carmassi, C., Foghi, C., Dell'Oste, V., Cordone, A., Bertelloni, C. A., Bui, E., & Dell'Osso, L. (2020). PTSD symptoms in healthcare workers facing the three coronavirus outbreaks: What can we expect after the COVID-19 pandemic. *Psychiatry Research, 292*, 113312. doi:10.1016/j.psychres.2020.113312 PMID:32717711

Charon, R. (2001). Narrative medicine: A model for empathy, reflection, profession, and trust. *Journal of the American Medical Association, 286*(15), 1897–1902. doi:10.1001/jama.286.15.1897 PMID:11597295

Chast, R. (2014). *Can't we talk about something more pleasant?* Bloomsbury.

Chen, K., Chen, Y., Ling, Y., & Lin, J. (2020). The individual experience of online chemistry teacher education in China: Coping with COVID-19 pandemic. *Journal of Chemical Education, 97*(9), 3265–3270. doi:10.1021/acs.jchemed.0c00581

Cheung, V. K.-L., So, E. H.-K., Ng, G. W.-Y., So, S.-S., Hung, J. L.-K., & Chia, N.-H. (2020). Investigating effects of healthcare simulation on personal strengths and organizational impacts for healthcare workers during COVID-19 pandemic: A cross-sectional study. *Integrative Medicine Research, 9*(3), 100476. doi:10.1016/j.imr.2020.100476 PMID:32802743

Cipriano, P. F., Boston-Leary, K., Mcmillan, K., & Peterson, C. (2020). The U.S. COVID-19 crises: Facts, science and solidarity. *International Nursing Review, 67*(4), 437–444. doi:10.1111/inr.12646 PMID:33428227

Colak, R. (2020). *The vitals: True nurse stories.* Marvel Comics.

Cole-King, A., & Dykes, L. (2020). *Wellbeing for HCWs during COVID19*. https://www.lindadykes.org/covid19

Conklin, E. J. (2006). *Dialogue mapping: Building shared understanding of wicked problems*. Wiley.

COVID Trauma Response Working Group. (2020). https://www.traumagroup.org

Crouch, M. (2021, May 11). What nurses want you to know about the past year. *AARP*. https://www.aarp.org/health/conditions-treatments/info-2021/nurses-reflect-on- pandemic.html

Czerwiec, M. K. (2017). *Taking turns: Stories from HIV/AIDS care Unit 371*. The Pennsylvania State University Press.

Czerwiec, M. K., & Huang, M. N. (2017). Hospice comics: Representations of patient and family experience of illness and death in graphic novels. *The Journal of Medical Humanities*, *38*(2), 95–113. doi:10.100710912-014-9303-7 PMID:25138207

Czerwiec, M. K., & Williams, I. (2015). Introduction. In *Graphic Medicine Manifesto* (pp. 1–20). The Pennsylvania State University Press.

Czerwiec, M. K., Williams, I., Squier, S. M., Green, M. J., Myers, K. R., & Smith, S. T. (2015). *Graphic medicine manifesto*. The Pennsylvania State University Press.

De Kock, J. H., Latham, H. A., Leslie, S. J., Grindle, M., Munoz, S.-A., Ellis, L., Polson, R., & O'Malley, C. M. (2021). A rapid review of the impact of COVID-19 on the mental health of healthcare workers: Implications for supporting psychological well-being. *BMC Public Health*, *21*(1), 104. doi:10.118612889-020-10070-3 PMID:33422039

Dean, W., Talbot, S., & Dean, A. (2019). Reframing clinician distress: Moral injury not burnout. *Federal Practitioner: For the Health Care Professionals of the VA, DoD, and PHS*, *36*(9), 400–402. PMID:31571807

Dennis, W. (Ed.). (2018). *Where we live: A benefit for the survivors in Las Vegas*. Image Comics.

DePierro, J., Katz, C. L., Marin, D., Feder, A., Bevilacqua, L., Sharma, V., Hurtado, A., Ripp, J., Lim, S., & Charney, D. (2020). Mount Sinai's Center for Stress, Resilience, and Personal Growth as a model for responding to the impact of COVID-19 on health care workers. *Psychiatry Research*, *29*, 113426. doi:10.1016/j.psychres.2020.113426 PMID:32861094

Doheny, K. (2021, Feb. 1). *Moral injury: Pandemic's fallout for healthcare workers*. WebMD Health News. https://www.webmd.com/lung/news/20210201/moral-injury-pandemics-fallout-for-health-care-workers

Donnelly, P. D., Davidson, M., Dunlop, N., McGale, M., Milligan, E., Worrall, M., Wylie, J., & Kidson, C. (2020). Well-being during coronavirus disease 2019: A PICU practical perspective. *Pediatric Critical Care Medicine*, *21*(8), e584–e586. doi:10.1097/PCC.0000000000002434 PMID:32412984

Easter, M. (2021, March 12). "Hamilton" cookie portraits? See how healthcare workers make art to cope with COVID-19. *Los Angeles Times*. https://www.latimes.com/entertainment-arts/story/2021-03-12/healthcare-workers-and-creativity-callout-responses

Fernandez, R., Lord, H., Halcomb, E., Moxham, L., Middleton, R., Alananzeh, I., & Ellwood, L. (2020). Implications for COVID-19: A systematic review of nurses' experiences of working in acute care hospital settings during a respiratory pandemic. *International Journal of Nursing Studies*, *111*, 103637. doi:10.1016/j.ijnurstu.2020.103637 PMID:32919358

Fies, B. (2008). *Mom's cancer*. Abrams Comicarts.

Fies, B. (2019). *A fire story*. Abrams ComicArts.

Galvin, J., Richards, G., & Smith, A. P. (2020). A longitudinal cohort study investigating inadequate preparation and death and dying in nursing students: Implications for the aftermath of the COVID-19 pandemic. *Frontiers in Psychology*, *11*, 2206. doi:10.3389/fpsyg.2020.02206 PMID:32982890

Gao, J., Wang, F., Guo, S., & Hu, F. (2021). Mental health of nursing students amid coronavirus disease 2019 pandemic. *Frontiers in Psychology*, *12*, 699558. doi:10.3389/fpsyg.2021.699558 PMID:34475837

Geoffroy, P. A., Le Goanvic, V., Sabbagh, O., Richoux, C., Weinstein, A., Dufayet, G., & Lejoyeux, M. (2020). Psychological support system for hospital workers during the Covid-19 outbreak: Rapid design and implementation of the Covid-Psy hotline. *Frontiers in Psychiatry*, *11*, 511. doi:10.3389/fpsyt.2020.00511 PMID:32670100

George, D. R., & Green, M. J. (2015). Lessons learned from comics produced by medical students: Art of darkness. *Journal of the American Medical Association*, *314*(22), 2345. doi:10.1001/jama.2015.13652 PMID:26647249

Goffman, E. (1963). Stigma: Notes on the management of spoiled identity. *Touchstone (Nashville, Tenn.)*.

Green, M. J., & Myers, K. R. (2010). Graphic medicine: Use of comics in medical education and patient care. *BMJ*, *340*(2), c863–c863. doi:10.1136/bmj.c863

Greenberg, N., & Tracy, D. (2020). What healthcare leaders need to do to protect the psychological well-being of frontline staff in the COVID-19 pandemic. *BMJ Leader*, *4*(3), 101–102. doi:10.1136/leader-2020-000273

Haddad, L., Annamaraju, P., & Toney-Butler, T. (2021). *Nursing Shortage*. StatPearls Publishing. https://www.ncbi.nlm.nih.gov/books/NBK493175/

Havsteen-Franklin, D., Tjasink, M., Kottler, J. W., Grant, C., & Kumari, V. (2020). Arts-based interventions for professionals in caring roles during and after crisis: A systematic review of the literature. *Frontiers in Psychology*, *11*, 589744. doi:10.3389/fpsyg.2020.589744 PMID:33414746

Heesakkers, H., Zegers, M., van Mol, M. M. C., & van den Boogaard, M. (2021). The impact of the first COVID-19 surge on the mental well-being of ICU nurses: A nationwide survey study. *Intensive & Critical Care Nursing*, *65*, 103034. doi:10.1016/j.iccn.2021.103034 PMID:33863609

Hershler, A., Hughes, L., Nguyen, P., & Wall, S. (Eds.). (2021). *Looking at trauma: A toolkit for clinicians*. The Pennsylvania University Press. doi:10.1515/9780271092287

Hinshaw, S. P. (2010). *The mark of shame: Stigma of mental illness and an agenda for change*. Oxford University Press.

Hong, Z., Li, N., Li, D., Li, J., Li, B., Xiong, W., Lu, L., Li, W., & Zhou, D. (2020). Telemedicine during the COVID-19 pandemic: Experiences from western China. *Journal of Medical Internet Research, 22*(5), e19577. doi:10.2196/19577 PMID:32349962

Jaggers, A. (2020, March 12). *COVID-19 Comics*. Graphic Medicine International Collective. https://www.graphicmedicine.org/covid-19-comics/

Johnson, J. (2010). The skeleton on the couch: The eagleton affair, rhetorical disability, and the stigma of mental illness. *Rhetoric Society Quarterly, 40*(5), 459–478. doi:10.1080/02773945.2010.517234

Kelly, L. A., Gee, P. M., & Butler, R. J. (2021). Impact of nurse burnout on organizational and position turnover. *Nursing Outlook, 69*(1), 96–102. doi:10.1016/j.outlook.2020.06.008 PMID:33023759

Khajuria, A., Tomaszewski, W., Liu, Z., Chen, J., Mehdian, R., Fleming, S., Vig, S., & Crawford, M. J. (2021). Workplace factors associated with mental health of healthcare workers during the COVID-19 pandemic: An international cross-sectional study. *BMC Health Services Research, 21*(1), 262. doi:10.118612913-021-06279-6 PMID:33743674

Knaak, S., Mantler, E., & Szeto, A. (2017). Mental illness-related stigma in healthcare: Barriers to access and care and evidence-based solutions. *Healthcare Management Forum, 30*(2), 111–116. doi:10.1177/0840470416679413 PMID:28929889

Kuttner, P. J., Weaver-Hightower, M. B., & Sousanis, N. (2021). Comics-based research: The affordances of comics for research across disciplines. *Qualitative Research, 21*(2), 195–214. doi:10.1177/1468794120918845

Lefèvre, H., Stheneur, C., Cardin, C., Fourcade, L., Fourmaux, C., Tordjman, E., Touati, M., Voisard, F., Minassian, S., Chaste, P., Moro, M. R., & Lachal, J. (2021). The Bulle: Support and prevention of psychological decompensation of health care workers during the trauma of the COVID-19 epidemic. *Journal of Pain and Symptom Management, 61*(2), 416–422. doi:10.1016/j.jpainsymman.2020.09.023 PMID:32961219

Litz, B. T., Stein, N., Delaney, E., Lebowitz, L., Nash, W. P., Silva, C., & Maguen, S. (2009). Moral injury and moral repair in war veterans: A preliminary model and intervention strategy. *Clinical Psychology Review, 29*(8), 695–706. doi:10.1016/j.cpr.2009.07.003 PMID:19683376

Logie, C. H. (2020). Lessons learned from HIV can inform our approach to COVID-19 stigma. *Journal of the International AIDS Society, 23*(5), e25504. doi:10.1002/jia2.25504 PMID:32365283

LoGiudice, J. A., & Bartos, S. (2021). Experiences of nurses during the COVID-19 pandemic: A mixed-methods study. *AACN Advanced Critical Care, 32*(1), 14–26. doi:10.4037/aacnacc2021816 PMID:33450763

Maben, J., & Bridges, J. (2020). Covid-19: Supporting nurses' psychological and mental health. *Journal of Clinical Nursing, 29*(15–16), 2742–2750. doi:10.1111/jocn.15307 PMID:32320509

Marvaldi, M., Mallet, J., Dubertret, C., Moro, M. R., & Guessoum, S. B. (2021). Anxiety, depression, trauma-related, and sleep disorders among healthcare workers during the COVID-19 pandemic: A systematic review and meta-analysis. *Neuroscience and Biobehavioral Reviews, 126*, 252–264. doi:10.1016/j.neubiorev.2021.03.024 PMID:33774085

McClendon, S. (2020, September 1). *New survey findings from 21K US nurses: PPE shortages persist, re-use practices on the rise amid COVID-19 pandemic.* American Nurses Association. https://www.nursingworld.org/news/news-releases/2020/new-survey-findings-from-21k-us-nurses--ppe-shortages-persist-re-use-practices-on-the-rise-amid-covid-19-pandemic/

McNicol, S., & Leamy, C. (2020). Co-creating a graphic illness narrative with people with dementia. *Journal of Applied Arts & Health, 11*(3), 267–280. doi:10.1386/jaah_00040_1

Mental Health America. (2021). *The mental health of healthcare workers in COVID-19.* https://mhanational.org/mental-health-healthcare-workers-covid-19

Molloy, C. (2019). *Rhetorical ethos in health and medicine: Patient credibility, stigma, and misdiagnosis.* Routledge. doi:10.4324/9780429291074

Muller, A. E., Hafstad, E. V., Himmels, J. P. W., Smedslund, G., Flottorp, S., Stensland, S. Ø., Stroobants, S., Van de Velde, S., & Vist, G. E. (2020). The mental health impact of the covid-19 pandemic on healthcare workers, and interventions to help them: A rapid systematic review. *Psychiatry Research, 293*, 113441. doi:10.1016/j.psychres.2020.113441 PMID:32898840

Mulvale, G., Wilson, F., Jones, S., Green, J., Johansen, K.-J., Arnold, I., & Kates, N. (2019). Integrating mental health peer support in clinical settings: Lessons from Canada and Norway. *Healthcare Management Forum, 32*(2), 68–72. doi:10.1177/0840470418812495 PMID:30744437

Noe, M. (2021, May 11). *Calling all frontline workers and comic artists!* Graphic Medicine International Collective. https://www.graphicmedicine.org/calling-all-frontline-workers-and-comics-artists/

Noe, M., & Levin, L. (2020). *Mapping the use of comics in health education: A scoping review of the graphic medicine literature*. Graphic Medicine.

Nyblade, L., Stockton, M. A., Giger, K., Bond, V., Ekstrand, M. L., Lean, R. M., Mitchell, E. M. H., Nelson, L. R. E., Sapag, J. C., Siraprapasiri, T., Turan, J., & Wouters, E. (2019). Stigma in health facilities: Why it matters and how we can change it. *BMC Medicine, 17*(1), 25. doi:10.118612916-019-1256-2 PMID:30764806

Obuobi, S., Vela, M. B., & Callender, B. (2021). Comics as anti-racist education and advocacy. *Lancet, 397*(10285), 1615–1617. doi:10.1016/S0140-6736(21)00940-5 PMID:33933198

Owens, I. T. (2020). Supporting nurses' mental health during the pandemic. *Nursing, 50*(10). https://journals.lww.com/nursing/Fulltext/2020/10000/Supporting_nurses__mental_health_during_the.13aspx

Palmer, E. (2020, May 11). Voices from the pandemic's front lines. *New York Times*. https://www.nytimes.com/2020/05/11/reader-center/coronavirus-healthcare-workers.html

Providence Health Care. (2021, May 12). Nurses express hope, anxiety around COVID-19 in new study. *The Daily Scan.* https://thedailyscan.providencehealthcare.org/2021/05/nurses-express-hope-anxiety-around-covid-19-in-new-study/

Rattner, N., & Towey, R. (2021, September 22). Average daily U.S. Covid deaths climb above 2,000 for the first time since March. *CNBC.* https://www.cnbc.com/2021/09/22/average-daily-us-covid-deaths-cross-2000.html

Rolling, J., Mengin, A. C., Palacio, C., Mastelli, D., Fath, M., Gras, A., Von Hunolstein, J.-J., Schröder, C. M., & Vidailhet, P. (2021). COVID-19: Mental health prevention and care for healthcare professionals. *Frontiers in Psychiatry*, *12*, 566740. doi:10.3389/fpsyt.2021.566740 PMID:33833696

Ryan, S. (2020). *The vitals: True nurse stories.* Marvel Comics. https://www.marvel.com/comics/issue/93069/the_vitals_true_nurse_stories_2020

Sacks, E., Talajic, D., & Kim, B. (2020). *Covid chronicles.* NBC News and Upshot Studios. https://www.nbcnews.com/think/opinion/covid-chronicles-series

Saji, S., Venkatesan, S., & Callender, B. (2021). Comics in the time of a pan(dem)ic: COVID- 19, graphic medicine, and metaphors. *Perspectives in Biology and Medicine*, *64*(1), 136–154. doi:10.1353/pbm.2021.0010 PMID:33746135

Schubert, M., Ludwig, J., Freiberg, A., Hahne, T. M., Romero Starke, K., Girbig, M., Faller, G., Apfelbacher, C., von dem Knesebeck, O., & Seidler, A. (2021). Stigmatization from work-related COVID-19 exposure: A systematic review with meta-analysis. *International Journal of Environmental Research and Public Health*, *18*(12), 6183. doi:10.3390/ijerph18126183 PMID:34201024

Schulte, E. E., Bernstein, C. A., & Cabana, M. D. (2020). Addressing faculty emotional responses during the coronavirus 2019 pandemic. *The Journal of Pediatrics*, *222*, 13–14. doi:10.1016/j.jpeds.2020.04.057 PMID:32387715

Shamia, N. A., Thabet, A. A. M., & Vostanis, P. (2015). Exposure to war traumatic experiences, post-traumatic stress disorder and post-traumatic growth among nurses in Gaza: War impact on nurses in Gaza. *Journal of Psychiatric and Mental Health Nursing*, *22*(10), 749–755. doi:10.1111/jpm.12264 PMID:26283005

Shapiro, G. K., Schulz-Quach, C., Matthew, A., Mosher, P., Rodin, G., de Vries, F., Hales, S., Korenblum, C., Black, S., Beck, L., Miller, K., Morita, J., Li, M., & Elliot, M. (2021, March 12). An institutional model for health care workers' mental health during COVID- 19. *NEJM Catalyst.* https://catalyst.nejm.org/doi/full/10.1056/CAT.20.0684

Sockalingam, S., Clarkin, C., Serhal, E., Pereira, C., & Crawford, A. (2020). Responding to health care professionals' mental health needs during COVID-19 through the rapid implementation of Project ECHO. *The Journal of Continuing Education in the Health Professions*, *40*(3), 211–214. doi:10.1097/CEH.0000000000000311 PMID:32658015

Stangl, A. L., Earnshaw, V. A., Logie, C. H., van Brakel, W. C., Simbayi, L., Barré, I., & Dovidio, J. F. (2019). The Health Stigma and Discrimination Framework: A global, crosscutting framework to inform research, intervention development, and policy on health-related stigmas. *BMC Medicine*, *17*(1), 31. doi:10.118612916-019-1271-3 PMID:30764826

Stockton, A., & King, L. (2021, February 24). Death, through a nurse's eyes. *New York Times*. https://www.nytimes.com/video/opinion/100000007578176/covid-icu-nurses-arizona.html

Stokes-Parish, J., Elliott, R., Rolls, K., & Massey, D. (2020). Angels and heroes: The unintended consequence of the hero narrative. *Journal of Nursing Scholarship*, *52*(5), 462–466. doi:10.1111/jnu.12591 PMID:32856396

Stower, H., & Guennot, M. (2021, March 15). Art in a pandemic: A digital gallery. *Nature Medicine*. https://www.nature.com/articles/d41591-021-00009-5

Sun, L., Gao, Y., Yang, J., Zang, X.-Y., & Wang, Y.-G. (2016). The impact of professional identity on role stress in nursing students: A cross-sectional study. *International Journal of Nursing Studies*, *63*, 1–8. doi:10.1016/j.ijnurstu.2016.08.010 PMID:27565423

Sutherland, T., Choi, D., & Yu, C. (2021). "Brought to life through imagery" – animated graphic novels to promote empathic, patient-centred care in postgraduate medical learners. *BMC Medical Education*, *21*(1), 66. doi:10.118612909-021-02491-4 PMID:33478483

ten Hoeve, Y., Jansen, G., & Roodbol, P. (2014). The nursing profession: Public image, self- concept and professional identity. A discussion paper. *Journal of Advanced Nursing*, *70*(2), 295–309. doi:10.1111/jan.12177 PMID:23711235

Teti, M., Epping, S., Myroniuk, T. W., & Evans-Agnew, R. (2021). HIV stigma and its metaphors: Photos, symbols, and solutions. *Journal of HIV/AIDS & Social Services*, *20*(1), 97–114. doi:10.1080/15381501.2021.1911903

Traynor, M. (2018). Guest editorial: What's wrong with resilience. *Journal of Research in Nursing*, *23*(1), 5–8. doi:10.1177/1744987117751458 PMID:34394401

Tsao, P., & Yu, C. H. (2016). "There's no billing code for empathy" - Animated comics remind medical students of empathy: A qualitative study. *BMC Medical Education*, *16*(1), 204. doi:10.118612909-016-0724-z PMID:27520824

Turan, B., Hatcher, A. M., Weiser, S. D., Johnson, M. O., Rice, W. S., & Turan, J. M. (2017). Framing Mechanisms Linking HIV-Related Stigma, Adherence to Treatment, and Health Outcomes. *American Journal of Public Health*, *107*(6), 863–869. doi:10.2105/AJPH.2017.303744 PMID:28426316

University of Colorado Anschutz Medical Campus. (2020, May 18). *Tell your story with COVID-19 narratives*. https://medschool.cuanschutz.edu/physical-medicine-and-rehabilitation/newsdetail/news-and-media-2020/tell-your-story-with-covid-19-narratives

Vagni, M., Maiorano, T., Giostra, V., & Pajardi, D. (2020). Hardiness, stress and secondary trauma in italian healthcare and emergency workers during the COVID-19 pandemic. *Sustainability*, *12*(14), 5592. doi:10.3390u12145592

Waterman, S., Hunter, E. C. M., Cole, C. L., Evans, L. J., Greenberg, N., Rubin, G. J., & Beck, A. (2018). Training peers to treat Ebola centre workers with anxiety and depression in Sierra Leone. *The International Journal of Social Psychiatry*, *64*(2), 156–165. doi:10.1177/0020764017752021 PMID:29432085

Weaver-Hightower, M. (2013). Sequential art for qualitative research: Making comics to make meaning of the social world. In C. Syma & R. Weiner (Eds.), *Graphic novels, comics, and education* (pp. 260–273). McFarland.

Williams, I. (2007). *What is "graphic medicine"?* Graphic Medicine International Collective. https://www.graphicmedicine.org/why-graphic-medicine/

Williams, I. (2011). Autography as auto-therapy: Psychic pain and the graphic memoir. *The Journal of Medical Humanities*, *32*(4), 353–366. doi:10.100710912-011-9158-0 PMID:21898054

Williams, I. C. (2012). Graphic medicine: Comics as medical narrative. *Medical Humanities*, *38*(1), 21–27. doi:10.1136/medhum-2011-010093 PMID:22282425

Williamson, V., Murphy, D., Phelps, A., Forbes, D., & Greenberg, N. (2021). Moral injury: The effect on mental health and implications for treatment. *The Lancet. Psychiatry*, *8*(6), 453–455. doi:10.1016/S2215-0366(21)00113-9 PMID:33743196

Williamson, V., Stevelink, S. A. M., & Greenberg, N. (2018). Occupational moral injury and mental health: Systematic review and meta-analysis. *The British Journal of Psychiatry*, *212*(6), 339–346. doi:10.1192/bjp.2018.55 PMID:29786495

Yong, E. (2020, November 13). No one is listening to us. *The Atlantic*. https://www.theatlantic.com/health/archive/2020/11/third-surge-breaking-healthcare-workers/617091/

Yu, M. (2018). Roles of graphic pathographies in clinical training. *AMA Journal of Ethics*, *20*(2), 115–121. doi:10.1001/journalofethics.2018.20.2.peer1-1802 PMID:29460763

Zaçe, D., Hoxhaj, I., Orfino, A., Viteritti, A. M., Janiri, L., & Di Pietro, M. L. (2021). Interventions to address mental health issues in healthcare workers during infectious disease outbreaks: A systematic review. *Journal of Psychiatric Research*, *136*, 319–333. doi:10.1016/j.jpsychires.2021.02.019 PMID:33636688

ADDITIONAL READING

Czerwiec, M. K., Williams, I., Squier, S. M., Green, M. J., Myers, K. R., & Smith, S. T. (2015). *Graphic medicine manifesto*. The Pennsylvania State University Press.

Jaggers, A., & Noe, M. (2018). *Essential graphic medicine: An annotated bibliography*. https://www.graphicmedicine.org/essentialgm/

McCloud, S. (1994). *Understanding comics: The invisible art*. William Morrow.

ENDNOTE

1 Much the same as his real-time work on *Mom's Cancer*, Fies drew his frantic experiences with the California wildfires on hotel stationary with whatever pens and markers he had packed before leaving. Those initial sketches documented not only the author's own traumatic experience, but also the larger experience of so many others who were—at that very moment—worried about their home or discovering that their homes were gone entirely. The sketches gained national attention on CNN and were later re-drawn as part of *A Fire Story* (2019), which told the more complete saga of the destructive wildfires and hellish aftermath for those who lost their homes.

Chapter 13
Mindfulness-Based Approaches to Reduce Injuries Among Nurses and Nursing Aides

William H. OBrien
https://orcid.org/0000-0001-6620-1401
Bowling Green State University, USA

Jennifer Chavanovanich
Chulalongkorn University, Thailand

Somboon Jarukasemthawee
Chulalongkorn University, Thailand

Kullaya Pisitsungkagarn
Chulalongkorn University, Thailand

Maria A. Kalantzis
Bowling Green State University, USA

ABSTRACT

Physical and psychological injuries occur at a high rate among nurses and nursing assistants (NNAs). The humanitarian and economic costs associated with injuries to these vulnerable workers is a global health concern. The characteristics and organization of work are major determinants of injuries. Individual differences are also important determinants with mindfulness skills being particularly relevant for injury prevention. There is a developing and promising literature examining mindfulness-based behavior therapy (MBBTs) for NNA psychological and physical injuries. Most research has been limited to Western countries and Western NNAs using MBBT interventions that use concepts and techniques from Eastern philosophy, religion, and cultures. The borrowing of these concepts and techniques was haphazard and incomplete which may limit their effectiveness. There is a pressing need to develop and evaluate MBBTs for NNAs that more thoughtfully and carefully integrate Eastern concepts and techniques. Interventions that better integrate East-West concepts and techniques are acceptable, feasible, and effective.

DOI: 10.4018/978-1-7998-8813-0.ch013

INTRODUCTION

Epidemiology of Nursing and Nursing Aide Injuries

Nurses and nursing aides (NNAs) working in healthcare settings are a vulnerable population of workers who experience some of the highest rates of work-related injuries relative to any other occupation. These work-related injuries and illnesses can be physical such as musculoskeletal pain and suffering as well as psychological such as emotional pain and suffering. Addressing work-related injuries among NNAs is an important health, social, economic, and humanitarian concern.

Surveillance data from the Bureau of Labor Statistics shed light on the impact of injury in the healthcare industry. NNAs experience high rates of physical injuries compared to other occupations. Approximately 249 out of 10,000 nursing aids report experiencing a significant musculoskeletal symptom due to work and approximately 104 nursing aides per 10,000 report missing one or more days of work due to a work-related injury (BLS, 2010, 2018). A national survey of NNAs working in long-term care found that 58% experienced a serious work-related physical injury in the prior year, with an average of 4.5 injuries per person per year (Khatutsky, et al., 2012).

Our survey of 229 NNAs working in long-term healthcare settings in Ohio and found that 66% reported one or more work-related physical injuries in the month prior to the survey (O'Brien et al., 2019a). The average number of work-related physical injuries per month was 5.44 ($sd = 12.08$) and 9% of the study participants reported missing one or more days of work in the prior month due to injury. These data are consistent with reports from Stanev and colleagues (2012) who found that the median rate of physical injury among Ohio NNAs was 5.7 serious incidents per 100 workers which was 200% higher than the combined incidence of work-related injuries among workers in other occupations.

In addition to physical injuries, NNAs also report high levels of psychological injuries which include stress, burnout, trauma, post-traumatic stress symptoms, and other work-related mental health problems (O'Brien et al., 2019a; Schuster & Dwyer, 2020; Woo et al., 2020). Data from Ohio NNAs indicated that these workers reported high levels of work-burnout, work-withdrawal, and a lower quality of life (O'Brien et al., 2019a). The psychological injuries experienced by NNAs is not confined to the USA. Woo et al. (2020) conducted a systematic review and meta-analysis focused on studies reporting the global prevalence of burnout symptoms among NNAs. They located 113 studies for the systematic review and 61 studies that could be coded for the meta-analysis. Woo et al. (2020) reported that across the 49 countries included in their meta-analysis, 11.23% of NNAs reported experiencing high levels of burnout symptoms. Heterogeneity was observed across global regions with the highest levels of burnout being reported in Southeast Asia and the Pacific Islands (13.68%) and the lowest levels of burnout being reported in Europe and Central Asia (10.06%). North America and Latin American/Caribbean countries fell between the two extremes (10.27% and 10.51% respectively). These high levels of burnout were associated with other adverse outcomes such as sleep disruption, depressive symptoms, job withdrawal, absenteeism, and intent to leave.

Work-stress and burnout are more than adverse work-related psychological injuries. Work stress and burnout are also significant risk factors for additional work-related physical and psychological injuries (Ahola et al., 2013). Furthermore, higher levels of psychological distress have been associated with an increased risk of exposure to aggression from patients. Indeed, NNAs are exposed to violent events at rates that are 300% higher than any other occupation (BLS, 2018). The cost of NNA injuries is most frequently measured in lost workdays, which average to about 5 days per work injury (BLS, 2010, 2018).

Lost workdays can then amplify the already problematic staffing shortages. Beyond lost workdays, NNA injuries can result in corporate insurance coverage increases, regulatory fines, settlement costs, legal fees, and additional intangible costs such as diminished employee morale, compassion fatigue, and less empathic patient care (Teleghani, et al., 2017). Finally, NNAs with work-related injuries are more prone to experience voluntary and involuntary job loss (Okechukwu et al., 2016), make medical errors, injure patients, and receive lower ratings of patient satisfaction (Jun et al., 2021).

Determinants of NNA Injury

Table 1 provides a summary of injury types and their determinants. NNA injuries partially occur as a function of the physically demanding workload, low staffing levels, irregular hours, long shifts, rotating shifts, limited access to assistive devices, limited access to personal protective equipment, a nonsupportive organizational climate, limited training, and exposure to pathogens (e.g., Chang et al., 2013; Woo et al., 2020). NNAs also experience work-related injuries as a function of the complex intersections among gender, social class, and ethno-racial minority status. Using Crenshaw's (1989) framework on intersectionality, NNA work settings are characterized by hiring practices, work assignments, and working conditions that expose the workers (who tend to be female, from lower SES backgrounds, and members of ethno-racial minorities; Morgan, et al., 2013) to particularly high levels of work-stress and worksite risk exposures. These work-related stressors can interact with non-work family, financial, and social stressors resulting in intensified psychological and physiological effects (McGinn & Eunsil, 2017).

Beyond the external contextual factors described above, there are important internal contextual factors that are associated with NNA work-related injuries (Dekker, 2002; Richardson et al., 2019). NNAs who have been injured often report familiarity with the recommended, taught, and "correct" caregiving procedures, lifting/transferring procedures, and organizational policies articulating how to address problems at work (Burton et al., 2016; Khatutsky et al, 2012; Schoenfisch, 2009). Yet, NNAs report that they often feel unable to adhere to these procedures because of myriad internal contextual factors such as feeling overwhelmed, hurried, reluctant to assert a need for assistance, and burned out (O'Brien, et al., 2019b; Richardson et al., 2019). As an illustration, focus groups conducted with NNAs by O'Brien et al. (2019b) reported themes that can be summarized as follows: (a) NNAs receive education and training that focuses on how to carry out various caregiving procedures for an individual patient but (b) there is virtually no training on how to manage patient care under typical high stress work conditions where there are multiple patients simultaneously requiring assistance nor (c) how to develop and maintain effective teamwork with other NNAs which is essential for managing the workload. Richardson and colleagues (2019) also conducted a thematic analysis of focus group interviews with nursing and physiotherapist experts. They abstracted categories of causal factors related to musculoskeletal injury. They found that attitudes, beliefs, contextual factors (e.g., demands from other staff, hierarchies, ward culture) were barriers to NNA implementation of injury prevention skills that they learned in training. These types of findings have led to calls for the development and testing of interventions that are focused on acquiring stress management skills as a means for reducing work-related injury among NNAs (Bernal et al, 2015; Bos, et al., 2006; Chang et al., 2013). Mindfulness approaches have been shown to be effective for managing stress across diverse populations and problem areas.

Evidence of the potential of mindfulness interventions for NNA injury was observed in a study of the 152 Ohio NNAs (O'Brien, et al., 2019a). All of the NNAs in the study had completed state mandated training that consisted of at least 52 classroom hours of focused on safety, patient care, basic nursing, and

Table 1. NNA injuries and determinants/predictors of injuries

Types of Injuries		Determinants and Predictors	Examples of Research
Physical	Overall	Individual characteristics (e.g. tenure, sex, ethnicity, race), health conditions and stress, work scheduling characteristics (e.g. night shift, overtime), job roles, workload, job characteristics, bullying, psychological hardiness, work environments (e.g. availability of resources and lifts), organizational climate, mindfulness.	D' Archy et al. (2011), De Castro et al. (2010); Hemingway & Smith (1999), Teo et al. (2021), Vecchio et al. (2011)
	Needle-stick injury	Age, department, gender, number of shifts, working hours, mental workload	Hosseinabadi et al. (2019), Ilhan et al. (2006), Xujun et al. (2015)
	Slips, trips and falls	Gender, age, job position, shift work, mental workload	Hosseinabadi et al. (2019)
Psychological	Overall mental health	Individual characteristics (living with spouse, gender, personal health), work-family conflict, sleeping problems, night shifts	McElroy et al. (2020), Perry et al. (2015)
	Stress	Tenure, workplace bullying and violence, mindfulness	Teo et al. (2021)
	Burnout	Age, individual coping strategy, conflicts with colleagues, death and dying of patients, mindfulness	Payne (2001), Zhang et al. (2020)
	PTSDs and trauma	Ineffective coping strategy and inadequate support after experiencing a disaster or traumatic event	Foli et al. (2021)

restorative care. The state mandated training provided no instruction on stress management, burnout, or coping. The NNAs reported the number of injuries experienced at work in the prior month. They also completed measures of safety and environmental resources (e.g., equipment availability, room space), safety climate, training in occupational safety and health, patient care training (e.g., bathing, communication, documentation), unit characteristics (e.g., staffing levels, type of unit), and demographic characteristics. Finally, they completed measures of psychological distress, coping, and mindfulness.

The results of the survey indicated that among the many potential external and internal contextual predictors, mindfulness accounted for a significant and unique proportion of variance in the frequency of reported injuries. Mindfulness was also the most consistent and significant correlate of the most common injury causes (e.g., slips, trips, patient aggression). Specifically, higher levels of mindfulness were associated with lower levels of reported injuries and lower exposure to the main causes of injury causes.

Mindfulness and the Work: Injury Relationship

The ways that mindfulness can be associated with work-related injury is illustrated in Figure 1 which is a cognitive-behavioral functional analytic model (O'Brien, et al., 2019b; O'Brien & Carhart, 2011). Based on the model, a patient's caregiving need may trigger a negative cognitive appraisal by a NNA (e.g., "I am overwhelmed, I don't have time, I can't take this."). Based on contemporary learning theory frameworks (Hayes & Hofman, 2017; Zettle, et al., 2016), when the NNA is cognitively "fused" with these appraisals (meaning that the appraisal is accepted uncritically and believed it to be literally true),

Figure 1. A functional analytic casual model of stress and risk for injury, assault, and abuse

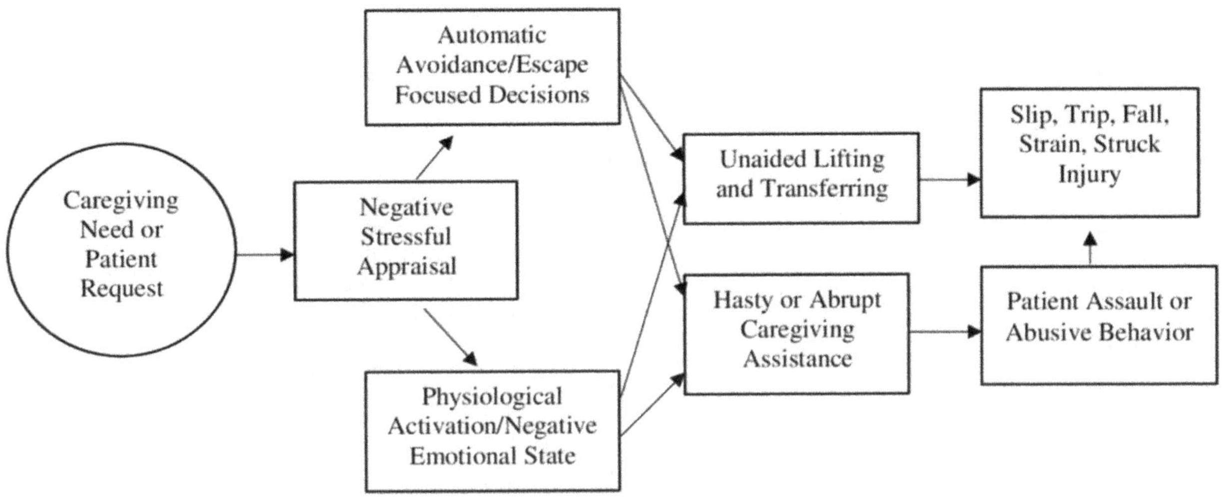

they will experience the patient's request as a threat to well-being. This perception of threat will then prompt psychophysiological activation patterns associated with defensive reactivity (e.g., sympathetic activation, vagal withdrawal), negative emotional states, cognitive interference, poorer problem solving, and less elaborative decision making (Petrocchi & Cheli, 2019). These cognitive and psychophysiological reactions can then lead to behavioral responses that are designed to avoid or escape from the stressor (interaction with the patient). These avoidance and escape responses can take the form of rushing through a medical procedure, not engaging in effective precautions, non-responding to a call light, unaided patient lifting or transfers, waiting for another staff member to provide care, and/or abrupt communications with the patient. These avoidance and escape responses are negatively reinforced (via reduction in negative affect and psychophysiological states) and can increase risk for work-related injuries as well as interpersonal conflict with the patient who may react to NNA behavior.

Based on the model, NNA work-related injuries can be reduced via mindfulness which can promote more effective management of the moment-to-moment experiences of stressful appraisals, physiological activation, automatic decision making, and avoidance behaviors. The functional analytic model in Figure 2 identifies logical and important cognitive, physiological, and behavioral intervention points for Mindfulness-Based Behavioral Therapy (MBBT. Note: There are many variations of mindfulness-based behavioral therapies that have been developed in the past two decades such as Mindfulness-Based Stress Reduction, Dialectical Behavior Therapy, Acceptance and Commitment Therapy, Functional Analytic Psychotherapy. We use the term MBBT as an umbrella term for the programs that include mindfulness as a central component of treatment). The acceptance, nonreactivity, and present-moment focus elements of MBBT target problematic cognitive appraisals. The breathing and meditation components of MBBT also target stressful appraisals as well as physiological activation. Finally, training in mindfulness-based skills related to communication and patient care targets problematic caregiving behaviors.

Figure 2. Mindfulness-based behavior therapy intervention points for NNAs

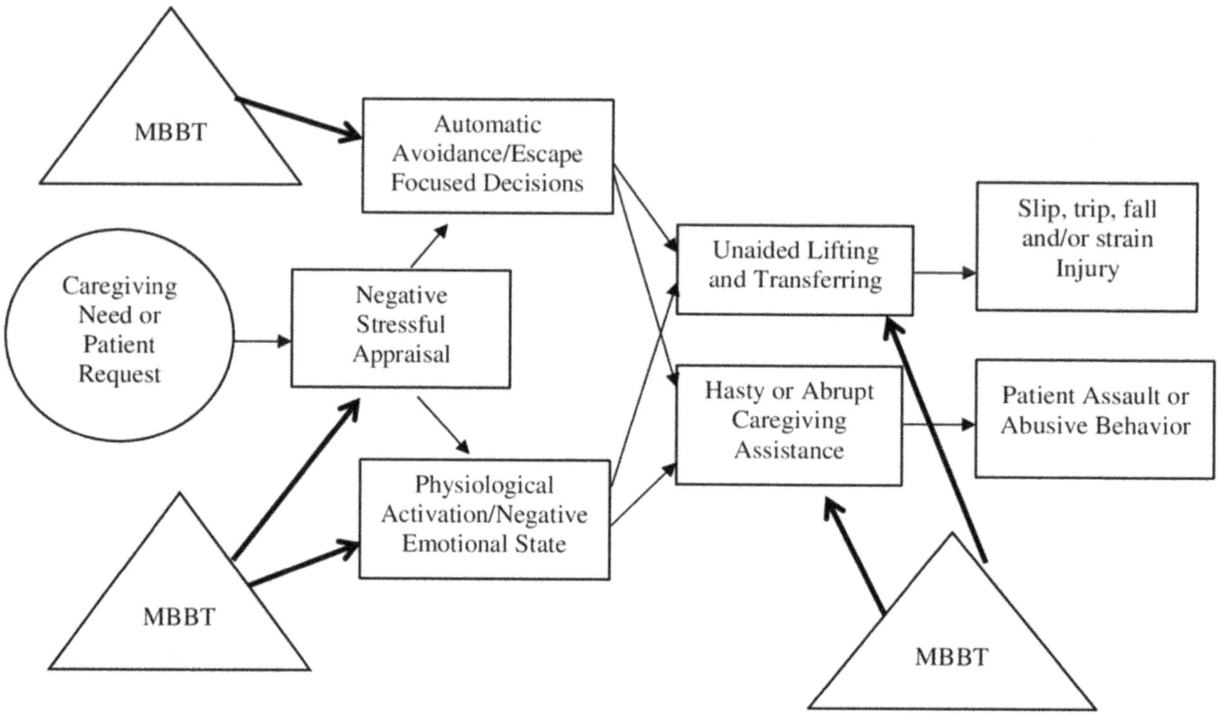

Mindfulness-Based Interventions: Characteristics and Effectiveness

There is a limited and developing literature investigating the effectiveness of MBBT interventions for NNAs in healthcare settings. Klein and colleagues (2019) conducted a systematic review of mindfulness-based interventions for burnout among healthcare providers (not specifically NNAs). A total of 34 studies were located. Nine of the studies provided interventions for 9 medical doctors exclusively, 7 for nurses exclusively, and 18 for general healthcare workers. The interventions varied in terms of length, number of sessions, duration of sessions, and session content. Overall, 68% of the articles reported participant improvement. However, this overall effect averaged across pre-post studies with no control group and RCTs. An examination of the RCTs alone (k = 9 studies) indicated that 4 reported significant treatment effects and 5 reported nonsignificant treatment effects. Klein et al., (2019) concluded that the methodological quality of the literature was limited by: Low power, few RCTs, no systematic examination of variation of treatment effects among subgroups (e.g., ethnicity, race, settings, professions), inadequate training (or unspecified training) of the therapists, a lack of transcultural validity.

The Klein et al. (2019) conclusions are consistent those offered by Ghawadra et al. (2019) who evaluated intervention studies using MBSR for RNs only. They located 9 treatment outcome studies. All of the studies measured psychological distress with results showing generally favorable outcomes with short follow-up periods. Using the Quality Assessment Tool for Quantitative Studies, the authors rated each study on selection bias, design, confounding variables, blinding, data collection, dropout rates, treatment integrity, and analysis. Results indicated that the methodology ratings classified most studies as weak due to selection bias, nonblinding, and the presence of confounds. Additionally, the typical study was underpowered due to a small sample size.

Halm (2017) conducted a systematic review of mindfulness-related interventions for nurses. In their study 11 articles were identified. Similar to Ghawadra, Halm found that the interventions generally provided benefit for participants on measures of stress, anxiety, depression, and burnout. Halm suggested that the reviewed studies had relatively good methodological features with inadequate sample sizes.

For this chapter we conducted an exhaustive literature search and in order to gather more contemporary information on the characteristics and effectiveness of MBBTs for NNAs. We searched Medline, Pubmed, and PsycInfo for articles that had combinations of the terms "nursing aid", "nurse", "certified nursing assistant", "nursing", "stress", "injury", "workplace violence", "health", "burnout", "acceptance and commitment therapy", "ACT", "mindfulness" in the title or abstract. Studies that met the following criteria were included for review: Quantitative data were reported; a MBBT intervention was provided); pre and post data were reported; a validated measurement of stress, burnout, or related psychological outcome was used; and participants were nurses or nursing aides.

Table 2 provides a summary of the 26 studies that were located and reviewed. Most articles reported on participants working in the USA or Western countries with two studies based in Asia and one in the Middle East. The sample sizes ranged from 13 to 91with nearly all studies (n = 22) being underpowered given a reasonable expectation of a moderate effect size (d = .60). Necessary demographic data were rarely reported and analyses of intervention responses among subgroups of participants were not presented. A median of 6 sessions were offered with 7 and 8 sessions being the most common. MBSR or a MBSR variant was the most common approach (k = 15, 60%). The interventions were primarily cognitively focused (mindfulness) and with some physiologically focused components (e.g., breathing). Importantly, only two studies had intervention components focused on developing NNA work-related skills (e.g., communication, patient care, managing interpersonal conflict). The most common outcomes were burnout, anxiety, depression, and stress. Injury and physical symptoms were measured in only one study (described below). A RCT design was used in 13 studies. Of the 13 RCTs, 10 reported significant reductions in psychological distress and 3 reported nonsignificant outcomes.

O'Brien and colleagues (2019a, 2019b) conducted a series of studies to explore the role of mindfulness in injuries and the effectiveness of a MBBT (ACT, Acceptance and Commitment Therapy) for injury reduction among NNAs in long-term care residential settings. The goal of the three-step project was to accurately measure, predict, and reduce work-related injury, stress, and burnout among NNAs using mindfulness measures. In step 1 focus groups were conducted and coded to develop a measurement tool that would capture important mindfulness, organizational, and individual predictors of NNA physical and psychological injuries. Focus group data were also used to design a NNA specific ACT intervention. In step 2, the newly developed measure called the Risk for Nursing Assault and Injury Inventory (RNAII) was evaluated for psychometric characteristics. It was also used to evaluate the extent to which various mindfulness-related constructs predicted injuries across a six-month interval. The constructs and items in the RNAII are provided in Tables 3 and 4.

As described earlier in this chapter, the results of the prediction study indicated that mindfulness was a significant predictor of injury. These results supported the hypothesis that an ACT intervention could yield significant effects on NNA injuries. In step 3, an NNA protocol based on ACT was developed and evaluated using a RCT (O'Brien et al., 2019b). ACT was selected because it is an empirically supported MBBT that has demonstrated effectiveness in over 500 treatment outcome studies (Gloster et al., 2020). The NNA ACT protocol consisted of two 2.5-hour sessions spaced one week apart. The first session focused on acceptance and mindfulness. The second session focused on identification and clarification

Table 2. Mindfulness Based Behavior Therapy for NNAs

Author (year)	Nationality	Sample Size (E/C), Job Position(s)	Racial/Ethnic Breakdown (sample)	Participants	# Sessions	Design of Intervention	Intervention period/week	Content of Sessions	Outcome Variable(s)	Results
Alsareireh et al. (2017)	Jordan*	91/90, Nurses	N/A	62% Female, Mean Age=22 Years	10	RCT	1 hour/3 days per week	Mindfulness breathing, body scan, and walking	Depression (CESD-R)	Both control and treatment groups showed a significant decrease in depression scores. Participants in the mindfulness group showed significantly more declines in their depression score than the control group, t (179) = 5.2; p = .00.
Ando et al. (2011)	Japan*	15/13, Nurses	N/A	Age Inclusion <20	2	RCT	1 session per week	Modified MSBR	Stress (GHQ)	The GHQ scores for the intervention group showed a significantly greater decrease relative to the control group (p<.05).
Bazarko et al. (2013)	USA	36, Nurses	N/A**	100% Female; Mean Age= 52.2 Years	8	Nonrandomized pre–post intervention study	Online	MBSR combined classroom and telephone delivery methods	Burnout, health & wellbeing (CBI)	Participants showed significant (p < .05) improvements in general health and decreases in stress and work burnout
Cohen-Katz et al. (2005)	USA	7/11, Nurses	96% White	100% Female; Mean Age = 46 Years	8	RCT	2 hour/1 day per week	MBSR	Burnout (ProQOL)	Participants reported positive changes in their relationships with spouses, children, and colleagues.
Ceravolo and Raines (2018)	USA	12, Nurse Managers	N/A**	N/A	8	Pre-post quasi experimental design	1 hour (1 day)	MBSR combined with aromatherapy, soft music, a singing bowl, and other enhancements to create a tranquil environment	Burnout (ProQOL)	There were significant (all p < .05) pre-post changes on satisfaction and burnout measures.
Delaney et al. (2018)	Ireland, N/A	13, N/A	N/A**	100% Female	8	Observational Pilot Study	2.5 hours (1 day)	Mindfulness Meditation (MM), Loving Kindness Meditation (LKM), and Compassion Meditation (CM).	Burnout (ProQOL)	The pre-post burnout significantly (p < .05) declined and changes were negatively associated with self-compassion (r = -.62, p = .02) (r = -.55, p = .05) and mindfulness (r = -.54, p = .05). (r = -.60, p = .03), respectively. Resilience and compassion satisfaction scores significantly increased.
Duchemin et al. (2013)	USA	32, SICU Nurses	N/A**	N/A	8	RCT	N/A	MBSR	Burnout (N/A)	Significant decrease in work stress and burnout in both groups (p<.05). Salivary amylase decreased in MBSR group at 8 weeks (p<.05).
Craigie et al. (2016)	West Australia	25, Nurses	N/A**	95.2% Female; Mean age=48.6 years	4	Pre-post quasi experimental design	3 hours (1 day)	MBSR combined with compassion and fatigue prevention educational workshop	Burnout (ProqQoL5), Depression and Anxiety symptoms (DASS), trait-negative anxiety (STAI-Y2)	Significant improvements were observed following the intervention for compassion, satisfaction, burnout, negative anxiety, and stress scores.
Dos Santos et al. (2016)	Brazil*	13, Nurses	N/A**	Mean Age=47.38	6	Pilot study, pre-post quasi experimental design	1 hour (4 days)	MBSR	Perceived stress (PSS), Burnout (MBI), Depression (BDI), Anxiety (STAI), Work Stress (WSS),	Significant reduction (p <.05) between pre-intervention and postintervention scores for perceived stress, burnout, depression, and anxiety.

continued on following page

Table 2. Continued

Author (year)	Nationality	Sample Size (E/C), Job Position(s)	Racial/Ethnic Breakdown (sample)	Participants	# Sessions	Design of Intervention	Intervention period/week	Content of Sessions	Outcome Variable(s)	Results
Duarte and Pinto-Gouveia (2016)	Portugal	29/19, Nurses	N/A**	88.4% Female; Mean Age=38.9 (Experimental Group)	6	RCT	2 hours (1 day)	Mindful breathing and mindful awareness of emotions and thoughts,, mindful communication loving kindness meditation practice.	Burnout (PRoQOL), Depression and Anxiety (DASS)	Nurses in the intervention reported significant decreases in burnout and stress (p<.05).
Hevezi (2016)	N/A	15, Oncology Nurses	N/A**	N/A	4	Observational pilot, pre-post design	10 minutes/5 days per week	Meditation designed to establish a sense of calm, and self-compassion.	Burnout (PROQOL)	Paired t-test expressed a significant decrease in burnout post-intervention (p<.05).
Gauthier et al. (2015)	USA	45, Nurses	Asian: 20%, Native Hawaiian or Pacific Islander: 2.2%, American Indian or Alaska Native: 2.2%**	93% Female	4	Pre-post quasi experimental design	30 minute group sessions/1 day per week, 10 minute CD-guided mindfulness/1 day per week	MBSR	Burnout (MBI)	A repeated measures ANOVA revealed significant decreases in stress from baseline to post intervention and maintained 1 month following the intervention (p<.05).
Foureur et al. (2013)	Australia	45, Nurses and Midwives		100% Female	8	RCT	1 day/week	MSBR	Burnout (GHQ-12), anxiety and depression (DASS)	Significant improvements in burnout, anxiety, and depressive symptomatology were observed in the intervention group (p<.05).
Hee et al. (2014)	Malaysia*	41, Critical Care Nurses	N/A	N/A	5	Pre-post, quasi experimental design	2 hours per week	Mindfulness-based Cognitive Therapy (b-MBCT)	Burnout, Anxiety, Depression (DASS)	Participants reported significant (all p < .05) improvement in the level of perceived stress, anxiety, and depression.
Horner et al. (2014)	USA	43, Child Nursing Staff	N/A**	N/A	10	Pre-post quasi experimental design	30 min/1 day per week	Mindful breathing, developing awareness of thoughts and feelings, and tips on how to be fully present during patient interactions.	Burnout (ProQOL)	Non-significant improvement in levels of mindfulness, burnout and stress for the treatment.
LaRose et al. (2010	USA	105, Nurses	N/A	N/A	4	Observational study	6 hours/across 6 months	Breathing meditation, biofeedback, compassion training	Emotional Exhaustion (N/A)	Emotional exhaustion significantly improved.
Mackenzie et al. (2006)	USA	16/14, Nurses, Nursing Aids	N/A**	94% Female (Experimental) 100% Female (Control)	4	RCT	30 minute (1 day)	Shortened MBSR	Burnout, emotional exhaustion (MBI)	The only significant finding was a preintervention difference where intervention participants were more emotionally exhausted than control participants (p = .01)
Mealer et al. (2014)	USA	13/14, Nurses	100% White	92% Female (Experimental); 86% Female (Control)	12	RCT	2 hour (1 day)	Educational Workshop combined with, day MBSR f	Anxiety and depression (HADS), Trauma sypmtoms (PDS),	A significant decrease in PTSD symptoms were observed for the intervention participants (p<.05).

continued on following page

Table 2. Continued

Author (year)	Nationality	Sample Size (E/C), Job Position(s)	Racial/Ethnic Breakdown (sample)	Participants	# Sessions	Design of Intervention	Intervention period/week	Content of Sessions	Outcome Variable(s)	Results
Montanari et al. (2018)	USA	55, Inpatient Nursing Staff	N/A**	N/A	6	Single arm, pre/ post test design	N/A	N/A	Perceived Stress Scale (PSS), Maslach Burnout Inventory (MBI)	Significant (p < .05) pre-post reductions in in emotional exhaustion and depersonalization were observed. Additionally, personal accomplishment increased from pre to post (p<.05).
O'Brien et al. (2019)	USA	37/34, Nurses, Nursing Aids	69% Caucasian/ White 14% African American 10% Hispanic/ Latino 2% Asian/ Pacific Islander 3% American Indian/ Alaskan Native	84% Female	2	RCT	2.5 hours/1 per week	ACT Intervention	Mental health symptoms (GHQ)	Participants in the treatment group reported a significant reduction in mental health symptoms (p = 0.005). Intervention group participants also reported fewer days missed due to injury than the control group (p < .-05).
Poulin et al. (2008)	Canada	16/10, Nursing Students	N/A**	78% Female; Mean age=26.2	8	RCT	2 hour/1 per biweekly	Brief MSBR	Distress (K-10 distress scale, OAO subscale)	Students in MBWE program experienced significantly less distress following the intervention (p<.05).
Pipe et al. (2009)	USA	15/17, Nurses	N/A**	96% Female; Mean age=50.2	4	RCT	2 hours/1 per week	Mindfulness mediation course	Stress, Distress (PSDI, SC-90-R)	Change scores on several sub-scales of the Symptom Checklist 90-Revised showed significantly more improvement for the treatment group relative to the control group. Treatment participants had significantly more improvement in a Positive Symptom Distress Index relative to the control group (p = 0.01).
Watanabe et al. (2019)	Japan*	40/40, Nurses	N/A**	Mean Age=30.1	52	factorial design RCT with brief mindfulness management program	30 min/1 per week	MBSR and Psychoeducation on Mindfulness	Anxiety and depression (HADS)	No significant treatment related outcome was observed.
Wylde et al. (2017)	USA	49/46, Pediatric, Novice Nurses	52% White, 27% Asian, 13% Latino, 3% Black/ African American*	92% Female	4	QCT	30 min/1 per week	MSBR	Post-traumatic symptoms, burnout (PCL-C)	Found a significant reduction in burnout and post-traumatic symptoms for the intervention group relative to the control group (p<.05)
Shapiro et al. (1998)	USA	18/20, Nursing Students	79% Caucasian, 8% Hispanic, 5% Indian, 3% African, 3% Asia	Age Range=18-65	8	RCT	2 hours/1per biweekly	MBSR	Distress, Stress (BSI, HAD)	Significant between-group differences were observed at post-treatment for Perceived Stress (p= .04). Additionally, the intervention group demonstrated a significant pre-post reduction in perceived stress.
Song & Lundquist	Korea*	21/23, Nurses	N/A	81% Female, Mean Age=19.6 years	8	RCT	2 hours/1per week	MSBR	Depression, anxiety, and stress (DASS-21)	Compared with WL participants, treatment participants reported significantly greater decreases in depression, anxiety and stress, and a greater increase in mindfulness (p<.05).

Table 3. RNAII Predictor Constructs

Construct	Description	Source	Number of Items
Mindfulness	Present-moment awareness.	Mindful Attention and Awareness Scale (Brown & Ryan, 2003)	15
Acceptance	Psychological flexibility, or willingness to experience uncomfortable and unwanted thoughts and feelings.	Acceptance and Action Questionnaire – II (Bond et al., 2011)	7
Resilience	Capacity to recover quickly from difficulties.	Brief Resilience Scale (Smith et al., 2008)	6
Staffing	Perceptions of adequate staffing at their facility	Alberta Context Tool (Estabrooks, et al., 2009)	3
Space	Perceptions of adequate space at facility.	Alberta Context Tool (Estabrooks et al., 2009)	2
Connections	Perceptions of an environment that is conducive to communication about patient care.	Alberta Context Tool (Estabrooks et al., 2009)	6
Training	Perceptions of adequate training in areas such as core job duties, workload management, and coworker interaction.	National Nursing Assistant Survey (Squillace, et al., 2007)	10
Time	Perceptions that the job allows sufficient time to perform tasks that would benefit patient care.	Alberta Context Tool (Estabrooks et al., 2009)	4
Formal Interactions	Frequency of formal meetings related to patient care and educational opportunities outside of their facility.	Alberta Context Tool (Estabrooks et al., 2009)	4
Structural Resources	Frequency of educational opportunities in their facility.	Alberta Context Tool (Estabrooks et al., 2009)	1
Physical Environment	Satisfaction with the quality of the physical work environment.	Adapted from Physical Work Environment Satisfaction Questionnaire (Carlopio, 1996)	6
Physical Work Task Risk	Frequency core job duties that requires performance of physical movements associated with injury.	(Muldoon, et al., (2012)	
Resources	Perception of adequate physical and nonphysical resources to complete job duties.	(Rousseau & Aube, 2010)	
Communication Openness	Perceptions of an environment that promotes communication about issues that may negatively impact patient care.	AHRQ Hospital Survey on Patient Safety Culture (Jones, et al., 2008)	3
Punitive Response to Errors	Perceptions of an environment that punishes mistakes rather than treating them as learning opportunities.	AHRQ Hospital Survey on Patient Safety Culture (Jones et al., 2008)	3
Handoffs and Transitions	Loss of information or accountability across shift or unit changes.	AHRQ Hospital Survey on Patient Safety Culture (Jones et al., 2008)	4
Organizational Constraints	Obstacles that prevent employees from translating effort to performance.	Adapted from NLSS Organizational Constraints Scale (unpublished manuscript)	8
Resident Aggression	Verbal or physical threatening or sexual behavior from a resident.	Adapted from the Workplace Violence Tool (Bostrom et al., 2011)	
Lift Availability, Use, and Training	Availability and typical use of lifting assistive devices and training to use such devices.	National Nursing Assistant Survey (Squillace et al., 2007)	3
Interpersonal Conflict	Disagreements among coworkers.	(Spector & Jex, 1998)	4
Incivility	Subtle behaviors that violate workplace norms for courteous or civil behavior	(Cortina, et al., 2013)	4
Work-Family Conflict	Work demands interfering with family demands.	(Grzywacz, et al., 2006)	3
Family-Work Conflict	Family demands interfering with work demands.	(Grzywacz, et al., 2006)	3
Safety Climate	Perceptions of policies and procedures that promote a safe work environment.	(Neal & Griffin, 2006)	3
Work-pace Safety	Perceptions that the speed of work is conducive to safety.	(Mueller, 1991)	3
Organizational Justice	Perception that the workplace outcomes and interactions are fair.	(Ambrose & Schminke, 2009)	6
Perceived Organizational Support	The degree to which the participant feels their organization values their contributions and cares about their well-being.	Eisenberger, et al., 2002)	3
Perceived Respect	Level of perceived respect as a healthcare professional from multiple sources.	National Nursing Assistant Survey (Squillace et al., 2007)	4
Supervisor Stress Management Focus	Perception that their supervisor prioritizes employee stress management.	Kath et al., 2012	4
Job Satisfaction	Level of contentment with their job.	Michigan Organizational Assessment Questionnaire (Cammann, et al., 1983)	1
Affective Commitment	The degree to which the employee likes their organization and desires to remain a part of it.	(Griffin, et al., 2007)	3

Table 4. RNAII outcome constructs

Construct	Description	Source	Number of Items
Work Frustration	Experience of upset or annoyance while trying to complete job duties.	(Peters, et al., 1980)	3
Work Burnout	Experience of emotional exhaustion related to work.	Copenhagen Burnout Inventory (Kristensen, et al., 2005)	7
Withdrawal	Intentionally limiting work time through behaviors such as tardiness or absence.	Withdrawal subscale of Workplace Counterproductive Behavior Checklist (Spector et al., 2006)	4
Musculoskeletal Symptoms	Pain in bones, joints, muscles, tendons, ligaments, or nerves associated with injury or overuse.	(Kourinka et al., 1987)	9
Injuries	The frequency of various injuries (e.g. muscle strain), the source of the injury (e.g. slips, trips, and falls), and the consequence (e.g. missed days).	National Nursing Assistant Survey (Squillace et al., 2009)	6

of values as they pertain to work and life combined with making a commitment to changing behaviors in order to promote more effective functioning.

Seventy-one NNAs participated in the study. The participants were primarily female with racial and ethnic characteristics that approximated Ohio census data (U.S. Census Bureau, 2016). Clinical psychology faculty and trained graduate clinical psychology students provided the ACT intervention. All graduate student therapists completed a semester-long seminar in the research, theory, and application of mindfulness and ACT therapies.

A total of 37 participants were randomly assigned to the NNA ACT group intervention and 34 were assigned to a waitlist control group. Participants completed measures at pretreatment, posttreatment, and at one-month follow-up. At the one-month follow-up, 32 NNA ACT participants completed measures yielding an 87% retention rate and 26 control group participants completed measures yielding a 77% retention rate. There were no significant differences in dropout rates between the NNA ACT and control groups. The retention rate for the NNA ACT group was higher than the average retention rate of 71% for MBBT randomized control trials (Nam & Toneatto, 2016). An analysis of treatment acceptability indicated that the NNAs perceived the ACT intervention to be supportive, task-focused, and without adverse experiences. A significant group-by-time interaction was observed for days missed due to injury which indicated that NNAs in the treatment group reported a decline in days missed due to injury relative to the control group. Between-group comparisons at one month follow-up indicated that the treatment group continued to report significantly fewer days missed due to injury relative to the control group (O'Brien et al, 2019b).

A significant group by time interaction with mental health symptomology was also observed. Follow-up comparisons indicated that that participants in the treatment group reported a significant reduction in mental health symptoms. In contrast, there were no significant changes across time for the control group participants. An analysis of individual mental health items indicated that NNA ACT participants reported significant declines sleep difficulties, feeling pressured, depression, and feelings of worthlessness (O'Brien et al, 2019b). Importantly, Horan et al. (2018) found that perceived supervisor support for this ACT intervention was a significant predictor of NNA perceptions of intervention helpfulness.

In summary, there is a limited research literature that has evaluated the effectiveness of mindfulness-based approaches for NNAs. The results from these investigations point towards positive effects for psychological distress which was commonly measured with burnout questionnaires. Measurement of other outcomes are rare. There is only one investigation of MBBT for NNA job-related injuries. The contact hours for interventions vary widely and most interventions used a variant of MBSR. The participants and researchers are principally from Western countries and information about variation in treatment responsiveness across cultures and minority status have not been examined.

EXPANDING THEORIES AND TECHNIQUES: MOVING FROM "WEIRD" PSYCHOLOGICAL SCIENCE IN NNA RESEARCH AND TREATMENT

Henrich et al. (2010) coined the term WEIRD – Western, Educated, Industrialized, Rich, and Democratic in their paper examining the "peculiarities" of the WEIRD subset of the human population that has exerted an inordinate impact on psychological theories, principles, and research findings. The authors presented a compelling argument that behavioral data collected from WEIRD samples are not normative and do not generalize to global populations. They also noted that WEIRD researchers, and by extension psychology intervention designers, were biased toward Western values and outcomes that are not always congruent with nonWestern cultures. We argue that WEIRD interventions are also using an excessively narrow set of techniques that may be limiting effectiveness. Health psychology training for the 21st century requires that research-practitioners gain global perspectives and skills in cross-cultural research, intervention design, and intervention delivery.

ACT and other MBBT approaches expanded Western cognitive behavioral therapy from its limited WEIRD roots by including concepts derived from Eastern Cultures such as acceptance, mindfulness, present-moment focus, and distancing oneself from thoughts through mindful meditation and non-judgmental/nonreactive observation of thoughts and feelings. MBBT interventions have gained strong empirical support for many different psychological problems (Gloster et al., 2020).

Juraskasemthawee and colleagues (2019) recognized that the incorporation of Eastern concepts created synergy between Eastern and Western therapy approaches. However, they also noted that important Eastern concepts were lost in the translation, secularization, treatment development, and application process. Jurawkasemthawee et al. (2019) also questioned why only a subset of Eastern concepts were selected for MBBTs noting that the selection process did not appear to be based on theoretical or even logical considerations. Finally, they argue that using a small subset of secularized Eastern concepts in Western MBBTs may yield suboptimal intervention effects because critically important and effective concepts and techniques are missing.

Pisitsungkagarn and colleagues (Neff et al., 2008; Uthayaratana et al., 2019) raised similar concerns in their research on the relevance of Eastern concepts such self-compassion and as the "Four Noble Truths" in problem solving therapy. They further noted that the processes of Eastern and Western approaches to therapy have different characteristics. Western approaches tend to use a mechanistic, sequential, and oftentimes didactic approach that is focused on symptom reduction. In contrast, Eastern approaches tend to use a more wholistic, nonlinear, and experiential approach more focused on insight and acceptance of suffering.

The integration of Eastern and Western theories, therapy approaches, and intervention techniques is an emerging and important topic that is relevant to NNA research. The promise of developing innovative and more complete theories of human behavior that generalize beyond WEIRD populations is an important driver of this zeitgeist. With approximately 6 billion of the 7.8 billion people on earth not living in WEIRD countries and a vast majority of NNAs not working in WEIRD countries, the need for culturally sensitive and research-supported techniques of therapy is an ethical and humanitarian issue. Furthermore, researchers have demonstrated that within WEIRD counties persons in low-income, urban, and minority communities have unique cultural values that are not always aligned with WEIRD values and that WEIRD psychological interventions can yield suboptimal outcomes for these persons (Henrich, et al., 2010). Notably, many NNAs hail from low-income, urban, and minority communities. Finally, East-West research collaborations are yielding new insights into many aspects of clinically relevant behaviors such as symptom perception and reporting, treatment-seeking, client-therapist relationship patterns, acceptability of treatments, and the moderating effects of culture on treatment effectiveness.

The Promise of East-West Integration in Mindfulness-Based Behavior Therapy

Jarukasemthawee, et al. (2019) proposed that reintroducing critically important Eastern and Buddhist elements into MBBTs would yield improved outcomes. They designed an East-West cognitive behavioral intervention that added three Buddhist principles to a traditional Western intervention: (a) "Dukkha" (suffering is an inevitable aspect of living), "Anicca" (all things and experiences are impermanent), and "Anatta" (there is no true existence of a separate self). The 8-session East-West MBBT intervention consisted of mindfulness training, meditation, and concentration, present-moment awareness, mindful living, acceptance of suffering, living harmoniously with suffering, cultivating self-compassion and compassion for others, loving-kindness, breathing training, insight into impermanence, interconnectedness of all living things, and understanding of self as a construction.

The researchers recruited 141 student participants in Thailand. Half of the participants were randomly assigned to the intervention and the other half were assigned to a waitlist control group. Results indicated that the intervention significantly increased well-being, mindfulness, and insight into Dukka, Anicca, and Anatta. Significant reductions in depression and anxiety were also observed. Jarukasemthawee et al. (2019) then provided the same intervention to 96 Western participants in Australia. Pre to post comparisons on all outcome measures yielded significant improvements with large effect sizes (Hedges' g ranging from .72 to 1.67).

Uthayaratana, Taephant, and Pisitsungkagarn (2019) combined a traditional WEIRD problem-solving therapy with concepts and techniques based on Eastern philosophy and Buddhism. The intervention, named Four Noble Truths Based Problem Solving, contained concepts of Dukka, Samudāya (examine, identify, and change the psychological processes that cause suffering), Nirodha (goal setting and formulating a plan to address suffering), and Magga (enacting the plan using the "Eightfold Path"). The researchers illustrated how the East-West intervention could be applied in a case study. They also provided a theoretical view of how this approach aligns with, and enhances, traditional Western problem-solving approaches.

Considering the unique identities and characteristics of NNAs combined the nature of NNA work, the promise of integrating Eastern and Western approaches is clear. MBBT training in present-moment awareness, acceptance of suffering, living harmoniously with suffering, cultivating self-compassion and other-compassion, loving-kindness, impermanence, and human interconnectedness have particular salience for NNAs. These concepts can be added to traditional MBBTs in an effort to promote better self and patient care in order to reduce frequency and intensity of NNA injuries.

CONCLUSION

Physical and psychological injuries occur at a high rate among NNAs. The humanitarian and economic costs to these vulnerable workers is a global health concern. The organization of work is a major contributor to injuries. Inadequate staffing, unpredictable work hours, and unsupportive organizational cultures are important determinants of injury. Individual differences are also important with mindfulness skills being particularly relevant for injury prevention. A functional analysis of the mindfulness – injury relationship suggests that appraisals, psychophysiological reactivity, and avoidance-based responding to patient caregiving needs may increase risk for injury. MBBTs focused on these three sets of NNA responses can be beneficial.

There is developing literature examining MBBTs for NNA psychological and physical injuries. Most of the studies have inadequate power and limitations that adversely affect internal, construct, and external validity. Most studies focus on burnout and psychological distress. The results of these studies do support the effectiveness of MBBTs for NNA psychological distress. Only one study examined a MBBT for NNA injury and found benefit in terms of lost workdays due to injury. This is a promising start, but more research using well-designed methods with more adequate power is very much needed.

WEIRD psychological science has severe limitations that are relevant to NNA research. Many NNAs working in Western countries have polycultural backgrounds. Furthermore, a large majority of global NNAs are working in non-western countries. Developing interventions that are more culturally sensitive is a significant additional research need in the NNA literature.

Western MBBT research borrowed concepts and techniques from Eastern philosophy, religion, and cultures. However, the borrowing of these concepts and techniques was haphazard and incomplete. Furthermore, the secularization of the concepts and techniques may have hampered their effectiveness. More thoughtful and careful integration of Eastern concepts and techniques can improve intervention effectiveness for NNAs.

There is a pressing need to develop and evaluate interventions that can promote reductions in injury rates among NNAs. Emerging research suggests that WEIRD clinical science, clinician training, and clinical interventions need to be augmented with more global and inclusive approaches that integrate philosophies, theories, and techniques of behavior change from diverse cultures. Interventions that combine Eastern and Western concepts and behavior change techniques have been demonstrated to be acceptable, feasible, and effective. Future directions point toward designing interventions that are more well-integrated with Eastern historical and cultural roots, better methodology, and training in specific skills needed to prevent NNA injury across cultures.

REFERENCES

Ahola, K., Salminen, S., Toppinen-Tanner, S., Koskinen, A., & Väänänen, A. (2013). Occupational Burnout and Severe Injuries: An Eight-year Prospective Cohort Study among Finnish Forest Industry Workers. *Journal of Occupational Health*, *55*(6), 450–457. doi:10.1539/joh.13-0021-OA PMID:24162145

Al Seraireh, F. A., & Aloush, S. M. (2017). Mindfulness meditation versus physical exercise in the management of depression among nursing students. *The Journal of Nursing Education*, *56*(10), 599–604. doi:10.3928/01484834-20170918-04 PMID:28972629

Ambrose, M. L., & Schminke, M. (2009). The role of overall justice judgments in organizational justice research: A test of mediation. *The Journal of Applied Psychology, 94*(2), 491–500. doi:10.1037/a0013203 PMID:19271803

Ando, M., Natsume, T., Kukihara, H., Shibata, H., & Ito, S. (2011). Efficacy of mindfulness-based meditation therapy on the sense of coherence and mental health of Nurses. *Health, 03*(02), 118–122. doi:10.4236/health.2011.32022

Bazarko, D., Cate, R. A., Azocar, F., & Kreitzer, M. J. (2013). The impact of an innovative mindfulness-based Stress Reduction Program on the health and well-being of nurses employed in a corporate setting. *Journal of Workplace Behavioral Health, 28*(2), 107–133. doi:10.1080/15555240.2013.779518 PMID:23667348

Bernal, D., Campos-Serna, J., Tobias, A., Vargas-Prada, S., Benavides, F. G., & Serra, C. (2015). Work-related psychosocial risk factors and musculoskeletal disorders in hospital nurses and nursing aides: a systematic review and meta-analysis. *International Journal of Nursing Studies, 52(*2), 635-648. doi/. doi:10.1016/j.ijnurstu.2014.11.003

Bond, F. W., Hayes, S. C., Baer, R. A., Carpenter, K., Guenole, N., Orcutt, H. K., Waltz, T., & Zettle, R. D. (2011). Preliminary Psychometric Properties of the Acceptance and Action Questionnaire–II: A Revised Measure of Psychological Inflexibility and Experiential Avoidance. *Behavior Therapy, 42*(4), 676–688. doi:10.1016/j.beth.2011.03.007 PMID:22035996

Bos, E. H., Krol, B., Van Der Star, A., & Groothoff, J. W. (2006). The effects of occupational interventions on reduction of musculoskeletal symptoms in the nursing profession. *Ergonomics, 49*(7), 706-723. doi:10.1080/00140130600578005

Bostrom, A., Squires, J., Mitchell, A., Sales, A., & Estabrooks, C. (2012). Workplace aggression experienced by frontline staff in nursing dementia care. *Journal of Clinical Nursing, 21*(10), 1453–1465. doi:10.1111/j.1365-2702.2011.03924.x PMID:22151034

Brown, K. W., & Ryan, R. M. (2003). The benefits of being present: Mindfulness and its role in psychological well-being. *Journal of Personality and Social Psychology, 84*(4), 822–848. doi:10.1037/0022-3514.84.4.822 PMID:12703651

Bureau of Labor Statistics. (2010). *Employer-reported workplace injuries and illnesses – 2013*. Retrieved from www.bls.gov

Bureau of Labor Statistics. (2018). *Employer-reported workplace injuries and illnesses – 2018*. Retrieved from www.bls.gov

Burton, A., Burgess, C., Dean, S., Koutsopoulou, G. Z., & Hugh-Jones, S. (2016). How Effective are Mindfulness-Based Interventions for Reducing Stress Among Healthcare Professionals? A Systematic Review and Meta-Analysis. *Stress and Health, 33*(1), 3–13. doi:10.1002mi.2673 PMID:26916333

Cammann, C., Fichman, M., Jenkins, G. D., & Klesh, J. (1983). Michigan organizational assessment questionnaire. In S. E. Seashore, E. E. Lawler, P. H. Mirvis, & C. Cammann (Eds.), *Assessing organizational change: a guide to methods, measures, and practices* (pp. 71–138). John Wiley & Sons.

Carlopio, J. R. (1996). Construct validity of a physical work environment satisfaction questionnaire. *Journal of Occupational Health Psychology*, *1*(3), 330–344. doi:10.1037/1076-8998.1.3.330 PMID:9547055

Ceravolo, D., & Raines, D. A. (2018). The impact of a mindfulness intervention for nurse managers. *Journal of Holistic Nursing*, *37*(1), 47–55. doi:10.1177/0898010118781620 PMID:29909707

Chang, Y.-J., Kwon, Y. C., Lee, W. J., Do, Y. R., Lee, K. S., Kim, H. T., Park, S. R., Hong, Y. S., Chung, I.-J., & Yun, Y. H. (2013). Burdens, Needs and Satisfaction of Terminal Cancer Patients and their Caregivers. *Asian Pacific Journal of Cancer Prevention*, *14*(1), 209–215. doi:10.7314/APJCP.2013.14.1.209 PMID:23534725

Cohen-Katz, J., Wiley, S., Capuano, T., Baker, D. M., Deitrick, L., & Shapiro, S. (2005). The effects of mindfulness-based stress reduction on nurse stress and burnout: A qualitative and quantitative study, part III. *Holistic Nursing Practice*, *19*(2), 78–86. doi:10.1097/00004650-200503000-00009 PMID:15871591

Cortina, L. M., Kabat-Farr, D., Leskinen, E. A., Huerta, M., & Magley, V. J. (2013). Selective Incivility as Modern Discrimination in Organizations: Evidence and Impact. *Journal of Management*, *39*(6), 1579–1605. doi:10.1177/0149206311418835

Craigie, M., Slatyer, S., Hegney, D., Osseiran-Moisson, R., Gentry, E., Davis, S., Dolan, T., & Rees, C. (2016). A pilot evaluation of a mindful self-care and resiliency (MSCR) intervention for Nurses. *Mindfulness*, *7*(3), 764–774. doi:10.100712671-016-0516-x

Crenshaw, K. (1989). *Demarginalizing the Intersection of Race and Sex: A Black* Feminist Critique of Antidiscrimination Doctrine, Feminist Theory and Antiracist Politics. University of Chicago Legal Forum.

D'Archy, L. P., Sasai, Y., & Stearns, S. C. (2011). Do assistive devices, training, and workload affect injury incidence?Prevention efforts by nursing homes and back injuries among nursing assistants? *Journal of Advanced Nursing*, *68*(4), 836–845. doi:10.1111/j.1365-2648.2011.05785.x

de Castro, A. B., Fujishiro, K., Tagalog, E. A., Samaco-Paquiz, L. P. G., & Gee, G. C. (2010). Associations between work schedule characte20ristics and occupational injury and illness. *International Nursing Review*, *57*(2), 188–194. doi:10.1111/j.1466-7657.2009.00793.x PMID:20579153

Dekker, S. W. A. (2002). Reconstructing human contributions to accidents: The new view on error and performance. *Journal of Safety Research, 33*(3), 371–385. . doi:10.1016/S0022-4375(02)00032-4

Delaney, L. J., Currie, M. J., Huang, H.-C. C., Lopez, V., & Van Haren, F. (2018). "They can rest at home": An observational study of patients' quality of sleep in an australian hospital. *BMC Health Services Research*, *18*(1), 524. Advance online publication. doi:10.118612913-018-3201-z PMID:29976191

dos Santos, T. M., Kozasa, E. H., Carmagnani, I. S., Tanaka, L. H., Lacerda, S. S., & Nogueira-Martins, L. A. (2016). Positive effects of a stress reduction program based on mindfulness meditation in Brazilian nursing professionals: Qualitative and quantitative evaluation. *Explore (New York, N.Y.)*, *12*(2), 90–99. doi:10.1016/j.explore.2015.12.005 PMID:26778081

Duarte, J., & Pinto-Gouveia, J. (2016). Effectiveness of a mindfulness-based intervention on oncology nurses' burnout and compassion fatigue symptoms: A non-randomized study. *International Journal of Nursing Studies*, *64*, 98–107. doi:10.1016/j.ijnurstu.2016.10.002 PMID:27744228

Duchemin, A.-M., Steinberg, B. A., Marks, D. R., Vanover, K., & Klatt, M. (2015). A small randomized pilot study of a workplace mindfulness-based intervention for Surgical Intensive Care Unit Personnel. *Journal of Occupational and Environmental Medicine*, *57*(4), 393–399. doi:10.1097/JOM.0000000000000371 PMID:25629803

Eisenberger, R., Stinglhamber, F., Vandenberghe, C., Sucharski, I. L., & Rhoades, L. (2002). Perceived supervisor support: Contributions to perceived organizational support and employee retention. *The Journal of Applied Psychology*, *87*(3), 565–573. doi:10.1037/0021-9010.87.3.565 PMID:12090614

Estabrooks, C., Squires, J., Cummings, G., Birdsell, J., & Norton, P. (2009). Development and assessment of the Alberta Conext Tool. *BMC Health Services Research*, *9*(1), 1–12. doi:10.1186/1472-6963-9-234 PMID:20003531

Foli, K. J., Reddick, B., Zhang, L., & Krcelich, K. (2020). Nurses' psychological trauma: "They leave me lying awake at night. *Archives of Psychiatric Nursing*, *34*(3), 86–95. doi:10.1016/j.apnu.2020.04.011 PMID:32513472

Foureur, M., Besley, K., Burton, G., Yu, N., & Crisp, J. (2013). Enhancing the resilience of nurses and midwives: Pilot of a mindfulnessbased program for increased health, sense of coherence and decreased depression, anxiety and stress. *Contemporary Nurse*, *45*(1), 114–125. doi:10.5172/conu.2013.45.1.114 PMID:24099232

Gauthier, T., Meyer, R. M. L., Grefe, D., & Gold, J. I. (2015). An on-the-job mindfulness-based intervention for pediatric ICU Nurses: A pilot. *Journal of Pediatric Nursing*, *30*(2), 402–409. doi:10.1016/j.pedn.2014.10.005 PMID:25450445

Ghawadra, S. F., Abdullah, K. L., Choo, W. Y., & Phang, C. K. (2019, November). Mindfulness-based stress reduction for psychological distress among nurses: A systematic review. *Journal of Clinical Nursing*, *28*(21-22), 3747–3758. doi:10.1111/jocn.14987 PMID:31267619

Gloster, A. T., Walder, N., Levin, M. E., Twohig, M. P., & Karekla, M. (2020). The empirical status of acceptance and commitment therapy: A review of meta-analyses. *Journal of Contextual Behavioral Science*, *18*, 181–192. doi:10.1016/j.jcbs.2020.09.009

Grzywacz, J. G., Frone, M. R., Brewer, C. S., & Kovner, C. T. (2006). Quantifying work–family conflict among registered nurses. *Research in Nursing & Health*, *29*(5), 414–426. doi:10.1002/nur.20133 PMID:16977647

Halm, M. (2017). The Role of Mindfulness in Enhancing Self-Care for Nurses. *American Journal of Critical Care*, *26*(4), 344–348. doi:10.4037/ajcc2017589 PMID:28668922

Hayes, S. C., & Hofmann, S. G. (2017). The third wave of cognitive behavioral therapy and the rise of process-based care. *World Psychiatry, 16*(3), 245-246. doi:10.1002/wps.20442

Hee, K. L., Pathmawati, S., Norsiah, R., & Phang, C. K. (2014). The effects of mindfulness training program on reducing stress and promoting well-being among nurses in critical care units. *The Australian Journal of Advanced Nursing*, *31*, 22–31.

Hemingway, M. A., & Smith, C. S. (1999). Organizational climate and occupational stressors as predictors of withdrawal behaviours and injuries in nurses. *Journal of Occupational and Organizational Psychology*, *72*(3), 285–299. doi:10.1348/096317999166680

Henrich, J., Heine, S. J., & Norenzayan, A. (2010). The weirdest people in the world? *Behavioral and Brain Sciences*, *33*(2), 61–83. doi:10.1017/S0140525X0999152X PMID:20550733

Hevezi, J. A. (2016). Evaluation of a Meditation Intervention to Reduce the Effects of Stressors Associated With Compassion Fatigue Among Nurses. *Journal of Holistic Nursing*, *34*(4), 343–350. doi:10.1177/0898010115615981 PMID:26598000

Horan, K. A., Moeller, M. T., Singh, R. S., Wasson, R., O'Brien, W. H., Matthews, R. A., Jex, S. M., & Barratt, C. L. (2018). Supervisor support for stress management and intervention process. *International Journal of Workplace Health Management*, *11*(4), 260–272. doi:10.1108/IJWHM-12-2017-0113

Horner, J. K., Piercy, B. S., Eure, L., & Woodard, E. K. (2014). A pilot study to evaluate mindfulness as a strategy to improve inpatient nurse and patient experiences. *Applied Nursing Research*, *27*(3), 198–201. doi:10.1016/j.apnr.2014.01.003 PMID:24602399

Hosseinabadi, M. B., Khanjani, N., Etemadinezhad, S., Samaei, S. E., Raadabadi, M., & Mostafaee, M. (2017). The associations of workload, individual and organisational factors on nurses' occupational injuries. *Journal of Clinical Nursing*, *28*(5-6), 902–911. doi:10.1111/jocn.14699 PMID:30357967

Ilhan, M. N., Durukan, E., Aras, E., Türkçüoğlu, S., & Aygün, R. (2006). Long working hours increase the risk of sharp and needlestick injury in nurses: The need for new policy implication. *Journal of Advanced Nursing*, *56*(5), 563–568. doi:10.1111/j.1365-2648.2006.04041.x PMID:17078831

Jarukasemthawee, S., Halford, W. K., & McLean, J. P. (2019). When East meets West: A randomized controlled trial and pre- to postprogram evaluation replication of the effects of insight-based mindfulness on psychological well-being. *Journal of Psychotherapy Integration*, *29*(3), 307–323. doi:10.1037/int0000179

Jones, K. J., Skinner, A., Xu, L., Sun, J., & Keith Muelleet, K. (2008). The AHRQ Hospital Survey on Patient Safety Culture: A Tool to Plan and Evaluate Patient Safety Programs. In *Advances in Patient Safety: New Directions and Alternative Approaches (Vol. 2: Culture and Redesign)*. Agency for Healthcare Research and Quality (US). ncbi.nlm.nih.gov/books/NBK43699/

Jun, J., Ojemeni, M. M., Kalamani, R., Tong, J., & Crecelius, M. L. (2021). Relationship between nurse burnout, patient and organizational outcomes: Systematic review. *International Journal of Nursing Studies*, *119*, 103933. doi:10.1016/j.ijnurstu.2021.103933 PMID:33901940

Kath, L. M., Ehrhart, M. E., Gates, M. G., & Stichler, J. F. (2012). *Nurse Leader Stress Study: Final Feedback Report Round 2 Survey* [Proprietary feedback reports prepared for 34 acute-care hospitals participating in the study.]. San Diego State University.

Khatutsky, G., Wiener, J., Anderson, W., & Porell, F. (2012). Work-related injuries among certified nursing assistants in nursing homes. RTI Press publication No. RR-0017-1204. Research Triangle Park, NC: RTI Press. doi:10.3768/rtipress.2012.rr.0017.1204

Klein, A., Taieb, O., Xavier, S., Baubet, T., & Reyre, A. (2019). The benefits of mindfulness-based interventions on burnout among health professionals: A systematic review. *Explore (New York, N.Y.), 16*(1), 35–43. doi:10.1016/j.explore.2019.09.002 PMID:31727578

Kristensen, T. S., Borritz, M., Villadsen, E., & Christensen, K. B. (2005). The Copenhagen Burnout Inventory: A new tool for the assessment of burnout. *Work & Stress, 19*(3), 192-207. doi/doi:10.1080/02678370500297720

Kuorinka, I., Jonsson, B., Kilbom, A., Vinterberg, H., Biering-Sørensen, F., Andersson, G., & Jørgensen, K. (1987). Standardised Nordic questionnaires for the analysis of musculoskeletal symptoms. *Applied Ergonomics, 18*(3), 233–237. doi:10.1016/0003-6870(87)90010-X PMID:15676628

LaRose, A., Danhauer, S. C., Feldman, J., Evans, G. W., & Kemper, K. J. (2010). Brief Stress-Reduction Training in an Academic Health Center. *Journal of Alternative and Complementary Medicine (New York, N.Y.), 16*(9), 935–936. doi:10.1089/acm.2010.0338 PMID:20715979

Mackenzie, C. S., Poulin, P. A., & Seidman-Carlson, R. (2006). A brief mindfulness-based stress reduction intervention for nurses and nurse aides. *Applied Nursing Research, 19*(2), 105–109. doi:10.1016/j.apnr.2005.08.002 PMID:16728295

McElroy, S. F., Olney, A., Hunt, C., & Glennon, C. (2020). Shift work and hospital employees: A descriptive multi-site study. *International Journal of Nursing Studies, 112*, 103746. doi:10.1016/j.ijnurstu.2020.103746 PMID:32928504

McGinn, K., & Eunsil, O. (2017). Gender, Social Class, and Women's Employment. *Current Opinion in Psychology, 18*, 84–88. Advance online publication. doi:10.1016/j.copsyc.2017.07.012 PMID:28866434

Mealer, M., Conrad, D., Evans, J., Jooste, K., Solyntjes, J., Rothbaum, B., & Moss, M. (2014). Feasibility and acceptability of a resilience training program for Intensive Care Unit Nurses. *American Journal of Critical Care, 23*(6), e97–e105. Advance online publication. doi:10.4037/ajcc2014747 PMID:25362680

Montanari, K. M., Bowe, C. L., Chesak, S. S., & Cutshall, S. M. (2018). Mindfulness: Assessing the feasibility of a pilot intervention to reduce stress and Burnout. *Journal of Holistic Nursing, 37*(2), 175–188. doi:10.1177/0898010118793465 PMID:30152244

Mueller, W. S. (1991). New Technology and Flexible Working. In J. Hartley & G. Stephenson (Eds.), *The Psychology of Employment Relations*. Basil Blackwell.

Muldoon, J., Matthews, R. A., & Foley, C. (2012). Mediated Effects of Physical Risk Factors, Leader–Member Exchange and Empowerment in Predicting Perceived Injury Risk. *Stress and Health, 28*(2), 149–162. doi:10.1002mi.1415 PMID:22282314

Nam, S., & Toneatto, T. (2016). The Influence of Attrition in Evaluating the Efficacy and Effectiveness of Mindfulness-Based Interventions. *International Journal of Mental Health and Addiction, 14*(6), 969–981. doi:10.100711469-016-9667-1

Neal, A., & Griffin, M. A. (2006). A study of the lagged relationships among safety climate, safety motivation, safety behavior, and accidents at the individual and group levels. *The Journal of Applied Psychology, 91*(4), 946–953. doi:10.1037/0021-9010.91.4.946 PMID:16834517

Neff, K. D., Pisitsungkagarn, K., & Hsieh, Y. P. (2008). Self-Compassion and Self-Construal in the United States, Thailand, and Taiwan. *Journal of Cross-Cultural Psychology*, *39*(3), 267–285. doi:10.1177/0022022108314544

O'Brien, W. H., & Carhart, V. (2011). Functional analysis in behavioral medicine settings. *European Journal of Psychological Assessment, 27*(1), 4-16. doi/. doi:10.1027/1015-5759/a000052

O'Brien, W. H., Horan, K. A., Singh, S., Moeller, M. A., Wasson, R. S., Jex, S. M., Matthews, R. A., & Barratt, C. L. (2019a). Relationships among training, mindfulness, and workplace injuries among nurse aides working in long-term care settings. *Occupational Health Science*, *3*(1), 45–58. doi:10.100741542-018-0031-7

O'Brien, W. H., Singh, S., Horan, K. A., Moeller, M. A., Wasson, R. S., & Jex, S. M. (2019b). Group-Based Acceptance and Commitment Therapy for Nurses and Nurse Aides Working in Long-Term Care Residential Settings. *Journal of Alternative and Complementary Medicine (New York, N.Y.)*, *25*(7), 753–761. doi:10.1089/acm.2019.0087 PMID:31314564

Okechukwu, C. A., Bacic, J., Velasquez, E., & Hammer, L. B. (2016). Marginal structural modelling of associations of occupational injuries with voluntary and involuntary job loss among nursing home workers. *Occupational and Environmental Medicine*, *73*(3), 175–182. doi:10.1136/oemed-2015-103067 PMID:26786757

Payne, N. (2001). Occupational stressors and coping as determinants of burnout in female hospice nurses. *Journal of Advanced Nursing*, *33*(3), 396–405. doi:10.1046/j.1365-2648.2001.01677.x PMID:11251727

Perry, L., Lamont, S., Brunero, S., Gallagher, R., & Duffield, C. (2015). The mental health of nurses in acute teaching hospital settings: A cross-sectional survey. *BMC Nursing*, *14*(1), 1–8. doi:10.118612912-015-0068-8 PMID:25904820

Peters, L. H., O'Connor, E. J., & Rudolf, C. J. (1980). The behavioral and affective consequences of performance-relevant situational variables. *Organizational Behavior and Human Performance*, *25*(1), 79–96. doi:10.1016/0030-5073(80)90026-4

Petrocchi, N., & Cheli, S. (2019). The social brain and heart rate variability: Implications for psychotherapy. *Psychology and Psychotherapy: Theory, Research and Practice*, *92*(2), 208–223. doi:10.1111/papt.12224 PMID:30891894

Pipe, T. B., Bortz, J. J., Dueck, A., Pendergast, D., Buchda, V., & Summers, J. (2009). Nurse Leader Mindfulness Meditation Program for Stress Management a Randomized Controlled Trial. *The Journal of Nursing Administration*, *39*(3), 130–137. doi:10.1097/NNA.0b013e31819894a0 PMID:19590469

Poulin, P. A., Mackenzie, C. S., Soloway, G., & Karayolas, E. (2008). Mindfulness training as an evidenced-based approach to reducing stress and promoting well-being among Human Services Professionals. *International Journal of Health Promotion and Education*, *46*(2), 72–80. doi:10.1080/14635240.2008.10708132

Ramos-Morcillo, A. J., Fernández-Salazar, S., Ruzafa-Martínez, M., & Del-Pino-Casado, R. (2015). Effectiveness of a Brief, Basic Evidence-Based Practice Course for Clinical Nurses. *Worldviews on Evidence-Based Nursing*, *12*(4), 199–207. doi:10.1111/wvn.12103 PMID:26220505

Richardson, A., Gurung, G., Derrett, S., & Harcombe, H. (2019). Perspectives on preventing musculoskeletal injuries in nurses: A qualitative study. *Nursing Open*, *6*(3), 915–929. doi:10.1002/nop2.272 PMID:31367415

Schoenfisch, A. L., & Lipscomb, H. J. (2009). Job characteristics and work organization factors associated with patient-handling injury among nursing personnel. *Work (Reading, Mass.)*, *33*(1), 117–128. doi:10.3233/WOR-2009-0847 PMID:19597289

Schuster, M., & Dwyer, P. A. (2020). Post-traumatic stress disorder in nurses: An integrative review. *Journal of Clinical Nursing*, *29*(15–16), 2769–2787. doi:10.1111/jocn.15288 PMID:32372541

Shapiro, S., Schwartz, G., & Bonner, G. (1998). Effects of mindfulness-based stress reduction on medical and premedical students. *Journal of Behavioral Medicine*, *21*(6), 581–599. doi:10.1023/A:1018700829825 PMID:9891256

Smith, B.W., Dalen, J., & Wiggins, K. (n.d.). The brief resilience scale: Assessing the ability to bounce back. *International Journal of Behavioral Medicine, 15,* 194–200. doi:10.1080/10705500802222972

Song, Y., & Lindquist, R. (2015). Effects of mindfulness-based stress reduction on depression, anxiety, stress and mindfulness in Korean nursing students. *Nurse Education Today*, *35*(1), 86–90. doi:10.1016/j.nedt.2014.06.010 PMID:25066651

Spector, P. E., Fox, S., Penney, L. M., Bruursema, K., Goh, A., & Kessler, S. (2006). The dimensionality of counterproductivity: Are all counterproductive behaviors created equal? *Journal of Vocational Behavior*, *68*(3), 446–460. doi:10.1016/j.jvb.2005.10.005

Spector, P. E., & Jex, S. M. (1998). Development of four self-report measures of job stressors and strain: Interpersonal Conflict at Work Scale, Organizational Constraints Scale, Quantitative Workload Inventory, and Physical Symptoms Inventory. *Journal of Occupational Health Psychology*, *3*(4), 356–367. doi:10.1037/1076-8998.3.4.356 PMID:9805281

Spector, P. E., Yang, L. Q., & Zhou, Z. E. (2015). A longitudinal investigation of the role of violence prevention climate in exposure to workplace physical violence and verbal abuse. *Work and Stress*, *29*(4), 325–340. doi:10.1080/02678373.2015.1076537

Squillace, M. R., Remsburg, R. E., Bercovitz, A., Rosenoff, E., & Branden, L. (2007). An introduction to the National Nursing Assistant Survey. *Vital and health statistics. Ser. 1, Programs and collection procedures*, (44), 1-54.

Stanev, S., Bailer, J., Straker, J. K., Mehdizadeh, S., Park, R. M., & Li, H. (2012). Worker injuries and safety equipment in Ohio nursing homes. *Journal of Gerontological Nursing*, *38*(6), 47–56. doi:10.3928/00989134-20120508-01 PMID:22774234

Teleghani, F., Ashouri, E., & Saburi, M. (2017). Empathy, burnout, demographic variables and their relationships in oncology nurses. *Iranian Journal of Nursing and Midwifery Research*, *22*(1), 41–45. doi:10.4103/ijnmr.IJNMR_66_16 PMID:28382057

Teo, S. T. T., Nguyen, D., Trevelyan, F., Lamm, F., & Boocock, M. (2021). Workplace bullying, psychological hardiness, and accidents and injuries in nursing: A moderated mediation model. *PLoS ONE, 16*(1), 1–15. doi:10.1371/journal.pone.0244426

U.S. Census Bureau. (2016). *US census bureau QuickFacts: Ohio*. Retrieved from www.census.gov/search-results.html?q=ohio&page=1&stateGeo=none&searchtype=web&cssp=SERP&_charset_=UTF-8

Uthayaratana, T., Taephant, N., & Pisitsungkagarn, K. (2019). Four Noble Truths based problem solving: A therapeutic view. *Mental Health, Religion & Culture*, *22*(2), 119–129. doi:10.1080/13674676.2018.1512565

Watanabe, N., Horikoshi, M., Shinmei, I., Oe, Y., Narisawa, T., Kumachi, M., Matsuoka, Y., Hamazaki, K., & Furukawa, T. A. (2019). Brief mindfulness-based stress management program for a better mental state in working populations - happy nurse project: A randomized controlled trial¶¶. *Journal of Affective Disorders*, *251*, 186–194. doi:10.1016/j.jad.2019.03.067 PMID:30927579

Woo, T., Ho, R., Tang, A., & Tam, W. (2019). Global prevalence of burnout symptoms among nurses: A systematic review and meta-analysis. *Journal of Psychiatric Research*, *123*, 9–20. doi:10.1016/j.jpsychires.2019.12.015 PMID:32007680

Wylde, C. M., Mahrer, N. E., Meyer, R. M. L., & Gold, J. I. (2017). Mindfulness for novice pediatric nurses: Smartphone application versus traditional intervention. *Journal of Pediatric Nursing*, *36*, 205–212. doi:10.1016/j.pedn.2017.06.008 PMID:28888505

Xujun, Z., Yue, G., Mengjing, C., Lorann, S., & Huiyun, X. (2015). Needlestick and sharps injuries among nurses at a teaching hospital in China. *Workplace Health & Safety*, *63*(5), 219–225. doi:10.1177/2165079915580035 PMID:26031696

Zettle, R. D., Hayes, S. C., Barnes-Holmes, D., & Biglan, A. (2016). *The Wiley handbook of contextual behavioral science*. John Wiley & Sons.

Zhang, Y., Wang, C., Pan, W., Zheng, J., Gao, J., Huang, X., Cai, S., Zhai, Y., Latour, J. M., & Zhu, C. (2020). Stress, Burnout, and Coping Strategies of Frontline Nurses During the COVID-19 Epidemic in Wuhan and Shanghai, China. *Frontiers in Psychiatry*, *11*(October), 1–9. doi:10.3389/fpsyt.2020.565520 PMID:33192686

Chapter 14
Working With Medical Personnel in the Aftermath of a Mass Shooting:
Lessons Learned From Nickel Mines

Ashley T. Winch
University of Central Florida, USA

Kathryn Sunderman
University of Central Florida, USA

Deborah C. Beidel
University of Central Florida, USA

ABSTRACT

The rising number of mass casualty incidents in the United States has exposed hospital personnel to more traumatic events on the job than ever before, with research citing a lack of mental health support following such events. It is often assumed that the advanced training of medical professionals serves as a protective factor against PTSD and other mental health disorders resulting from occupational trauma. However, this notion is false, and if left untreated, these mental health issues may extend beyond personal distress and negatively impact patient care. Furthermore, not all hospital personnel who are directly exposed to mass casualty incidents have advanced medical training, and many of these individuals have had no experience with these types of traumas. This chapter outlines planning and implementation measures that hospitals can take prior to a mass casualty incident occurring, followed by steps, strategies, and supports that can be deployed once a hospital has become a treating facility for victims of a mass casualty incident.

DOI: 10.4018/978-1-7998-8813-0.ch014

INTRODUCTION

On October 2, 2006, Charles Carl Roberts entered a one-room schoolhouse in the Amish community of Nickel Mines, Pennsylvania. He lined up the ten young girls who were in the schoolhouse and shot them each in the head at point blank range. The result was five girls died and five were severely wounded. The shooter then killed himself. The Amish community asked for privacy during that time. As a psychologist working at one of the medical centers where some of those girls were sent for treatment, one of the authors of this chapter (DCB) was called to help the staff and the community deal with this horrific event. What follows is a personal assessment of the medical center's response and some personal lessons learned.

It is fair to say that at the time of this event, the medical center was caught by surprise. School shootings were not as prevalent in 2006 as they have become. Psychiatric and psychological services had never discussed a response plan for such an event. Some actions went well – the medical center protected the affected families from the press. But as a whole, the medical center was not prepared to deal with the incident's complicated aftermath. There was no plan to deal with the number of members of the Amish community that would come to the hospital to await news of the children's condition. Keeping the press away from the community became a challenge.

Likewise, there was no plan to deal with the psychological reaction of the first responders and the medical center staff. Even individuals who might be assumed to have experience dealing with gunshot wounds were overwhelmed by the number and nature of the injuries, not to mention the ages of the children. Additionally, there was minimal attention given at the time to the non-medical members of the hospital community – such as chaplains and environmental services staff- who were unprepared for what they would see and hear.

Furthermore, initially, there was no coordinated plan to reach out and work with the hospital staff who were affected by the trauma. Independent efforts were occurring with emergency room personnel and critical care units, but certain departments such as radiology and environmental services were completely overlooked. By the time that a comprehensive plan was in place, it was too late – many hospital staff felt unsupported and ignored. Difficult lessons were learned. First, there is a need to expect the unexpected and prepare for the unthinkable. Second, communication needed to be swift and there needed to be a planned outreach to all staff, both at the time of the event and in the weeks and months afterwards. Below we discuss the sparse literature that is available for working with medical personnel after the occurrence of mass shootings/mass casualty events and we propose a plan for assessment/intervention to maintain staff mental wellness in the aftermath of these events.

BACKGROUND

The public tends to assume that individuals who are in the medical field, because of their medical training, are more resilient to traumatic events and the resultant medical casualties, such as the often horrific nature of gunshot wounds, than the general population. Certainly, clinical training emphasizes the need to be objective, and perhaps even detached, when engaged in clinical care. This assumption, however, is not absolute. For example, Dr. Albert Wu, a professor of health policy and management at Johns Hopkins School of Public Health notes that "it's not a matter of if clinicians are going to experience trauma while providing care, but when and how often" (Paturel, 2019).

Mass casualty incidents would seem to be among the ones most likely to meet criteria for the "when" and "how often." Mass casualty incidents are defined as "an event wherein the number and severity of injuries exceeds the resources immediately available to treat them effectively" (p. 3, Hodgson, 2021). Previously, if not war-related, most mass casualty incidents were accidents, and were often caused by weather or natural events (e.g., earthquakes or sunken ships). Today however, many mass casualty incidents are caused by intentional acts of violence (e.g., improvised explosions such as the Boston Marathon Bombing, vehicle rammings, and mass stabbings; Hodgson, 2021). Unfortunately, the aggressive intent behind these acts coupled with today's more powerful weapons are creating what has been termed "mega-mass casualty incidents." These events are becoming more frequent and resulting in death and injury rates higher than ever before (Hodgson, 2021). Since 2013, there have been 3,978 mass shootings (defined as 4 or more people killed or injured) in the United States, with 414 of those mass shootings occurring in the first half of 2021 (Mass Shooting Tracker [MST], 2021) and the data from 2021 are not an anomaly. For example, in comparison to 2014, in 2020 there was a 126.3% increase in the number of mass shootings that took place in the United States (Gun Violence Archive [GVA], 2021).

With each mass shooting comes an influx of deceased and injured victims and while it is recognized that some first responders (fire, emergency medical services, law enforcement) face an enormous burden when providing aid in these circumstances, others (emergency room hospital personnel and hospital support staff) are often overlooked. Experiencing a traumatic event on the job has always been an occupational hazard of emergency medicine. However, the data makes it clear that traumatic experiences in emergency medicine are occurring more often and with more devastation than ever before. It is important to acknowledge and conceptualize the hospital as a second trauma location following a mass casualty incident and provide the necessary mental health support needed so that hospital personnel can do their jobs on the day of the event and also months and years later.

The current prevalence of posttraumatic stress disorder (PTSD) amongst physicians is 14.8%, which is approximately two times greater than the prevalence amongst the general population (Vanyo, 2017). The specific rate among emergency room personnel is 15.1% (Delucia, 2016 as cited in Vanyo, 2017), and when the sample is restricted to EM residents only, there is a two-fold increase, with 30% endorsing PTSD symptoms (Mills & Mills, 2005; Vanyo, 2017). Even so, most experts agree that PTSD is underdiagnosed in this population and that underreporting is due to (a) the inability of some to identify a specific traumatic event and (b) the stigma surrounding a PTSD diagnosis (Vanyo, 2017).

These rates are similar to that of other first responders and are, ironically, not all that different from rates for combat veterans; the demographic group perhaps most commonly associated with PTSD (Jones, 2017; U.S. Department of Veterans Affairs, 2018). From a clinical perspective, this is not surprising given that, in many ways, the types of experiences and decisions physicians face in the emergency department (ED) during a mass casualty incident are not all that different from the traumatic experiences reported by combat veterans seeking treatment for PTSD – the majority of which entail death or extensive injuries to fellow personnel. Yet, there are important differences. First, emergency room personnel likely experience trauma on a regular, if not daily, basis and likely see more trauma over their lifetime than the average veteran. Second, it appears that awareness and understanding of PTSD resulting from emergency medical practice lags behind the extant literature for combat PTSD. Third, and perhaps equally concerning, is that current data suggest that seeking help for PTSD amongst physicians is very low (Sendler et al., 2016). At the organizational level, this is problematic as untreated PTSD can impact patient care. Common symptoms of PTSD, such as flashbacks and difficulty sleeping, can result in lack of energy and difficulty concentrating, which in turn can lead to difficulty managing patients and an increase in errors, complications, and even death (Sendler et al., 2016). To a field whose Hippocratic Oath is partly rooted in the concept of "primum non nocere" (translated from Latin to English, this phrase means "first, do no harm"), the possibility that patient care could be negatively impacted should be enough reason to propose a structure to address the prevention, mitigation, and treatment of PTSD in medical personnel (Schmerling, 2020). Below, we will address ways to help reduce risk of hospital personnel developing adverse mental health outcomes associated with an mass casualty incident.

PLANNING AND PREPARATION

Preparation Starts in the Classroom

Before discussing preparation for stress management during and after a mass casualty incident, it is worth noting that preparation should begin in the classroom. Rates of PTSD amongst medical personnel are high, but seeking professional help is low. It is clear that there is, at the very least, a culture issue, often referred to as stigma, that prevents medical personnel from reaching out for help from a behavioral health professional (Sendler et al., 2016). Aware of this issue, several medical schools and teaching hospitals have implemented a number of strategies with the goal of decreasing stigma and promoting a healthier culture for both physicians and nurses. Some of these measures include establishing a "chief wellness officer" position and starting peer support programs (Connors et al., 2019; Paturel, 2019). Note that, for the purpose of this chapter, we define peer support programs as those that are based on formal training experiences. Johns Hopkins, for example, has a 24/7 peer support program called Resilience in Stressful Events (RISE) where peer volunteers are trained in Psychological First Aid (PFA). In addition, Johns Hopkins offers a patient safety course in which there is a 1.5-hour small group session where second-year students learn how to handle adverse events, how to disclose their experiences to others, and consequently how to move on (Paturel, 2019). Introducing these topics during graduate school education begins to educate future medical personnel that (a) traumatic events will be part of their career, and (b) taking steps to understand, acknowledge and mitigate is a proactive, reasoned approach to having a long and successful career. This training also helps to combat the stigma that developing PTSD means you are weak or can't handle the job. It is likely that students who receive these messages and instructional content will be better equipped to recognize and respond to their own emotional distress and provide emotional support to their medical colleagues.

Pre-Incident Planning

According to Hodgson (2021), the nature of an mass casualty incident implies there are more victims than resources available to save everyone. If so, this puts medical personnel in the difficult position of triage, meaning that personnel may need to decide who is too grievously wounded to receive limited resources and aid (Hodgson, 2021). These decisions can be traumatic as personnel may later "second-guess" themselves, leading to psychological distress and perhaps long-term mental health problems. When training leads to solid preparation, the result can be a better allocation of needed resources to save more lives. As one example, over 60 patients were admitted to the University Medical Center of Southern Nevada at the time of the mass shooting at the Harvest Music Festival. This hospital had engaged in extensive disaster response planning prior to the 2017 shooting, and this preparation was cited by the medical personnel as the reason they were able to treat so many victims with no warning (Sofer, 2018). Rarely however, do these drills ever include psychoeducation on the emotional effects on personnel either during or after the event (Brondolo et al., 2008), although clearly one's emotional status can impact a myriad of cognitive functions necessary for optimal job performance..

Key to this preparation is educating personnel on the typical physical, emotional, and behavioral responses that follow traumatic events and educating or reminding employees of the available company and community resources. Crisis Response Planning (CRP) is one model that may be appropriate for this task. A CRP is written on a small card that individuals can carry on their person or keep close by. The CRP begins with warning signs of emotional distress, followed by coping strategies, social supports, and accessing professional services (Bryan et al., 2017; Stanley & Brown, 2012). Originally developed to help individuals with suicidal ideation, its simple format and individual adaptability make it ideal for pre-incident planning for mass casualty incidents.

Mental Health Awareness Training to Assist Others

Creation of a Psychological First Aid Team. Psychological First Aid (PFA) was developed by the National Child Traumatic Stress Network in partnership with the National Center for PTSD (Ruzek et al., 2007). The purpose of PFA is to provide immediate psychosocial aid to those who have just experienced a traumatic event in an effort to reduce distress and facilitate coping (Brymer et al., 2006). For PFA to be deployed during or in the immediate aftermath of a mass casualty event, creation and training of the PFA team must already be in place. While a PFA can consist of people from a variety of disaster response backgrounds (Brymer et al., 2006), it may be beneficial for various medical settings within a community to each have their own PFA team, one or more of which would be deployed to the hospital(s) working the mass casualty event. There are two reasons for this recommendation. First, this allows all personnel at the hospital where mass casualty incidents patients are being treated to attend to those patients and their families. Second, because employees may be less willing to speak to peers or supervisors about negative mental health symptoms, a PFA team external to the agency may be more approachable. Such reciprocal arrangements often exist between hospitals and first responder communities when a first responder requires hospitalization for psychological distress. Rather than hospitalizing a first responder where he/she typically brings other emergency patients, hospitalization outside of the district provides a level of confidentiality that allows individuals to accept their need for treatment. A similar reciprocal arrangement for PFA in the time of crisis could be equally beneficial.

Creation of a Peer Support Program. Peer support has a variety of definitions, but the basic foundation is that peers are the first line of support for other peers with mental health problems associated with their specific line of work (Cyr et al., 2016). A qualitative study of nurses (Lavoie et al., 2010) found that a supportive social network and an environment where nurses could discuss negative hospital-based experiences with colleagues were judged as very helpful following traumatic work experiences. Across a variety of outcomes measures, engagement in peer support for first responders and health care workers has yielded beneficial outcomes (Anderson et al., 2020). Peer support teams should cross all levels of staff and should, at the minimum, consist of individuals with empathy and a desire to undergo specific training in procedures such as recognizing psychological distress, having difficult conversations with peers, effective listening skills, and knowledge/facilitation to a higher level of care when necessary.

Personal Emergency Plans

When a hospital becomes a main treatment facility for a mass casualty incident, there is typically no or minimal warning. While it is important to prepare at an organizational level, it is equally important for employees to prepare at a personal level. Employees may also be parents or guardians, babysitters, caretakers to elderly or disabled relatives, neighbors, or friends, etc. When victims of a mass casualty incident arrive at the hospital, shifts get extended and other employees get called in early. As a result, personal emergency plans may need to be created and updated regularly. Personal emergency plans should include consideration of child care/ adult care arrangements (Sabbath et al., 2018) and the contact information of people who would need to be alerted in the event of an emergency. These contacts can be registered into an automated emergency communication system and serve to keep the staff's loved ones informed of their status without diverting time/attention from the emergency duties. Documentation of pre-existing medical conditions that may need to be monitored during a crisis, such as diabetes, heart and blood pressure related complications, etc. could also be advantageous so that the hospital pharmacy can supply the potential needs of the employees. Such advance planning will alleviate stress during an emergency situation. Plans should be established regardless of one's job description, perhaps by creating the plan during the hiring/on-boarding process and then updating these plans during their yearly reviews.

Within Incident Planning

During the initial response to a mass casualty incident, care of the victims is paramount and the most important action that ancillary services (such as mental wellness counselors) can take is not to get in the way of critical care. Therefore, even though the PFA team should be notified as quickly as possible of deployment to a site, until given permission to enter the hospital, the PFA team should focus on gathering supplies and preparing for engagement. This means that any interactions would only take place when a member of the hospital personnel is coming off of a shift or on a break.

Post-Incident

Dispatching the PFA Team

Once contacted, the PFA team should become visible to hospital personnel, victims' families, and survivors. Given the topic of this book, we will focus on interventions for medical personnel. The core actions of PFA are designed to be used at the site of an event in order to provide emotional stabilization and assure the presence of emotional support when individuals leave the scene. For a full description of PFA and an online training program, see the National Child Traumatic Stress Network website at nctsn.org.

Contact and Engagement. The goal is "to respond to contacts initiated by survivors, or to initiate contacts in a non-intrusive, compassionate and helpful manner" (Brymer et al., 2006, p. 19). Contact should never be made with individuals during the provision of medical services. Contact should be with personnel when they are leaving the hospital or are currently on break. Contact is as simple as offering food or something to drink.

Safety and Comfort. The goal is "to enhance immediate and ongoing safety and provide physical and emotional comfort" (Brymer et al., 2006, p.19). Therefore, an increase in security is imperative to ensure that only victims and designated support staff are entering the hospital. It is understandable that victims' families will be doing everything that they can to search for their loved ones, but in acts of desperation these family members may act rashly and potentially impact the safety of those attempting to save the lives of the victims. Here, a PFA team could assist in the coordination of designated media and family areas where other community support teams can be of assistance.

Stabilization. The goal is to "to calm and orient emotionally overwhelmed or distraught survivors" (Brymer et al., 2006, p.19). In the scope of this chapter, hospital personnel are conceptualized as survivors of the traumatic event as they are the ones witnessing and attending to the severity of the victim's injuries. As suggested previously, other community support teams should be dispatched to help victims and their families. The members of the PFA team should focus on assisting and monitoring the mental status following staff members being relieved of their duties, or while on break. It is especially important to look for signs of distress following the death of a pediatric case since these events often precipitate the most distress (Mishra et al., 2010). It is also critically important to remember that hospital personnel are not just first line medical workers but support staff and custodial services, who might have to clean the emergency room or operating rooms. It is custodial staff that are responsible for cleaning the blood from the floors, cafeteria staff are overhearing distressed victims' families and medical staff's stories, and medical examiners are facing extreme demands that they may have never experienced before (Brondolo et al., 2008). Thus, defining hospital personnel with this broad brush will often reveal individuals who may be overlooked or who have not had the prior training of physicians and nurses to deal with this level of trauma.

Information Gathering: Current Needs and Concerns. The goal is "to identify immediate needs and concerns, gather additional information, and tailor Psychological First Aid interventions" (Brymer et al., 2006, p.19). Translating this to the case of hospital personnel in the wake of a mass casualty event, the PFA member may offer to contact family members to advise of their status or offer to check on vulnerable family members, etc.

Practical Assistance. The goal is "to offer practical assistance to [hospital personnel] in addressing immediate needs and concerns" (Brymer et al., 2006, p. 19). Assistance is often in the form of tangible items, such as more hospital scrubs being brought in for both the medical personnel and the custodial staff so that they are not in blood-stained clothes any longer than they need to be. While food is essential, it is also important for everyone's dietary restrictions to be met. Setting up spaces for members of staff to allow for religious/spiritual activities may also be important.

Connection with Social Support. The goal is "to help establish brief or ongoing contact with primary support persons and other sources of support, including family members, friends, and community helping resources" (Brymer et al., 2006, p. 19). This could include assuring everyone's phones are fully charged. There may be situations in which cell phone towers are down or being overloaded with calls, therefore the members of the PFA team may need to come up with creative solutions in order to assist in getting in touch with loved ones. Additionally, it may be helpful to alert social supports of when a hospital worker's work break occurs so that they can be available to take the call.

Information on Coping. The goal is "to provide information about stress reactions and coping to reduce distress and promote adaptive functioning" (Brymer et al., 2006, p.19). It is important to convey the message that it is okay to not be okay, it is okay to be okay now and not be okay later, and it is okay to be unaffected.

Linkage with Collaborative Services. The goal is "to link [hospital personnel] with available services needed at the time or in the future" (Brymer et al., 2006, p.19).

Post Incident Planning

The first few days after an MCI are probably the most critical for establishing the availability and distribution of services for hospital personnel.

Debriefing

Debriefing, often conducted with law enforcement and fire personnel, is most often delivered between 24-72 hours of the traumatic event. During this session, trained peers assist in providing education about stress reactions and facilitate the discussion about the event (Neisler et al., 2020). While it may seem obvious to incorporate debriefing into post incident planning for medical personnel, debriefings should not be conducted with the goal of preventing posttraumatic stress disorder [PTSD; National Institute for Health and Care Excellence (NICE), 2018]. Scientific reviews (Anderson et al., 2020) indicate that debriefing can potentially make mental health symptoms worse over time or have no effect on mental health symptoms. Other organizations such as the North Atlantic Treaty Organization (NATO) also find that asking those who have just undergone a trauma to engage in a single-session intervention designed to elicit people's emotional reactions to the event poses the risk of re-traumatizing those affected and may impede the advantages of engaging in social support (NATO, 2009). An alternative to debriefings is Psychological First Aid, as referenced above.

Community Psychoeducation

Debriefings and PFA are most often directed toward people in direct contact with the mass casualty incident. However, the broader hospital or medical community may also feel the impact of these tragic events and may benefit from psychoeducation regarding trauma and its aftermath. Even if they were not directly affected by the event, they may be in close contact with someone who was impacted. Understanding the impact of such an event may allow them to provide support to affected family and friends. The content of psychoeducation efforts should include:

1. Basic information about traumatic events including how they are defined, types of traumas, and who are most likely to be affected by traumatic events.
2. Typical reactions to trauma – symptoms that are characteristic and expected to occur in the short term after a traumatic event. Most people are surprised that difficulty sleeping or eating, nightmares, and spending a lot of time thinking about the traumatic event are common and expected reactions to trauma in the days and weeks that follow the event.
3. The fact that some people will recover over the next few weeks or months and that some people recover without intervention.
4. How to talk to children about the event – broken down by age groups.
5. Simple things that friends and family can do. Offer childcare, shop for their groceries, take their dog for a walk. Simple things that can help alleviate their stress and show care and concern.

Peer Support

The utilization of peer support has a significant scientific literature supporting its use (Anderson et al., 2020) and has gained acceptance by some professions in the emergency healthcare field, such as nurses (Lavoie et al., 2010). Peer support should begin as soon as possible following an incident. Peer support teams offer assistance individually and in a group environment and are trained to determine if someone needs additional mental health assistance beyond what the team can provide. That team member can then assist the individual with referrals for a higher level of care. Peer support is so beneficial because it allows for members of the support team to normalize what the staff is experiencing and helps to improve social functioning (Repper & Carter, 2011), promote hope (Repper & Carter, 2011), and reduce the stigma around disclosure of negative mental health symptoms one may be experiencing (Milliard, 2020).

Follow-Up Screening

Exposure to trauma results in a variety of potential responses and initially, those reactions may help the individual adapt and cope. For example, engagement in emotional avoidance can aid in the ability to focus on the provision of medical care without emotional interference (Minnie et al., 2015). However, for some, these responses become intrusive and distressing (Center for Substance Abuse Treatment, 2015), particularly over time. In order to monitor employee reactions over time, psychological screenings, conducted at standard intervals may be effective in allowing employees, as well as healthcare professionals, to monitor their own symptoms. Screenings can be voluntary, or in some cases, mandated by employers. One way to screen individuals is through the use of web-based surveys that may be conducted by a third-party, such as an EAP mental wellness partner. Arrangements can be made where only the third party has knowledge of the participant completing the survey and therefore can reach out confidentially to the individual should the survey responses indicate severe distress or the intention to harm self or others. Individuals who decide to participate in monthly surveys could provide a personal email where the survey link could be sent, thus eliminating the need to use an employer-provided email. Emergency contacts, such as suicide crisis telephone lines or text lines can be embedded within the surveys to be sure that individuals in crisis have immediate access to emergency mental wellness resources. Consistent monitoring, perhaps for the first-year post-incident, could potentially mitigate the most severe reactions and prevent the onset of disorders such as PTSD, substance abuse or severe depression.

FUTURE RESEARCH DIRECTIONS

Given that the prevalence of mass casualty incidents is not expected to decline, preparation for these events in medical settings is paramount. Adoption of education around signs and symptoms of trauma, as well as mitigation of trauma symptoms should become a standard part of the curriculum for all those pursuing an advanced degree in the healthcare field. This training should also be continuously provided at hospitals and medical settings that have the potential to treat victims of a mass casualty incident. Additionally, national standards should be implemented with respect to trauma mitigation efforts and treatment plans for hospital personnel.

CONCLUSION

In conclusion, while mass casualty incidents are unpredictable, there are preparations that can be taken to mitigate the potential negative emotional impacts on medical staff. These preparations start during a health care worker's training to enter the profession, with education about emotional responses to traumatic events and how to mitigate them. It is recommended that preparations then continue into employment for all hospital personnel through pre-incident drills, the creation of PFA and Peer Support teams, and the development of personal emergency plans. Once an MCI has occurred, the PFA and peer support teams should be mobilized to establish the multi-step plan outlined above, with continued implementation in the following days. In conjunction, psychoeducation should be offered to the broader medical staff community, providing information on trauma and how to help those affected. Finally, follow-up screenings at regular intervals should be offered to monitor the long-term effects in the aftermath of these traumatic events.

REFERENCES

Anderson, G. S., Di Nota, P. M., Groll, D., & Carleton, R. N. (2020). Peer support and crisis-focused psychological interventions designed to mitigate post-traumatic stress injuries among public safety and frontline healthcare personnel: A systematic review. *International Journal of Environmental Research and Public Health, 17*(20), 7645. doi:10.3390/ijerph17207645 PMID:33092146

Brondolo, E., Wellington, R., Brady, N., Libby, D., & Brondolo, T. J. (2008). Mechanism and strategies for preventing post-traumatic stress disorder in forensic workers responding to mass fatality incidents. *Journal of Forensic and Legal Medicine, 15*(2), 78–88. doi:10.1016/j.jflm.2007.04.007 PMID:18206823

Bryan, C. J., Mintz, J., Clemans, T. A., Leeson, B., Burch, T. S., Williams, S. R., Maney, E., & Rudd, M. D. (2017). Effect of crisis response planning vs. contracts for safety on suicide risk in U.S. Army Soldiers: A randomized clinical trial. *Journal of Affective Disorders, 212*, 64–72. doi:10.1016/j.jad.2017.01.028 PMID:28142085

Brymer, M., Layne, C., Jacobs, A., Pynoos, R., Ruzek, J., Steinberg, A., . . . Watson, P. (2006). *Psychological first aid field operations guide.* National Child Traumatic Stress Network. Available from: https://www.nctsn.org/resources/psychological-first-aid-pfa-field-operations-guide-2nd-edition

Center for Substance Abuse Treatment (US), Trauma-Informed Care in Behavioral Health Services, Substance Abuse and Mental Health Services Administration (US). (2014). *Treatment Improvement Protocol (TIP) Series, No. 57. Chapter 3, Understanding the Impact of Trauma.* Available from: https://www.ncbi.nlm.nih.gov/books/NBK207191/

Connors, C. A., Dukhanin, V., March, A. L., Parks, J. A., Norvell, M., & Wu, A. W. (2020). Peer support for nurses as second victims: Resilience, burnout, and job satisfaction. *Journal of Patient Safety and Risk Management, 25*(1), 22–28. doi:10.1177/2516043519882517

Cyr, C., McKee, H., O'Hagan, M., & Priest, R. (2016). *Making the Case for Peer Support: Report to the Peer Support Project Committee of the Mental Health Commission of Canada*. Mental Health Commission of Canada. Available online https://www.mentalhealthcommission.ca/sites/default/files/2016-07/MHCC_Making_the_Case_for_Peer_Support_2016_Eng.pdf

Delucia, J. (2016, May 10-13) *Rate of post-traumatic stress disorder in emergency medicine physicians*. Society of Academic Emergency Medicine meeting, New Orleans, LA.

Gun Violence Archive. (2021). Retrieved from https://www.gunviolencearchive.org/

Hodgson, L. (2021). How violent attacks are changing the demands of mass casualty incidents: A review of the challenges associated with intentional mass casualty incidents. *The Journal of the NPS Center for Homeland Defense and Security*, *17*(1). https://www.hsaj.org/articles/16880

Jones, S. (2017). Describing the mental health profile of first responders: A systematic review. *Journal of the American Psychiatric Nurses Association*, *23*(3), 200–214. doi:10.1177/1078390317695266 PMID:28445653

Lavoie, S., Talbot, L. R., & Mathieu, L. (2011). Post-traumatic stress disorder symptoms among emergency nurses: Their perspective and a 'tailor-made' solution. *Journal of Advanced Nursing*, *67*(7), 1514–1522. doi:10.1111/j.1365-2648.2010.05584.x PMID:21323975

Mass Shooting Tracker. (2021). Retrieved from https://www.massshootingtracker.site/

Milliard, B. (2020). Utilization and impact of peer-support programs on police officers' mental health. *Frontiers in Psychology*, *11*, 1686. doi:10.3389/fpsyg.2020.01686 PMID:32765375

Mills, L., & Mills, T. (2005). Symptoms of post-traumatic stress disorder among emergency medicine residents. *The Journal of Emergency Medicine*, *28*(1), 1–4. doi:10.1016/j.jemermed.2004.05.009 PMID:15656996

Minnie, L., Goodman, S., & Wallis, L. (2015). Exposure to daily trauma: The experiences and coping mechanism of Emergency Medical Personnel. A cross-sectional study. *African Journal of Emergency Medicine*, *5*(1), 12–18. doi:10.1016/j.afjem.2014.10.010 PMID:30456058

Mishra, S., Goebert, D., Char, E., Dukes, P., & Ahmed, I. (2010). Trauma exposure and symptoms of post-traumatic stress disorder in emergency medical services personnel in Hawaii. *Emergency Medicine Journal, 27*(9), 708–711. doi:10.1136/emj.2009.080622

National Collaborating Centre for Mental Health (UK). (2005). *Post-Traumatic Stress Disorder: The Management of PTSD in Adults and Children in Primary and Secondary Care*. Gaskell. Available from: https://www.ncbi.nlm.nih.gov/books/NBK56494/

Neisler, K., Rosado, N., & Beidel, D. C. (2020). Changing Hearts and Minds: Getting Administrative Support for Delivery of Care. In C. Bowers, D. Beidel, & M. Marks (Eds.), *Mental Health Intervention and Treatment of First Responders and Emergency Workers* (pp. 291–301). IGI Global. doi:10.4018/978-1-5225-9803-9.ch017

Paturel, A. (2019). *When physicians are traumatized.* American Association of Medical Colleges News. Available from: https://www.aamc.org/news-insights/when-physicians-are-traumatized

Repper, J., & Carter, T. (2011). A review of the literature on peer support in mental health services. *Journal of Mental Health (Abingdon, England)*, *20*(4), 392–411. doi:10.3109/09638237.2011.583947 PMID:21770786

Ruzek, J. I., Brymer, M. J., Jacobs, A. K., Layne, C. M., Vernberg, E. M., Patricia, J., & Watson, P. J. (2007). Psychological First Aid. *Journal of Mental Health Counseling*, *29*(1), 17–49. doi:10.17744/mehc.29.1.5racqxjueafabgwp

Sabbath, E. L., Shaw, J., Stidsen, A., & Hashimoto, D. (2018). Protecting Mental Health of Hospital Workers after Mass Casualty Events: A Social Work Imperative. *Social Work*, *63*(3), 272–275. doi:10.1093wwy029 PMID:29701847

Schmerling, R. H. (2020). *First, do no harm.* Harvard Health Publishing. https://www.health.harvard.edu/blog/first-do-no-harm-201510138421

Sendler, D., Rutkowska, A., & Makara-Studzinska, M. (2016). How the exposure to trauma has hindered physician's capacity to heal: Prevalence of PTSD among healthcare workers. *European Journal of Psychiatry*, *30*(4), 321–334. doi:10.7490/f1000research.1111861.1

Sofer, D. (2018). Responding to Mass Shootings: Are Hospitals and Nurses Fully Prepared? *The American Journal of Nursing*, *118*(9), 18–19. doi:10.1097/01.NAJ.0000544970.28486.90 PMID:30138194

Stanley, B., & Brown, G. K. (2012). Safety planning intervention: A brief intervention to mitigate suicide risk. *Cognitive and Behavioral Practice*, *19*(2), 256–264. doi:10.1016/j.cbpra.2011.01.001

U.S. Department of Veterans Affairs. (2018, September 24). *How Common is PTSD in Veterans.* National Center for PTSD. https://www.ptsd.va.gov/understand/common/common_veterans.asp

Vanyo, L., Sorge, R., Chen, A., & Lakoff, D. (2017). Posttraumatic stress disorder in emergency medicine residents. *Annals of Emergency Medicine*, *70*(6), 898–903. doi:10.1016/j.annemergmed.2017.07.010 PMID:28826753

KEY TERMS AND DEFINITIONS

Crisis Response Plan (CRP): A behavioral intervention plan that is personalized to the individual to be used when they are experiencing a crisis.

Debriefing: An organized meeting that takes place 24-72 hours after a traumatic event in which trained peers facilitate education about stress reactions and facilitate discussions about the event.

Mass Casualty Incident: An event where the number and severity of injured victims exceeds the resources available to treat the victims.

Hospital Personnel: Any staff member of a hospital that is treating victims of an MCI.

Peer-Support: Peers formally trained to provide support around mental health needs to those of equal employment status following exposure to a traumatic event.

Posttraumatic Stress Disorder (PTSD): A mental health disorder that can result from exposure, or repeated exposures to traumatic events.

Traumatic Event: An event in which someone is exposed to death, injury, sexual violence, or the threat of any of these. The event can either be through direct exposure, such as witnessing the event, or it can be through learning of such an event happening to someone the person is close to.

Chapter 15
Team Resilience in Healthcare

Jonah Swinson
University of Central Florida, USA

Clint Bowers
University of Central Florida, USA

Jan Canon-Bowers
Cannon-Bowers Consulting, USA

ABSTRACT

This chapter focuses on the broader topic of team resiliency within the healthcare profession. Specifically, the authors discuss the current body of literature relating to healthcare teams, the concept of team resilience, and its potential application within the field of healthcare. Moreover, the authors propose different means of developing team resilience within healthcare teams including the theoretical application of an existing team resilience model to the healthcare profession. Lastly, suggestions are provided for future research that could help to develop the body of knowledge related to the topic.

INTRODUCTION

Although healthcare has always been a stressful environment, the Covid pandemic has not only increased that stress dramatically but revealed the mental health consequences of the hospital work environment. A variety of negative mental health outcomes have been linked to the stress of the healthcare work environment (Schreffler, Petrey, & Huecker, 2020). These include depression and anxiety (Liang et al, 2020), burnout (Wu, et al., 2020), and sleep disturbance (Huang & Zhao, 2020). Even prior to the pandemic researchers feared that the psychological consequences of the stress associated with healthcare presented an upcoming crisis (Mateen & Dorji, 2009). This concern has risen exponentially due to Covid.

While maintaining the health of frontline workers is of paramount importance, it is equally important to maintain their performance. Healthcare workers perform critical activities. Even small errors can have disastrous consequences. The stressors noted above can lead to an increase in medical errors. Furthermore, changes to the work environment necessitated by Covid further increase the risk of error.

DOI: 10.4018/978-1-7998-8813-0.ch015

Hospital personnel have been moved to settings with which they may be unfamiliar. Furthermore, workers have been re-assigned to positions with which they may be unfamiliar. This increases the risk of both individual and team-based errors (Ellis, Hay-David, & Brennan, 2020). The effects of workplace on the health and performance of medical teams have gone largely overlooked during the pandemic, but there can be little doubt that the pandemic has increased the challenges confronted by these teams. Furthermore, changes due to the pandemic may also have increased the difficulty of using the team processes that have been shown to mitigate stress effects. Therefore, in this chapter we will explore these issues with an eye towards identifying factors that may help healthcare teams to be resilient during these difficult times.

HEALTHCARE TEAMS

Teamwork has emerged as an important factor in increasing the quality of healthcare, as well as a critical element in reducing medical error (Rosen, et al., 2018). Team members must be able to coordinate their activities to provide effective, efficient care. Communication is critical during many phases of care such as transitioning from one unit to another, communication among team members during surgery, and when providing information to the patient.

Over and above communication, effective teamwork behaviors such as leadership, planning, situation awareness, and assertiveness are all critical in identifying and preventing errors and allowing team members to all work using a "shared mental model" (Cannon-Bowers, 2007). In so doing team members can work together effectively in the absence of explicit communication.

The recent Covid-19 pandemic has shed further light on the potential benefits of healthcare teams (Cheng,et. al., 2020). During the pandemic, an intervention was implemented within a medical team consisting of doctors, nurses, and staff members where the team could rely on one another through means such as peer support, after work social gatherings (i.e., sporting events), and daily measurements of the team members' mood. Despite the demands of the pandemic, the team reported a generally positive outlook over the course of six weeks. Through these means, the team was able to rely on one another as a means of monitoring one another's mental well-being in a difficult circumstance.

While there are benefits to working in healthcare teams, teamwork can also be difficult. Team members often come together relatively quickly and may be unfamiliar with one another. Many healthcare workers have not had specific training in effective teamwork. Furthermore, the Covid pandemic has made team processes more difficult in many cases. For example, personal protective equipment such as masks and face shields may make it harder to speak. Additionally, non-verbal communication may be severely curtailed. Reduced communication can result in downstream issues such as poorer decision making and reduced situation awareness (Ellis, Hay-David, & Brennan, 2020). New settings may induce role ambiguity, leading a breakdown of team processes

Bosch and Mansell (2015) point to the notion that adversity is going to be present anytime people are going to work together in healthcare teams. However, a team should be able to overcome difficulties without inhibiting performance (Bowers et. al, 2017). Alliger et. al (2015) argue resilience is necessary for a team to be able to perform consistently in a difficult environment. Considering the number of adverse events faced in healthcare, the propensity to work in teams, and the necessity of resilience to ensure team's performance in troublesome environments, it appears to be vital to take steps aimed at fostering team resilience for healthcare professionals.

RESILIENCE

Prior to understanding the concept of team resilience, it is useful to understand the broader concept of resilience as a whole. In an effort to conceptualize resilience, Fletcher and Sarkar (2013) identified two foundational concepts, adversity and positive adaptation, that appear in the literature to be crucial in understanding resilience. The authors went further in defining resilience as the "role of mental processes and behavior in promoting personal assets and protecting an individual from the potential negative effect of stressors (Fletcher & Sarkar, 2013, p. 16).

In more recent attempts to further clarify key characteristics of resilience, Ijntema, Burger, & Shaufeli (2019) distinguish psychological resilience as a cognitive process that does not incorporate physical characteristics. Essentially, in discussing resilience in this capacity, researchers are only interested in the mental aspects related to resilience rather than the physical characteristics. For example, if a bodybuilder is attempting to get stronger by deadlifting, and he or she has an injury that results from a ripped callous. The researcher studying psychological resilience would not be interested in the physical response from adversity (i.e., the new, tougher callous that forms on the lifter's hand.) Rather, the researcher is interested in the cognitive response required from the lifter in order to continue improving despite the new adversity of the hand injury.

Stovernik et. al (2020) highlight the difference between being resilient and demonstrating resiliency. Demonstrations of resiliency require adversity whereas being resilience does not. Remember, adversity was identified as one of the key foundational concepts of resiliency according to Fletcher and Sarkar (2013). Relating back to our previous example of the bodybuilder. The lifter was resilient prior to his or her injury. He or she had the capacity to successfully overcome the injury to his or her hand. However, the resiliency was not demonstrated until the injury (i.e., the adversity) was introduced into the equation.

Team Resilience

With a rudimentary understanding of the broader topic of resilience, team resilience can likely be more easily understood. Team resilience research is in its earlier stages (Chapman et. al, 2020). Moreover, Alliger et. al (2015) indicate that more research has been devoted to individual resilience as opposed to team resilience. First, it is important to understand that collections of individually resilient people do not necessarily result in a resilient team (Alliger et. al, 2015). For example, the team could be horrendous at communicating with one another or there could be consistent quarrels over who gets to be the team leader.

Furthermore, Alliger et. al (2015) note key actions taken by resilient teams that help to lay an early foundation of what it means for a team to be resilient and to potentially become more resilient. The authors argue that the actions of resilient teams can be dissected into three distinct parts (minimizing, managing, and mending). These three actions can be categorized based on when they occur in relation to the adverse scenario. Minimizing actions are anticipatory and result from foresight and planning in order to prevent adverse scenarios or significantly mitigate their effects. An example of this sort of action would be a surgery team sitting down prior to a pending surgery to discuss the necessary actions to take in order to ensure that a foreign object does not accidentally get left inside the patient.

The second class of actions performed by resilient teams can be described as managing actions (Alliger et. al, 2015). These sorts of actions occur during the adverse situation in order to effectively navigate whatever obstacle the team is facing. For example, if the hospital is overrun with patients and one nurse is becoming overwhelmed by the massive patient load, another nurse on the team with a lighter load could step in and help his or her overwhelmed teammate. The final classification of actions of a resilient team identified by Alliger et. al (2015) is labeled as mending actions. These represent the means to which a team will go in order to recover from and prevent future adverse scenarios. In the example of the overwhelmed nursing team, mending actions could include going through a debrief in order to make sure that the team does not become overwhelmed in future scenarios.

Stovernik et. al (2020) further discuss the actions of resilient teams by indicating two forms of effective responses to setbacks taken by teams. Those two forms are adapting current actions and perseverance. Interestingly, those two actions are in direct contrast to one another, yet according to the authors, can both produce an effective response. Again, imagine a team of nurses that is facing an unusually high demand due to the number of patients admitted at the hospital. The team is under a great deal of stress, and there is little time between patients to do any sort of decompression. In responding to this adversity, the solution to the circumstance is either to continue operating how they normally operate and trusting the system that is in place, or making adjustments to their normal operating procedures in order to effectively address their unusually large patient load. However, the authors also discuss the potential for conflict to arise when teams must decide whether to persist or adapt.

Development of Team Resilience

Following establishing an understanding of the concept of team resilience as well as providing a justification as to why it is important to a population of healthcare professionals, the attention can then be shifted towards how team resilience in healthcare can be developed. Unfortunately, the body of research devoted to fostering team resilience in healthcare is rather limited. This is not surprising considering that team resilience remains in its earlier stages (Chapman et. al, 2020). However, there have been findings from examinations of team resilience in other contexts that could prove to be useful. For example, a narrative analysis of world championship rugby athletes identified characteristics that helped to foster team resilience in a sporting capacity (Morgan, Fletcher, & Sarkar, 2015). Some of the key factors in developing team resilience that the authors found included learning from previous experiences, sharing leadership responsibilities, maintaining positive emotions, and developing a social identity.

Also from the sporting context, Sarkar and Page (2020) outlined recommendations for developing team resilience in sport. These recommendations included transformational leadership, sharing leadership tasks, developing an identity, learning as a team, and bolstering team enjoyment. In looking at team resilience in the workplace, Vera, Rodriguez-Sanchez, and Salanova (2017) posit that crucial factors for developing team resilience are teamwork, collective efficacy, and transformational leadership. While this research is derived from a context outside of healthcare, there is considerable overlap in the key areas proposed as targets for interventions across different contexts that could prove useful to the healthcare setting.

Conceptual Model of Team Resilience

While understanding certain actions or characteristics of resilient teams can serve as a useful starting point for fully understanding the topic and deciphering ways in which to actually foster team resilience in a given population, it still leaves unknown factors such as causes, methods of development, or moderating variables. In an effort to provide further clarity on the topic, Bowers et. al (2017) formulate a conceptual model of team resilience in which team resilience is conceptualized as a second order emergent state (see Fig. 1). This conceptualization signifies that team resilience can be best understood as something that is prone to fluctuation and comprised by lower order factors.

The model Bowers et. al (2017) propose is comprised of five different levels. Those levels consist of inputs at the individual, team, and organizational level, processes at the individual, team, and organizational level, first order emergent states), second order emergent state (team resilience), and outcome variables at the individual, team, and organizational level. Individual factors include issues such personality, coping ability, faith, and mental toughness. Team-level inputs include variables such as trust, implicit and explicit communication, psychological safety, and assertiveness. Organizational factors include adaptive capacity, attitudes towards failure, and situation awareness. Bowers et al. (2017) argue that these factors interact with individual and team processes to create an environment where certain helpful first-order states might emerge. These first-order states include important pre-conditions for team resilience. They include important states such as team cohesion, collective efficacy, shared mental models, and adaptability. These first-order states combine to create conditions favorable to the emergence of team resilience. The emergence of the team resilience state is hypotheses to lead to positive outcomes for the individual (e.g., increased perceived social support, improved psychological health), the team (e.g., improved performance, error avoidance), and the organization (e.g. goal attainment).

IMPLEMENTING THE CONCEPTUAL MODEL IN HEALTHCARE

While the previously provided means of developing team resilience are somewhat vague and theoretical, the second order emergent state model provided by Bowers et. al (2017) can potentially provide insight into the development of team resilience and its desired effects through intervening at the lower levels and hoping for a downstream effect. The following are some potential approaches that, drawing from the model, could facilitate the emergence of team resilience in healthcare teams.

Individual Inputs

Personality

Researchers from a variety of disciplines have attempted to identify personality variables that are associated with the ability to remain resilient in the face of stressors. The goal of this work is to, potentially, identify personality factors that would either allow us to select personnel that are best able to cope with the demands of the healthcare workplace or identify those that may need additional support during times of stress. For example, a study of emergency room nurses found that those high in extroversion were best able to cope with workplace stress, while those high in neuroticism were at risk for adverse impacts (Hsieh et al., 2015). Neuroticism was also identified as a risk factor in a study of paramedics (Froutan et al., 2017). These researchers also found that extraversion and conscientiousness were positively related to resilience. Recently, researchers have also implicated “Type D” personality traits as factors in individual resilience (cf. Cho & Kang, 2017; Lim, Noh, & Jeong 2016). Type D personality involves a constellation of factors that indicate a predisposition towards feelings of distress (e.g., worry, irritability; Denollet, 2005). Although this construct requires more research, it might be useful in accomplishing the goals stated above.

Perseverance

As previously discussed, Stovernik et. al (2020) identify two distinct ways in which a team with resilience could respond to an adverse scenario: adapting the current behaviors of the team and persevering through the particular hardship. Therefore, it stands to reason that an individual within the healthcare team should display a certain level of competency in his or her ability to persevere in adverse scenarios. A qualitative study consisting of 30 individuals with experience in interprofessional healthcare teams within the military identified six ways in which perseverance was displayed within these healthcare teams including humility, maintaining focus on the team's mission, working together as a team, refusing failure, being comfortable in uncomfortable situations, and focusing on improving (Meyer et. al, 2021). While the initial characteristics refer to the team's functioning as a whole, the latter three characteristics represent tasks on which an individual working within the team can focus. Identifying individuals that possess these characteristics as well as improving upon these aspects in current team members could potentially improve the individual's perseverance and potentially have downstream effects on the team's resiliency.

Future research related to perseverance in healthcare could build upon the findings of Meyer et. al, (2021). While Meyer et. al (2021) identify key characteristics associated with military healthcare teams, researchers could further this line of inquiry to determine if those characteristics remain consistent in civilian healthcare teams. Moreover, it could be useful to understand if certain factors are more conducive to developing perseverance than others. Lastly, researchers could identify if certain characteristics related to the broader factor of perseverance are better suited for addressing certain adverse scenarios. Then, interventions designed to foster perseverance could target an individual's perseverance related deficiencies and tailor interventions to his or her needs.

Hardiness

Research has shown that nurses that are found to have increased hardiness report that they have less perceived stress and higher satisfaction from their occupation in comparison to nurses with less hardiness (Judkins & Rind, 2005). Moreover, in a sample of nurses working during the Mers-Cov epidemic, hardiness was found to have an effect on mental health. In order to actually develop this characteristic, Judkins and Rind (2005) suggest that understanding hardiness levels in employees can aid in understanding which individuals may need special attention regarding areas such as job satisfaction, strategies to reduce perceived stress levels, and developing abilities to problem solve. Moreover, it was suggested those who are hardier could assist their colleagues who are not.

Regarding future research directions for hardiness in healthcare, Judkins and Rind (2005) posit that those who have higher levels of hardiness could assist colleagues with less hardiness. This could potentially be facilitative to hospitals due to the potential ease and lowered cost relative to hiring outside individuals to foster hardiness in healthcare staff. Future research could devote itself to finding ways in which this sort of peer mentorship could be developed and implemented within healthcare settings. For example, educational interventions could be developed that are aimed at teaching staff how to identify those who are not as hardy as well as ways for mentors to encourage that characteristics' development.

Self-Esteem

Valizadeh et. al (2016) identified such factors as gaining knowledge, spirituality, and a desire to be involved in a nursing career as assets that protected the self-esteem of a sample of nursing students as well as students who had recently graduated. Moreover, self-esteem was presented as something that was a dynamic characteristic (Valizadeh et. al, 2016). Therefore, the identified protective factors, like many of the previously identified characteristics, could be used as potential screening or for identifying individuals who may be at elevated risk. However, these could also be areas in which one encourages improvement. Rather than merely accepting the current self-esteem levels of healthcare team members, the development of that characteristic could be encouraged and modeled.

While Valizadeh et. al (2016) argue that self-esteem is a characteristic that can be fostered in healthcare workers, future research could be devoted to actually developing this particular factor. Researchers could potentially focus their attention to certain questions such as if certain occupations within the field tend to derive self-esteem from different sources than others. Moreover, are certain factors that contribute to self-esteem more valuable than others? Lastly, what are the most effective methods of fostering this trait in the given population? Answering these questions could elevate the current body of literature as well as provide useful information for the field.

Optimism

Luthans et. al (2008) found that nurses with higher levels of optimism received better performance evaluations from their supervisors as well as being reported as more committed to the hospital's overall mission. Moreover, more proactive coping and optimistic views have shown to be related to lower reported levels of burnout (Chang & Chan, 2015). Chang and Chan (2015) report that those with higher levels of optimism indicate less emotional exhaustion in comparison to those with less optimism. Interestingly, Luthans et. al (2008) found higher levels of optimism to be related with more years of education. The authors argue that this relationship points to the idea that rather than optimism being a stable trait, it is a characteristic that can be improved upon through further training and development. As a means of developing levels of optimism, Chang and Chan (2015) posit that optimism should be encouraged within healthcare staff and even proposed education interventions geared towards enhancing optimism amongst healthcare professionals.

While the outcome measures provided by Luthans et. al (2008) yield promising results in reference to the outcomes afforded through optimism in healthcare workers, these outcomes were based on subjective reporting. Future research should seek to provide a more objective means of evaluating the benefits that optimism can provide. For example, are there less incidents, an ability to take on more patients, or less complaints filed against those employees with more as opposed to less optimism? Providing objective reports could enhance the current body of literature relating to optimism in healthcare.

Coping

Research has identified multiple means in which healthcare professionals cope with the stress of their occupations (Anton et. al, 2015; Healy & McKay, 2000). Anton et. al (2015) report that a sample of surgeons indicated a wide range of coping strategies as a means of coping with stress ranging from facilitative strategies such as deep breathing to non-facilitative coping strategies such as yelling. Moreover,

Healy and McKay (2000) note that in a sample of nurses, the primary coping strategy employed was problem solving. The next most popular strategy was attempting to find some means of social support, and the least commonly implemented coping strategy used by the nurses was avoiding the issue altogether. Furthermore, the type of coping strategy that one employs is related to how he or she views the adverse scenario, and not all coping strategies lead to the same outcomes (Healy and McKay 2000). For example, the authors found that use of avoidance as a means of coping with stress was related to worse outcomes relative to the participants' mood. Therefore, identification and encouragement of effective coping strategies within the healthcare workers could be an effective means of ensuring the members within the team are effectively responding to stress.

The coping strategies employed by surgeons provided by Anton et. al (2015) did not directly mirror the strategies employed by nurses as indicated by Healy and McKay (2000). Moreover, Healy and McKay (2000) argue that different strategies did not all result in identical outcomes. Therefore, future research could be devoted to understanding which particular coping strategies are ideal for producing the desired outcomes within the profession. Moreover, it could be helpful to understand if different strategies are better suited to certain circumstances or certain occupations within the broader field. For example, is there a coping strategy that helps a surgeon who hit an artery that may not be as helpful for a physician that is forced to treat an unusually large number of patients?

Mental Toughness

While the current literature focusing on developing mental toughness within a population of healthcare professionals appears somewhat limited, literature from other contexts could provide useful information regarding development. In providing recommendations for fostering mental toughness in athletes, Crust and Clough (2011) encourage the individual to be challenged. Through these challenging situations, the individual is able to manufacture coping skills for difficult situations (Crust & Clough, 2011). Furthermore, Crust and Clough (2011), encourage leaders not to merely provide top-down solutions but to allow for the individual to learn through problem-solving, and the authors advise that mistakes made should be seen as a chance to learn and grow as a healthcare professional. Interestingly, many of the individual input factors discussed serve as a means for selection and identification of employees who may need additional assistance. Contrastingly, mental toughness could be an area for growth and development within the individual as well as the healthcare team.

While borrowing recommendations from other contexts could be useful, further research would be required in order to tailor the recommendations to the healthcare field. For example, Crust and Clough (2011) advise introducing challenging situations as a means of fostering mental toughness. However, more information would likely be required in how to do this in an ethical and practical manner within the healthcare field in order to not cause unnecessary harm to the patients. Furthermore, it would be essential to understand if recommendations provided for another context and population truly carry over to the healthcare profession. If not, future research could identify means of fostering mental toughness more suited to the healthcare profession.

Overall, many of the individual input factors affect how the member of the healthcare team both views and reacts to the adverse scenarios that he or she will encounter on the job (e.g., Kuiper et. al, 1995; Healy & McKay, 2000). Some of the input factors, such as personality, represent more solidified traits that could be the object of initial screenings and identification of employees who are at increased risk. Conversely, some of the other factors, such as mental toughness, have been described as characteristics that are able to be fostered and developed over time (Crust and Clough, 2011). Given the implicit flow in. the Bowers et. al (2017) secondary order emergent state model of team resilience, identification and enhancement of these characteristics have the potential for downstream effect in order to reach the desired outcome goals by means of fostering team resilience.

Individual Processes

Contrasting the individual input factors that primarily comprise individual characteristics or traits, the individual processes comprise tasks or actions that an individual healthcare professional could complete (Bowers et.al, 2017). While not encompassing the entire list of individual processes, the following list serves to provide further examples of potential points of intervention that could potentially serve the overarching purpose of fostering team resilience by impacting first order and second order emergent states.

Mindfulness

In a systematic review examining the effects of mindfulness on healthcare workers Lomas et. al (2018) found that mindfulness could be beneficial in addressing a number of factors contributing to overall mental well-being in healthcare workers including anxiety, depression, and stress levels. Burton et. al (2017) completed a meta-analysis revealing that mindfulness has been shown to have a medium effect on stress levels within the population of healthcare professionals. However, Burton et. al (2017) continue by indicating that mindfulness is a practice that requires a considerable amount of buy-in on behalf of the participant. This combined with the medium effect size suggests that mindfulness might not be a solution that is proscribed to the entire population. Rather, it could potentially be a solution for individuals who have been identified, through means previously discussed, as being particularly at risk for harmful effects of workplace stress and adverse scenarios.

Burton et. al (2017) recommend that future research concerning mindfulness in healthcare professionals should focus attention towards the development of means of implementing mindfulness in a manner that does not require the amount of time that it currently does. From a policy standpoint, this could reduce the amount of time that valuable workers are taken away from their position in order to develop the skill. Moreover, Lomas et. al (2018) argue that the effects of mindfulness on burnout in a sample of healthcare workers are somewhat vague. Future research could dedicate efforts towards increased understanding of this particular relationship in order to understand if mindfulness can be implemented in order to combat the negative impacts of burnout.

Social Support

Research has suggested that social support has the potential to mitigate the harmful effects of burnout in populations of healthcare workers (Woodhead et. al, 2016; Jenkins & Elliot, 2004). Jenkins and Elliot (2004) found that more support from colleagues resulted in less perceived emotional exhaustion. Moreover, Woodhead et. al (2016) found that support for healthcare workers came from both within the job (i.e., supervisors) as well as outside the job (i.e., families and friends). This implies that those members of the healthcare team that may not have adequate available social support outside the workplace might require additional social support while on the job due to a lack of social support from other areas. It was also argued that when dealing with populations of healthcare professionals, it may be insufficient to merely have the means of social support available. Woodhead et. al (2016) contend that people might require learning on how to actually accept the social support when it is available to them. Lastly, Jenkins and Elliot (2004) posit that it is important that social groups consisting of fellow colleagues need to reduce the level of discussing the job in a negative manner as opposed to addressing the issues more productively in order to achieve the desired results.

While this research can serve as preliminary understanding of social support within healthcare populations, future research could seek to further the existing literature to answer key questions about the topic. While Woodhead et. al (2016) identified that social support for healthcare workers can come from multiple different sources, it could be beneficial to understand how the different sources relate to one another in their ability to foster social support. For example, is support coming from supervisors more facilitative than support coming from friends? Moreover, when Jenkins and Elliot (2004) advise against negativity in social support circles, but how can this be implemented at a policy level without becoming overbearing and overly restricting the staff? Answers to these questions could increase current understanding of the topic.

Mental Simulation

As it relates to the overarching goal of fostering team resilience, Alliger et. al (2015) provide means in which mental simulation can be employed in order to improve resilience. While the recommendations provided are directed at a team level, certain behaviors could be implemented individually. One such recommendation for improving resiliency through mental simulation would be contingency planning (Alliger et. al, 2015). This involves devising plans for ways to resolve issues that have either happened previously or could potentially occur in the future. For example, the individual could imagine being overextended with the number of patients to whom he or she has to attend or having insufficient sleep due to being on call. The individual would then be forced to imagine ways to effectively respond to the adverse scenario. In this manner, the individual employs his or imagination to develop methods for coping with issues before they actually occur.

Regarding the implementation of contingency planning as a means of mental stimulation geared towards fostering resilience in healthcare workers, the action itself is somewhat broad and theoretical. Future research could be aimed at developing specific plans not only to implement this activity, but to develop the ability within personnel. Within the population of healthcare workers, future research could seek to identify if there are any specific issues that arise as well as specific complications for contingency planning within given subsets of the population (e.g., nurses, surgeons, or physicians). Moreover, are certain training or educational programs more effective in developing this capability than others? Nevertheless, contingency planning through the implementation of mental simulation remains a cost-efficient option with the potential to foster team resilience in healthcare professionals (Alliger et. al, 2015).

Stress Management

Some of the previously discussed factors related to individual inputs and processes have already touched on the topic of stress management (e.g., coping skills, humor, and mindfulness). Nevertheless, it remains a topic that warrants further consideration. In a study related to coping strategies in a population of surgeons, the majority of participants reported that there was a particular need for training related to managing stress (Anton et. al, 2015). Relative to the type of stress for which stress management training is potentially required, Woodhead et. al (2016) found that a sample of nurses reported higher levels of stress related to their everyday lives in comparison to the perceived stress relative to their jobs. Therefore, means of managing stress should not be solely directed to stress faced due to their occupation. Specific means and characteristics related to effectively managing stress in a healthcare population can be seen in other sections devoted to individual input and processes such as coping skills, social support, and mindfulness.

Team Inputs

Trust

Bowers et al. (2017) suggest several input factors at the team level that may contribute to the emergence of team resilience. One of these is the degree of trust among teammates. Trust has long been thought to be an important factor in team performance (Costa, 2003; Erdem, Ozen, & Atlan, 2003). This assertion has received substantial empirical support (see De Jong, Dirks, & Gillepsie (2016) for a meta-analytic review). Although this is a new area of research, trust has also been shown to be an important predictor of resilience in work teams (e.g., Pavez et al., 2021; Varajao et al., 2021). Unfortunately, how best to increase trust among team members (beyond simple experience together) is unclear. Composing teams of members that share demographic characteristics may lead to greater trust (Chowdhury, 2005), but this may be impractical in the healthcare setting.

Although some researchers have suggested that rewarding specific team behaviors can increase trust (e.g., Hertel, Geister, & Konradt, 2005), others have cautioned that these rewards can have de-motivating effects in some types of teams (DeMatteo, Eby, & Sundstrom, 1998). Other researchers have associated job autonomy with increased trust among team members (Collins & Clark, 2003), but there are relatively few empirical studies investigating this hypothesis.

Norms

Team norms serve as a set of "unwritten rules" that create standards for acceptable and unacceptable performance. Although these norms may not directly influence performance, they have been associated with some of the first-order emergent states that lead to team resilience. For example, widely accepted norms may lead to increased team cohesion (Patterson, Carron, & Loughead, 2005), shared mental models (Converse, Cannon-Bowers, & Salas, 1991), and adaptability (Kozlowski & Bell, 2007).

The development of team norms can be facilitated through appropriate leadership behaviors. Some team norms can be articulated during the on-boarding process. Norms can also emerge from a specific process asking members to establish them early in the team's development (Friedkin, 2001). Norms can be strengthened and refined by having specific time set aside for that purpose (Colman & Carron, 2001). It is also helpful to ensure that accepted norms are communicated as new members join the team (Taggar & Ellis, 2007).

Redundancy/Bench Strength

A factor that is frequently mentioned as a factor in team functioning relates to reliance upon a single member to perform a critical task. This creates a situation where said individual is in a very stressful position, and the team is at risk for poor performance if that member is unable to perform their task. To alleviate this problem, it has been suggested that the team deepen it's "bench strength" by specifically developing high-value skills so that several members can fill any given role. Obviously, members of healthcare teams have specialized training that does not lend itself to informal training. However, it has been demonstrated that even "cross-training" experiences that provide awareness of the demands of other member's roles allow team members to assist one another (Blickensderfer, Cannon-Bowers, & Salas, 1998). Even if they can't perform the role themselves, cross-training may allow teammates to recognize cues that spawn behaviors such as increased error monitoring or dynamic role reassignment.

Team Processes

Perhaps the most important determinants of team resilience are the specific team process behaviors that have often been associated with team performance (Hartwig et. al., 2020). Many processes have been proposed in this regard - some of the most promising are described below.

Communication

Of all of the team processes, communication appears to be a chief driver of team performance. Proper communication allows team members to share information and other resources that are needed in the execution of a task. Bowers et al. (2017) also hypothesize that communication is an important factor in creating the first-order emergent states that lead to team resilience. This hypothesis was recently tested by Brykman & King (2021). These researchers conducted a longitudinal field study of startup teams with the goal of identifying predictors of team resilience. The results supported the hypothesis lead to down-stream emergence of resilience.

Communication is most often improved through training. It's important to note, though, that this training should be focused not just on communicating *more,* but *better*. Fortunately, several effective communication training programs for healthcare teams already exist. For example, the TEAMSTEPPS program (King et al., 2008) has been implemented throughout the world and appears to be effective in improving communication to reduce medical errors (Parker, Forsyth, & Kohlmorgan, 2019). This type of training could be easily adapted to encourage the emergence of team (and individual) resilience.

Monitoring and Backup

A unique benefit of team-based work is that members can often monitor the progress of their teammates and provide backup when needed. This results in increased performance and fewer errors (Burke et al., 2004). For example, Burtscher et al. (2011), studied the role of monitoring in a simulated anesthesia task. They found that the frequency of monitoring behaviors was a strong predictor of performance on the simulated task.

Monitoring is equally important in maintaining psychological resilience. Team members can assess their colleagues for cues indicating fatigue, burnout or even psychological illness. In fact, teaching teammates about these cues is a foundation of many peer support programs used to support mental health in high-risk occupations. For example, the REACT peer support program (Marks et al., 2017) for first responders focuses on teaching peer supports key behavioral cues of stress and mental illness. Peers are then taught appropriate intervention and referral skills for dealing with observed problems.

Leadership

Leadership is another factor that is frequently mentioned in regards to both team performance and eventual team resilience. Leadership subsumes several behaviors that can allow the team to be resilient in the face of stressors. For example, leaders can facilitate resilience by making plans (and alternate contingency plans) to allow the team to have a shred mental model while performing. Leaders can also enhance resilience by fostering an environment of empowerment. Finally, Leaders can hold post-performance debriefings to allow the team to correct misunderstandings going forward (Stoverink et al., 2020). Furthermore, leaders can increase individual psychological resilience through empathy, emotional support, and coaching.

FUTURE DIRECTIONS IN RESEARCH

Chapman et. al (2020) mentioned that the body of research related to team resilience is rather new, and that implies that there are many different avenues for future research. Hartwig et al (2020) argue that team resilience has not yet successfully made itself distinct from other concepts such as team adaptation. Stovernik et. al (2020) sought to clarify this distinction by explaining how resilient teams can also select to persevere rather than being forced adapt. Moreover, simply electing to adapt does not sufficiently encapsulate the concept of resilience. However, it does stand to reason that there could be significant overlap when looking at the operationalization of the two concepts, so further clarity could be useful in future research.

Macedo et. al (2014) discussed the benefit of research populations such as first responders that routinely undergo dangerous situations in order to allow for measurements at baseline and following an adverse scenario. Considering the adverse scenarios previously discussed in the healthcare population, it stands to reason that healthcare professionals could potentially fulfill that role. Similarly, King, Newman, & Luthans (2016) posited that longitudinal research could be beneficial in resilience-based research to allow for a fuller understanding of how resiliency is developed and fluctuates over time.

Lastly, incorporating the Bowers et. al (2017) conceptual model of team resilience, future research should seek to test the model to ensure that the implicit flow from input to output follows in a naturalistic setting. Essentially, does intervening in the lower order domains, such as the inputs or processes, result in improvement at the higher-level domains. Moreover, is there a hierarchy within the varying levels of the conceptual model? For example, does development of group cohesion at the first order emergent state level have a stronger effect than the development of shared mental models? Also, despite them being separate constructs, how do the varying levels of resilience (individual, team, and organizational) interact with and affect one another?

CONCLUSION

Due to the difficulty of the environment in which healthcare professionals operate as well as the notion that hospital workers are inclined to work in teams, it appears that team resilience is an area that should be granted considerable attention for healthcare professionals. The implementation of Bowers et. al (2017) second order emergent state model could help to provide the means of not only addressing key areas in the healthcare profession, but also having downstream effects resulting in improved team resilience. Ultimately, these concepts can help to provide a launching point for future research.

REFERENCES

Alliger, G. M., Cerasoli, C. P., Tannenbaum, S. I., & Vessey, W. B. (2015). Team resilience. *Organizational Dynamics, 44*(3), 176–184. doi:10.1016/j.orgdyn.2015.05.003

Anton, N. E., Montero, P. N., Howley, L. D., Brown, C., & Stefanidis, D. (2015). What stress coping strategies are surgeons relying upon during surgery? *American Journal of Surgery, 210*(5), 846–851. doi:10.1016/j.amjsurg.2015.04.002 PMID:26105802

Blickensderfer, E., Cannon-Bowers, J. A., & Salas, E. (1998). Cross-training and team performance. In J. A. Cannon-Bowers & E. Salas (Eds.), *Making decisions under stress: Implications for individual and team training*. American Psychological Association. doi:10.1037/10278-011

Bosch, B., & Mansell, H. (2015). Interprofessional collaboration in health care: Lessons to be learned from competitive sports. *Canadian Pharmacists Journal. Revue des Pharmaciens du Canada, 148*(4), 176–179. doi:10.1177/1715163515588106 PMID:26448769

Bowers, C., Kreutzer, C., Cannon-Bowers, J., & Lamb, J. (2017). Team resilience as a second order emergent state: A theoretical model and research directions. *Frontiers in Psychology, 8*, 1–14. doi:10.3389/fpsyg.2017.01360 PMID:28861013

Brykman, K. M., & King, D. D. (2021). A Resource Model of Team Resilience Capacity and Learning. *Group & Organization Management, 46*(4). doi:10.1177/10596011211018008

Burke, C.S., Salas, E., Wilson-Donnelly, K., & Priest, H. (2004). How to turn a team of experts into an expert medical team: guidance from the aviation and military communities. *Quality & Safety in Health Care, 13*(1), 96-104. doi:10.1136/qshc.2004.009829

Burton, A., Burgess, C., Dean, S., Koutsopoulou, G. Z., & Hugh-Jones, S. (2017). How effective are mindfulness-based interventions for reducing stress among healthcare professionals? A systematic review and meta-analysis. *Stress and Health, 33*(1), 3–13. doi:10.1002mi.2673 PMID:26916333

Burtscher, M. J., Kolbe, M., Wacker, J., & Manser, T. (2011). Interactions of team mental models and monitoring behaviors predict team performance in simulated anesthesia inductions. *Journal of Experimental Psychology. Applied, 17*(3), 257–269. doi:10.1037/a0025148 PMID:21942315

Cannon-Bowers, J. (2007). Fostering mental model convergence through training. In *Multi-level issues in organizations and time*. Emerald Group Publishing Limited. doi:10.1016/S1475-9144(07)06006-7

Chang, Y., & Chan, H. J. (2015). Optimism and proactive coping in relation to burnout among nurses. *Journal of Nursing Management, 23*(3), 401–408. doi:10.1111/jonm.12148 PMID:24112222

Chapman, M. T., Lines, R. L. J., Crane, M., Ducker, K. J., Ntoumanis, N., Peeling, P., Parker, S. K., Quested, E., Temby, P., Thøgersen-Ntoumani, C., & Gucciardi, D. F. (2020). Team resilience: A scoping review of conceptual and empirical work. *Work and Stress*, *34*(1), 57–81. doi:10.1080/02678373.2018.1529064

Cheng, W., Zhang, F., Liu, Z., Zhang, H., Lyu, Y., Xu, H., Hua, Y., Gu, J., Yang, Z., & Liu, J. (2020). A psychological health support scheme for medical teams in COVID-19 outbreak and its effectiveness. *General Psychiatry*, *33*(5), e100288. doi:10.1136/gpsych-2020-100288 PMID:34192236

Cho, G. J., & Kang, J. (2017). Type D personality and post-traumatic stress disorder symptoms among intensive care unit nurses: The mediating effect of resilience. *PLoS One*, *12*(4), e0175067. doi:10.1371/journal.pone.0175067 PMID:28380063

Chowdhury, S. (2005). Demographic diversity for building an effective entrepreneurial team: Is it important? *Journal of Business Venturing*, *20*(6), 727–746. doi:10.1016/j.jbusvent.2004.07.001

Collins, C. J., & Clark, K. D. (2003). Strategic human resource practices, top management team social networks, and firm performance: The role of human resource practices in creating organizational competitive advantage. *Academy of Management Journal*, *46*(6), 740–751.

Colman, M. M., & Carron, A. V. (2001). The nature of norms in individual sport teams. *Small Group Research*, *32*(2), 206–222. doi:10.1177/104649640103200204

Converse, S. A., Cannon-Bowers, J. A., & Salas, E. (1991, September). Team member shared mental models: A theory and some methodological issues. In *Proceedings of the Human Factors Society Annual Meeting* (Vol. 35, No. 19, pp. 1417-1421). SAGE Publications. 10.1177/154193129103501917

Costa, A. C. (2003). Work team trust and effectiveness. *Personnel Review*, *32*(5), 605–622. doi:10.1108/00483480310488360

Crust, L., & Clough, J. (2011). Developing mental toughness: From research to practice. *Journal of Sport Psychology in Action*, *2*(1), 21–32. doi:10.1080/21520704.2011.563436

De Jong, B. A., Dirks, K. T., & Gillespie, N. (2016). Trust and team performance: A meta-analysis of main effects, moderators, and covariates. *The Journal of Applied Psychology*, *101*(8), 1134–1150. doi:10.1037/apl0000110 PMID:27123697

DeMatteo, J. S., Eby, L. T., & Sundstrom, E. (1998). Team-based rewards: Current empirical evidence. *Research in Organizational Behavior*, *20*, 141–183.

Denollet, J. (2005). DS14: Standard assessment of negative affectivity, social inhibition, and Type D personality. *Psychosomatic Medicine*, *67*(1), 89–97. doi:10.1097/01.psy.0000149256.81953.49 PMID:15673629

Ellis, R., Hay-David, A. G. C., & Brennan, P. A. (2020). Operating during the COVID-19 pandemic: How to reduce medical error. *British Journal of Oral & Maxillofacial Surgery*, *58*(5), 577–580. doi:10.1016/j.bjoms.2020.04.002 PMID:32312584

Erdem, F., Ozen, J., & Atsan, N. (2003). The relationship between trust and team performance. *Work Study*, *52*(7), 337–340. doi:10.1108/00438020310502633

Fletcher, D., & Sarkar, M. (2013). Psychological resilience: A review and critique of definitions, concepts, and theory. *European Psychologist*, *18*(1), 12–23. doi:10.1027/1016-9040/a000124

Friedkin, N. E. (2001). Norm formation in social influence networks. *Social Networks*, *23*(3), 167–189. doi:10.1016/S0378-8733(01)00036-3

Froutan, R., Mazlom, R., Malekzadeh, J., & Mirhaghi, A. (2017). *Relationship between resilience and personality traits in paramedics. International Journal of Emergency Services.*

Hartwig, A., Clarke, S., Johnson, S., & Willis, S. (2020). Workplace team resilience: A systematic review and conceptual development. *Organizational Psychology Review*, *10*(3-4), 169–200. doi:10.1177/2041386620919476

Healy, C. M., & McKay, M. F. (2000). Nursing stress: The effects of coping strategies and job satisfaction in a sample of Australian nurses. *Journal of Advanced Nursing*, *31*(3), 681–688. doi:10.1046/j.1365-2648.2000.01323.x PMID:10718888

Hertel, G., Geister, S., & Konradt, U. (2005). Managing virtual teams: A review of current empirical research. *Human Resource Management Review*, *15*(1), 69–95. doi:10.1016/j.hrmr.2005.01.002

Hsieh, H. F., Hung, Y. T., Wang, H. H., Ma, S. C., & Chang, S. C. (2016). Factors of resilience in emergency department nurses who have experienced workplace violence in Taiwan. *Journal of Nursing Scholarship*, *48*(1), 23–30. doi:10.1111/jnu.12177 PMID:26580490

Huang, Y., & Zhao, N. (2020). Generalized anxiety disorder, depressive symptoms and sleep quality during COVID-19 outbreak in China: A web-based cross-sectional survey. *Psychiatry Research*, *288*, 112954–112954. doi:10.1016/j.psychres.2020.112954 PMID:32325383

Ijntema, R. C., Burger, Y. D., & Schaufeli, W. B. (2019). Reviewing the labyrinth of psychological resilience: Establishing criteria for resilience-building programs. *Consulting Psychology Journal*, *71*(4), 288–304. doi:10.1037/cpb0000147

Jenkins, R., & Elliot, P. (2004). Stressors, burnout and social support: Nurses in acute mental mental health settings. *Journal of Advanced Nursing*, *48*(6), 622–631. doi:10.1111/j.1365-2648.2004.03240.x PMID:15548253

Judkins, S. & Rind, R. (2005). Hardiness, job satisfaction, and stress among home health nurses. *Home Health Care Management & Practice, 17*(2), 113-118. DOI:70020 doi:10.1177/10848223042

King, D. D., Newman, A., & Luthans, F. (2016). Not if, but when we need resilience in the workplace. *Organizational Behavior*, *37*, 782–786. doi:10.1002/job

King, H. B., Battles, J., Baker, D. P., Alonso, A., Salas, E., Webster, J., ... Salisbury, M. (2008). TeamSTEPPS™: team strategies and tools to enhance performance and patient safety. *Advances in Patient Safety: new directions and alternative approaches (Vol. 3: performance and tools).*

Kozlowski, S. W., & Bell, B. S. (2007). Team learning, development, and adaptation. In *Work group learning* (pp. 39–68). Psychology Press.

Kuiper, N. A., McKenzie, S. D., & Belanger, K. A. (1995). Cognitive appraisals and individual differences in sense of humor: Motivational and affective implications. *Personality and Individual Differences, 19*(3), 359–372. https://doi.org/10.1016/0191-8869(95)00072-E

Liang, Y., Wu, K., Zhou, Y., Huang, X., Zhou, Y., & Liu, Z. (2020). Mental health in frontline medical workers during the 2019 novel coronavirus disease epidemic in China: A comparison with the general population. *International Journal of Environmental Research and Public Health, 17*(18), 6550. doi:10.3390/ijerph17186550

Lim, E. J., Noh, J. H., & Jeong, Y. S. (2016). The relationships among type D personality, self resilience, and health promoting behaviors in nursing students. *International Journal of Bio-Science and Bio-Technology, 8*(2), 341–352.

Lomas, T., Medina, J. C., Ivtzan, I., Rupprecht, S., & Eiroa-Orosa, F. J. (2018). A systematic review of the impact of mindfulness on the well-being of healthcare professionals. *Journal of Clinical Psychology, 74*(3), 319–355. doi:10.1002/jclop.22515

Luthans, K. W., Lebsack, S. A., & Lebsack, R. R. (2008). Positivity in healthcare: Relation of optimism to performance. *Journal of Health Organization and Management, 22*(2), 178–188. doi:10.1108/14777260810876330

Macedo, T., Wilheim, L., Gonçalves, R., Coutinjo, E. S. F., Vilete, L., Figueira, I., & Ventura, P. (2014). Building resilience for future adversity: A systematic review of interventions in non-clinical samples of adults. *BMC Psychiatry, 14*, 1–8.

Marks, M. R., Bowers, C., DePesa, N. S., Trachik, B., Deavers, F. E., & James, N. T. (2017). REACT: A paraprofessional training program for first responders – A pilot study. *Bulletin of the Menninger Clinc, 81*(2), 150-166. .81.2.150 doi:10.1521/bumc.2017

Mateen, F., & Dorji, C. (2009). Health-care worker burnout and the mental health imperative. *Lancet, 374*(9690), 595–597. doi:10.1016/S0140-6736(09)61483-5

Meyer, H. S., Durning, S. J., Bader-Larsen, K. S., Hamwey, M., & Varpio, L. (2021). Perseverance: An essential trait of military interprofessional healthcare teams. *Military Medicine, 186*(3), 29–34. https://doi.org/10.1093/milmed/usab185

Morgan, P. B. C., Fletcher, D., & Sarkar, M. (2015). Understanding team resilience in the world's best athletes: A case study of a rugby union World cup winning team. *Psychology of Sport and Exercise, 16*, 91-100. doi:10.1016/j.psychsport.2014.08.007

Parker, A. L., Forsythe, L. L., & Kohlmorgen, I. K. (2019). TeamSTEPPS®: An evidence-based approach to reduce clinical errors threatening safety in outpatient settings: An integrative review. *Journal of Healthcare Risk Management, 38*(4), 19–31.

Patterson, M. M., Carron, A. V., & Loughead, T. M. (2005). The influence of team norms on the cohesion–self-reported performance relationship: A multi-level analysis. *Psychology of Sport and Exercise, 6*(4), 479–493.

Pavez, I., Gómez, H., Laulié, L., & González, V. A. (2021). Project team resilience: The effect of group potency and interpersonal trust. *International Journal of Project Management, 39*(6), 697–708.

Rosen, M. A., Diazgranados, D., Dietz, A. S., Benishek, L. E., Thompson, D., Pronovost, P. J., & Weaver, S. J. (2018). Teamwork in healthcare: Key discoveries enabling safer, high-quality care. *American Psychologist, 73*(4), 433-450. 8 doi:10.1037/amp000029

Sarkar, M., & Page, A. E. (2020). Developing individual and team resilience in elite sport: Research to practice. *Journal of Sport Psychology in Action*. Advance online publication. doi:10.1080/21520704.2020.1861144

Schreffler, J., Petrey, J., & Huecker, M. (2020). The impact of COVID-19 on healthcare worker wellness: A scoping review. *The Western Journal of Emergency Medicine, 21*(5), 1059–1066. doi:10.5811/westjem.2020.7.48684

Stovernik, A. C., Kirkman, B. L., Mistry, S., & Rosen, B. (2020). Bouncing back together: Toward a theoretical model of work team resilience. *Academy of Management Review, 45*, 395–422. https://doi.org/10.5465/amr.2017.0005

Taggar, S., & Ellis, R. (2007). The role of leaders in shaping formal team norms. *The Leadership Quarterly, 18*(2), 105–120.

Valizadeh, L., Zamanzadeh, V., Gargari, R. B., Ghahramanian, A., Tabrizi, F. J., & Keogh, B. (2016). Pressure and protective factors influencing nursing students' self-esteem: A content analysis study. *Nurse Education Today, 36,* 468-472. .nedt.2015.10.019 doi:10.1016/j

Varajao, J., Fernandes, G., Amaral, A., & Gonçalves, A. M. (2021). Team Resilience Model: An Empirical Examination of Information Systems Projects. *Reliability Engineering & System Safety, 206*, 107303.

Vera, M., Rodríguez-Sánchez, A. M., & Salanova, M. (2017). May the force be with you: Looking for resources that build team resilience. *Journal of Workplace Behavioral Health, 32*, 119–138. doi:10.1080/15555240.2017.1329629

Woodhead, E.L., Northrop, L., & Edelstein, B. (2016). Stress, social support, and burnout among long-term care nursing staff. *Journal of Applied Gerontology, 35*(1), 84-105. DOI: 10.1177/0733464814542465

Wu, Y., Wang, J., Luo, C., Hu, S., Lin, X., Anderson, A. E., Bruera, E., Yang, X., Wei, S., & Qian, Y. (2020). A comparison of burnout frequency among oncology physicians and nurses working on the frontline and usual wards during the COVID-19 epidemic in Wuhan, China. *Journal of Pain and Symptom Management, 60*(1), e60-e65. .1016/j,painsymman.2020.04.008 doi:https://doi.org/10

Compilation of References

AACN. (2021, September 21). Hear us out campaign reports nurses' COVID-19 reality. *American Association of Critical Care Nurses*. https://www.aacn.org/newsroom/hear-us-out-campaign-reports-nurses-covid-19-reality

Abbasi, K. (2019). A workforce crisis in the NHS. *Journal of the Royal Society of Medicine*, *112*(9), 363–363. doi:10.1177/0141076819875444 PMID:31496348

Abildgaard, J. S., Nielsen, K., & Sverke, M. (2018). Can job insecurity be managed? Evaluating an organizational-level intervention addressing the negative effects of restructuring. *Work and Stress*, *32*(2), 105–123. doi:10.1080/02678373.2017.1367735

Abraham, J. M., Feldman, R., Nyman, J. A., & Barleen, N. (2011). What factors influence participation in an exercise-focused, employer-based wellness program? *INQUIRY: The Journal of Health Care Organization, Provision, and Financing*, *48*(3), 221–241. doi:10.5034/inquiryjrnl_48.03.01 PMID:22235547

Abramovitz, M., Zelnick, J. (2010). Double jeopardy: the impact of neoliberalism on care workers in the United States and South Africa. *International Journal of Health Services: Planning, Administration, Evaluation*, *40*(1), 97–117. . doi:10.2190/HS.40.1.f

Abuhashesh, M., Al-Khasawneh, M., Al-Dmour, R., & Masa'deh, R. (2019). The impact of Facebook on Jordanian consum-ers' decision process in the hotel selection. *IBIMA Business Review*, 1-16.

Adams, J. G., & Walls, R. M. (2020). Supporting the health care workforce during the COVID- 19 global epidemic. *Journal of the American Medical Association*, *323*(15), 1439. doi:10.1001/jama.2020.3972 PMID:32163102

Adler, A. B., Saboe, K. N., Anderson, J., Sipos, M. L., & Thomas, J. L. (2014). Behavioral Health Leadership: New Directions in Occupational Mental Health. *Current Psychiatry Reports*, *16*(10), 1–7. doi:10.100711920-014-0484-6 PMID:25160794

Agarwal, S., Goel, D., & Sharma, A. (2013). Evaluation of the factors which contribute to the ocular complaints in computer users. *Journal of Clinical and Diagnostic Research: JCDR*, *7*(2), 331–335. doi:10.7860/JCDR/2013/5150.2760 PMID:23543722

Ahmad, W., Taggart, F., Shafique, M. S., Muzafar, Y., Abidi, S., Ghani, N., Malik, Z., Zahid, T., Waqas, A., & Ghaffar, N. (2015). Diet, exercise and mental-wellbeing of healthcare professionals (doctors, dentists and nurses) in Pakistan. *PeerJ*, *3*, e1250. doi:10.7717/peerj.1250 PMID:26401460

Ahmed, A., & Ramzan, M. (2013). Effects of job stress on employees job performance: A study on banking sector of Pakistan. *IOSR Journal of Business and Management*, *11*(6), 61–68. doi:10.9790/487X-1166168

Ahola, K., & Hakanen, J. (2007). Job strain, burnout, and depressive symptoms: A prospective study among dentists. *Journal of Affective Disorders*, *104*(1-3), 103–110. doi:10.1016/j.jad.2007.03.004 PMID:17448543

Ahola, K., Hakanen, J., Perhoniemi, R., & Mutanen, P. (2014). Relationship between burnout and depressive symptoms: A study using the person-centred approach. *Burnout Research*, *1*(1), 29–37. doi:10.1016/j.burn.2014.03.003

Ahola, K., Salminen, S., Toppinen-Tanner, S., Koskinen, A., & Väänänen, A. (2013). Occupational Burnout and Severe Injuries: An Eight-year Prospective Cohort Study among Finnish Forest Industry Workers. *Journal of Occupational Health*, *55*(6), 450–457. doi:10.1539/joh.13-0021-OA PMID:24162145

Aiken, L. H., Clarke, S. P., Sloane, D. M., Sochalski, J., & Silber, J. H. (2002). Hospital nurse staffing and patient mortality, nurse burnout, and job dissatisfaction. *Journal of the American Medical Association*, *288*(16), 1987–1993. doi:10.1001/jama.288.16.1987 PMID:12387650

Aiken, L. H., Sloane, D., Griffiths, P., Rafferty, A. M., Bruyneel, L., McHugh, M., Maier, C. B., Moreno-Casbas, T., Ball, J. E., Ausserhofer, D., & Sermeus, W. (2017). Nursing skill mix in European hospitals: Cross-sectional study of the association with mortality, patient ratings, and quality of care. *BMJ Quality & Safety*, *26*(7), 559–568. doi:10.1136/bmjqs-2016-005567 PMID:28626086

Ajzen, I. (1991). The Theory of Planned Behavior. *Organizational Behavior and Human Decision Processes*, *50*(2), 179–211. doi:10.1016/0749-5978(91)90020-T

Al Hazmi, T. M., Alghamdi, A., & Abdulmajeed, I. (2018). Eating habits among healthcare providers during working hours at National Guard Health Affairs-Riyadh, Saudi Arabia. *International Journal of Medical Research & Health Sciences*, *7*(9), 1–14.

Al Seraireh, F. A., & Aloush, S. M. (2017). Mindfulness meditation versus physical exercise in the management of depression among nursing students. *The Journal of Nursing Education*, *56*(10), 599–604. doi:10.3928/01484834-20170918-04 PMID:28972629

Albert, N. M., Butler, R., & Sorrell, J. (2014). Factors related to healthy diet and physical activity in hospital-based clinical nurses. *OJIN: The Online Journal of Issues in Nursing*, *19*(3).

Albertson, K., Nielsen, M., & Borg, V. (2001). The Danish psychosocial work environment and symptoms of stress, the main, mediating, and moderating role of sense of coherence. *Work and Stress*, *15*(3), 241–253. doi:10.1080/02678370110066562

Albott, C. S., Wozniak, J. R., McGlinch, B. P., Wall, M. H., Gold, B. S., & Vinogradov, S. (2020). Battle Buddies: Rapid deployment of a psychological resilience intervention for health care workers during the COVID-19 pandemic. *Anesthesia and Analgesia*, *131*(1), 43–54. doi:10.1213/ANE.0000000000004912 PMID:32345861

Aldana, S. G., Anderson, D. R., Adams, T. B., Whitmer, R. W., Merrill, R. M., George, V., & Noyce, J. (2012). A review of the knowledge base on healthy worksite culture. *Journal of Occupational and Environmental Medicine*, *54*(4), 414–419. doi:10.1097/JOM.0b013e31824be25f PMID:22446571

Alegría, M., Fortuna, L. R., Lin, J. Y., Norris, F. H., Gao, S., Takeuchi, D. T., Jackson, J. S., Shrout, P. E., & Valentine, A. (2013). Prevalence, risk, and correlates of posttraumatic stress disorder across ethnic and racial minority groups in the United States. *Medical Care*, *51*(12), 1114–1123. doi:10.1097/MLR.0000000000000007 PMID:24226308

Alexandrova-Karamanova, A., Todorova, I., Montgomery, A., Panagopoulou, E., Costa, P., Baban, A., Davas, A., Milosevic, M., & Mijakoski, D. (2016). Burnout and health behaviors in health professionals from seven European countries. *International Archives of Occupational and Environmental Health*, *89*(7), 1059–1075. doi:10.100700420-016-1143-5 PMID:27251338

Allen, R., Judkins-Cohn, T., deVelasco, R., Forges, E., Lee, R., Clark, L., & Procunier, M. (2013). Moral Distress Among Healthcare Professionals at a Health System. *JONA'S Healthcare Law, Ethics and Regulation*, *15*(3), 111–118. doi:10.1097/NHL.0b013e3182a1bf33 PMID:23963112

Allen, T. D., & Armstrong, J. (2006). Further examination of the link between work-faimly conflict and physical health: The role of health-related behaviors. *The American Behavioral Scientist*, *49*, 1204–1221. doi:10.1177/0002764206286386

Alliger, G. M., Cerasoli, C. P., Tannenbaum, S. I., & Vessey, W. B. (2015). Team resilience. *Organizational Dynamics*, *44*(3), 176–184. doi:10.1016/j.orgdyn.2015.05.003

Allisey, A. F., Noblet, A. J., Lamontagne, A. D., & Houdmont, J. (2014). Testing a model of officer intentions to quit: The mediating effects of job stress and job satisfaction. *Criminal Justice and Behavior*, *41*(6), 751–771. doi:10.1177/0093854813509987

Al-Mohannadi, A. S., Albuflasa, A. M., Sayegh, S., Salman, A., & Farooq, A. (2020). A cross-sectional study exploring motivators and barriers to physical activity participation among hospital workers. *Global Journal of Health Science*, *12*(9), 76–85. doi:10.5539/gjhs.v12n9p76

Altman, M. (2020, April 10). Shifting ethic in a crisis: Responding to COVID-19. *American Association of Critical Care Nurses*. https://www.aacn.org/blog/shifting-ethics-in-a-crisis-responding-to-covid-19

Amandolare, S., Gallagher, L., Bowles, J., & Dvorkin, E. (2020). *Under Threat & Left Out: NYC's Immigrants and the Coronavirus Crisis*. Academic Press.

Ambrose, M. L., & Schminke, M. (2009). The role of overall justice judgments in organizational justice research: A test of mediation. *The Journal of Applied Psychology*, *94*(2), 491–500. doi:10.1037/a0013203 PMID:19271803

American Academy of Pediatrics. (2012). Patient- and family-centered care and the pediatrician's role. *Pediatrics*, *129*(2), 394–404. doi:10.1542/peds.2011-3084 PMID:22291118

American Association of Colleges of Nursing. (n.d.). *Nursing Fact Sheet*. https://www.aacnnursing.org/News-Information/Fact-Sheets/Nursing-Fact-Sheet

American College of Physicians. (2021). *Annals graphic medicine*. https://www.acpjournals.org/topic/web-exclusives/annals-graphic-medicine

American Hospital Association. (n.d.). *Stories from the front lines*. https://www.aha.org/issue-landing-page/2020-06-02-stories-front-lines

American Nurses Association. (2011). *The ANA Health & Safety Survey: Hazards of the RN work environment*. www.NursingWorld.org

American Nurses Association. (2021, October 14). Well-being inititative. *Nursing World*. https://www.nursingworld.org/practice-policy/work-environment/health-safety/disaster-preparedness/coronavirus/what-you-need-to-know/the-well-being-initiative/

American Nurses Credentialing Center. (n.d.). *Magnet recognition program®*. Nursing World. https://www.nursingworld.org/organizational-programs/magnet/

American Psychiatric Association. (2013). *Diagnostic and statistical manual of mental disorders (DSM-5®)*. American Psychiatric Pub.

American Psychological Association (APA). (2008). *Stress in America*. Accessed on March 12, 2022 from https://www.apa.org/news/press/releases/2008/10/stress-in-america.pdf

Anderson, G. S., Di Nota, P. M., Groll, D., & Carleton, R. N. (2020). Peer support and crisis-focused psychological interventions designed to mitigate post-traumatic stress injuries among public safety and frontline healthcare personnel: A systematic review. *International Journal of Environmental Research and Public Health, 17*(20), 7645. doi:10.3390/ijerph17207645 PMID:33092146

Andolhe, R., Barbosa, R. L., de Oliveira, E. M., Costa, A. L. S., & Padilha, K. G. (2015). Estresse, coping e burnout da Equipe de Enfermagem de Unidades de Terapia Intensiva: Fatores associados. *Revista Da Escola de Enfermagem Da USP, 49*(spe), 58–64. doi:10.1590/S0080-623420150000700009

Ando, M., Natsume, T., Kukihara, H., Shibata, H., & Ito, S. (2011). Efficacy of mindfulness-based meditation therapy on the sense of coherence and mental health of Nurses. *Health, 03*(02), 118–122. doi:10.4236/health.2011.32022

Andreyko, M., Gaydos, S., & Rich, J. (Eds.). (2017). *Love is love: A comic book anthology to benefit the survivors of the Orlando Pulse shooting*. IDW Publishing.

Anton, N. E., Montero, P. N., Howley, L. D., Brown, C., & Stefanidis, D. (2015). What stress coping strategies are surgeons relying upon during surgery? *American Journal of Surgery, 210*(5), 846–851. doi:10.1016/j.amjsurg.2015.04.002 PMID:26105802

APA. (2020). *COVID-19 pandemic guidance document: moral injury during the COVID-19 pandemic*. Retrieved from American Psychiatric Association: https://www.psychiatry.org/File%20Library/Psychiatrists/APA-Guidance-COVID-19-Moral-Injury.pdf

Appleby, J. (2018). *70 years of NHS spending*. Nuffield Trust. Retrieved from https://ww.nuffieldtrust.org.uk/news-item/70-year-of-nhs-spending

Arain, G. A., Bhatti, Z. A., Ashraf, N., & Fang, Y. H. (2020). Top-down knowledge hiding in organizations: An empirical study of the consequences of supervisor knowledge hiding among local and foreign workers in the Middle East. *Journal of Business Ethics, 164*(3), 611–625. doi:10.100710551-018-4056-2

Araujo, L. A., Veloso, C. F., Souza, M. C., Azevedo, J. M. C., & Tarro, G. (2021). The potential impact of the COVID-19 pandemic on child growth and development: A systematic review. *Jornal de Pediatria, 97*(4), 369–377. doi:10.1016/j.jped.2020.08.008 PMID:32980318

Arefi, M. F., & Poursadeqiyan, M. (2020). A review of studies on the epidemic crisis of COVID-19 disease with a preventive approach. *Work*, 1-13.

Armitage, C. J., & Christian, J. (2003). From attitudes to behaviour: Basic and applied research on the theory of planned behaviour. *Current Psychology (New Brunswick, N.J.), 22*(3), 187–195. doi:10.100712144-003-1015-5

Armitage, C. J., & Conner, M. (1999). Distinguishing perceptions of control from self-efficacy: Predicting consumption of a low-fat diet using the theory of planned behavior. *Journal of Applied Social Psychology, 29*(1), 72–90. doi:10.1111/j.1559-1816.1999.tb01375.x

Arnetz, J. E., Goetz, C. M., Sudan, S., Arble, E., Janisse, J., & Arnetz, B. B. (2020). Personal protective equipment and mental health symptoms among nurses during the COVID-19 pandemic. *Journal of Occupational and Environmental Medicine, 62*(11), 892–897. doi:10.1097/JOM.0000000000001999 PMID:32804747

Arnold, T. C. (2020). Moral distress in emergency and critical care nurses: A metaethnography. *Nursing Ethics, 27*(8), 1681–1693. doi:10.1177/0969733020935952 PMID:32700649

Aronsson, G., & Lindh, T. (2004). *Långtidsfriskas arbetsvillkor: En populationsstudie. Arbete och Hälsa, 10*. Arbetslivsinstitutet.

Atkinson, G., Fullick, S., Grindey, C., & Maclaren, D. (2008). Exercise, energy balance and the shift worker. *Sports Medicine (Auckland, N.Z.), 38*(8), 671–685. doi:10.2165/00007256-200838080-00005 PMID:18620467

Azoulay, E., Cariou, A., Bruneel, F., Demoule, A., Kouatchet, A., Reuter, D., Souppart, V., Combes, A., Klouche, K., Argaud, L., Barbier, F., Jourdain, M., Reignier, J., Papazian, L., Guidet, B., Géri, G., Resche-Rigon, M., Guisset, O., Labbé, V., ... Kentish-Barnes, N. (2020). Symptoms of anxiety, depression, and peritraumatic dissociation in critical care clinicians managing patients with COVID-19. A cross-sectional study. *American Journal of Respiratory and Critical Care Medicine, 202*(10), 1388–1398. doi:10.1164/rccm.202006-2568OC PMID:32866409

B., D. (2006). *Epileptic*. Pantheon.

Babore, A., Lombardi, L., Viceconti, M. L., Pignataro, S., Marino, V., Crudele, M., Candelori, C., Bramanti, S. M., & Trumello, C. (2020). Psychological effects of the COVID-2019 pandemic: Perceived stress and coping strategies among healthcare professionals. *Psychiatry Research, 293*, 113366. doi:10.1016/j.psychres.2020.113366 PMID:32798932

Badanta, B., Acevedo-Aguilera, R., Lucchetti, G., & de Diego-Cordero, R. (2021). "A picture is worth a thousand words": A photovoice study exploring health professionals' experiences during the COVID-19 pandemic. *Journal of Clinical Nursing, 30*(10.1111), 1-13. doi:10.1111/jocn.15887

Bagcchi, S. (2020). Stigma during the COVID-19 pandemic. *The Lancet. Infectious Diseases, 20*(7), 782. doi:10.1016/S1473-3099(20)30498-9 PMID:32592670

Baird, J., Davies, B., Hinds, P. S., Baggott, C., & Rehm, R. S. (2015). What impact do hospital and unit-based rules have upon patient- and family-centered care in the pediatric intensive care unit? *Journal of Pediatric Nursing, 30*(1), 133–142. doi:10.1016/j.pedn.2014.10.001 PMID:25450441

Bakker, A. B., & Demerouti, E. (2017). Job demands-resources theory: Taking stock and looking forward. *Journal of Occupational Health Psychology, 22*(3), 273–285. doi:10.1037/ocp0000056 PMID:27732008

Bakker, A. B., & Demerouti, E. (2018). Multiple levels in job demands-resources theory: Implications for employee well-being and performance. In E. Diener, S. Oishi, & L. Tay (Eds.), *Handbook of Well-Being* (pp. 1–13). DEF Publishers. https://nobascholar.com

Baldisseri, M. R. (2007). Impaired healthcare professional. *Critical Care Medicine, 35*(2, Suppl), S106–S116. doi:10.1097/01.CCM.0000252918.87746.96 PMID:17242598

Bandura, A. (1977). Self-efficacy: Toward a unifying theory of behavioral change. *Psychological Review, 84*(2), 191–215. doi:10.1037/0033-295X.84.2.191 PMID:847061

Bandura, A. (1986). The explanatory and predictive scope of self-efficacy theory. *Journal of Social and Clinical Psychology, 4*(3), 359–373. doi:10.1521/jscp.1986.4.3.359

Banerjee, A., Mukherjee, K., Bhattacharjee, D., Garai, D., & Chakraborty, R. (2020). Status of Healthcare Workers in Relation to COVID-19 Infection: A Retrospective Study in a Level 4 COVID Hospital in Eastern India. *The Journal of the Association of Physicians of India, 68*(12), 55–57. PMID:33247643

Bani-Issa, W., Radwan, H., Al Marzooq, F., Al Awar, S., Al-Shujairi, A. M., Samsudin, A. R., Khasawneh, W., & Al-bluwi, N. (2020). Salivary cortisol, subjective stress and quality of sleep among female healthcare professionals. *Journal of Multidisciplinary Healthcare, 13*, 125–140. doi:10.2147/JMDH.S229396 PMID:32103972

Barr-Anderson, D., AuYoung, M., Whitt-Glover, M. C., Glenn, B. A., & Yancey, A. K. (2011). Integration of short bouts of physical activity into organizational routine. *American Journal of Preventive Medicine, 40*(1), 76–93. doi:10.1016/j.amepre.2010.09.033 PMID:21146772

Barry, L. (2014). *Syllabus: Notes from an accidental professor*. Drawn and Quarterly.

Barsade, S. G. (2002). The ripple effect: Emotional contagion and its influence on group behavior. *Administrative Science Quarterly*, *47*(4), 644–675. doi:10.2307/3094912

Barzideh, M., Choobineh, A. R., & Tabatabaee, H. R. (2014). Job stress dimensions and their relationship to musculoskeletal disorders in Iranian nurses. *Work (Reading, Mass.)*, *47*(4), 423–429. doi:10.3233/WOR-121585 PMID:23324727

Bass, B. M. (1985). *Leadership and performance beyond expectations*. Free Press.

Batalova, J. (2020). *Immigrant Health-Care Workers in the United States*. Academic Press.

Bauer, J., Stamm, A., Virnich, K., Wissing, K., Müller, U., Wirsching, M., & Schaarschmidt, U. (2006). Correlation between burnout syndrome and psychological and psychosomatic symptoms among teachers. *International Archives of Occupational and Environmental Health*, *79*(3), 199–204. doi:10.100700420-005-0050-y PMID:16258752

Bauldry, S., & Szaflarski, M. (2017). Immigrant-based disparities in mental health care utilization. *Socius: Sociological Research for a Dynamic World*, *3*. doi:10.1177/2378023116685718 PMID:28845455

Baumeister, R. F. (2014). Self-regulation, ego depletion, and inhibition. *Neuropsychologia*, *65*, 313–319. doi:10.1016/j.neuropsychologia.2014.08.012 PMID:25149821

Bazarko, D., Cate, R. A., Azocar, F., & Kreitzer, M. J. (2013). The impact of an innovative mindfulness-based Stress Reduction Program on the health and well-being of nurses employed in a corporate setting. *Journal of Workplace Behavioral Health*, *28*(2), 107–133. doi:10.1080/15555240.2013.779518 PMID:23667348

Bazeley, P., & Jackson, K. (2013). *Qualitative Data Analysis with NVivo* (2nd ed.). SAGE Publications Ltd.

BBC. (2020). *Coronavirus: NHS workers who died in the pandemic*. Retrieved from https://www.bbc.co.uk/news/av/uk-53914546

Beauvais, A., Andreychik, M., & Henkel, L. A. (2017). The role of emotional intelligence and empathy in compassionate nursing care. *Mindfulness & Compassion*, *2*(2), 92–100. doi:10.1016/j.mincom.2017.09.001

Becker, J. E., Smith, J. R., & Hazen, E. P. (2020). Pediatric consultation-liaison psychiatry: An update and review. *Psychosomatics*, *61*(5), 467–480. doi:10.1016/j.psym.2020.04.015 PMID:32482345

Beheshtifar, M., Hoseinifar, H., & Moghadam, M. (2011). Effect procrastination on work-related stress. *European JOurnal of Economics Finance Administration Science*, 38-59.

Bellchambers, A. S. (2020). One of my demons: Crying (or a lack of). *Annals Graphic Medicine*. https://www.acpjournals.org/doi/10.7326/G19-0054

Bender, A. E., Berg, K. A., Miller, E. K., Evans, K. E., & Holmes, M. R. (2021). "Making sure we are all okay": Healthcare workers' strategies for emotional connectedness during the COVID-19 pandemic. *Clinical Social Work Journal*, *49*(4), 445–455. Advance online publication. doi:10.100710615-020-00781-w PMID:33456094

Benfante, A., Di Tella, M., Romeo, A., & Castelli, L. (2020). Traumatic stress in healthcare workers during COVID-19 pandemic: A review of the immediate impact. *Frontiers in Psychology*, *11*, 2816. doi:10.3389/fpsyg.2020.569935 PMID:33192854

Benziman, Y. (2020). "Winning" the "battle" and "beating" the COVID-19 "enemy": Leaders' use of war frames to define the pandemic. *Peace and Conflict*, *26*(3), 247–256. doi:10.1037/pac0000494

Bergsträsser, E., Cignacco, E., & Luck, P. (2017). Health care professionals' experiences and needs when delivering end-of-life care to children: A qualitative study. *Palliative Care, 10*. Advance online publication. doi:10.1177/1178224217724770 PMID:28835736

Berken, J. A., Heard-Garris, N., & Wakschlag, L. S. (2021). Guardians at the gate: Early adversity, neurocognitive development, and the role of the pediatrician in the era of COVID-19. *Frontiers in Pediatrics, 9*, 1–6. doi:10.3389/fped.2021.665335 PMID:33937157

Bernal, D., Campos-Serna, J., Tobias, A., Vargas-Prada, S., Benavides, F. G., & Serra, C. (2015). Work-related psychosocial risk factors and musculoskeletal disorders in hospital nurses and nursing aides: a systematic review and meta-analysis. *International Journal of Nursing Studies, 52(*2), 635-648. doi/. doi:10.1016/j.ijnurstu.2014.11.003

Bernburg, M., Vitzthum, K., Groneberg, D. A., & Mache, S. (2016). Physicians' occupational stress, depressive symptoms and work ability in relation to their working environment: A cross-sectional study of differences among medical residents with various specialties working in German hospitals. *BMJ Open*, *6*(6), e011369. doi:10.1136/bmjopen-2016-011369 PMID:27311909

Berry, J. (1997). Immigration, acculturation, and adaptation. *Applied Psychology*, *46*(1), 5–34.

Bhandari, D., Kotera, Y., Ozaki, A., Abeysinghe, S., Kosaka, M., & Tanimoto, T. (2021). COVID-19: challenges faced by Nepalese migrants living in Japan. *BMC Public Health, 21*(1), 1–14.

Bianchi, R., Schonfeld, I. S., & Laurent, E. (2014). Is burnout a depressive disorder? A reexamination with special focus on atypical depression. *International Journal of Stress Management*, *21*(4), 307–324. doi:10.1037/a0037906

Bier, D. J. (2020). Immigrants aid America during COVID-19 crisis. Cato Institute.

Bischoff, L. L., Otto, A. K., Hold, C., & Wollesen, B. (2019). The effect of physical activity interventions on occupational stress for health personnel – a systematic review. *International Journal of Nursing Studies*. doi:10.1016/j.ijnurstu.2019.06.002

Blackburn, P., McAuliffe, D., & Johns, L. (2020, May 18). Health-care workers share our trauma during the coronavirus pandemic-on top of their own. *The Conversation*. https://theconversation.com/health-care-workers-share-our-trauma-during-the-coronavirus-pandemic-on-top-of-their-own-137887

Blackford, K., Jancey, J., Howat, P., Ledger, M., & Lee, A. H. (2013). Office-Based physical activity and nutrition intervention: Barriers, enablers, and preferred strategies for workplace obesity prevention, Perth, Western Australia, 2012. *Preventing Chronic Disease*, *10*(1), 1–11. doi:10.5888/pcd10.130029 PMID:24028834

Blair, S. N. (2009). Physical inactivity: The biggest public health problem of the 21st century. *British Journal of Sports Medicine*, *43*(1), 1–2. PMID:19136507

Blake, H., Bermingham, F., Johnson, G., & Tabner, A. (2020). Mitigating the psychological impact of COVID-19 on healthcare workers: A digital learning package. *International Journal of Environmental Research and Public Health*, *17*(9), E2997. doi:10.3390/ijerph17092997 PMID:32357424

Blickensderfer, E., Cannon-Bowers, J. A., & Salas, E. (1998). Cross-training and team performance. In J. A. Cannon-Bowers & E. Salas (Eds.), *Making decisions under stress: Implications for individual and team training*. American Psychological Association. doi:10.1037/10278-011

BMA. (2020). *Almost half of UK doctors suffering from burnout, depression or anxiety, BMA survey reveals*. Retrieved from https://www.bma.org.uk/bma-media-centre/almost-half-of-uk-doctors-suffering-from-burnout-depression-or-anxiety-bma-survey-reveals

Bodenheimer, T., & Sinsky, C. (2014). From triple to quadruple aim: Care of the patient requires care of the provider. *Annals of Family Medicine, 12*(6), 573–576. doi:10.1370/afm.1713 PMID:25384822

Boehm, S. A., Baumgärtner, M. K., & Kreissner, L. M. (2016). The relationship between leadership and health: A comparison of general and health-focused leadership approaches. In M. Wiencke, M. Cacace, & S. Fischer (Eds.), *Healthy at Work*. Springer. doi:10.1007/978-3-319-32331-2_7

Bolieau, K., & Johnson, R. (Eds.). (2021). *COVID chronicles: A comics anthology*. Graphic Mundi. doi:10.1515/9780271091723

Bond, F. W., Hayes, S. C., Baer, R. A., Carpenter, K., Guenole, N., Orcutt, H. K., Waltz, T., & Zettle, R. D. (2011). Preliminary Psychometric Properties of the Acceptance and Action Questionnaire–II: A Revised Measure of Psychological Inflexibility and Experiential Avoidance. *Behavior Therapy, 42*(4), 676–688. doi:10.1016/j.beth.2011.03.007 PMID:22035996

Boorman, S. (2010). Health and well-being of the NHS workforce. *Journal of Public Mental Health, 9*(1), 4-7.

Borges, L. M., Barnes, S. M., Farnsworth, J. K., Bahraini, N. H., & Brenner, L. A. (2020). A commentary on moral injury among health care providers during the COVID-19 pandemic. *Psychological Trauma: Theory, Research, Practice, and Policy, 12*(S1), S138–S140. doi:10.1037/tra0000698 PMID:32496101

Bos, E. H., Krol, B., Van Der Star, A., & Groothoff, J. W. (2006). The effects of occupational interventions on reduction of musculoskeletal symptoms in the nursing profession. *Ergonomics, 49*(7), 706-723. doi:10.1080/00140130600578005

Bos, C., van der Lans, I. A., van Kleef, E., & van Trijp, H. C. (2018). Promoting healthy choices from vending machines: Effectiveness and consumer evaluations of four types of interventions. *Food Policy, 79*, 247–255. doi:10.1016/j.foodpol.2018.07.001

Bosch, B., & Mansell, H. (2015). Interprofessional collaboration in health care: Lessons to be learned from competitive sports. *Canadian Pharmacists Journal. Revue des Pharmaciens du Canada, 148*(4), 176–179. doi:10.1177/1715163515588106 PMID:26448769

Bostrom, A., Squires, J., Mitchell, A., Sales, A., & Estabrooks, C. (2012). Workplace aggression experienced by frontline staff in nursing dementia care. *Journal of Clinical Nursing, 21*(10), 1453–1465. doi:10.1111/j.1365-2702.2011.03924.x PMID:22151034

Böttche, M., Stammel, N., & Knaevelsrud, C. (2016). Psychotherapeutic treatment of traumatized refugees in Germany. *Der Nervenarzt, 87*(11), 1136–1143. doi:10.100700115-016-0214-x PMID:27649983

Bowers, C., Kreutzer, C., Cannon-Bowers, J., & Lamb, J. (2017). Team resilience as a second order emergent state: A theoretical model and research directions. *Frontiers in Psychology, 8*, 1–14. doi:10.3389/fpsyg.2017.01360 PMID:28861013

Bozdağ, F., & Ergün, N. (2020). Psychological resilience of healthcare professionals during COVID-19 pandemic. *Psychological Reports*. PMID:33050800

Brady, J. M., Hammer, L. B., Mohr, C. D., & Bodner, T. E. (2021). Supportive supervisor training improves family relationships among employee and spouse dyads. *Journal of Occupational Health Psychology, 26*(1), 31–48. doi:10.1037/ocp0000264 PMID:33119332

Branch, C., & Klinkerberg, D. (2015). Compassion fatigue among pediatric healthcare providers. *The American Journal of Maternal/Child Nursing, 40*(3), 160–166. doi:10.1097/NMC.0000000000000133

Brandenburg, J. E., Holman, L. K., Apkon, S. D., Houtrow, A. J., Rinaldi, R., & Sholas, M. G. (2020). School reopening during COVID-19 pandemic: Considering students with disabilities. *Journal of Pediatric Rehabilitation Medicine: An Interdisciplinary Approach*, *13*(3), 425–431. doi:10.3233/PRM-200789 PMID:33136082

Brand, S. L., Thompson Coon, J., Fleming, L. E., Carroll, L., Bethel, A., & Wyatt, K. (2017). Whole-system approaches to improving the health and wellbeing of healthcare workers: A systematic review. *PLoS One*, *12*(12), 1–26. doi:10.1371/journal.pone.0188418 PMID:29200422

Branson, D. C. (2019). Vicarious trauma, themes in research, and terminology: A review of literature. *Traumatology*, *25*(1), 2–10. doi:10.1037/trm0000161

Bredahl, T. V. G., Særvoll, C. A., Kirkelund, L., Sjøgaard, G., & Andersen, L. L. (2015). When intervention meets organisation: A qualitative study of motivation and barriers to physical exercise at the workplace. *TheScientificWorldJournal*, *2015*, 1–12. doi:10.1155/2015/518561 PMID:26380361

Bressi, C., Porcellana, M., Gambini, O., Madia, L., Muffatti, R., Peirone, A., Zanini, S., Erlicher, A., Scarone, S., & Altamura, A. C. (2009). Burnout Among Psychiatrists in Milan: A Multicenter Survey. *Psychiatric Services (Washington, D.C.)*, *60*(7), 985–988. doi:10.1176/ps.2009.60.7.985 PMID:19564233

Bride, B. E., & Kintzle, S. (2011). Secondary traumatic stress, job satisfaction, and occupational commitment in substance abuse counselors. *Traumatology*, *17*(1), 22–28. doi:10.1177/1534765610395617

Bride, B. E., Robinson, M. M., Yegidis, B., & Figley, C. R. (2004). Development and validation of the secondary traumatic stress scale. *Research on Social Work Practice*, *14*(1), 27–35. doi:10.1177/1049731503254106

Bridger, R. S., Day, A. J., & Morton, K. (2013). Occupational stress and employee turnover. *Ergonomics*, *56*(11), 1629–1639. doi:10.1080/00140139.2013.836251 PMID:24047248

Bright, M. A., Thompson, L., Esernio-Jenssen, D., Alford, S., & Shenkman, E. (2015). Primary care pediatricians' perceived prevalence and surveillance of adverse childhood experiences in low-income children. *Journal of Health Care for the Poor and Underserved*, *26*(3), 686–700. doi:10.1353/hpu.2015.0080 PMID:26320905

Broetje, S., Jenny, G. J., & Bauer, G. F. (2020). The key job demands and resources of nursing staff: An integrative review of reviews. *Frontiers in Psychology*, *11*, 84. doi:10.3389/fpsyg.2020.00084 PMID:32082226

Brogan, E., Rossiter, C., Duffield, C., & Denney-Wilson, E. (2021). Healthy eating and physical activity among new graduate nurses: A qualitative study of barriers and enablers during their first year of clinical practice. *Collegian (Royal College of Nursing, Australia)*, *28*(5), 489–497. doi:10.1016/j.colegn.2020.12.008

Brondolo, E., Wellington, R., Brady, N., Libby, D., & Brondolo, T. J. (2008). Mechanism and strategies for preventing post-traumatic stress disorder in forensic workers responding to mass fatality incidents. *Journal of Forensic and Legal Medicine*, *15*(2), 78–88. doi:10.1016/j.jflm.2007.04.007 PMID:18206823

Bronkhorst, B., Tummers, L., & Steijn, B. (2018). Improving safety climate and behavior through a multifaceted intervention: Results from a field experiment. *Safety Science*, *103*, 293–304. doi:10.1016/j.ssci.2017.12.009

Brooks, S. K., Dunn, R., Amlôt, R., Greenberg, N., & Rubin, G. J. (2016). Social and occupational factors associated with psychological distress and disorder among disaster responders: a systematic review. *BMC Psychology*, *4*(1), 1–13. doi:10.1186/s40359-016-0120-9

Brooks, S. K., Webster, R. K., Smith, L. E., Woodland, L., Wessely, S., Greenberg, N., & Rubin, G. J. (2020). The psychological impact of quarantine and how to reduce it: Rapid review of the evidence. *Lancet*, *395*(10227), 912–920. doi:10.1016/S0140-6736(20)30460-8 PMID:32112714

Brotheridge, C. M., & Grandey, A. A. (2002). Emotional Labor and Burnout: Comparing Two Perspectives of "People Work". *Journal of Vocational Behavior*, *60*(1), 17–39. doi:10.1006/jvbe.2001.1815

Browall, M., Henoch, I., Melin-Johansson, C., Strang, S., & Danielson, E. (2014). Existential encounters: Nurses' descriptions of critical incidents in end-of-life cancer care. *European Journal of Oncology Nursing*, *18*(6), 636–644. doi:10.1016/j.ejon.2014.06.001 PMID:24996512

Brown, T., & Rushton, C. (n.d.). *Frontline Nurses WikiWisdom Forum.* https://nurses.wikiwisdomforum.com/

Brown, J. P., Martin, D., Nagaria, Z., Verceles, A. C., Jobe, S. L., & Wickwire, E. M. (2020). Mental health consequences of shift work: An updated review. *Current Psychiatry Reports*, *22*(7), 1–7. doi:10.100711920-020-1131-z PMID:31955278

Brown, K. W., & Ryan, R. M. (2003). The benefits of being present: Mindfulness and its role in psychological well-being. *Journal of Personality and Social Psychology*, *84*(4), 822–848. doi:10.1037/0022-3514.84.4.822 PMID:12703651

Bryan, C. J., Mintz, J., Clemans, T. A., Leeson, B., Burch, T. S., Williams, S. R., Maney, E., & Rudd, M. D. (2017). Effect of crisis response planning vs. contracts for safety on suicide risk in U.S. Army Soldiers: A randomized clinical trial. *Journal of Affective Disorders*, *212*, 64–72. doi:10.1016/j.jad.2017.01.028 PMID:28142085

Bryant, D. J., Oo, M., & Damian, A. J. (2020). The rise of adverse childhood experiences during the COVID-19 pandemic. *Psychological Trauma: Theory, Research, Practice, and Policy*, *12*(S1), S193–S194. doi:10.1037/tra0000711 PMID:32551773

Bryce, I. (2020). Responding to the accumulation of adverse childhood experiences in the wake of the COVID-19 pandemic: Implications for practice. *Children Australia*, *45*(2), 80–87. doi:10.1017/cha.2020.27

Brykman, K. M., & King, D. D. (2021). A Resource Model of Team Resilience Capacity and Learning. *Group & Organization Management*, *46*(4). doi:10.1177/10596011211018008

Brymer, M., Layne, C., Jacobs, A., Pynoos, R., Ruzek, J., Steinberg, A., . . . Watson, P. (2006). *Psychological first aid field operations guide.* National Child Traumatic Stress Network. Available from: https://www.nctsn.org/resources/psychological-first-aid-pfa-field-operations-guide-2nd-edition

Buckley, L., Berta, W., Cleverley, K., Medeiros, C., & Widger, K. (2020). What is known about paediatric nurse burnout: A scoping review. *Human Resources for Health*, *18*(1), 1–23. doi:10.118612960-020-0451-8 PMID:32046721

Budhwani, H., & Sun, R. (2020). Creating COVID-19 stigma by referencing the novel coronavirus as the "Chinese virus" on Twitter: Quantitative analysis of social media data. *Journal of Medical Internet Research*, *22*(5), e19301. doi:10.2196/19301 PMID:32343669

Budiman, A. (2020, August 20). *Key findings about U.S. immigrants.* Pew Research Center.

Burdick, L., Mielke, G. I., Parra, D. C., Gomes, G., Florindo, A., Bracco, M., Lobelo, F., Simoes, E. J., Pratt, M., Ramos, L. R., Moura, L., Brownson, R. C., & Hallal, P. C. (2015). Physicians', nurses' and community health workers' knowledge about physical activity in Brazil: A cross-sectional study. *Preventive Medicine Reports*, *2*, 467–472. doi:10.1016/j.pmedr.2015.06.001 PMID:26844104

Bureau of Labor Statistics. (2010). *Employer-reported workplace injuries and illnesses – 2013.* Retrieved from www.bls.gov

Bureau of Labor Statistics. (2018). *Employer-reported workplace injuries and illnesses – 2018.* Retrieved from www.bls.gov

Bureau of Labor Statistics. (2020). *Foreign-born workers: Labor force characteristics - 2019.* Author.

Burke, C.S., Salas, E., Wilson-Donnelly, K., & Priest, H. (2004). How to turn a team of experts into an expert medical team: guidance from the aviation and military communities. *Quality & Safety in Health Care, 13*(1), 96-104. doi:10.1136/qshc.2004.009829

Burton, A., Burgess, C., Dean, S., Koutsopoulou, G. Z., & Hugh-Jones, S. (2017). How effective are mindfulness-based interventions for reducing stress among healthcare professionals? A systematic review and meta-analysis. *Stress and Health, 33*(1), 3–13. doi:10.1002mi.2673 PMID:26916333

Burtscher, M. J., Kolbe, M., Wacker, J., & Manser, T. (2011). Interactions of team mental models and monitoring behaviors predict team performance in simulated anesthesia inductions. *Journal of Experimental Psychology. Applied, 17*(3), 257–269. doi:10.1037/a0025148 PMID:21942315

Bylander, J. (2020). How COVID-19 threatens the safety net for US children. *Health Affairs, 39*(10), 1668–1671. doi:10.1377/hlthaff.2020.01576 PMID:33017239

Cabarkapa, S., Nadjidai, S. E., Murgier, J., & Ng, C. H. (2020). The psychological impact of COVID-19 and other viral epidemics on frontline healthcare workers and ways to address it: A rapid systematic review. *Brain, Behavior, & Immunity - Health, 8*, 100144.

Cai, B., Tu, J., Ma, L., Chen, L., Fu, Y., & Jiang, Q. (2020). Psychological impact and coping strategies of frontline medical staff in Hunan between January and March 2020 during the outbreak of coronavirus disease 2019 (COVID19) in Hubei. *China Med. Sci. Monit., 26*, e924171. PMID:32291383

Callary, B., Rathwell, S., & Young, B. W. (2015). Insights on the Process of Using Interpretive Phenomenological Analysis in a Sport Coaching Research Project. *Qualitative Report, 20*(2), 63–75. doi:10.46743/2160-3715/2015.2096

Cammann, C., Fichman, M., Jenkins, G. D., & Klesh, J. (1983). Michigan organizational assessment questionnaire. In S. E. Seashore, E. E. Lawler, P. H. Mirvis, & C. Cammann (Eds.), *Assessing organizational change: a guide to methods, measures, and practices* (pp. 71–138). John Wiley & Sons.

Campbell, J. P. (1990). Modeling the performance prediction problem in industrial and organizational psychology. In M. D. Dunnette & L. M. Hough (Eds.), *Handbook of industrial and organizational psychology* (pp. 687–732). Consulting Psychologists Press.

Canepa, C. M. (2020). COVID Blues. *Annals graphic medicine.* https://www.acpjournals.org/doi/10.7326/G20-0053

Cannon-Bowers, J. (2007). Fostering mental model convergence through training. In *Multi-level issues in organizations and time*. Emerald Group Publishing Limited. doi:10.1016/S1475-9144(07)06006-7

Carlopio, J. R. (1996). Construct validity of a physical work environment satisfaction questionnaire. *Journal of Occupational Health Psychology, 1*(3), 330–344. doi:10.1037/1076-8998.1.3.330 PMID:9547055

Carmassi, C., Foghi, C., Dell'Oste, V., Cordone, A., Bertelloni, C. A., Bui, E., & Dell'Osso, L. (2020). PTSD symptoms in healthcare workers facing the three coronavirus outbreaks: What can we expect after the COVID-19 pandemic. *Psychiatry Research, 292*, 113312. doi:10.1016/j.psychres.2020.113312 PMID:32717711

Carubia, B., Becker, A., & Levine, B. H. (2016). Child psychiatric emergencies: Updates on trends, clinical care, and practice challenges. *Current Psychiatry Reports, 18*(4), 41. doi:10.100711920-016-0670-9 PMID:26932516

Casper, W. J., Fox, K. E., Sitzmann, T. M., & Landy, A. L. (2004). Supervisor referrals to work-family programs. *Journal of Occupational Health Psychology, 9*(2), 136–151. doi:10.1037/1076-8998.9.2.136 PMID:15053713

Cavanagh, N., Cockett, G., Heinrich, C., Doig, L., Fiest, K., Guichon, J. R., Page, S., Mitchell, I., & Doig, C. J. (2019). Compassion fatigue in healthcare providers: A systematic review and meta-analysis. *Nursing Ethics*, *27*(3), 639–665. doi:10.1177/0969733019889400 PMID:31829113

Center for Substance Abuse Treatment (US), Trauma-Informed Care in Behavioral Health Services, Substance Abuse and Mental Health Services Administration (US). (2014). *Treatment Improvement Protocol (TIP) Series, No. 57. Chapter 3, Understanding the Impact of Trauma*. Available from: https://www.ncbi.nlm.nih.gov/books/NBK207191/

Center for Translational Neuroscience. (n.d.). *Rapid assessment of pandemic impact on development–early childhood (RAPID-EC)*. University of Oregon. https://www.uorapidresponse.com/latest-data-and-trends

Centers for Disease Control and Prevention. (2018). *Workplace Health in America 2017*. Centers for Disease Control and Prevention, U.S. Department of Health and Human Services.

Centers for Disease Control. (2021). *Preventing child abuse and neglect*. https://www.cdc.gov/violenceprevention/childabuseandneglect/fastfact.html

Ceravolo, D., & Raines, D. A. (2018). The impact of a mindfulness intervention for nurse managers. *Journal of Holistic Nursing*, *37*(1), 47–55. doi:10.1177/0898010118781620 PMID:29909707

Chang, M., Nitzke, S., Guilford, E., Adair, C. H., & Hazard, D. L. (2008). Motivators and barriers to healthful eating and physical activity among low-income overweight and obese mothers. *Journal of the American Dietetic Association*, *108*(6), 1023–1028. doi:10.1016/j.jada.2008.03.004 PMID:18502238

Chang, Y., & Chan, H. J. (2015). Optimism and proactive coping in relation to burnout among nurses. *Journal of Nursing Management*, *23*(3), 401–408. doi:10.1111/jonm.12148 PMID:24112222

Chang, Y.-J., Kwon, Y. C., Lee, W. J., Do, Y. R., Lee, K. S., Kim, H. T., Park, S. R., Hong, Y. S., Chung, I.-J., & Yun, Y. H. (2013). Burdens, Needs and Satisfaction of Terminal Cancer Patients and their Caregivers. *Asian Pacific Journal of Cancer Prevention*, *14*(1), 209–215. doi:10.7314/APJCP.2013.14.1.209 PMID:23534725

Chan, J. F. W., Yuan, S., Kok, K. H., To, K. K. W., Chu, H., Yang, J., Xing, F., Liu, J., Yip, C. C.-Y., Poon, R. W.-S., Tsoi, H.-W., Lo, S. K.-F., Chan, K.-H., Poon, V. K.-M., Chan, W.-M., Ip, J. D., Cai, J.-P., Cheng, V. C.-C., Chen, H., ... Yuen, K. Y. (2020). A familial cluster of pneumonia associated with the 2019 novel coronavirus indicating person-to-person transmission: A study of a family cluster. *Lancet*, *395*(10223), 514–523. doi:10.1016/S0140-6736(20)30154-9 PMID:31986261

Chan, Z. C., Fung, Y., & Chien, W. (2013). Bracketing in Phenomenology: Only Undertaken in the Data Collection and Analysis Process. *Qualitative Report*, *18*(30), 1–9. doi:10.46743/2160-3715/2013.1486

Chapman, M. T., Lines, R. L. J., Crane, M., Ducker, K. J., Ntoumanis, N., Peeling, P., Parker, S. K., Quested, E., Temby, P., Thøgersen-Ntoumani, C., & Gucciardi, D. F. (2020). Team resilience: A scoping review of conceptual and empirical work. *Work and Stress*, *34*(1), 57–81. doi:10.1080/02678373.2018.1529064

Chappel, S. E., Verswijveren, S. J. J. M., Aisbett, B., Considine, J., & Ridgers, N. D. (2017). Nurses' occupational physical activity levels: A systematic review. *International Journal of Nursing Studies*, *73*, 52–62. doi:10.1016/j.ijnurstu.2017.05.006 PMID:28535398

Charon, R. (2001). Narrative medicine: A model for empathy, reflection, profession, and trust. *Journal of the American Medical Association*, *286*(15), 1897–1902. doi:10.1001/jama.286.15.1897 PMID:11597295

Chast, R. (2014). *Can't we talk about something more pleasant?* Bloomsbury.

Chattu, V. K., Sakhamuri, S. M., Kumar, R., Spence, D. W., BaHammam, A. S., & Pandi-Perumal, S. R. (2018). BaHammam AS, Pandi-Perumal SR. Insufficient Sleep Syndrome: Is it time to classify it as a major noncommunicable disease? *Sleep Science*, *11*(2), 56. doi:10.5935/1984-0063.20180013 PMID:30083291

Chauhan, P. (2020). Gendering COVID-19: Impact of the Pandemic on Women's Burden of Unpaid Work in India. *Gender Issues*. Advance online publication. doi:10.100712147-020-09269-w PMID:33132690

Chen, D., Jaenicke, E. C., & Volpe, R. J. (2016). Food environments and obesity: Household diet expenditure versus food deserts. *American Journal of Public Health*, *106*(5), 881–889. doi:10.2105/AJPH.2016.303048 PMID:26985622

Cheng, H., Yang, H., Ding, Y., & Wang, B. (2020). Nurses' mental health and patient safety: An extension of the job demands-resources model. *Journal of Nursing Management*, *28*(3), 653–663. doi:10.1111/jonm.12971 PMID:32052511

Cheng, W., Zhang, F., Liu, Z., Zhang, H., Lyu, Y., Xu, H., Hua, Y., Gu, J., Yang, Z., & Liu, J. (2020). A psychological health support scheme for medical teams in COVID-19 outbreak and its effectiveness. *General Psychiatry*, *33*(5), e100288. doi:10.1136/gpsych-2020-100288 PMID:34192236

Chen, H.-M., & Hu, H.-M. (2019). Randomized trial of modified stretching exercise program for menstrual low back pain. *Western Journal of Nursing Research*, *41*(2), 238–257. doi:10.1177/0193945918763817 PMID:29529975

Chen, K., Chen, Y., Ling, Y., & Lin, J. (2020). The individual experience of online chemistry teacher education in China: Coping with COVID-19 pandemic. *Journal of Chemical Education*, *97*(9), 3265–3270. doi:10.1021/acs.jchemed.0c00581

Chen, P. G., Auerbach, D. I., Muench, U., Curry, L. A., & Bradley, E. H. (2013). Policy solutions to address the foreign-educated and foreign-born health care workforce in the United States. *Health Affairs*, *32*(11), 1906–1913. doi:10.1377/hlthaff.2013.0576 PMID:24191079

Chen, S.-L., Shih, C.-T., & Chi, N.-W. (2018). A multilevel job demands-resources model of work engagement: Antecedents, consequences, and boundary conditions. *Human Performance*, *31*(5), 282–304. doi:10.1080/08959285.2018.1531867

Cheong, Z. Y., Lopez, V., & Tam, W. S. W. (2021). Barriers to healthy eating among nurses working in hospitals: A meta-synthesis. *Journal of Advanced Nursing*. PMID:34477228

Cheung, T., Wong, S. Y., Wong, K. Y., Law, L. Y., Ng, K., Tong, M. T., Wong, K. Y., Ng, M. Y., & Yip, P. S. (2016). Depression, anxiety and symptoms of stress among baccalaureate nursing students in Hong Kong: A cross-sectional study. *International Journal of Environmental Research and Public Health*, *13*(8), 779. doi:10.3390/ijerph13080779 PMID:27527192

Cheung, V. K.-L., So, E. H.-K., Ng, G. W.-Y., So, S.-S., Hung, J. L.-K., & Chia, N.-H. (2020). Investigating effects of healthcare simulation on personal strengths and organizational impacts for healthcare workers during COVID-19 pandemic: A cross-sectional study. *Integrative Medicine Research*, *9*(3), 100476. doi:10.1016/j.imr.2020.100476 PMID:32802743

Child Welfare Information Gateway. (2021). Child maltreatment 2019: *Summary of key findings*. U.S. Department of Health and Human Services. https://www.childwelfare.gov/pubs/factsheets/canstats/

Chishti, M., & Bolter, J. (2020, April 24). *Vulnerable to COVID-19 and in frontline job, immigrants are mostly shut out of U.S. relief*. Migration Policy Institute.

Cho, G. J., & Kang, J. (2017). Type D personality and post-traumatic stress disorder symptoms among intensive care unit nurses: The mediating effect of resilience. *PLoS One*, *12*(4), e0175067. doi:10.1371/journal.pone.0175067 PMID:28380063

Choi, S., Hong, J. Y., Kim, Y. J., & Park, H. (2020). Predicting psychological distress amid the COVID-19 pandemic by machine learning: Discrimination and coping mechanisms of Korean immigrants in the U.S. *International Journal of Environmental Research and Public Health*, *17*(17), 1–14. doi:10.3390/ijerph17176057 PMID:32825349

Chokshi, M., Patil, B., Khanna, R., Neogi, S. B., Sharma, J., Paul, V. K., & Zodpey, S. (2016). Health systems in India. *Journal of Perinatology*, *36*(3), S9–S12. doi:10.1038/jp.2016.184 PMID:27924110

Chowdhury, S. (2005). Demographic diversity for building an effective entrepreneurial team: Is it important? *Journal of Business Venturing*, *20*(6), 727–746. doi:10.1016/j.jbusvent.2004.07.001

Christensen, M., Innstrand, S. T., & Saksvik, P. Ø. (2020). Healthy workplaces: Designing and implementing health-promoting organizational interventions in healthcare. In L. Tevik Løsveth & A. de Lange (Eds.), *Integrating the Organization of Health Services, Worker Wellbeing and Quality of Care* (pp. 1–15). Springer. doi:10.1007/978-3-030-59467-1_14

Christensen, M., Innstrand, S. T., Saksvik, P. Ø., & Nielsen, K. (2019). The line manager's role in implementing successful organizational interventions. *The Spanish Journal of Psychology*, *22*(e5), 1–11. doi:10.1017jp.2019.4 PMID:30819272

Christian, C. W., Crawford-Jakubiak, J. E., Flaherty, E. G., Leventhal, J. M., Lukefahr, J. L., Sege, R. D., MacMillan, H., Nolan, C. M., Valley, L. A., & Hurley, T. P. (2015). The evaluation of suspected child physical abuse. *Pediatrics*, *135*(5), e1337–e1354. doi:10.1542/peds.2015-0356 PMID:25917988

Cipriano, P. F., Boston-Leary, K., Mcmillan, K., & Peterson, C. (2020). The U.S. COVID-19 crises: Facts, science and solidarity. *International Nursing Review*, *67*(4), 437–444. doi:10.1111/inr.12646 PMID:33428227

Clark, E., Fredricksid, K., Woc-Colburn, L., Bottazzi, M. E., & Weatherheadid, J. (2020). Disproportionate impact of the COVID-19 pandemic on immigrant communities in the United States. *PLoS Neglected Tropical Diseases*, *14*(7), 1–9. doi:10.1371/journal.pntd.0008484 PMID:32658925

Clay, R. A. (2020, June 11). *Are you experiencing compassion fatigue?* American Psychological Association. http://www.apa.org/topics/covid-19/compassion-fatigue

Clegg, A. (2001). Occupational stress in nursing: A review of the literature. *Journal of Nursing Management*, *9*(2), 101–106. doi:10.1046/j.1365-2834.2001.00216.x PMID:11879452

Coetzee, S. K., & Klopper, H. C. (2010). Compassion fatigue within nursing practice: A concept analysis. *Nursing & Health Sciences*, *12*(2), 235–243. doi:10.1111/j.1442-2018.2010.00526.x PMID:20602697

Cohen, C. I., Lo, P., Nzodom, C., & Sahlu, S. (2018). Culture, heritage, and diversity in older adult mental health care. In Migration, acculturation, and mental health (pp. 53–180). Academic Press.

Cohen-Katz, J., Wiley, S., Capuano, T., Baker, D. M., Deitrick, L., & Shapiro, S. (2005). The effects of mindfulness-based stress reduction on nurse stress and burnout: A qualitative and quantitative study, part III. *Holistic Nursing Practice*, *19*(2), 78–86. doi:10.1097/00004650-200503000-00009 PMID:15871591

Cohen, S., Janicki-Deverts, D., & Miller, G. E. (2007). Psychological stress and disease. *Journal of the American Medical Association*, *298*(14), 1685–1687. doi:10.1001/jama.298.14.1685 PMID:17925521

Cohen, S., Kamarck, T., & Mermelstein, R. (1983). A global measure of perceived stress. *Journal of Health and Social Behavior*, *24*(4), 385–396. doi:10.2307/2136404 PMID:6668417

Colak, R. (2020). *The vitals: True nurse stories.* Marvel Comics.

Cole-King, A., & Dykes, L. (2020). *Wellbeing for HCWs during COVID19.* https://www.lindadykes.org/covid19

Cole-King, A., & Gilbert, P. (2011). Compassionate care: The theory and the reality. *Journal of Holistic Healthcare*, *8*(3).

Collins, C. J., & Clark, K. D. (2003). Strategic human resource practices, top management team social networks, and firm performance: The role of human resource practices in creating organizational competitive advantage. *Academy of Management Journal*, *46*(6), 740–751.

Collins, K., & Nicolson, P. (2002). The meaning of 'satisfaction for people with dermatological problems: Re-assessing approaches to qualitative health psychology research. *Journal of Health Psychology*, *7*(5), 615–629. doi:10.1177/1359105302007005681 PMID:22113145

Colman, M. M., & Carron, A. V. (2001). The nature of norms in individual sport teams. *Small Group Research*, *32*(2), 206–222. doi:10.1177/104649640103200204

Colville, G. A., & Smith, J. G. (2017). The overlap between burnout and depression in ICU staff. *Critical Care Medicine*, *45*(10), e1102–e1103. doi:10.1097/CCM.0000000000002546 PMID:28915199

Colville, G., Dawson, D., Rabinthiran, S., Chaudry-Daley, Z., & Perkins-Porras, L. (2019). A survey of moral distress in staff working in intensive care in the UK. *The Journal of the Intensive Care Society*, *20*(3), 196–203. doi:10.1177/1751143718787753 PMID:31447911

Compassion Fatigue Awareness Project. (2013). *The Caregiver's Bill of Rights*. https://compassionfatigue.org/pages/TheBillOfRights.pdf

Conklin, E. J. (2006). *Dialogue mapping: Building shared understanding of wicked problems*. Wiley.

Connor, D. B. O., Jones, F., Conner, M., Mcmillan, B., & Ferguson, E. (2008). Effects of daily hassles and eating style on eating behavior. *Health Psychology*, *27*(1), 20–31. doi:10.1037/0278-6133.27.1.S20 PMID:18248102

Connors, C. A., Dukhanin, V., March, A. L., Parks, J. A., Norvell, M., & Wu, A. W. (2020). Peer support for nurses as second victims: Resilience, burnout, and job satisfaction. *Journal of Patient Safety and Risk Management*, *25*(1), 22–28. doi:10.1177/2516043519882517

Conrad, P. (1987). The experience of illness: recent and new directions. Research in the sociology of health care. Vol. 6: the experience and management of chronic illness, 1-31.

Converse, S. A., Cannon-Bowers, J. A., & Salas, E. (1991, September). Team member shared mental models: A theory and some methodological issues. In *Proceedings of the Human Factors Society Annual Meeting* (Vol. 35, No. 19, pp. 1417-1421). SAGE Publications. 10.1177/154193129103501917

Cook, C., & Burgess-Limerick, R. (2003). Guidelines for computer workstations. *Ergonomics Australia*, *17*(1), 19–37. doi:10.1080/00140139.2015.1076528

Cooper, C. L., Dewe, P. J., & O'Driscoll, M. P. (2001). Organizational Stress: A Review and Critique of Theory, Research, and Applications. *Sage (Atlanta, Ga.)*.

Corley, M. C. (2002). Nurse moral distress: A proposed theory and research agenda. *Nursing Ethics*, *9*(6), 636–650. doi:10.1191/0969733002ne557oa PMID:12450000

Cortina, L. M., Kabat-Farr, D., Leskinen, E. A., Huerta, M., & Magley, V. J. (2013). Selective Incivility as Modern Discrimination in Organizations: Evidence and Impact. *Journal of Management*, *39*(6), 1579–1605. doi:10.1177/0149206311418835

Costa, A. C. (2003). Work team trust and effectiveness. *Personnel Review*, *32*(5), 605–622. doi:10.1108/00483480310488360

Coughlan, B., Powell, D., & Higgins, M. F. (2017). The second victim: A review. *European Journal of Obstetrics, Gynecology, and Reproductive Biology*, *213*, 11–16. doi:10.1016/j.ejogrb.2017.04.002 PMID:28526169

COVID Trauma Response Working Group. (2020). https://www.traumagroup.org

Cox, T., & Rial-Gonzalez, E. (2002). Work-related stress: the European picture. *Magazine of the European Agency for Safety and Health at Work*, *5*, 4-6. https://osha.europa.eu/en/publications/magazine/5

Craigie, M., Slatyer, S., Hegney, D., Osseiran-Moisson, R., Gentry, E., Davis, S., Dolan, T., & Rees, C. (2016). A pilot evaluation of a mindful self-care and resiliency (MSCR) intervention for Nurses. *Mindfulness, 7*(3), 764–774. doi:10.100712671-016-0516-x

Crenshaw, K. (1989). *Demarginalizing the Intersection of Race and Sex: A Black* Feminist Critique of Antidiscrimination Doctrine, Feminist Theory and Antiracist Politics. University of Chicago Legal Forum.

Crimi, C., & Carlucci, A. (2021). Challenges for the female healthcare workers during the COVID-19 pandemic: The need for protection beyond the mask. *Pulmonology, 27*(1), 1–3. doi:10.1016/j.pulmoe.2020.09.004 PMID:33087308

Cropanzano, R., Rupp, D. E., & Byrne, Z. S. (2003). The relationship of emotional exhaustion to work attitudes, job performance, and organizational citizenship behaviors. *The Journal of Applied Psychology, 88*(1), 160–169. doi:10.1037/0021-9010.88.1.160 PMID:12675403

Crouch, M. (2021, May 11). What nurses want you to know about the past year. *AARP*. https://www.aarp.org/health/conditions-treatments/info-2021/nurses-reflect-on- pandemic.html

Crust, L., & Clough, J. (2011). Developing mental toughness: From research to practice. *Journal of Sport Psychology in Action, 2*(1), 21–32. doi:10.1080/21520704.2011.563436

Cubrich, M., & Tengesdal, J. (2021). Precarious work during precarious times: Addressing the compounding effects of race, gender, and immigration status. *Industrial and Organizational Psychology: Perspectives on Science and Practice, 14*(1–2), 133–138. doi:10.1017/iop.2021.42

Cull, W. L., Frintner, M. P., Starmer, A. J., & Leslie, L. K. (2019). Longitudinal analyses of pediatrician burnout. *Academic Pediatrics, 19*(3), 256–262. doi:10.1016/j.acap.2018.11.006 PMID:30412766

Curtis, J. R., Sprung, C. L., & Azoulay, E. (2014). The importance of word choice in the care of critically ill patients and their families. *Intensive Care Medicine, 40*(4), 606–608. doi:10.100700134-013-3201-8 PMID:24441669

Cyr, C., McKee, H., O'Hagan, M., & Priest, R. (2016). *Making the Case for Peer Support: Report to the Peer Support Project Committee of the Mental Health Commission of Canada*. Mental Health Commission of Canada. Available online https://www.mentalhealthcommission.ca/sites/default/files/2016-07/MHCC_Making_the_Case_for_Peer_Support_2016_Eng.pdf

Czerwiec, M. K. (2017). *Taking turns: Stories from HIV/AIDS care Unit 371*. The Pennsylvania State University Press.

Czerwiec, M. K., & Huang, M. N. (2017). Hospice comics: Representations of patient and family experience of illness and death in graphic novels. *The Journal of Medical Humanities, 38*(2), 95–113. doi:10.100710912-014-9303-7 PMID:25138207

Czerwiec, M. K., & Williams, I. (2015). Introduction. In *Graphic Medicine Manifesto* (pp. 1–20). The Pennsylvania State University Press.

Czerwiec, M. K., Williams, I., Squier, S. M., Green, M. J., Myers, K. R., & Smith, S. T. (2015). *Graphic medicine manifesto*. The Pennsylvania State University Press.

D'Archy, L. P., Sasai, Y., & Stearns, S. C. (2011). Do assistive devices, training, and workload affect injury incidence?Prevention efforts by nursing homes and back injuries among nursing assistants? *Journal of Advanced Nursing, 68*(4), 836–845. doi:10.1111/j.1365-2648.2011.05785.x

D'Rozario, A. (2021, September 7). *Supporting India's Healthcare Workers. New Asia Perspective*. Retrieved from https://www.csis.org/blogs/new-perspectives-asia/supporting-indias-healthcare-workers

Dale, M., & Bell, J. (1999). *Informal learning in the workplace, Research Brief, Number 134*. Department for Education and Employment. www.dfes.gov.uk/research/data/uploadfiles/RB134.doc

Dall'Ora, C., Ball, J., Redfern, O., Recio, S. A., Maruotti, A., Meredith, P., & Griffiths, P. (2019). Are long nursing shifts on hospital wards associated with sickness absence? A longitudinal retrospective observational study. *Journal of Nursing Management*, *27*(1), 19–26. doi:10.1111/jonm.12643 PMID:29978584

Dasborough, M. T., Ashkanasy, N. M., Tee, E. Y., & Herman, H. M. (2009). What goes around comes around: How meso-level negative emotional contagion can ultimately determine organizational attitudes toward leaders. *The Leadership Quarterly*, *20*(4), 571–585. doi:10.1016/j.leaqua.2009.04.009

Day, A., & Nielsen, K. (2017). What does our organization do to help our well-being? Creating healthy workplaces and workers. In N. Chmiel, F. Fraccaroli, & M. Sverke (Eds.), *An Introduction to Work and Organizational Psychology: An International Perspective* (pp. 295–314). Wiley-Blackwell. doi:10.1002/9781119168058.ch16

de Castro, A. B., Fujishiro, K., Tagalog, E. A., Samaco-Paquiz, L. P. G., & Gee, G. C. (2010). Associations between work schedule characte20ristics and occupational injury and illness. *International Nursing Review*, *57*(2), 188–194. doi:10.1111/j.1466-7657.2009.00793.x PMID:20579153

De Hert, S. (2020). Burnout in healthcare workers: Prevalence, impac and preventative strategies. *Local and Regional Anesthesia*, *13*, 171–183. doi:10.2147/LRA.S240564 PMID:33149664

De Jong, B. A., Dirks, K. T., & Gillespie, N. (2016). Trust and team performance: A meta-analysis of main effects, moderators, and covariates. *The Journal of Applied Psychology*, *101*(8), 1134–1150. doi:10.1037/apl0000110 PMID:27123697

De Kock, J. H., Latham, H. A., Leslie, S. J., Grindle, M., Munoz, S.-A., Ellis, L., Polson, R., & O'Malley, C. M. (2021). A rapid review of the impact of COVID-19 on the mental health of healthcare workers: Implications for supporting psychological well-being. *BMC Public Health*, *21*(1), 104. doi:10.118612889-020-10070-3 PMID:33422039

de Moor, M. H. M., Beem, A. L., Stubbe, J. H., Boomsma, D. I., & de Geus, E. J. C. (2006). Regular exercise, anxiety, depression and personality: A population-based study. *Preventive Medicine*, *42*(4), 273–279. doi:10.1016/j.ypmed.2005.12.002 PMID:16439008

Dean, W., Jacobs, B., & Manfredi, R. A. (2020). Moral Injury: The Invisible Epidemic in COVID Health Care Workers. *Annals of Emergency Medicine*, *76*(4), 385–386. doi:10.1016/j.annemergmed.2020.05.023 PMID:32586634

Dean, W., Talbot, S., & Dean, A. (2019). Reframing clinician distress: Moral injury not burnout. *Federal Practitioner: For the Health Care Professionals of the VA, DoD, and PHS*, *36*(9), 400–402. PMID:31571807

Dekker, S. W. A. (2002). Reconstructing human contributions to accidents: The new view on error and performance. *Journal of Safety Research, 33*(3), 371–385. . doi:10.1016/S0022-4375(02)00032-4

Delaney, L. J., Currie, M. J., Huang, H.-C. C., Lopez, V., & Van Haren, F. (2018). "They can rest at home": An observational study of patients' quality of sleep in an australian hospital. *BMC Health Services Research*, *18*(1), 524. Advance online publication. doi:10.118612913-018-3201-z PMID:29976191

Dellve, L., & Eriksson, A. (2017). Health-promoting managerial work: A theoretical framework for a leadership program that supports knowledge and capability to craft sustainable work practices in daily practice and during organizational change. *Societies (Basel, Switzerland)*, *7*(2), 12. doi:10.3390oc7020012

Deloitte. (2018). *2019 Global health care outlook: The evolution of smart health care*. Deloitte Touche Thomtsu Limited.

Delucia, J. (2016, May 10-13) *Rate of post-traumatic stress disorder in emergency medicine physicians*. Society of Academic Emergency Medicine meeting, New Orleans, LA.

DeMatteo, J. S., Eby, L. T., & Sundstrom, E. (1998). Team-based rewards: Current empirical evidence. *Research in Organizational Behavior*, *20*, 141–183.

Demerouti, E., Bakker, A. B., Vardakou, I., & Kantas, A. (2003). The convergent validity of two burnout instruments: A multitrait-multimethod analysis. *European Journal of Psychological Assessment*, *19*(1), 12–23. doi:10.1027//1015-5759.19.1.12

Dennis, W. (Ed.). (2018). *Where we live: A benefit for the survivors in Las Vegas*. Image Comics.

Denollet, J. (2005). DS14: Standard assessment of negative affectivity, social inhibition, and Type D personality. *Psychosomatic Medicine*, *67*(1), 89–97. doi:10.1097/01.psy.0000149256.81953.49 PMID:15673629

DePierro, J., Katz, C. L., Marin, D., Feder, A., Bevilacqua, L., Sharma, V., Hurtado, A., Ripp, J., Lim, S., & Charney, D. (2020). Mount Sinai's Center for Stress, Resilience, and Personal Growth as a model for responding to the impact of COVID-19 on health care workers. *Psychiatry Research*, *29*, 113426. doi:10.1016/j.psychres.2020.113426 PMID:32861094

Derr, A. S. (2016). Mental health service use among immigrants in the United States: A systematic review. *Psychiatric Services (Washington, D.C.)*, *67*(3), 265–274. doi:10.1176/appi.ps.201500004 PMID:26695493

Devries, S., Agatston, A., Aggarwal, M., Aspry, K. E., Esselstyn, C. B., Kris-Etherton, P., Miller, M., O'Keefe, J. H., Ros, E., Rzeszut, A. K., White, B. A., Williams, K. A., & Freeman, A. M. (2017). A deficiency of nutrition education and practice in cardiology. *The American Journal of Medicine*, *130*(11), 1298–1305. doi:10.1016/j.amjmed.2017.04.043 PMID:28551044

Dhanani, L. Y., & Franz, B. (2021). Why public health framing matters: An experimental study of the effects of COVID-19 framing on prejudice and xenophobia in the United States. *Social Science & Medicine*, *269*, 113572. doi:10.1016/j.socscimed.2020.113572 PMID:33321405

DHSC. (2020). *Patients admitted to hospital*. Retrieved from https://coronavirus.data.gov.uk/details/healthcare

Di Tecco, C., Nielsen, K., Ghelli, M., Ronchetti, M., Marzocchi, I., Persechino, B., & Iavicoli, S. (2020). Improving working conditions and job satisfaction in healthcare: A study concept design on a participatory organizational level intervention in psychosocial risks management. *International Journal of Environmental Research and Public Health*, *17*(10), 3677. doi:10.3390/ijerph17103677 PMID:32456147

Di Tella, M., Romeo, A., Benfante, A., & Castelli, L. (2020). Mental health of healthcare workers during the COVID-19 pandemic in Italy. *Journal of Evaluation in Clinical Practice*, *26*(6), 1583–1587. doi:10.1111/jep.13444 PMID:32710481

Díaz Ramiro, E. M., Rubio Valdehita, S., López Núñez, M. I., & Aparicio García, M. E. (2020). *Sleep habits as predictors of psychological health in healthcare professionals*. Academic Press.

DiBenedetto, D. V. (1995). Occupational hazards of the health care industry: Protecting health care workers. *AAOHN Journal*, *43*(3), 131–137. doi:10.1177/216507999504300303 PMID:7702679

DiMaria-Ghalili, R. A., Mirtallo, J. M., Tobin, B. W., Hark, L., Van Horn, L., & Palmer, C. A. (2014). Challenges and opportunities for nutrition education and training in the health care professions: Intraprofessional and interprofessional call to action. *The American Journal of Clinical Nutrition*, *99*(5), 1184S–1193S. doi:10.3945/ajcn.113.073536 PMID:24646823

Doheny, K. (2021, Feb. 1). *Moral injury: Pandemic's fallout for healthcare workers*. WebMD Health News. https://www.webmd.com/lung/news/20210201/moral-injury-pandemics-fallout-for-health-care-workers

Donald, I., Taylor, P., Johnson, S., Cooper, C., Cartwright, S., & Robertson, S. (2005). Work environments, stress, and productivity: An examination using ASSET. *International Journal of Stress Management*, *12*(4), 409–423. doi:10.1037/1072-5245.12.4.409

Donnelly, P. D., Davidson, M., Dunlop, N., McGale, M., Milligan, E., Worrall, M., Wylie, J., & Kidson, C. (2020). Well-being during coronavirus disease 2019: A PICU practical perspective. *Pediatric Critical Care Medicine, 21*(8), e584–e586. doi:10.1097/PCC.0000000000002434 PMID:32412984

Dormann, C., & Zapf, D. (1999). Social support, social stressors at work, and depressive symptoms: Testing for main and moderating effects with structural equations in a three-wave longitudinal study. *The Journal of Applied Psychology, 84*(6), 874–884. doi:10.1037/0021-9010.84.6.874 PMID:10639907

dos Santos, T. M., Kozasa, E. H., Carmagnani, I. S., Tanaka, L. H., Lacerda, S. S., & Nogueira-Martins, L. A. (2016). Positive effects of a stress reduction program based on mindfulness meditation in Brazilian nursing professionals: Qualitative and quantitative evaluation. *Explore (New York, N.Y.), 12*(2), 90–99. doi:10.1016/j.explore.2015.12.005 PMID:26778081

Dowd, M. D. (2019). The relevance of parental adverse childhood experiences in pediatric patients. *Pediatric Annals, 48*(12), e463–e465. doi:10.3928/19382359-20191118-03 PMID:31830283

Duarte, J., & Pinto-Gouveia, J. (2016). Effectiveness of a mindfulness-based intervention on oncology nurses' burnout and compassion fatigue symptoms: A non-randomized study. *International Journal of Nursing Studies, 64*, 98–107. doi:10.1016/j.ijnurstu.2016.10.002 PMID:27744228

Duchemin, A.-M., Steinberg, B. A., Marks, D. R., Vanover, K., & Klatt, M. (2015). A small randomized pilot study of a workplace mindfulness-based intervention for Surgical Intensive Care Unit Personnel. *Journal of Occupational and Environmental Medicine, 57*(4), 393–399. doi:10.1097/JOM.0000000000000371 PMID:25629803

Dyrbye, L. N., Shanafelt, T. D., Sinsky, C. A., Cipriano, P. F., Bhatt, J., Ommaya, A., ... & Meyers, D. (2017). Burnout among health care professionals: A call to explore and address this underrecognized threat to safe, high-quality care. *NAM Perspectives*.

Dzeng, E., Colaianni, A., Roland, M., Levine, D., Kelly, M. P., Barclay, S., & Smith, T. J. (2016). Moral distress amongst American physician trainees regarding futile treatments at the end of life: A qualitative study. *Journal of General Internal Medicine, 31*(1), 93–99. doi:10.100711606-015-3505-1 PMID:26391029

Easter, M. (2021, March 12). "Hamilton" cookie portraits? See how healthcare workers make art to cope with COVID-19. *Los Angeles Times*. https://www.latimes.com/entertainment-arts/story/2021-03-12/healthcare-workers-and-creativity-callout-responses

Eberz, S., & Antoni, C. H. (2018). The TIMP-inventory – a contribution to the identification of core-factors of salutogenic leadership. *Zeitschrift für angewandte Organisationspsychologie, 1*, 69-80. doi:10.1007/s11612-017-0384-4

Eberz, S., & Antoni, C. H. (2016). The Systemic Salutogenic Interaction Modell (SSIM) - A holistic approach for explanation and development of health-promoting interactions between leaders and employees. Gruppe. Interaktion. Organisation. *Zeitschrift für Angewandte Organisationspsychologie, 47*(3), 265–273. doi:10.1007/11612.1862-2615

Eisenberger, R., Stinglhamber, F., Vandenberghe, C., Sucharski, I. L., & Rhoades, L. (2002). Perceived supervisor support: Contributions to perceived organizational support and employee retention. *The Journal of Applied Psychology, 87*(3), 565–573. doi:10.1037/0021-9010.87.3.565 PMID:12090614

Ellis, R., Hay-David, A. G. C., & Brennan, P. A. (2020). Operating during the COVID-19 pandemic: How to reduce medical error. *British Journal of Oral & Maxillofacial Surgery, 58*(5), 577–580. doi:10.1016/j.bjoms.2020.04.002 PMID:32312584

Embriaco, N., Papazian, L., Kentish-Barnes, N., Pochard, F., & Azoulay, E. (2007). Burnout syndrome among critical care healthcare workers. *Current Opinion in Critical Care, 13*(5), 482–488. doi:10.1097/MCC.0b013e3282efd28a PMID:17762223

Emmons, K. M., Linnan, L., Shadel, W. G., Marcus, B., & Abrams, D. B. (1999). The Working Healthy Project: A worksite health-promotion trial targeting physical activity, diet, and smoking. *Journal of Occupational and Environmental Medicine, 41*(7), 545–555. doi:10.1097/00043764-199907000-00003 PMID:10412096

Epstein, E. G., & Hamric, A. B. (2009). Moral distress, moral residue, and the crescendo effect. *The Journal of Clinical Ethics, 20*(4), 330–342. PMID:20120853

Erdem, F., Ozen, J., & Atsan, N. (2003). The relationship between trust and team performance. *Work Study, 52*(7), 337–340. doi:10.1108/00438020310502633

Esmee van Steijn, M., Scheepstra, K. W. F., Yasar, G., Olff, M., Charlotte de Vries, M., & Gabriel van Pampus, M. (2019). Occupational well-being in pediatricians: A survey about work-related posttraumatic stress, depression, and anxiety. *European Journal of Pediatrics, 178*(5), 681–693. doi:10.100700431-019-03334-7 PMID:30783762

Esquivel, M. K. (2021). Nutrition strategies for reducing risk of burnout among physicians and health care professionals. *American Journal of Lifestyle Medicine, 15*(2), 126–129. doi:10.1177/1559827620976538 PMID:33790697

Estabrooks, C., Squires, J., Cummings, G., Birdsell, J., & Norton, P. (2009). Development and assessment of the Alberta Conext Tool. *BMC Health Services Research, 9*(1), 1–12. doi:10.1186/1472-6963-9-234 PMID:20003531

Fairbrother, K., & Warn, J. (2003). Workplace dimensions, stress and job satisfaction. *Journal of Managerial Psychology, 18*(1), 8–21. doi:10.1108/02683940310459565

Falatah, R. (2021). The Impact of the Coronavirus Disease (COVID-19) Pandemic on Nurses' Turnover Intention: An Integrative Review. *Nursing Reports, 11*(4), 787–810. doi:10.3390/nursrep11040075 PMID:34968269

Fan, J., Jiang, Y., Hu, K., Chen, X., Xu, Q., Qi, Y., Yin, H., Gou, X., & Liang, S. (2020). Barriers to using personal protective equipment by healthcare staff during the COVID-19 outbreak in China. *Medicine, 99*(48), e23310. doi:10.1097/MD.0000000000023310 PMID:33235088

Faragher, E. B., Cass, M., & Cooper, C. L. (2005). The relationship between job satisfaction and health: A meta-analysis. *Occupational and Environmental Medicine, 62*(2), 105–112. doi:10.1136/oem.2002.006734 PMID:15657192

Farnsworth, J. K. (2014). Dialogical tensions in heroic military and military-related moral injury. *International Journal for Dialogical Science, 8*(1), 13–37.

Farquharson, B., Bell, C., Johnston, D., Jones, M., Schofield, P., Allan, J., Ricketts, I., Morrison, K., & Johnston, M. (2013). Nursing stress and patient care: real-time investigation of the effect of nursing tasks and demands on psychological stress, physiological stress, and job performance: study protocol. *Journal of Advanced Nursing, 69*(10), 2327–2335. doi:10.1111/jan.12090 PMID:23387943

Faulkner, S. L., & Trotter, S. P. (2017). *Theoretical saturation. In The International Encyclopedia of Communication Research Methods*. John Wiley & Sons.

Fazio, R. H. (1990). Multiple processes by which attitudes guide behavior: The MODE model as an integrative framework. In Advances in experimental social psychology (Vol. 23, pp. 75–109). Academic Press. doi:10.1016/S0065-2601(08)60318-4

Fazio, R. H. (1995). Attitudes as object-evaluation associations: Determinants, consequences, and correlates of attitude accessibility. *Attitude strength: Antecedents and consequences, 4*, 247-282.

Fazio, R. H. (1986). How do attitudes guide behavior? In R. M. Sorrentino & E. T. Higgins (Eds.), *Handbook of motivation and cognition: Foundations of social behavior* (pp. 204–243). Guilford Press.

Feeney, S., O'Brien, K., O'Keeffe, N., Iomaire, A. N. C., Kelly, M. E., McCormack, J., McGuire, G., & Evans, D. S. (2016). Practise what you preach: Health behaviours and stress among non-consultant hospital doctors. *Clinical Medicine*, *16*(1), 12–18. doi:10.7861/clinmedicine.16-1-12 PMID:26833509

Felitti, V. J., Anda, R. F., Nordenberg, D., Williamson, D. F., Spitz, A. M., Edwards, V., Koss, M. P., & Marks, J. S. (1998). Relationship of childhood abuse and household dysfunction to many of the leading causes of death in adults: The adverse childhood experiences (ACS) study. *American Journal of Preventive Medicine*, *14*(4), 245–258. doi:10.1016/S0749-3797(98)00017-8 PMID:9635069

Fernandez, R., Lord, H., Halcomb, E., Moxham, L., Middleton, R., Alananzeh, I., & Ellwood, L. (2020). Implications for COVID-19: A systematic review of nurses' experiences of working in acute care hospital settings during a respiratory pandemic. *International Journal of Nursing Studies*, *111*, 103637. doi:10.1016/j.ijnurstu.2020.103637 PMID:32919358

Ferri, P., Guadi, M., Marcheselli, L., Balduzzi, S., Magnani, D., & Di Lorenzo, R. (2016). The impact of shift work on the psychological and physical health of nurses in a general hospital: A comparison between rotating night shifts and day shifts. *Risk Management and Healthcare Policy*, *9*, 203–211. doi:10.2147/RMHP.S115326 PMID:27695372

Fies, B. (2008). *Mom's cancer*. Abrams Comicarts.

Fies, B. (2019). *A fire story*. Abrams ComicArts.

Figley, C. R. (1995). Compassion fatigue: Toward a new understanding of the costs of caring. In B. H. Stamm (Ed.), *Secondary traumatic stress: Self-care issues for clinicians, researchers, and educators* (pp. 3–28). The Sidran Press.

Figley, C. R. (Ed.). (1995). *Compassion fatigue: Coping with secondary traumatic stress disorder in those who treat the traumatized*. Brunner/Mazel.

Finne, L. B., Christensen, J. O., & Knardahl, S. (2014). Psychological and social work factors as predictors of mental distress: A prospective study. *PLoS One*, *9*(7), e102514. doi:10.1371/journal.pone.0102514 PMID:25048033

Flaherty, E. G., Schwartz, K., Jones, R. D., & Sege, R. D. (2012). Child abuse physicians: Coping with challenges. *Evaluation & the Health Professions*, *36*(2), 163–173. doi:10.1177/0163278712459196 PMID:22960291

Fletcher, D., & Sarkar, M. (2013). Psychological resilience: A review and critique of definitions, concepts, and theory. *European Psychologist*, *18*(1), 12–23. doi:10.1027/1016-9040/a000124

Fletcher, K. A., & Bedwell, W. L. (2017). Cognitive Aids in Emergency Medical Services. In J. R. Keebler, E. H. Lazzara, & P. Misasi (Eds.), *Human Factors and Ergonomics of Prehospital Emergency Care* (pp. 123–140). CRC Press. doi:10.1201/9781315280172-9

Flynn, M., & Mercer, D. (2013). Is compassion possible in a market-led NHS? *Nursing Times*, *109*(7), 12–14. PMID:23513933

Foli, K. J., Reddick, B., Zhang, L., & Krcelich, K. (2020). Nurses' psychological trauma: "They leave me lying awake at night. *Archives of Psychiatric Nursing*, *34*(3), 86–95. doi:10.1016/j.apnu.2020.04.011 PMID:32513472

Fortenberry, K. T., Jansen, K. L., & Clark, M. S. (2017). Positive Affectivity. In M. D. Gellman & J. R. Turner (Eds.), *Encyclopedia of behavioral medicine*. Springer. doi:10.1007/978-1-4614-6439-6_977-2

Foureur, M., Besley, K., Burton, G., Yu, N., & Crisp, J. (2013). Enhancing the resilience of nurses and midwives: Pilot of a mindfulnessbased program for increased health, sense of coherence and decreased depression, anxiety and stress. *Contemporary Nurse*, *45*(1), 114–125. doi:10.5172/conu.2013.45.1.114 PMID:24099232

Franke, F., & Felfe, J. (2011). Diagnose gesundheitsförderlicher führung - Das instrument "health-oriented leadership". In B. Badura, A. Ducki, H. Schröder, J. Klose, & K. Macco (Eds.), *Fehlzeiten-Report 2011* (pp. 3–13). Springer. doi:10.1007/978-3-642-21655-8_1

Franke, F., Felfe, J., & Pundt, A. (2014). The impact of health-oriented leadership on follower health: Development and test of a new instrument measuring health-promoting leadership. *German Journal of Human Resource Management, 28*(1–2), 139–161. doi:10.1177/239700221402800108

Frates, B. (2019). *Lifestyle medicine handbook: An introduction to the power of healthy habits*. Healthy Learning.

Frear, K. A., Donsbach, J., Theilgard, N., & Shanock, L. R. (2018). Supported supervisors are more supportive, but why? A multilevel study of mechanisms and outcomes. *Journal of Business and Psychology, 33*(1), 55–69. doi:10.100710869-016-9485-2

French, K. A., & Shockley, K. M. (2020). Formal and informal supports for managing work and family. *Current Directions in Psychological Science, 29*(2), 207–216. doi:10.1177/0963721420906218

Freudenberger, H. J. (1974). Staff burn-out. *The Journal of Social Issues, 30*(1), 159–165. doi:10.1111/j.1540-4560.1974.tb00706.x

Fridrich, A., Jenny, G. J., & Bauer, G. F. (2015). The context, process, and outcome evaluation model for organisational health interventions. *BioMed Research International, 414832*, 1–12. doi:10.1155/2015/414832 PMID:26557665

Friedkin, N. E. (2001). Norm formation in social influence networks. *Social Networks, 23*(3), 167–189. doi:10.1016/S0378-8733(01)00036-3

Fried, Y., Laurence, G. A., Shirom, A., Melamed, S., Toker, S., Berliner, S., & Shapira, I. (2013). The relationship between job enrichment and abdominal obesity: A longitudinal field study of apparently healthy individuals. *Journal of Occupational Health Psychology, 18*(4), 458–468. doi:10.1037/a0033730 PMID:24001329

Froutan, R., Mazlom, R., Malekzadeh, J., & Mirhaghi, A. (2017). *Relationship between resilience and personality traits in paramedics. International Journal of Emergency Services.*

Gagne, R. M. (1984). Learning outcomes and their effects: Useful categories of human performance. *The American Psychologist, 39*(4), 377. doi:10.1037/0003-066X.39.4.377

Galal, Y. S., Labib, J. R., & Abouelhamd, W. A. (2014). Impact of an infection-control program on nurses' knowledge and attitude in pediatric intensive care units at Cairo University hospitals. *The Journal of the Egyptian Public Health Association, 89*(1), 22–28. doi:10.1097/01.EPX.0000444562.71691.06 PMID:24717397

Galpin, K., Sikka, N., King, S. L., Horvath, K. A., & Shipman, S. A.AAMC Telehealth Advisory Committee. (2021). Expert consensus: Telehealth skills for health care professionals. *Telemedicine Journal and e-Health, 27*(7), 820–824. doi:10.1089/tmj.2020.0420 PMID:33236964

Galuska, L., Hahn, J., Polifroni, E. C., & Crow, G. (2018). A narrative analysis of nurses' experiences with meaning and joy in nursing practice. *Nursing Administration Quarterly, 42*(2), 154–163. doi:10.1097/NAQ.0000000000000280 PMID:29494451

Galvin, J., Richards, G., & Smith, A. P. (2020). A longitudinal cohort study investigating inadequate preparation and death and dying in nursing students: Implications for the aftermath of the COVID-19 pandemic. *Frontiers in Psychology, 11*, 2206. doi:10.3389/fpsyg.2020.02206 PMID:32982890

Gama, G., Barbosa, F., & Vieira, M. (2014). Personal determinants of nurses' burnout in end of life care. *European Journal of Oncology Nursing, 18*(5), 527–533. doi:10.1016/j.ejon.2014.04.005 PMID:24888265

Gameiro, M., Chambel, M. J., & Carvalho, V. S. (2020). A person-centered approach to the job demands–control model: A multifunctioning test of additive and buffer hypotheses to explain burnout. *International Journal of Environmental Research and Public Health, 17*(23), 8871. doi:10.3390/ijerph17238871 PMID:33260306

Ganster, D. C., Crain, T. L., & Brossoit, R. M. (2018). Physiological Measurement in the Organizational Sciences: A Review and Recommendations for Future Use. *Annual Review of Organizational Psychology and Organizational Behavior, 5*(1), 267–293. doi:10.1146/annurev-orgpsych-032117-104613

Gao, J., Wang, F., Guo, S., & Hu, F. (2021). Mental health of nursing students amid coronavirus disease 2019 pandemic. *Frontiers in Psychology, 12*, 699558. doi:10.3389/fpsyg.2021.699558 PMID:34475837

Gao, W., Ping, S., & Liu, X. (2020). Gender differences in depression, anxiety, and stress among college students: A longitudinal study from China. *Journal of Affective Disorders, 263*, 292–300. doi:10.1016/j.jad.2019.11.121 PMID:31818792

García-Fernández, L., Romero-Ferreiro, V., López-Roldán, P., Padilla, S., Calero-Sierra, I., Monzó-García, M., Perez-Martin, J., & Rodriguez-Jimenez, R. (2020). Mental health impact of COVID-19 pandemic on Spanish healthcare workers. *Psychological Medicine, 51*, 1–3. doi:10.1017/S0033291720002019 PMID:32456735

Garman, A. N., Corrigan, P. W., & Morris, S. (2002). Staff burnout and patient satisfaction: Evidence of relationships at the care unit level. *Journal of Occupational Health Psychology, 7*(3), 235–241. doi:10.1037/1076-8998.7.3.235 PMID:12148955

Gauthier, T., Meyer, R. M. L., Grefe, D., & Gold, J. I. (2015). An on-the-job mindfulness-based intervention for pediatric ICU Nurses: A pilot. *Journal of Pediatric Nursing, 30*(2), 402–409. doi:10.1016/j.pedn.2014.10.005 PMID:25450445

Gayed, A., Milligan-Saville, J. S., Nicholas, J., Bryan, B. T., LaMontagne, A. D., Milner, A., Madan, I., Calvo, R. A., Christensen, H., Mykletun, A., Glozier, N., & Harvey, S. B. (2018). Effectiveness of training workplace managers to understand and support the mental health needs of employees: A systematic review and meta-analysis. *Occupational and Environmental Medicine, 75*(6), 462–470. doi:10.1136/oemed-2017-104789 PMID:29563195

Geaney, F., Kelly, C., Di Marrazzo, J. S., Harrington, J. M., Fitzgerald, A. P., Greiner, B. A., & Perry, I. J. (2016). The effect of complex workplace dietary interventions on employees' dietary intakes, nutrition knowledge and health status: A cluster controlled trial. *Preventive Medicine, 89*, 76–83. doi:10.1016/j.ypmed.2016.05.005 PMID:27208667

Geaney, F., Kelly, C., Greiner, B. A., Harrington, J. M., Perry, I. J., & Beirne, P. (2013). The effectiveness of workplace dietary modification interventions: A systematic review. *Preventive Medicine, 57*(5), 438–447. doi:10.1016/j.ypmed.2013.06.032 PMID:23850518

Gelatt, J. (2020). *Immigrant Workers: Vital to the U.S. COVID-19 Response, Disproportionately Vulnerable.* Migration Policy Institute.

Geoffroy, P. A., Le Goanvic, V., Sabbagh, O., Richoux, C., Weinstein, A., Dufayet, G., & Lejoyeux, M. (2020). Psychological support system for hospital workers during the Covid-19 outbreak: Rapid design and implementation of the Covid-Psy hotline. *Frontiers in Psychiatry, 11*, 511. doi:10.3389/fpsyt.2020.00511 PMID:32670100

George, C. E., Inbaraj, L. R., Rajukutty, S., & de Witte, L. P. (2020). Challenges, experience and coping of health professionals in delivering healthcare in an urban slum in India during the first 40 days of COVID-19 crisis: A mixed method study. *BMJ Open, 10*(11), e042171. doi:10.1136/bmjopen-2020-042171 PMID:33208338

George, D. R., & Green, M. J. (2015). Lessons learned from comics produced by medical students: Art of darkness. *Journal of the American Medical Association, 314*(22), 2345. doi:10.1001/jama.2015.13652 PMID:26647249

Gerson, R., Malas, N., & Mroczkowski, M. (2018). Crisis in the emergency department: The evaluation and management of acute agitation in children and adolescents. *Child and Adolescent Psychiatric Clinics of North America, 27*(3), 367–386. doi:10.1016/j.chc.2018.02.002 PMID:29933788

Ghawadra, S. F., Abdullah, K. L., Choo, W. Y., & Phang, C. K. (2019, November). Mindfulness-based stress reduction for psychological distress among nurses: A systematic review. *Journal of Clinical Nursing, 28*(21-22), 3747–3758. doi:10.1111/jocn.14987 PMID:31267619

Ghosh, S., Moledina, N., Hasan, M. M., Jain, S., & Ghosh, A. (2021). Colossal Challenges to the healthcare workers combating the second wave of COVID-19 in India. *Infection Control and Hospital Epidemiology, 1-5*. Advance online publication. doi:10.1017/ice.2021.257 PMID:34075871

Gibbons, S. W., Shafer, M., Hickling, E. J., & Ramsey, G. (2013). How Do Deployed Health Care Providers Experience Moral Injury? *Narrative Inquiry in Bioethics, 3*(3), 247–259. doi:10.1353/nib.2013.0055 PMID:24407133

Gibbs, T., Pauselli, L., Vieux, U., Solan, M., & Rosenfield, P. (2020). Mental Health Disparities Among Black Americans During the COVID-19 Pandemic. *Psychiatric Times*.

Gibson, C. B., Conger, J. A., & Cooper, C. (2001). Perceptual distance: The impact of differences in team leader and member perceptions across cultures. In J. Osland, M. E. Mendenhall, R. S. Reiche, & B. Szkudlarek (Eds.), *Advances in Global Leadership* (Vol. 2, pp. 245–276). Emerald Group Publishing Limited. doi:10.1016/S1535-1203(01)02122-0

Gibson, C. B., Cooper, C. D., & Conger, J. A. (2009). Do you see what we see? The complex effects of perceptual distance between leaders and teams. *The Journal of Applied Psychology, 94*(1), 62–76. doi:10.1037/a0013073 PMID:19186896

Gifford, V., Niles, B., Rivkin, I., Koverola, C., & Polaha, J. (2012). Continuing education training focused on the development of behavioral telehealth competencies in behavioral healthcare providers. *Rural and Remote Health, 12*, 1–15. doi:10.22605/RRH2108 PMID:23240871

Gilbert, P. (2010). Compassion Focused Therapy: Distinctive Features. Routledge.

Gilbert, P., Catarino, F., Duarte, C., Matos, M., Kolts, R., Stubbs, J., Ceresatto, L., Duarte, J., Pinto-Gouveia, J., & Basran, J. (2017). The development of compassionate engagement and action scales for self and others. *Journal of Compassionate Health Care, 4*(1), 4. doi:10.118640639-017-0033-3

Gilbreath, B., & Benson, P. G. (2004). The contribution of supervisor behaviour to employee psychological well-being. *Work and Stress, 18*(3), 255–266. doi:10.1080/02678370412331317499

Given, L. M. (2015). *100 Questions (and Answers) about Qualitative Research*. SAGE publications.

Gjerde, S., & Alvesson, M. (2020). Sandwiched: Exploring role and identity of middle managers in the genuine middle. *Human Relations, 73*(1), 124–151. doi:10.1177/0018726718823243

Glasø, L., & Einarsen, S. (2008). Emotion regulation in leader-follower relationships. *European Journal of Work and Organizational Psychology, 17*(4), 482–500. doi:10.1080/13594320801994960

Gloster, A. T., Walder, N., Levin, M. E., Twohig, M. P., & Karekla, M. (2020). The empirical status of acceptance and commitment therapy: A review of meta-analyses. *Journal of Contextual Behavioral Science, 18*, 181–192. doi:10.1016/j.jcbs.2020.09.009

Goel, S. (2020, January 31). The doctor-population ratio in India is 1:1456 against WHO recommendation. *Deccan Herald*. Retrieved from https://www.deccanherald.com/business/budget-2020/the-doctor-population-ratio-in-india-is-11456-against-who-recommendation-800034.html

Goetzel, R. Z., & Ozminkowski, R. J. (2008). The health and cost benefits of work site programs. *Annual Review of Public Health*, *29*(1), 303–323. doi:10.1146/annurev.publhealth.29.020907.090930 PMID:18173386

Goffman, E. (1963). Stigma: Notes on the management of spoiled identity. *Touchstone (Nashville, Tenn.)*.

Gold, J. A. (2020). Covid-19: Adverse mental health outcomes for healthcare workers. *BMJ (Clinical Research Ed.)*, 369. doi:10.1136/bmj.m1815 PMID:32371465

Golubic, R., Milosevic, M., Knezevic, B., & Mustajbegovic, J. (2009). Work-related stress, education and work ability among hospital nurses. *Journal of Advanced Nursing*, *65*(10), 2056–2066. doi:10.1111/j.1365-2648.2009.05057.x PMID:19627386

Gómez-Urquiza, J. L., Albendín-García, L., Velando-Soriano, A., Ortega-Campos, E., Ramírez-Baena, L., Membrive-Jiménez, M. J., & Suleiman-Martos, N. (2020). Burnout in palliative care nurses, prevalence and risk factors: A systematic review and meta-analysis. *International Journal of Environmental Research and Public Health*, *17*(20), 7672. doi:10.3390/ijerph17207672 PMID:33096682

Goode, S., Diefendorf, M., & Colgan, S. (2011). *The importance of early intervention for infants and toddlers with developmental disabilities and their families*. National Early Childhood Technical Assistance Center. https://ectacenter.org/~pdfs/pubs/importanceofearlyintervention.pdf

Graber, J. E., Huang, E. S., Drum, M. L., Chin, M. H., Walters, A. E., Heuer, L., Tang, H., Schaefer, C. T., & Quinn, M. T. (2008). Predicting Changes in Staff Morale and Burnout at Community Health Centers Participating in the Health Disparities Collaboratives: Staff Morale and Burnout at Community Health Centers. *Health Services Research*, *43*(4), 1403–1423. doi:10.1111/j.1475-6773.2007.00828.x PMID:18248402

Grauerholz, K. R., Fredenburg, M., Jones, P. T., & Jenkins, K. N. (2020). Fostering vicarious resilience for perinatal palliative care professionals. *Frontiers in Pediatrics*, *8*, 572933. Advance online publication. doi:10.3389/fped.2020.572933 PMID:33134232

Green, M. J., & Myers, K. R. (2010). Graphic medicine: Use of comics in medical education and patient care. *BMJ*, *340*(2), c863–c863. doi:10.1136/bmj.c863

Greenberg, N., Docherty, M., Gnanapragasam, S., & Wessely, S. (2020). Managing mental health challenges faced by healthcare workers during covid-19 pandemic. *BMJ (Clinical Research Ed.)*, *m1211*, m1211. doi:10.1136/bmj.m1211 PMID:32217624

Greenberg, N., & Tracy, D. (2020). What healthcare leaders need to do to protect the psychological well-being of frontline staff in the COVID-19 pandemic. *BMJ Leader*, *4*(3), 101–102. doi:10.1136/leader-2020-000273

Grimm, C. A. (2020). *Hospital experiences responding to the COVID-19 pandemic: Results of a national pulse survey March 23-27, 2020*. U.S. Department of Health and Human Services Office of Inspector general. Retrieved on March 12, 2022 from https://oig.hhs.gov/oei/reports/oei-06-20-00300.pdf

Griswold, D. T., & Salmon, J. (2020). Lower Barriers to Immigrant Healthcare Workers to Help Combat the COVID-19 Pandemic. SSRN *Electronic Journal*. doi:10.2139/ssrn.3592978

Grzywacz, J. G. (2000). Work-family spillover and health during midlife: Is managing conflict everything? *American Journal of Health Promotion*, *14*(4), 236–243. doi:10.4278/0890-1171-14.4.236 PMID:10915535

Grzywacz, J. G., Casey, P. R., & Jones, F. A. (2007). The effects of workplace flexibility on health behaviors: A cross-sectional and longitudinal analysis. *Journal of Occupational and Environmental Medicine*, *49*(12), 1302–1309. doi:10.1097/JOM.0b013e31815ae9bc PMID:18231077

Grzywacz, J. G., Frone, M. R., Brewer, C. S., & Kovner, C. T. (2006). Quantifying work–family conflict among registered nurses. *Research in Nursing & Health*, *29*(5), 414–426. doi:10.1002/nur.20133 PMID:16977647

Guadagno, L. (2020). *Migrants and the COVID-19 pandemic: An initial analysis*. International Organization for Migration.

Gun Violence Archive. (2021). Retrieved from https://www.gunviolencearchive.org/

Gunia, B. C., Sipos, M. L., LoPresti, M., & Adler, A. B. (2015). Sleep leadership in high-risk occupations: An investigation of soldiers on peacekeeping and combat missions. *Military Psychology*, *27*(4), 197–211. doi:10.1037/mil0000078

Gupta, S., & Sahoo, S. (2020). Pandemic and mental health of the frontline healthcare workers: A review and implications in the Indian context amidst COVID-19. *General Psychiatry*, *33*(5), 1–10. doi:10.1136/gpsych-2020-100284 PMID:34192235

Gurt, J., Schwennen, C., & Elke, G. (2011). Health-specific leadership: Is there an association between leader consideration for the health of employees and their strain and well-being? *Work and Stress*, *25*(2), 108–127. doi:10.1080/02678373.2011.595947

Gustin, T. S., Kott, K., & Rutledge, C. (2020). Telehealth etiquette training: A guideline for preparing interprofessional teams for successful encounters. *Nurse Educator*, *45*(2), 88–92. doi:10.1097/NNE.0000000000000680 PMID:31022072

Hacimusalar, Y., Kahve, A. C., Yasar, A. B., & Aydin, M. S. (2020). Effects of coronavirus disease 2019 (COVID-19) pandemic on anxiety and hopelessness levels: A cross-sectional study in healthcare workers and community sample in Turkey. *Journal of Psychiatric Research*, *129*, 181–188. doi:10.1016/j.jpsychires.2020.07.024 PMID:32758711

Haddad, L., Annamaraju, P., & Toney-Butler, T. (2021). *Nursing Shortage*. StatPearls Publishing. https://www.ncbi.nlm.nih.gov/books/NBK493175/

Haight, W., Sugrue, E. P., & Calhoun, M. (2017). Moral injury among Child Protection Professionals: Implications for the ethical treatment and retention of workers. *Children and Youth Services Review*, *82*, 27–41. doi:10.1016/j.childyouth.2017.08.030

Hall, G. B., Dollard, M. F., & Coward, J. (2010). Psychosocial safety climate: Development of the PSC-12. *International Journal of Stress Management*, *17*(4), 353–383. doi:10.1037/a0021320

Hall, L. H., Johnson, J., Watt, I., Tsipa, A., & O'Connor, D. B. (2016). Healthcare Staff Wellbeing, Burnout, and Patient Safety: A Systematic Review. *PLoS One*, *11*(7), e0159015. doi:10.1371/journal.pone.0159015 PMID:27391946

Hall, R. C., Hall, R. C., & Chapman, M. J. (2008). The 1995 Kikwit Ebola outbreak: Lessons hospitals and physicians can apply to future viral epidemics. *General Hospital Psychiatry*, *30*(5), 446–452. doi:10.1016/j.genhosppsych.2008.05.003 PMID:18774428

Halm, M. (2017). The Role of Mindfulness in Enhancing Self-Care for Nurses. *American Journal of Critical Care*, *26*(4), 344–348. doi:10.4037/ajcc2017589 PMID:28668922

Hammerback, K., Hannon, P. A., Harris, J. R., Clegg-Thorp, C., Kohn, M., & Parrish, A. (2015). Perspectives on workplace health promotion among employees in low-wage industries. *American Journal of Health Promotion*, *29*(6), 384–392. doi:10.4278/ajhp.130924-QUAL-495 PMID:25162321

Hammer, L., Brady, J. M., & Perry, M. (2020). Training supervisors to support veterans at work: Effects on supervisor attitudes and employee sleep and stress. *Journal of Occupational and Organizational Psychology*, *93*(2), 273–301. doi:10.1111/joop.12299

Hamouche, S. (2020). COVID-19 and employees' mental health: Stressors, moderators and agenda for organizational actions. *Emerald Open Research*, *2*, 15. doi:10.35241/emeraldopenres.13550.1

Hamric, A. B., & Blackhall, L. J. (2007). Nurse-physician perspectives on the care of dying patients in intensive care units: Collaboration, moral distress, and ethical climate*. *Critical Care Medicine*, *35*(2), 422–429. doi:10.1097/01.CCM.0000254722.50608.2D PMID:17205001

Hamric, A. B., Borchers, C. T., & Epstein, E. G. (2012). Development and Testing of an Instrument to Measure Moral Distress in Healthcare Professionals. *AJOB Primary Research*, *3*(2), 1–9. doi:10.1080/21507716.2011.652337

Han, K., Trinkoff, A. M., Storr, C. L., & Geiger-Brown, J. (2011). Job stress and work schedules in relation to nurse obesity. *JONA: The Journal of Nursing Administration*, *41*(11), 488-495. https://www.healthypeople.gov/2020/leading-health-indicators/2020-lhi-topics/Nutrition-Physical-Activity-and-Obesity

Hartwig, A., Clarke, S., Johnson, S., & Willis, S. (2020). Workplace team resilience: A systematic review and conceptual development. *Organizational Psychology Review*, *10*(3-4), 169–200. doi:10.1177/2041386620919476

Hasson, R., Stark, A. H., Constantini, N., Polak, R., Verbov, G., Edelstein, N., ... Soltz-Aharony, H. (2018). "Practice What You Teach" Public Health Nurses Promoting Healthy Lifestyles (PHeeL-PHiNe): Program Evaluation. *The Journal of Ambulatory Care Management*, *41*(3), 171–180. doi:10.1097/JAC.0000000000000243 PMID:29847404

Havsteen-Franklin, D., Tjasink, M., Kottler, J. W., Grant, C., & Kumari, V. (2020). Arts-based interventions for professionals in caring roles during and after crisis: A systematic review of the literature. *Frontiers in Psychology*, *11*, 589744. doi:10.3389/fpsyg.2020.589744 PMID:33414746

Hayes, S. C., & Hofmann, S. G. (2017). The third wave of cognitive behavioral therapy and the rise of process-based care. *World Psychiatry, 16*(3), 245-246. doi:10.1002/wps.20442

Hazarika, O. B., & Das, S. (2021). Paid and unpaid work during the Covid-19 pandemic: A study of the gendered division of domestic responsibilities during lockdown. *Journal of Gender Studies*, *30*(4), 429–439. doi:10.1080/09589236.2020.1863202

Healy, C. M., & McKay, M. F. (2000). Nursing stress: The effects of coping strategies and job satisfaction in a sample of Australian nurses. *Journal of Advanced Nursing*, *31*(3), 681–688. doi:10.1046/j.1365-2648.2000.01323.x PMID:10718888

Hearn, D., Schuh-Renner, A., Canham-Chervak, M., Hodges, E. U., & Evarts, L. (2018). Barriers to physical activity among military hospital employees. The United States Army Medical Department, 1(205), 76.

Heath, C., Sommerfield, A., & von Ungern-Sternberg, B. S. (2020). Resilience strategies to manage psychological distress among healthcare workers during the COVID-19 pandemic: A narrative review. *Anaesthesia*, *75*(10), 1364–1371. doi:10.1111/anae.15180 PMID:32534465

HEE. (2019). *NHS Staff and Learners' Mental Wellbeing Commission.* Retrieved from https://www.hee.nhs.uk/sites/default/files/documents/NHS%20%28HEE%29%20-%20Mental%20Wellbeing%20Commission%20Report.pdf

Hee, K. L., Pathmawati, S., Norsiah, R., & Phang, C. K. (2014). The effects of mindfulness training program on reducing stress and promoting well-being among nurses in critical care units. *The Australian Journal of Advanced Nursing*, *31*, 22–31.

Heesakkers, H., Zegers, M., van Mol, M. M. C., & van den Boogaard, M. (2021). The impact of the first COVID-19 surge on the mental well-being of ICU nurses: A nationwide survey study. *Intensive & Critical Care Nursing*, *65*, 103034. doi:10.1016/j.iccn.2021.103034 PMID:33863609

Heesch, K. C., Brown, D. R., & Blanton, C. J. (2000). Perceived barriers to exercise and stage of exercise adoption in older women of different racial/ethnic groups. *Women & Health*, *30*(4), 61–76. doi:10.1300/J013v30n04_05 PMID:10983610

Hellhammer, D., & Hellhammer, J. (Eds.). (2008). *Stress: the brain-body connection*. Karger Medical and Scientific Publishers. doi:10.1159/isbn.978-3-8055-7969-8

Hemingway, M. A., & Smith, C. S. (1999). Organizational climate and occupational stressors as predictors of withdrawal behaviours and injuries in nurses. *Journal of Occupational and Organizational Psychology*, *72*(3), 285–299. doi:10.1348/096317999166680

Henrich, J., Heine, S. J., & Norenzayan, A. (2010). The weirdest people in the world? *Behavioral and Brain Sciences*, *33*(2), 61–83. doi:10.1017/S0140525X0999152X PMID:20550733

Hensel, J. M., Ruiz, C., Finney, C., & Dewa, C. S. (2015). Meta-analysis of risk factors for secondary traumatic stress in therapeutic work with trauma victims. *Journal of Traumatic Stress*, *28*(2), 83–91. doi:10.1002/jts.21998 PMID:25864503

Hershler, A., Hughes, L., Nguyen, P., & Wall, S. (Eds.). (2021). *Looking at trauma: A toolkit for clinicians*. The Pennsylvania University Press. doi:10.1515/9780271092287

Hertel, G., Geister, S., & Konradt, U. (2005). Managing virtual teams: A review of current empirical research. *Human Resource Management Review*, *15*(1), 69–95. doi:10.1016/j.hrmr.2005.01.002

Hevezi, J. A. (2016). Evaluation of a Meditation Intervention to Reduce the Effects of Stressors Associated With Compassion Fatigue Among Nurses. *Journal of Holistic Nursing*, *34*(4), 343–350. doi:10.1177/0898010115615981 PMID:26598000

Hinchey, S. A., & Jackson, J. L. (2011). A cohort study assessing difficult patient encounters in a walk-in primary care clinic: Predictors and outcomes. *Journal of General Internal Medicine*, *26*(6), 588–594. doi:10.100711606-010-1620-6 PMID:21264521

Hines, S. E., Chin, K. H., Levine, A. R., & Wickwire, E. M. (2020). Initiation of a survey of healthcare worker distress and moral injury at the onset of the COVID-19 surge. *American Journal of Industrial Medicine*, *63*(9), 830–833. doi:10.1002/ajim.23157

Hinshaw, S. P. (2010). *The mark of shame: Stigma of mental illness and an agenda for change*. Oxford University Press.

Hoboubi, N., Choobineh, A., Ghanavati, F. K., Keshavarzi, S., & Hosseini, A. A. (2017). The impact of job stress and job satisfaction on workforce productivity in an Iranian petrochemical industry. *Safety and Health at Work*, *8*(1), 67–71. doi:10.1016/j.shaw.2016.07.002 PMID:28344843

Hodgson, L. (2021). How violent attacks are changing the demands of mass casualty incidents: A review of the challenges associated with intentional mass casualty incidents. *The Journal of the NPS Center for Homeland Defense and Security*, *17*(1). https://www.hsaj.org/articles/16880

Hoelscher, L., & Ravert, R. (2021). Workplace relationships and professional burnout among certified child life specialists. *The Journal of Child Life: Psychosocial Theory and Practice*, *2*(1), 15–25. doi:10.55591/001c.22523

Hoge, C. W., Castro, C. A., Messer, S. C., McGurk, D., Cotting, D. I., & Koffman, R. L. (2004). Combat Duty in Iraq and Afghanistan, Mental Health Problems, and Barriers to Care. *The New England Journal of Medicine*, *351*(1), 13–22. doi:10.1056/NEJMoa040603 PMID:15229303

Holdsworth, M. A. (2019). Health, wellness and wellbeing. *Revue Interventions Économiques. Papers in Political Economy*, (62).

Holtzclaw, L., Arlinghaus, K. R., & Johnston, C. A. (2021). The Health of Health Care Professionals. *American Journal of Lifestyle Medicine*, *15*(2), 130–132. doi:10.1177/1559827620977065 PMID:33790698

Hong, Z., Li, N., Li, D., Li, J., Li, B., Xiong, W., Lu, L., Li, W., & Zhou, D. (2020). Telemedicine during the COVID-19 pandemic: Experiences from western China. *Journal of Medical Internet Research*, *22*(5), e19577. doi:10.2196/19577 PMID:32349962

Horan, K. A., Moeller, M. T., Singh, R. S., Wasson, R., O'Brien, W. H., Matthews, R. A., Jex, S. M., & Barratt, C. L. (2018). Supervisor support for stress management and intervention process. *International Journal of Workplace Health Management*, *11*(4), 260–272. doi:10.1108/IJWHM-12-2017-0113

Horner, J. K., Piercy, B. S., Eure, L., & Woodard, E. K. (2014). A pilot study to evaluate mindfulness as a strategy to improve inpatient nurse and patient experiences. *Applied Nursing Research*, *27*(3), 198–201. doi:10.1016/j.apnr.2014.01.003 PMID:24602399

Horton, R. (2019). Offline: Touch—the first language. *Lancet*, *394*(10206), 1310. doi:10.1016/S0140-6736(19)32280-9 PMID:31609215

Hosseinabadi, M. B., Khanjani, N., Etemadinezhad, S., Samaei, S. E., Raadabadi, M., & Mostafaee, M. (2017). The associations of workload, individual and organisational factors on nurses' occupational injuries. *Journal of Clinical Nursing*, *28*(5-6), 902–911. doi:10.1111/jocn.14699 PMID:30357967

House, J. S. (1981). *Work stress and social support*. Addison-Wesley Series on Occupational Stress.

Houston, S., Casanova, M. A., Leveille, M., Schmidt, K. L., Barnes, S. A., Trungale, K. R., & Fine, R. L. (2013). The intensity and frequency of moral distress among different healthcare disciplines. *The Journal of Clinical Ethics*, *24*(2), 98–112.

Houtrow, A. J. (2020). Addressing burnout: Symptom management versus treating the cause. *The Journal of Pediatrics*, *224*, 18–19. doi:10.1016/j.jpeds.2020.04.068 PMID:32370952

Howard, K. J., Howard, J. T., & Smyth, A. F. (2012). The problem of absenteeism and presenteeism in the workplace. In R. J. Gatchel & I. Z. Schultz (Eds.), *Handbook of Occupational Health and Wellness* (pp. 151–917). Springer Science + Business Media. https://doi-org.proxy108.nclive.org/10.1007/978-1-4614-4839-6_8

Hsieh, H. F., Hung, Y. T., Wang, H. H., Ma, S. C., & Chang, S. C. (2016). Factors of resilience in emergency department nurses who have experienced workplace violence in Taiwan. *Journal of Nursing Scholarship*, *48*(1), 23–30. doi:10.1111/jnu.12177 PMID:26580490

Huang, Y., & Zhao, N. (2020). Generalized anxiety disorder, depressive symptoms and sleep quality during COVID-19 outbreak in China: A web-based cross-sectional survey. *Psychiatry Research*, *288*, 112954–112954. doi:10.1016/j.psychres.2020.112954 PMID:32325383

Hui, B. P., Ng, J. C., Berzaghi, E., Cunningham-Amos, L. A., & Kogan, A. (2020). Rewards of kindness? A meta-analysis of the link between prosociality and well-being. *Psychological Bulletin*, *146*(12), 1084–1116. doi:10.1037/bul0000298 PMID:32881540

Hummel, S., Oetjen, N., Du, J., Posenato, E., de Almeida, R. M. R., Losada, R., ... Schultz, J. H. (2021). Mental health among medical professionals during the COVID-19 pandemic in eight european countries: Cross-sectional survey study. *Journal of Medical Internet Research*, *23*(1), e24983. doi:10.2196/24983 PMID:33411670

Humpel, N., Owen, N., & Leslie, E. (2002). Environmental factors associated with adults' participation in physical activity: A review. *American Journal of Preventive Medicine*, *22*(3), 188–199. doi:10.1016/S0749-3797(01)00426-3 PMID:11897464

Hurtado, D. A., Nelson, C. C., Hashimoto, D., & Sorensen, G. (2015). Supervisors' Support for Nurses' Meal Breaks and Mental Health. *Workplace Health & Safety*, *63*(3), 107–115. doi:10.1177/2165079915571354 PMID:25994975

Hu, Y.-Y., Ellis, R. J., Hewitt, D. B., Yang, A. D., Cheung, E. O., Moskowitz, J. T., Potts, J. R. III, Buyske, J., Hoyt, D. B., Nasca, T. J., & Bilimoria, K. Y. (2019). Discrimination, Abuse, Harassment, and Burnout in Surgical Residency Training. *The New England Journal of Medicine*, *381*(18), 1741–1752. doi:10.1056/NEJMsa1903759 PMID:31657887

Hyman, P. (2020). The disappearance of the primary care physical examination—Losing touch. *JAMA Internal Medicine*, *180*(11), 1417–1418. doi:10.1001/jamainternmed.2020.3546 PMID:32832987

Igou, E. R., Blake, A. A., & Bless, H. (2020). Just-world beliefs increase helping intentions via meaning and affect. *Journal of Happiness Studies*, *22*(5), 2235–2253. doi:10.100710902-020-00317-6

Ijntema, R. C., Burger, Y. D., & Schaufeli, W. B. (2019). Reviewing the labyrinth of psychological resilience: Establishing criteria for resilience-building programs. *Consulting Psychology Journal*, *71*(4), 288–304. doi:10.1037/cpb0000147

Ilhan, M. N., Durukan, E., Aras, E., Türkçüoğlu, S., & Aygün, R. (2006). Long working hours increase the risk of sharp and needlestick injury in nurses: The need for new policy implication. *Journal of Advanced Nursing*, *56*(5), 563–568. doi:10.1111/j.1365-2648.2006.04041.x PMID:17078831

Iliffe, S., & Manthorpe, J. (2019). Job dissatisfaction, 'burnout' and alienation of labour: Undercurrents in England's NHS. *Journal of the Royal Society of Medicine*, *112*(9), 370–377. doi:10.1177/0141076819855956

Imboden, A., Sobczak, B. K., & Griffin, V. (2021). The impact of the COVID-19 pandemic on infant and toddler development. *Journal of the American Association of Nurse Practitioners*, 1–11. doi:10.1097/JXX.0000000000000653 PMID:34519673

Imo, U. O. (2017). Burnout and psychiatric morbidity among doctors in the UK: A systematic literature review of prevalence and associated factors. *BJPsych Bulletin*, *41*(4), 197–204. doi:10.1192/pb.bp.116.054247

Institute for healthcare improvement. (n.d.a). *The IHI Triple Aim*. Improving Health and Health Care Worldwide | IHI - Institute for Healthcare Improvement. https://www.ihi.org/Engage/Initiatives/TripleAim/Pages/default.aspx

Institute for healthcare improvement. (n.d.b). *Joy in work*. Improving Health and Health Care Worldwide | IHI - Institute for Healthcare Improvement. https://www.ihi.org/Topics/Joy-In-Work/Pages/default.aspx

Institute Of Medicine Committee on Quality Healthcare in America. (2001). *Crossing the quality chasm*. National Academies Press. What Physicians need to do to optimize telehealth after the pandemic.

Ives, J., Greenfield, S., Parry, J. M., Draper, H., Gratus, C., Petts, J. I., Sorell, T., & Wilson, S. (2009). Healthcare workers' attitudes to working during pandemic influenza: A qualitative study. *BMC Public Health*, *9*(1), 1–13. doi:10.1186/1471-2458-9-56 PMID:19216738

Iyengar, K. P., Jain, V. K., & Vaishya, R. (2020). Current situation with doctors and healthcare workers during COVID-19 pandemic in India. *Postgraduate Medical Journal*, *0*, 1–2. doi:10.1136/postgradmedj-2020-138496 PMID:32817496

Jacobsen, H. B., Reme, S. E., Sembajwe, G., Hopcia, K., Stiles, T. C., Sorensen, G., Porter, J. H., Marino, M., & Buxton, O. M. (2014). Work stress, sleep deficiency, and predicted 10-year cardiometabolic risk in a female patient care worker population. *American Journal of Industrial Medicine*, *57*(8), 940–949. doi:10.1002/ajim.22340 PMID:24809311

Jaggers, A. (2020, March 12). *COVID-19 Comics.* Graphic Medicine International Collective. https://www.graphicmedicine.org/covid-19-comics/

Jakobsen, M. D., Sundstrup, E., Brandt, M., & Andersen, L. L. (2018). Effect of physical exercise on musculoskeletal pain in multiple body regions among healthcare workers: Secondary analysis of a cluster randomized controlled trial. *Musculoskeletal Science & Practice, 34*, 89–96. doi:10.1016/j.msksp.2018.01.006 PMID:29414757

Jakobsen, M. D., Sundstrup, E., Brandt, M., Jay, K., Aagaard, P., & Andersen, L. L. (2015). Physical exercise at the workplace prevents deterioration of work ability among healthcare workers: Cluster randomized controlled trial. *BMC Public Health, 15*(1), 1–9. doi:10.118612889-015-2448-0 PMID:26607232

Jameton, A. (1984). *Nursing practice: The ethical issues.* Prentice Hall.

Jameton, A. (2017). What moral distress in nursing history could suggest about the future of health care. *AMA Journal of Ethics, 19*(6), 617–628. doi:10.1001/journalofethics.2017.19.6.mhst1-1706 PMID:28644792

Jarukasemthawee, S., Halford, W. K., & McLean, J. P. (2019). When East meets West: A randomized controlled trial and pre- to postprogram evaluation replication of the effects of insight-based mindfulness on psychological well-being. *Journal of Psychotherapy Integration, 29*(3), 307–323. doi:10.1037/int0000179

Jeffrey, R. W., French, S. A., Raether, C., & Baxter, J. E. (1994). An environmental intervention to increase fruit and salad purchases in a cafeteria. *Preventive Medicine, 23*(6), 788–792. doi:10.1006/pmed.1994.1135 PMID:7855111

Jenkins, R., & Elliot, P. (2004). Stressors, burnout and social support: Nurses in acute mental mental health settings. *Journal of Advanced Nursing, 48*(6), 622–631. doi:10.1111/j.1365-2648.2004.03240.x PMID:15548253

Jenkins, S. R., & Baird, S. (2002). Secondary traumatic stress and vicarious trauma: A validational study. *Journal of Traumatic Stress: Official Publication of The International Society for Traumatic Stress Studies, 15*(5), 423–432. doi:10.1023/A:1020193526843 PMID:12392231

Johnson, J. (2010). The skeleton on the couch: The eagleton affair, rhetorical disability, and the stigma of mental illness. *Rhetoric Society Quarterly, 40*(5), 459–478. doi:10.1080/02773945.2010.517234

Joinson, C. (1992). Coping with compassion fatigue. *Nursing, 22*(4), 116–121. doi:10.1097/00152193-199204000-00035 PMID:1570090

Jones, K. J., Skinner, A., Xu, L., Sun, J., & Keith Muelleet, K. (2008). The AHRQ Hospital Survey on Patient Safety Culture: A Tool to Plan and Evaluate Patient Safety Programs. In *Advances in Patient Safety: New Directions and Alternative Approaches (Vol. 2: Culture and Redesign).* Agency for Healthcare Research and Quality (US). ncbi.nlm.nih.gov/books/NBK43699/

Jones-Berry, S. (2020). COVID-19: nurses offered alternative housing to safeguard loved ones. Nursing Standard. *Nursing Standard.* Retrieved from https://rcni.com/nursing-standard/newsroom/news/covid-19-nurses-offered-alternative-housing-to-safeguard-loved-ones-159156

Jones, S. (2017). Describing the mental health profile of first responders: A systematic review. *Journal of the American Psychiatric Nurses Association, 23*(3), 200–214. doi:10.1177/1078390317695266 PMID:28445653

Joy, S. (2020, March 25). Amidst COVID-19 outbreak, landlords ask doctors, nurses to vacate houses; govt warns owners. *Deccan Herald.* Retrieved from https://www.deccanherald.com/national/amidst-covid-19-outbreak-landlords-ask-doctors-nurses-to-vacate-houses-govt-warns-owners-817435.html

Judd-Glossy, L., & Twohy, E. (2020). Distress parents and family issues. In B. D. Carter & K. A. Kullgren (Eds.), *Clinical Handbook of Psychological Consultation in Pediatric Medical Settings* (pp. 401–412). Springer Nature. doi:10.1007/978-3-030-35598-2_30

Judge, T. A., Piccolo, R. F., & Ilies, R. (2004). The forgotten ones? The validity of consideration and initiating structure in leadership research. *The Journal of Applied Psychology*, *89*(1), 36–51. doi:10.1037/0021-9010.89.1.36 PMID:14769119

Judkins, S. & Rind, R. (2005). Hardiness, job satisfaction, and stress among home health nurses. *Home Health Care Management & Practice, 17*(2), 113-118. DOI:70020 doi:10.1177/10848223042

Jun, J., Ojemeni, M. M., Kalamani, R., Tong, J., & Crecelius, M. L. (2021). Relationship between nurse burnout, patient and organizational outcomes: Systematic review. *International Journal of Nursing Studies*, *119*, 103933. doi:10.1016/j.ijnurstu.2021.103933 PMID:33901940

Juvanhol, L. L., Silva-Costa, A., Rotenberg, L., Moreno, A. B., Melo, E. C. P., Santos, I. S., Nunes, M. A. A., Toivanen, S., Chor, D., & Griep, R. H. (2022). Is work-family conflict a pathway between job strain components and binge eating? A cross-sectional analysis from the ELSA-Brasil study. *Journal of Eating Disorders*, *10*(1), 1–9. doi:10.118640337-022-00540-x PMID:35123594

Kahn-Marshall, J. L., & Gallant, M. P. (2012). Making healthy behaviors the easy choice for employees. *Health Education & Behavior*, *39*(6), 752–776. doi:10.1177/1090198111434153 PMID:22872583

Kakunje, A. (2011). Stress among health care professionals - The need for resiliency. *Online Journal of Health and Allied Sciences: OJHAS*, *10*, 1.

Kalmakis, K. A., & Chandler, G. E. (2013). Adverse childhood experiences: Towards a clear conceptual meaning. *Journal of Advanced Nursing*, *70*(7), 1489–1501. Advance online publication. doi:10.1111/jan.12329 PMID:24329930

Kanter, R. M., Stein, B. A., & Jick, T. D. (1992). *The Challenge of Organisational Change*. The Free Press.

Kasila, K., Hallman, M., Kautiainen, H., Vanhala, M., & Kettunen, T. (2018). The gap between behavioral risk status and willingness to change behavior among healthcare professionals. *Perspectives in Public Health*, *138*(6), 311–315. doi:10.1177/1757913917751564 PMID:29356601

Kath, L. M., Ehrhart, M. E., Gates, M. G., & Stichler, J. F. (2012). *Nurse Leader Stress Study: Final Feedback Report Round 2 Survey* [Proprietary feedback reports prepared for 34 acute-care hospitals participating in the study.]. San Diego State University.

Kawakami, N., Kobayashi, Y., Takao, S., & Tsutsumi, A. (2005). Effects of web-based supervisor training on supervisor support and psychological distress among workers: A randomized controlled trial. *Preventive Medicine*, *41*(2), 471–478. doi:10.1016/j.ypmed.2005.01.001 PMID:15917043

Kelly, L. A., Gee, P. M., & Butler, R. J. (2021). Impact of nurse burnout on organizational and position turnover. *Nursing Outlook*, *69*(1), 96–102. doi:10.1016/j.outlook.2020.06.008 PMID:33023759

Kenna, G. A., & Lewis, D. C. (2008). Risk factors for alcohol and other drug use by healthcare professionals. *Substance Abuse Treatment, Prevention, and Policy*, *3*(1), 1–8. doi:10.1186/1747-597X-3-3 PMID:18230139

Kerker, B. D., Storfer-Isser, A., Szilagyi, M., Stein, R. E. K., Garner, A. S., O'Connor, K. G., Hoagwood, K. E., & Horwitz, S. M. (2016). Do pediatricians ask about adverse childhood experiences in pediatric primary care? *Academic Pediatrics*, *16*(2), 154–160. doi:10.1016/j.acap.2015.08.002 PMID:26530850

Khajuria, A., Tomaszewski, W., Liu, Z., Chen, J., Mehdian, R., Fleming, S., Vig, S., & Crawford, M. J. (2021). Workplace factors associated with mental health of healthcare workers during the COVID-19 pandemic: An international cross-sectional study. *BMC Health Services Research, 21*(1), 262. doi:10.118612913-021-06279-6 PMID:33743674

Khamisa, N., Peltzer, K., & Oldenburg, B. (2013). Burnout in relation to specific contributing factors and health outcomes among nurses: A systematic review. *International Journal of Environmental Research and Public Health, 10*(6), 2214–2240. doi:10.3390/ijerph10062214 PMID:23727902

Khasne, R. W., Dhakulkar, B. S., & Mahajan, H. C. (2020). Burnout among Healthcare Workers during COVID-19 Pandemic in India: Results of a Questionnaire-based Survey. *Indian Journal of Critical Care Medicine, 24*(8), 664–671. doi:10.5005/jp-journals-10071-23518

Khatutsky, G., Wiener, J., Anderson, W., & Porell, F. (2012). Work-related injuries among certified nursing assistants in nursing homes. RTI Press publication No. RR-0017-1204. Research Triangle Park, NC: RTI Press. doi:10.3768/rtipress.2012.rr.0017.1204

Kim, E. J., Marrast, L., & Conigliaro, J. (2020). COVID-19: Magnifying the Effect of Health Disparities. *Journal of General Internal Medicine, 35*(8), 2441–2442. Advance online publication. doi:10.100711606-020-05881-4 PMID:32394141

Kim, J. J., Brookman-Frazee, L., Gellatly, R., Stadnick, N., Barnett, M. L., & Lau, A. S. (2018). Predictors of burnout among community therapists in the sustainment phase of a system-driven implementation of multiple evidence-based practices in children's mental health. *Professional Psychology, Research and Practice, 49*(2), 131–142. doi:10.1037/pro0000182 PMID:30270968

King, H. B., Battles, J., Baker, D. P., Alonso, A., Salas, E., Webster, J., ... Salisbury, M. (2008). TeamSTEPPS™: team strategies and tools to enhance performance and patient safety. *Advances in Patient Safety: new directions and alternative approaches (Vol. 3: performance and tools).*

King, D. D., Newman, A., & Luthans, F. (2016). Not if, but when we need resilience in the workplace. *Organizational Behavior, 37*, 782–786. doi:10.1002/job

Kirkcaldy, B., Wittig, U., Furnham, A., Merbach, M., & Siefen, R. G. (2006). Health and migration. Psychosocial determinants. *Bundesgesundheitsblatt, Gesundheitsforschung, Gesundheitsschutz, 49*(9), 873–883. doi:10.100700103-006-0021-9 PMID:16953359

Kitahara, C. M., Flint, A. J., Berrington de Gonzalez, A., Bernstein, L., Brotzman, M., MacInnis, R. J., Moore, S. C., Robien, K., Rosenberg, P. S., Singh, P. N., Weiderpass, E., Adami, H. O., Anton-Culver, H., Ballard-Barbash, R., Buring, J. E., Freedman, D. M., Fraser, G. E., Beane Freeman, L. E., Gapstur, S. M., ... Hartge, P. (2014). Association between Class III obesity (BMI of 40–59 kg/m2) and mortality: A pooled analysis of 20 prospective studies. *PLoS Medicine, 11*(7), 1–14. doi:10.1371/journal.pmed.1001673 PMID:25003901

Kitao, M., Setou, N., Yamamoto, A., & Takada, S. (2018). Associated factors of psychological distress among Japanese NICU nurses in supporting bereaved families who have lost children. *The Kobe Journal of Medical Sciences, 64*(1), E11–E19. PMID:30282893

Klebe, L., Felfe, J., & Klug, K. (2021). Healthy Leadership in Turbulent Times: The Effectiveness of Health-Oriented Leadership in Crisis. *British Journal of Management, 32*(4), 1203–1218. Advance online publication. doi:10.1111/1467-8551.12498

Klein, A., Taieb, O., Xavier, S., Baubet, T., & Reyre, A. (2019). The benefits of mindfulness-based interventions on burnout among health professionals: A systematic review. *Explore (New York, N.Y.), 16*(1), 35–43. doi:10.1016/j.explore.2019.09.002 PMID:31727578

Knaak, S., Mantler, E., & Szeto, A. (2017). Mental illness-related stigma in healthcare: Barriers to access and care and evidence-based solutions. *Healthcare Management Forum, 30*(2), 111–116. doi:10.1177/0840470416679413 PMID:28929889

Kochenderfer, A. (2021, February 11). *Immigrant Healthcare Workers Are Essential to the U.S. Comeback.* Think Immigration.

Koinis, A., Giannou, V., Drantaki, V., Angelaina, S., Stratou, E., & Saridi, M. (2015). The impact of healthcare workers job environment on their mental-emotional health. Coping strategies: The case of a local general hospital. *Health Psychology Research, 3*(1). Advance online publication. doi:10.4081/hpr.2015.1984 PMID:26973958

Kopacz, M. S., Ames, D., & Koenig, H. G. (2019). It's time to talk about physician burnout and moral injury. *The Lancet. Psychiatry, 6*(11), e28. doi:10.1016/S2215-0366(19)30385-2

Kotter, J. P. (1996). Why transformation efforts fail. *Harvard Business Review.*

Kottke, T., Baechler, C., Canterbury, M., Danner, C., Erickson, K., & Hayes, R. (2013). *ICSI Health Care Guideline: Healthy Lifestyles.* Institute for Clinical Systems Improvement (ICSI).

Koutsimani, P., Montgomery, A., & Georganta, K. (2019). The Relationship Between Burnout, Depression, and Anxiety: A Systematic Review and Meta-Analysis. *Frontiers in Psychology, 10*, 284. doi:10.3389/fpsyg.2019.00284

Kovner, C., Raveis, V. H., Van Devanter, N., Yu, G., Glassman, K., & Ridge, L. J. (2021). The psychosocial impact on frontline nurses of caring for patients with COVID-19 during the first wave of the pandemic in New York City. I-II, 1-11. *Nursing Outlook, 69*(5), 744–754. Advance online publication. doi:10.1016/j.outlook.2021.03.019 PMID:33894986

Kowalczyk, O., Roszkowski, K., Montane, X., Pawliszak, W., Tylkowski, B., & Bajek, A. (2020). Religion and Faith Perception in a Pandemic of COVID-19. *Journal of Religion and Health, 59*(6), 2671–2677. doi:10.100710943-020-01088-3 PMID:33044598

Kowalska, W., & Szwamel, K. (2021). Stress management strategies and quality of life in undergraduate nursing and midwifery students in Poland: A pilot study. *Nursing Open.* Advance online publication. doi:10.1002/nop2.982 PMID:34227744

Kozlowski, S. W., & Bell, B. S. (2007). Team learning, development, and adaptation. In *Work group learning* (pp. 39–68). Psychology Press.

Kraiger, K., Ford, J. K., & Salas, E. (1993). Application of cognitive, skill-based, and affective theories of learning outcomes to new methods of training evaluation. *The Journal of Applied Psychology, 78*(2), 311–328. doi:10.1037/0021-9010.78.2.311

Kristensen, T. S., Borritz, M., Villadsen, E., & Christensen, K. B. (2005). The Copenhagen Burnout Inventory: A new tool for the assessment of burnout. *Work and Stress, 19*(3), 192–207. doi:10.1080/02678370500297720

Kronsberg, S., Bouret, J., & Brett, A. (2017). Lived experiences of male nurses: Dire consequences for the nursing profession. *Journal of Nursing Education and Practice, 8*(46), 46. doi:10.5430/jnep.v8n1p46

Kruk, M. E., Myers, M., Varpilah, S. T., & Dahn, B. T. (2015). What is a resilient health system? Lessons from Ebola. *Lancet, 385*(9980), 1910–1912. doi:10.1016/S0140-6736(15)60755-3 PMID:25987159

Kuiper, N. A., McKenzie, S. D., & Belanger, K. A. (1995). Cognitive appraisals and individual differences in sense of humor: Motivational and affective implications. *Personality and Individual Differences, 19*(3), 359–372. https://doi.org/10.1016/0191-8869(95)00072-E

Kumar, K., Mehra, A., Sahoo, S., Nehra, R., & Grover, S. (2020). The psychological impact of COVID-19 pandemic and lockdown on the migrant workers: A cross-sectional survey. *Asian Journal of Psychiatry*, *53*, 102252. doi:10.1016/j.ajp.2020.102252 PMID:32593970

Kumar, R., & Pal, R. (2018). India achieves WHO recommended doctor population ratio: A call for paradigm shift in public health discourse! *Journal of Family Medicine and Primary Care*, *7*(5), 841–844. doi:10.4103/jfmpc.jfmpc_218_18 PMID:30598921

Kumar, S. (2016). Burnout and Doctors: Prevalence, Prevention and Intervention. *Health Care*, *4*(3), 37. doi:10.3390/healthcare4030037

Kuoppala, J., Lamminpää, A., Liira, J., & Vainio, H. (2008). Leadership, job well-being, and health effects—A systematic review and a meta-analysis. *Journal of Occupational and Environmental Medicine*, *50*(8), 904–915. doi:10.1097/JOM.0b013e31817e918d PMID:18695449

Kuorinka, I., Jonsson, B., Kilbom, A., Vinterberg, H., Biering-Sørensen, F., Andersson, G., & Jørgensen, K. (1987). Standardised Nordic questionnaires for the analysis of musculoskeletal symptoms. *Applied Ergonomics*, *18*(3), 233–237. doi:10.1016/0003-6870(87)90010-X PMID:15676628

Kuttner, P. J., Weaver-Hightower, M. B., & Sousanis, N. (2021). Comics-based research: The affordances of comics for research across disciplines. *Qualitative Research*, *21*(2), 195–214. doi:10.1177/1468794120918845

Kyle, R. G., Wills, J., Mahoney, C., Hoyle, L., Kelly, M., & Atherton, I. M. (2017). Obesity prevalence among healthcare professionals in England: A cross-sectional study using the Health Survey for England. *BMJ Open*, *7*(12), e018498. doi:10.1136/bmjopen-2017-018498 PMID:29203505

Lacagnina, S. (2019). The Triple Aim Plus More. *American Journal of Lifestyle Medicine*, *13*(1), 42–43. doi:10.1177/1559827618806183 PMID:30627077

Lachance, C. (2014). Nursing journal clubs: A literature review on the effective teaching strategy for continuing education and evidence-based practice. *Journal of Continuing Education in Nursing*, *45*(12), 559–565. doi:10.3928/00220124-20141120-01 PMID:25401339

Laharnar, N., Glass, N., Perrin, N., Hanson, G., & Anger, W. K. (2013). A training intervention for supervisors to support a work-life policy implementation. *Safety and Health at Work*, *4*(3), 166–176. doi:10.1016/j.shaw.2013.07.001 PMID:24106648

Lai, J., Ma, S., Wang, Y., Cai, Z., Hu, J., Wei, N., Wu, J., Du, H., Chen, T., Li, R., Tan, H., Kang, L., Yao, L., Huang, M., Wang, H., Wang, G., Liu, Z., & Hu, S. (2020). Factors associated with mental health outcomes among health care workers exposed to coronavirus disease 2019. *JAMA Network Open*, *3*(3), e203976–e203976. doi:10.1001/jamanetworkopen.2020.3976 PMID:32202646

Lambden, J. P., Chamberlin, P., Kozlov, E., Lief, L., Berlin, D. A., Pelissier, L. A., ... Prigerson, H. G. (2019). Association of Perceived Futile or Potentially Inappropriate Care With Burnout and Thoughts of Quitting Among Health-Care Providers. *The American Journal of Hospice & Palliative Care*, *36*(3), 200–206. doi:10.1177/1049909118792517

Lamiani, G., Borghi, L., & Argentero, P. (2017). When healthcare professionals cannot do the right thing: A systematic review of moral distress and its correlates. *Journal of Health Psychology*, *22*(1), 51–67. doi:10.1177/1359105315595120

Lancee, W. J., Maunder, R. G., & Goldbloom, D. S. (2008). Prevalence of psychiatric disorders among Toronto hospital workers one to two years after the SARS outbreak. *Psychiatric Services (Washington, D.C.)*, *59*(1), 91–95. doi:10.1176/ps.2008.59.1.91 PMID:18182545

Lancet. (2020). India under COVID-19 lockdown. *Lancet, 395*(10233), 1315. doi:10.1016/S0140-6736(20)30938-7 PMID:32334687

Langarizadeh, M., Tabatabaeim, M. S., Tavakol, K., Naghipour, M., Rostami, A., & Moghbeli, F. (2017). Telemental health care, an effective alternative to conventional mental care: A systematic review. *Acta Informatica Medica, 25*(4), 240–246. doi:10.5455/aim.2017.25.240-246 PMID:29284913

Lara, D. R. (2010). Caffeine, mental health, and psychiatric disorders. *Journal of Alzheimer's Disease, 20*(s1), S239–S248. doi:10.3233/JAD-2010-1378 PMID:20164571

LaRose, A., Danhauer, S. C., Feldman, J., Evans, G. W., & Kemper, K. J. (2010). Brief Stress-Reduction Training in an Academic Health Center. *Journal of Alternative and Complementary Medicine (New York, N.Y.), 16*(9), 935–936. doi:10.1089/acm.2010.0338 PMID:20715979

Larson, E. B., & Yao, X. (2005). Clinical empathy as emotional labor in the patient-physician relationship. *Journal of the American Medical Association, 293*(9), 1100–1106.

Laschinger, H. K. S., & Leiter, M. P. (2006). The impact of nursing work environments on patient safety outcomes: the mediating role of burnout/engagement. *JONA: The Journal of Nursing Administration, 36*(5), 259–267. https://doi-org.proxy108.nclive.org/10.1097/00005110-200605000-00019

Lavoie, S., Talbot, L. R., & Mathieu, L. (2011). Post-traumatic stress disorder symptoms among emergency nurses: Their perspective and a 'tailor-made' solution. *Journal of Advanced Nursing, 67*(7), 1514–1522. doi:10.1111/j.1365-2648.2010.05584.x PMID:21323975

Lavrakas, P. (2008). *Encyclopedia of Survey Research Methods*. SAGE Publications. doi:10.4135/9781412963947

Le, T. K., Cha, L., Han, H. R., & Tseng, W. (2020). Anti-asian xenophobia and Asian American COVID-19 disparities. In American Journal of Public Health (Vol. 110, Issue 9, pp. 1371–1373). American Public Health Association Inc. doi:10.2105/AJPH.2020.305846

Lee, C., Podury, A., Kaduthodil, J., & Graham, L. (2020). Long-term care facilities must prioritize immigrant workers' needs to contain COVID-19. *Health Affairs Blog*.

Lee, T., & Stoye, G. (2018). What does the NHS spend its money on? In A. Charlesworth & P. Johnson (Eds.), *Securing the Future: Funding Health and Social Care to the 2030s*. Institute for Fiscal Studies.

Lefèvre, H., Stheneur, C., Cardin, C., Fourcade, L., Fourmaux, C., Tordjman, E., Touati, M., Voisard, F., Minassian, S., Chaste, P., Moro, M. R., & Lachal, J. (2021). The Bulle: Support and prevention of psychological decompensation of health care workers during the trauma of the COVID-19 epidemic. *Journal of Pain and Symptom Management, 61*(2), 416–422. doi:10.1016/j.jpainsymman.2020.09.023 PMID:32961219

Leslie, J. H., Braun, K. L., Novotny, R., & Mokuau, N. (2013). Factors affecting healthy eating and physical activity behaviors among multiethnic blue-and white-collar workers: A case study of one healthcare institution. *Hawai'i Journal of Medicine & Public Health: a Journal of Asia Pacific Medicine & Public Health, 72*(9), 300. PMID:24069570

Leviyeva, E. (2021, April 13). *Proposed bipartisan bill to recapture 40,000 visas for physicians and nurses to remedy ongoing shortage, id Onogoing COVID-19 health response*. Inside Business Immigration.

Liang, Y., Wu, K., Zhou, Y., Huang, X., Zhou, Y., & Liu, Z. (2020). Mental health in frontline medical workers during the 2019 novel coronavirus disease epidemic in China: A comparison with the general population. *International Journal of Environmental Research and Public Health, 17*(18), 6550. doi:10.3390/ijerph17186550

Lianov, L. (2019). *Roots of Positive Change: Optimizing Health Care with Positive Psychology*. American College of Lifestyle Medicine.

Lianov, L. (2021). A Powerful Antidote to Physician Burnout: Intensive Healthy Lifestyle and Positive Psychology Approaches. *American Journal of Lifestyle Medicine*, *15*(5), 15598276211006626. doi:10.1177/15598276211006626 PMID:34646108

Lianov, L. S., Barron, G. C., Fredrickson, B. L., Hashmi, S., Klemes, A., Krishnaswami, J., Lee, J., Le Pertel, N., Matthews, J. A., Millstein, R. A., Phillips, E. M., Sannidhi, D., Purpur de Vries, P., Wallace, A., & Winter, S. J. (2020). Positive psychology in health care: Defining key stakeholders and their roles. *Translational Behavioral Medicine*, *10*(3), 637–647. doi:10.1093/tbm/ibz150 PMID:32766868

Lianov, L. S., Fredrickson, B. L., Barron, C., Krishnaswami, J., & Wallace, A. (2019). Positive psychology in lifestyle medicine and health care: Strategies for implementation. *American Journal of Lifestyle Medicine*, *13*(5), 480–486. doi:10.1177/1559827619838992 PMID:31523213

Liao, C., Wayne, S. J., & Rousseau, D. M. (2016). Idiosyncratic deals in contemporary organizations: A qualitative and meta-analytical review. *Journal of Organizational Behavior*, *37*, S9–S29. doi:10.1002/job.1959

Liaudanskiene, R., Varnas, N., & Ustinovichius, L. (2010). Modelling the application of workplace safety and health act in Lithuanian construction sector. *Technological and Economic Development*, *16*(2), 233–253. doi:10.3846/tede.2010.15

Lightbody-Warner, M. (2020, December 4). *Compassion satisfaction and compassion fatigue: Helpful tips for our frontline workers*. The Louis A. Faillace, MD, Department of Psychiatry and Behavioral Sciences, McGovern Medical School. https://med.uth.edu/psychiatry/2020/10/29/compassion-satisfaction-and-compassion-fatigue-helpful-tips-for-our-frontline-workers/

Lima Vilela, B., Benedito Silva, A. A., Barbosa de Lira, C. A., & dos Santos Andrade, M. (2015). Workplace exercise and educational program for improving fitness outcomes related to health in workers. *Journal of Occupational and Environmental Medicine*, *57*(3), 235–240. doi:10.1097/JOM.0000000000000393 PMID:25742529

Lim, E. J., Noh, J. H., & Jeong, Y. S. (2016). The relationships among type D personality, self resilience, and health promoting behaviors in nursing students. *International Journal of Bio-Science and Bio-Technology*, *8*(2), 341–352.

Lincoln, S. Y., & Guba, E. G. (1985). *Naturalistic inquiry*. Sage. doi:10.1016/0147-1767(85)90062-8

Lindwall, M., Gerber, M., Jonsdottir, I. H., Börjesson, M., & Ahlborg, G. Jr. (2014). The relationships of change in physical activity with change in depression, anxiety, and burnout: A longitudinal study of Swedish healthcare workers. *Health Psychology*, *33*(11), 1309–1339. doi:10.1037/a0034402 PMID:24245832

Linnan, L., Weiner, B., Graham, A., & Emmons, K. (2007). Manager Beliefs regarding Worksite Health Promotion: Findings from the Working Healthy Project 2. *American Journal of Health Promotion*, *21*(6), 521–528. doi:10.4278/0890-1171-21.6.521 PMID:17674640

Litz, B. T., Stein, N., Delaney, E., Lebowitz, L., Nash, W. P., Silva, C., & Maguen, S. (2009). Moral injury and moral repair in war veterans: A preliminary model and intervention strategy. *Clinical Psychology Review*, *29*(8), 695–706. doi:10.1016/j.cpr.2009.07.003

Liu, S., Yang, L., Zhang, C., Xiang, Y. T., Liu, Z., Hu, S., & Zhang, B. (2020). Online mental health services in China during the COVID-19 outbreak. *The Lancet. Psychiatry*, *7*(4), e17–e18. doi:10.1016/S2215-0366(20)30077-8 PMID:32085841

Liu, Y., Wheaton, A. G., Chapman, D. P., Cunningham, T. J., Lu, H., & Croft, J. B. (2016). Prevalence of Healthy Sleep Duration among Adults— United States, 2014. *Morbidity and Mortality; Weekly Report*, *65*(6), 137–141. doi:10.15585/mmwr.mm6506a1 PMID:26890214

Li, Y.-L., Li, R.-Q., Qiu, D., & Xiao, S.-Y. (2020). Prevalence of workplace physical violence against healthcare professionals by patients and visitors: A systematic review and meta-analysis. *International Journal of Environmental Research and Public Health*, *17*(1), 299. doi:10.3390/ijerph17010299 PMID:31906306

Li, Y., Scherer, N., Felix, L., & Kuper, H. (2021). Prevalence of depression, anxiety and post-traumatic stress disorder in health care workers during the COVID-19 pandemic: A systematic review and meta-analysis. *PLoS One*, *16*(3), e0246454. doi:10.1371/journal.pone.0246454 PMID:33690641

Logie, C. H. (2020). Lessons learned from HIV can inform our approach to COVID-19 stigma. *Journal of the International AIDS Society*, *23*(5), e25504. doi:10.1002/jia2.25504 PMID:32365283

LoGiudice, J. A., & Bartos, S. (2021). Experiences of nurses during the COVID-19 pandemic: A mixed-methods study. *AACN Advanced Critical Care*, *32*(1), 14–26. doi:10.4037/aacnacc2021816 PMID:33450763

Lomas, T., Medina, J. C., Ivtzan, I., Rupprecht, S., & Eiroa-Orosa, F. J. (2018). A systematic review of the impact of mindfulness on the well-being of healthcare professionals. *Journal of Clinical Psychology*, *74*(3), 319–355. doi:10.1002/jclop.22515

López Gómez, M. A., Gundersen, D. A., Boden, L. I., Sorensen, G., Katz, J. N., Collins, J. E., Wagner, G., Vriniotis, M. G., & Williams, J. A. R. (2021). Validation of the Workplace Integrated Safety and Health (WISH) assessment in a sample of nursing homes using Item Response Theory (IRT) methods. *BMJ Open*, *11*(6), e045656. doi:10.1136/bmjopen-2020-045656 PMID:34145013

Luceño-Moreno, L., Talavera-Velasco, B., García-Albuerne, Y., & Martín-García, J. (2020). Symptoms of posttraumatic stress, anxiety, depression, levels of resilience and burnout in Spanish health personnel during the COVID-19 pandemic. *International Journal of Environmental Research and Public Health*, *17*(15), 5514. doi:10.3390/ijerph17155514 PMID:32751624

Luecke, R. (2003). *Managing change and transition* (Vol. 3). Harvard Business Press.

Luftman, K., Aydelotte, J., Rix, K., Ali, S., Houck, K., Coopwood, T. B., Teixeira, P., Eastman, A., Eastridge, B., Brown, C. V. R., & Davis, M. (2017). PTSD in those who care for the injured. *Injury*, *48*(2), 293–296. doi:10.1016/j.injury.2016.11.001 PMID:27871770

Lu, H., While, A. E., & Barriball, K. L. (2005). Job satisfaction among nurses: A literature review. *International Journal of Nursing Studies*, *42*(2), 211–227. doi:10.1016/j.ijnurstu.2004.09.003 PMID:15680619

Luhmann, M. (2017). The development of subjective well-being. In J. Specht (Ed.), *Personality development across the lifespan* (pp. 197–218). Ruhr University Bochum. doi:10.1016/B978-0-12-804674-6.00013-2

Luthans, K. W., Lebsack, S. A., & Lebsack, R. R. (2008). Positivity in healthcare: Relation of optimism to performance. *Journal of Health Organization and Management*, *22*(2), 178–188. doi:10.1108/14777260810876330

Maben, J., & Bridges, J. (2020). Covid-19: Supporting nurses' psychological and mental health. *Journal of Clinical Nursing*, *29*(15–16), 2742–2750. doi:10.1111/jocn.15307 PMID:32320509

Macedo, T., Wilheim, L., Gonçalves, R., Coutinjo, E. S. F., Vilete, L., Figueira, I., & Ventura, P. (2014). Building resilience for future adversity: A systematic review of interventions in non-clinical samples of adults. *BMC Psychiatry*, *14*, 1–8.

Mackenzie, C. S., Poulin, P. A., & Seidman-Carlson, R. (2006). A brief mindfulness-based stress reduction intervention for nurses and nurse aides. *Applied Nursing Research, 19*(2), 105–109. doi:10.1016/j.apnr.2005.08.002 PMID:16728295

MacKinnon, M., & Murray, S. (2018). Reframing physician burnout as an organizational problem: A novel pragmatic approach to physician burnout. *Academic Psychiatry, 42*(1), 123–128. doi:10.100740596-017-0689-1 PMID:28247366

Maestripieri, L. (2021). The Covid-19 pandemics: Why intersectionality matters. *Frontiers in Sociology, 6*, 52. doi:10.3389/fsoc.2021.642662 PMID:33869589

Mahajan, A. (2020, December 12). *Heroes or aliens: The hidden dichotomy of immigrant physicians*. The Hill.

Maheu, M., Callan, J., & Hilty, D. M. (2020). *Telebehavioral health: foundations in theory and practice for graduate learners*. Cognella.

Malik, S., Blake, H., & Batt, M. (2011). How healthy are our nurses? New and registered nurses compared. *British Journal of Nursing (Mark Allen Publishing), 20*(8), 489–496. doi:10.12968/bjon.2011.20.8.489 PMID:21537281

Marchiondo, L. A., Verney, S. P., & Venner, K. L. (2021). Academic leaders' diversity attitudes: Their role in predicting faculty support for institutional diversity. *Journal of Diversity in Higher Education*. Advance online publication. doi:10.1037/dhe0000333

Marcy, R. T., & Mumford, M. D. (2010). Leader cognition: Improving leader performance through causal analysis. *The Leadership Quarterly, 21*(1), 1–19. doi:10.1016/j.leaqua.2009.10.001

Maria, S., Francesca, L., Massimiliano, P., & Mirco, F. (2020). Parents' Stress and Children's Psychological Problems in Families Facing the COVID-19 Outbreak in Italy. *Frontiers in Psychology*, 11. https://www.frontiersin.org/article/10.3389/fpsyg.2020.01713

Marie-Mitchell, A., & O'Connor, T. (2013). Adverse childhood experiences: Translating knowledge into identification of children at risk for poor outcomes. *Academic Pediatrics, 13*(1), 14–19. doi:10.1016/j.acap.2012.10.006 PMID:23312855

Marie-Mitchell, A., Studer, K. R., & O'Connor, T. G. (2016). How knowledge of adverse childhood experiences can help pediatricians prevent mental health problems. *Families, Systems & Health, 34*(2), 128–135. doi:10.1037/fsh0000179 PMID:26950476

Marks, M. R., Bowers, C., DePesa, N. S., Trachik, B., Deavers, F. E., & James, N. T. (2017). REACT: A paraprofessional training program for first responders – A pilot study. *Bulletin of the Menninger Clinc, 81*(2), 150-166. .81.2.150 doi:10.1521/bumc.2017

Marks, M., Mathieu, J., & Zaccaro, S. (2001). A temporally based framework and taxonomy of team processes. *Academy of Management Review, 26*(3), 356–376. doi:10.5465/amr.2001.4845785

Martin, A., Karanika-Murray, M., Biron, C., & Sanderson, K. (2016). The psychosocial work environment, employee mental health and organizational interventions: Improving research and practice by taking a multilevel approach. *Stress and Health, 32*(3), 201–215. doi:10.1002mi.2593 PMID:25044861

Martino, J., Pegg, J., & Frates, E. P. (2017). The connection prescription: Using the power of social interactions and the deep desire for connectedness to empower health and wellness. *American Journal of Lifestyle Medicine, 11*(6), 466–475. doi:10.1177/1559827615608788 PMID:30202372

Marvaldi, M., Mallet, J., Dubertret, C., Moro, M. R., & Guessoum, S. B. (2021). Anxiety, depression, trauma-related, and sleep disorders among healthcare workers during the COVID-19 pandemic: A systematic review and meta-analysis. *Neuroscience and Biobehavioral Reviews, 126*, 252–264. doi:10.1016/j.neubiorev.2021.03.024 PMID:33774085

Masa'deh, R., Obeidat, B. Y., & Tarhini, A. (2016). A Jordanian empirical study of the associations among transformational leadership, transactional leadership, knowledge sharing, job performance, and firm performance: A structural equation modelling approach. *Journal of Management Development, 35*(5), 681–705. doi:10.1108/JMD-09-2015-0134

Maslach, C., Jackson, S. E., Leiter, M. P., Schaufeli, W. B., & Schwab, R. L. (1986). Maslach burnout inventory (Vol. 21). Consulting Psychologists Press.

Maslach, C. (1982). *Burnout: The Cost of Caring*. Prentice-Hall.

Maslach, C., & Jackson, S. E. (1981). *Maslach Burnout Inventory: MBI.* Consulting Psychologists Press.

Maslach, C., Jackson, S. E., & Leiter, M. (1996). Maslach Burnout Inventory. In C. P. Zalaquett & R. J. Wood (Eds.), *Evaluating stress: A book of resources* (3rd ed., pp. 191–218). Scarecrow Education.

Maslach, C., Schaufeli, W. B., & Leiter, M. P. (2001). Job burnout. *Annual Review of Psychology, 52*(1), 397–422. doi:10.1146/annurev.psych.52.1.397 PMID:11148311

Mass Shooting Tracker. (2021). Retrieved from https://www.massshootingtracker.site/

Mateen, F., & Dorji, C. (2009). Health-care worker burnout and the mental health imperative. *Lancet, 374*(9690), 595–597. doi:10.1016/S0140-6736(09)61483-5

Mathema, S. (2019). Immigrant Doctors Can Help Lower Physician Shortages in Rural America. Center for American Progress.

Mathema, S. (2020, April 2). *Removing Barriers for Immigrant Medical Professionals Is Critical To Help Fight Coronavirus.* Center for Immigrant Progress.

Mathieu, F. (2012). *The compassion fatigue workbook: Creative tools for transforming compassion fatigue and vicarious traumatization.* Routledge/Taylor & Francis Group.

Matsuo, T., Kobayashi, D., Taki, F., Sakamoto, F., Uehara, Y., Mori, N., & Fukui, T. (2020). Prevalence of Health Care Worker Burnout During the Coronavirus Disease 2019 (COVID-19) Pandemic in Japan. *JAMA Network Open, 3*(8), e2017271. doi:10.1001/jamanetworkopen.2020.17271

Mays, V. M., Cochran, S. D., & Barnes, N. W. (2007). Race, race-based discrimination, and health outcomes among African Americans. *Annual Review of Psychology, 5*(1), 201–225. doi:10.1146/annurev.psych.57.102904.190212 PMID:16953796

Mazzola, J. J., Jackson, A., & Thiele, A. (2019). Obesity in the workplace: Physical, social, and environmental barriers and facilitators to healthy lifestyles. *Occupational Health Science, 3*, 239–264. doi:10.100741542-019-00046-0

Mazzola, J. J., Moore, J. T., & Alexander, K. A. (2017). Is work preventing us from acting healthy? The relationship between daily workplace barriers and facilitators on nutrition and exercise behaviors. *Stress and Health, 33*(5), 479–489. doi:10.1002mi.2731 PMID:27891758

McCain, R. S., McKinley, N., Dempster, M., Campbell, W. J., & Kirk, S. J. (2018). A study of the relationship between resilience, burnout and coping strategies in doctors. *Postgraduate Medical Journal, 94*(1107), 43–47.

McCarthy, A., Darcy, C., & Grady, G. (2010). Work-life balance policy and practice: Understanding line manager attitudes and behaviors. *Human Resource Management Review, 20*(2), 158–167. doi:10.1016/j.hrmr.2009.12.001

McClendon, S. (2020, September 1). *New survey findings from 21K US nurses: PPE shortages persist, re-use practices on the rise amid COVID-19 pandemic.* American Nurses Association. https://www.nursingworld.org/news/news-releases/2020/new-survey-findings-from-21k-us-nurses--ppe-shortages-persist-re-use-practices-on-the-rise-amid-covid-19-pandemic/

McCord, C., Bernhard, P., Walsh, M., Rosner, C., & Console, K. (2020). A consolidated model for telepsychology practice. *Journal of Clinical Psychology, 76*(6), 1060–1082. doi:10.1002/jclp.22954 PMID:32285940

McElroy, S. F., Olney, A., Hunt, C., & Glennon, C. (2020). Shift work and hospital employees: A descriptive multi-site study. *International Journal of Nursing Studies, 112*, 103746. doi:10.1016/j.ijnurstu.2020.103746 PMID:32928504

McGinn, K., & Eunsil, O. (2017). Gender, Social Class, and Women's Employment. *Current Opinion in Psychology, 18*, 84–88. Advance online publication. doi:10.1016/j.copsyc.2017.07.012 PMID:28866434

McGonigal, K. (2016). *The upside of stress: Why stress is good for you, and how to get good at it*. Penguin.

McKinley, N., McCain, R. S., Convie, L., Clarke, M., Dempster, M., Campbell, W. J., & Kirk, S. J. (2020). Resilience, burnout and coping mechanisms in UK doctors: A cross-sectional study. *BMJ Open, 10*(1), e031765. doi:10.1136/bmjopen-2019-031765

McKinley, T. F., Boland, K. A., & Mahan, J. D. (2017). Burnout and interventions in pediatric residency: A literature review. *Burnout Research, 6*, 9–17. doi:10.1016/j.burn.2017.02.003

McNeill, L. H., Wyrwich, K. W., Brownson, R. C., Clark, E. M., & Kreuter, M. W. (2006). Individual, social environmental, and physical environmental influences on physical activity among black and white adults: A structural equation analysis. *Annals of Behavioral Medicine, 31*(1), 36–44. doi:10.120715324796abm3101_7 PMID:16472037

McNicol, S., & Leamy, C. (2020). Co-creating a graphic illness narrative with people with dementia. *Journal of Applied Arts & Health, 11*(3), 267–280. doi:10.1386/jaah_00040_1

McVicar, A. (2003). Workplace stress in nursing: A literature review. *Journal of Advanced Nursing, 44*(6), 633–642. doi:10.1046/j.0309-2402.2003.02853.x PMID:14651686

Meadors, P., Lamson, A., Swanson, M., White, M., & Sira, N. (2010). Secondary traumatization in pediatric healthcare providers: Compassion fatigue, burnout, and secondary traumatic stress. *Omega, 60*(2), 103–128. doi:10.2190/OM.60.2.a PMID:20222232

Mealer, M., Conrad, D., Evans, J., Jooste, K., Solyntjes, J., Rothbaum, B., & Moss, M. (2014). Feasibility and acceptability of a resilience training program for Intensive Care Unit Nurses. *American Journal of Critical Care, 23*(6), e97–e105. Advance online publication. doi:10.4037/ajcc2014747 PMID:25362680

Medisauskaite, A., & Kamau, C. (2019). Does occupational distress raise the risk of alcohol use, binge-eating, ill health and sleep problems among medical doctors? A UK cross-sectional study. *BMJ Open, 9*(5), e027362. doi:10.1136/bmjopen-2018-027362 PMID:31092661

Mehta, S. (2014). *Acculturation and mental health: Asian Indian immigrants in the United States*. Academic Press.

Meltzer, L. S., & Huckabay, L. M. (2004). Critical Care Nurses' Perceptions of Futile Care and Its Effect on Burnout. *American Journal of Critical Care, 13*(3), 202–208. doi:10.4037/ajcc2004.13.3.202

Membrive-Jiménez, M. J., Pradas-Hernández, L., Suleiman-Martos, N., Vargas-Román, K., Cañadas-De la Fuente, G., Gomez-Urquiza, J. L., & De la Fuente-Solana, E. I. (2020). Burnout in nursing managers: A systematic review and meta-analysis of related factors, levels and prevalence. *International Journal of Environmental Research and Public Health, 17*(11), 3983. doi:10.3390/ijerph17113983 PMID:32512738

Mendes, A. (2014). Recognising and combating compassion fatigue in nursing. *British Journal of Nursing (Mark Allen Publishing), 23*(21), 1146–1146. doi:10.12968/bjon.2014.23.21.1146

Mendes, M., Bordignon, J. S., Menegat, R. P., Schneider, D. G., Vargas, M. A. D. O., Santos, E. K. A. D., & Cunha, P. R. D. (2021). Neither angels nor heroes: Nurse speeches during the COVID-19 pandemic from a Foucauldian perspective. *Revista Brasileira de Enfermagem*, 75. PMID:34614072

Menekay, M., & Celmece, N. (2017). Investigation of the quality of life scale improvement. *J. Econ. Manag. Perspect.*, *11*, 327–336.

Mental Health America. (2020). *The Mental Health of Healthcare Workers in COVID-19*. Mental Health America.

Mental Health America. (2021). *The mental health of healthcare workers in COVID-19*. https://mhanational.org/mental-health-healthcare-workers-covid-19

Merlo, G., & Rippe, J. (2021). Physician burnout: A lifestyle medicine perspective. *American Journal of Lifestyle Medicine*, *15*(2), 148–157.

Merlo, G., & Vela, A. (2021). Mental Health in Lifestyle Medicine: A Call to Action. *American Journal of Lifestyle Medicine*. PMID:35185421

Merrifield, N. (2017). Essex trust switches to 12-hour nursing shifts to alleviate staffing and cost concerns. *Nursing Times*. Retrieved from: https://www.nursingtimes.net/news/hospital/trust-makes-12- hour-shifts-standard-for-most-nursing-staff/7017911.article

Meyer, H. S., Durning, S. J., Bader-Larsen, K. S., Hamwey, M., & Varpio, L. (2021). Perseverance: An essential trait of military interprofessional healthcare teams. *Military Medicine*, *186*(3), 29–34. https://doi.org/10.1093/milmed/usab185

Miguel, K., Snyderman, C., Capasso, V., Walsh, M., Murphy, J., & Wang, X. (2021). Development of a prone team and exploration of staff perceptions during COVID-19. *AACN Advanced Critical Care*, *32*(2), 159–168. doi:10.4037/aacnacc2021848 PMID:33878151

Miller, P., & Haslam, C. (2009). Why employers spend money on employee health: Interviews with occupational health and safety professionals from British Industry. *Safety Science*, *47*(2), 163–169. doi:10.1016/j.ssci.2008.04.001

Milliard, B. (2020). Utilization and impact of peer-support programs on police officers' mental health. *Frontiers in Psychology*, *11*, 1686. doi:10.3389/fpsyg.2020.01686 PMID:32765375

Milligan-Saville, J. S., Paterson, H. M., Harkness, E. L., Marsh, A. M., Dobson, M., Kemp, R. I., Bryant, R. A., & Harvey, S. B. (2017). The amplification of common somatic symptoms by posttraumatic stress disorder in firefighters. *Journal of Traumatic Stress*, *30*(2), 142–148. doi:10.1002/jts.22166 PMID:28273379

Mills, L., & Mills, T. (2005). Symptoms of post-traumatic stress disorder among emergency medicine residents. *The Journal of Emergency Medicine*, *28*(1), 1–4. doi:10.1016/j.jemermed.2004.05.009 PMID:15656996

Mina, T. H., Lahti, M., & Drake, A. J. (2016). Maternal lipids in pregnancy are associated with. *Psychoneuroendocrinology*, *34*, 953–967. PMID:28599146

Ming, X., & De Jong, M. D. T. (2021). Mental well-being of Chinese immigrants in the Netherlands during the covid-19 pandemic: A survey investigating personal and societal antecedents. *Sustainability (Switzerland)*, *13*(8), 4198. doi:10.3390u13084198

Minnie, L., Goodman, S., & Wallis, L. (2015). Exposure to daily trauma: The experiences and coping mechanism of Emergency Medical Personnel. A cross-sectional study. *African Journal of Emergency Medicine*, *5*(1), 12–18. doi:10.1016/j.afjem.2014.10.010 PMID:30456058

Mishra, S., Goebert, D., Char, E., Dukes, P., & Ahmed, I. (2010). Trauma exposure and symptoms of post-traumatic stress disorder in emergency medical services personnel in Hawaii. *Emergency Medicine Journal, 27*(9), 708–711. doi:10.1136/emj.2009.080622

Mittal, M., & Bhakar, S. S. (2018). Examining the impact of role overload on job stress, job satisfaction and job performance: A study among married workingwomen in banking sector. *International Journal of Management Study, 7*(1), 2231–2528. doi:10.18843/ijms/v5i2(7)/01

Moberly, T. (2017). Five minutes with . . . Suzy Jordache. *BMJ (Clinical Research Ed.), j2371*. doi:10.1136/bmj.j2371

Moen, P., Kelly, E. L., Fan, W., Lee, S.-R., Almeida, D., Kossek, E. E., & Buxton, O. M. (2016). Does a flexibility/support organizational initiative improve high-tech employees' well-being? Evidence from the work, family, and health network. *American Sociological Review, 81*(1), 134–164. doi:10.1177/0003122415622391

Mohanty, A., Kabi, A., & Mohanty, A. P. (2019). Health problems in healthcare workers: A review. *Journal of Family Medicine and Primary Care, 8*(8), 2568–2572. doi:10.4103/jfmpc.jfmpc_431_19 PMID:31548933

Mohindra, R., Ravaki, R., Suri, V., Bhalla, A., & Singh, S. M. (2020). Issues relevant to mental health promotion in frontline health care providers managing quarantined/isolated COVID19 patients. *Asian Journal of Psychiatry, 51*(3), 102084. doi:10.1016/j.ajp.2020.102084 PMID:32289728

Mohindra, R., Soni, R. K., Suri, V., Bhalla, A., & Singh, S. M. (2021). The experience of social and emotional distancing among health care providers in the context of COVID-19: A study from North India. *Journal of Human Behavior in the Social Environment, 31*(1-4), 173–183. doi:10.1080/10911359.2020.1792385

Mohr, C. D., Hammer, L. B., Brady, J. M., Perry, M. L., & Bodner, T. (2021). Can supervisor support improve daily employee well-being? Evidence of supervisor training effectiveness in a study of veteran employee emotions. *Journal of Occupational and Organizational Psychology, 94*(2), 400–426. doi:10.1111/joop.12342

Molloy, C. (2019). *Rhetorical ethos in health and medicine: Patient credibility, stigma, and misdiagnosis*. Routledge. doi:10.4324/9780429291074

Monrouxe, L. V., Rees, C. E., Dennis, I., & Wells, S. E. (2015). Professionalism dilemmas, moral distress and the healthcare student: Insights from two online UK-wide questionnaire studies. *BMJ Open, 5*(5), e007518–e007518. doi:10.1136/bmjopen-2014-007518

Montanari, K. M., Bowe, C. L., Chesak, S. S., & Cutshall, S. M. (2018). Mindfulness: Assessing the feasibility of a pilot intervention to reduce stress and Burnout. *Journal of Holistic Nursing, 37*(2), 175–188. doi:10.1177/0898010118793465 PMID:30152244

Monti, K., Monti, J. D., & Thomas, D. (2021). Knowledge and Attitudes of Lifestyle Medicine–Based Care in a Military Community. *Military Medicine*, usab279. doi:10.1093/milmed/usab279 PMID:34254645

Moore, R. M. Jr, & Kaczmarek, R. G. (1990). Occupational hazards to health care workers: Diverse, ill-defined, and not fully appreciated. *American Journal of Infection Control, 18*(5), 316–327. doi:10.1016/0196-6553(90)90231-G PMID:2174654

Morgan, P. B. C., Fletcher, D., & Sarkar, M. (2015). Understanding team resilience in the world's best athletes: A case study of a rugby union World cup winning team. *Psychology of Sport and Exercise, 16*, 91-100. doi:10.1016/j.psychsport.2014.08.007

Morgantini, L. A., Naha, U., Wang, H., Francavilla, S., Acar, Ö., Flores, J. M., Crivellaro, S., Moreira, D., Abern, M., Eklund, M., Vigneswaran, H. T., & Weine, S. M. (2020). Factors contributing to healthcare professional burnout during the COVID-19 pandemic: A rapid turnaround global survey. *PLoS One*, *15*(9), e0238217. doi:10.1371/journal.pone.0238217 PMID:32881887

Morley, G. (2016). Efficacy of the nurse ethicist in reducing moral distress: What can the NHS learn from the USA? Part 2. *British Journal of Nursing (Mark Allen Publishing)*, *25*(3), 156–161. doi:10.12968/bjon.2016.25.3.156

Morley, G., Ives, J., & Bradbury-Jones, C. (2019). Moral Distress and Austerity: An Avoidable Ethical Challenge in Healthcare. *Health Care Analysis*, *27*(3), 185–201. doi:10.100710728-019-00376-8

Morse, G., Salyers, M. P., Rollins, A. L., Monroe-DeVita, M., & Pfahler, C. (2012). Burnout in mental health services: A review of the problem and its remediation. *Administration and Policy in Mental Health*, *39*(5), 341–352. doi:10.100710488-011-0352-1 PMID:21533847

Moura, I. H., Nobre, R., Cortez, R. M., Campelo, V., Macedo, S. F., & Silva, A. R. (2016). Quality of life of undergraduate nursing students. Qualidade de vida de estudantes de graduacao em enfermagem. *Revista Gaúcha de Enfermagem*, *37*(2), e55291. doi:10.1590/1983-1447.2016.02.55291 PMID:27253594

Mueller, W. S. (1991). New Technology and Flexible Working. In J. Hartley & G. Stephenson (Eds.), *The Psychology of Employment Relations*. Basil Blackwell.

Mukumbang, F. C., Ambe, A. N., & Adebiyi, B. O. (2020). Unspoken inequality: how COVID-19 has exacerbated existing vulnerabilities of asylum-seekers, refugees, and undocumented migrants in South Africa. *International Journal for Equity in Health, 19*(1), 1–7.

Muldoon, J., Matthews, R. A., & Foley, C. (2012). Mediated Effects of Physical Risk Factors, Leader–Member Exchange and Empowerment in Predicting Perceived Injury Risk. *Stress and Health*, *28*(2), 149–162. doi:10.1002mi.1415 PMID:22282314

Mullen, J. E., & Kelloway, E. K. (2009). Safety leadership: A longitudinal study of the effects of transformational leadership on safety outcomes. *Journal of Occupational and Organizational Psychology*, *82*(2), 253–272. doi:10.1348/096317908X325313

Muller, A. E., Hafstad, E. V., Himmels, J. P. W., Smedslund, G., Flottorp, S., Stensland, S. Ø., Stroobants, S., Van de Velde, S., & Vist, G. E. (2020). The mental health impact of the covid-19 pandemic on healthcare workers, and interventions to help them: A rapid systematic review. *Psychiatry Research*, *293*, 113441. doi:10.1016/j.psychres.2020.113441 PMID:32898840

Mulvale, G., Wilson, F., Jones, S., Green, J., Johansen, K.-J., Arnold, I., & Kates, N. (2019). Integrating mental health peer support in clinical settings: Lessons from Canada and Norway. *Healthcare Management Forum*, *32*(2), 68–72. doi:10.1177/0840470418812495 PMID:30744437

Mumford, M. D., Friedrich, T. L., Caughron, J. J., & Byrne, C. L. (2007). Leader cognition in real-world settings: How do leaders think about crises? *The Leadership Quarterly*, *18*(6), 515–543. doi:10.1016/j.leaqua.2007.09.002

Mursali, A., Basuki, E., & Dharmono, S. (2009). Relationship between noise and job stress at private thread spinning company. *University Medicine*, *28*, 8.

Myers, K., Nelson, E. L., Rabinowitz, T., Hilty, D., Baker, D., Barnwell, S. S., Boyce, G., Bufka, L. F., Cain, S., Chui, L., Comer, J. S., Cradock, C., Goldstein, F., Johnston, B., Krupinski, E., Lo, K., Luxton, D. D., McSwain, S. D., McWilliams, J., ... Bernard, J. (2017). American telemedicine association practice guidelines for telemental health with children and adolescents. *Telemedicine Journal and e-Health*, *23*(10), 779–804. doi:10.1089/tmj.2017.0177 PMID:28930496

Nachnani, E., & Bulchandani, D. (2019). Do doctors practice what they preach regarding nutrition, exercise and sleep. *Endocrine Practice*, *25*, 188–189. doi:10.1016/S1530-891X(20)46747-3

Nahm, E. S., Warren, J., Zhu, S., An, M., & Brown, J. (2012). Nurses' self-care behaviors related to weight and stress. *Nursing Outlook*, *60*(5), e23–e31. doi:10.1016/j.outlook.2012.04.005 PMID:22770679

Nam, S., & Toneatto, T. (2016). The Influence of Attrition in Evaluating the Efficacy and Effectiveness of Mindfulness-Based Interventions. *International Journal of Mental Health and Addiction*, *14*(6), 969–981. doi:10.100711469-016-9667-1

Narwal, S., & Jain, S. (2021). Building Resilient Health Systems: Patient Safety during COVID-19 and Lessons for the Future. *Journal of Health Management*, *23*(1), 166–181. doi:10.1177/0972063421994935

National Collaborating Centre for Mental Health (UK). (2005). *Post-Traumatic Stress Disorder: The Management of PTSD in Adults and Children in Primary and Secondary Care*. Gaskell. Available from: https://www.ncbi.nlm.nih.gov/books/NBK56494/

National Heart, Lung, and Blood Institute. (1998). *Clinical guidelines on the identification, evaluation, and treatment overweight and obesity in adults.* NIH Publication, No. 98-4083.

National Institute of Standards and Technology. (2021). *Malcolm Baldrige national quality award.* NIST. https://www.nist.gov/baldrige/baldrige-award

National Occupational Research Agenda Healthcare and Social Assistance Council (NORA HCSA Council). (2019). *National Occupational Research Agenda for Healthcare and Social Assistance*. Retrieved on March 11, 2022 from https://www.cdc.gov/nora/councils/hcsa/pdfs/National_Occpational_Agenda_for_HCSA_February_2019-508.pdf

National Traumatic Stress Network. (2021). https://www.nctsn.org

Nawrot, P., Jordan, S., Eastwood, J., Rotstein, J., Hugenholtz, A., & Feeley, M. (2003). Effects of caffeine on human health. *Food Additives and Contaminants*, *20*(1), 1–30. doi:10.1080/0265203021000007840 PMID:12519715

Nea, F. M., Kearney, J., Livingstone, M. B. E., Pourshahidi, L. K., & Corish, C. A. (2015). Dietary and lifestyle habits and the associated health risks in shift workers. *Nutrition Research Reviews*, *28*(2), 143–166. doi:10.1017/S095442241500013X PMID:26650243

Neal, A., & Griffin, M. A. (2006). A study of the lagged relationships among safety climate, safety motivation, safety behavior, and accidents at the individual and group levels. *The Journal of Applied Psychology*, *91*(4), 946–953. doi:10.1037/0021-9010.91.4.946 PMID:16834517

Neece, C., McIntyre, L. L., & Fenning, R. (2020). Examining the impact of COVID-19 in ethnically diverse families with young children with intellectual and developmental disabilities. *Journal of Intellectual Disability Research*, *64*(10), 739–749. doi:10.1111/jir.12769 PMID:32808424

Neff, K. D., Pisitsungkagarn, K., & Hsieh, Y. P. (2008). Self-Compassion and Self-Construal in the United States, Thailand, and Taiwan. *Journal of Cross-Cultural Psychology*, *39*(3), 267–285. doi:10.1177/0022022108314544

Negrini, A., Corbiere, M., Lecomte, T., Coutu, M. F., Nieuwenhuijsen, K., St-Arnaud, L., Durand, M.-J., Gragnano, A., & Berbiche, D. (2018). How can supervisors contribute to the return to work of employees who have experienced depression? *Journal of Occupational Rehabilitation*, *28*(2), 279–288. doi:10.100710926-017-9715-0 PMID:28660364

Neisler, K., Rosado, N., & Beidel, D. C. (2020). Changing Hearts and Minds: Getting Administrative Support for Delivery of Care. In C. Bowers, D. Beidel, & M. Marks (Eds.), *Mental Health Intervention and Treatment of First Responders and Emergency Workers* (pp. 291–301). IGI Global. doi:10.4018/978-1-5225-9803-9.ch017

Nepper, M. J., McAtee, J. R., & Chai, W. (2021). Effect of a workplace weight-loss program for overweight and obese healthcare workers. *American Journal of Health Promotion, 35*(3), 352–361. doi:10.1177/0890117120960393 PMID:32969262

Ness, M. M., Saylor, J., Di Fusco, L. A., & Evans, K. (2021). Healthcare providers' challenges during the coronavirus disease (COVID-19) pandemic: A qualitative approach. *Nursing & Health Sciences, 23*(2), 1–9. doi:10.1111/nhs.12820 PMID:33580590

New American Economy. (2020). *Asian Americans and Pacific Islander Americans on the Frontlines*. Author.

NHS. (2020). *Our NHS people: wellbeing support*. Retrieved from NHS Employers: https://www.nhsemployers.org/-/media/Employers/Documents/Retain-and-improve/Health-and-wellbeing/NHSSupportingOurPeople12.pdf?la=en&hash=D49FAA8660A94E578AC08B10553D61DEFC297EEE

Nicholls, R., Perry, L., Duffield, C., Gallagher, R., & Pierce, H. (2017). Barriers and facilitators to healthy eating for nurses in the workplace: An integrative review. *Journal of Advanced Nursing, 73*(5), 1051–1065. doi:10.1111/jan.13185 PMID:27732741

Nielsen, K., Abildgaard, J. S., & Daniels, K. (2014). Putting context into organizational intervention design: Using tailored questionnaires to measure initiatives for worker well-being. *Human Relations, 67*(12), 1537–1560. doi:10.1177/0018726714525974

Nielsen, K., Antino, M., Rodríguez-Muñoz, A., & Sanz-Vergel, A. (2021). Is it me or us? The impact of individual and collective participation on work engagement and burnout in a cluster-randomized organisational intervention. *Work and Stress, 35*(4), 374–397. Advance online publication. doi:10.1080/02678373.2021.1889072

Nielsen, K., & Christensen, M. (2021). Positive participatory organizational interventions: A multilevel approach for creating healthy workplaces. *Frontiers in Psychology, 12*, 696245. doi:10.3389/fpsyg.2021.696245 PMID:34262513

Nielsen, K., Nielsen, M. B., Ogbonnaya, C., Känsälä, M., Saari, E., & Isaksson, K. (2017). Workplace resources to improve both employee well-being and performance: A systematic review and meta-analysis. *Work and Stress, 31*(2), 101–120. doi:10.1080/02678373.2017.1304463

Nielsen, K., Randall, R., Holten, A.-L., & González, E. R. (2010). Conducting organizational-level occupational health interventions: What works? *Work and Stress, 24*(3), 234–259. doi:10.1080/02678373.2010.515393

Nielsen, K., Stage, M., Abildgaard, J. S., & Brauer, C. V. (2013). Participatory intervention from an organizational perspective: Employees as active agents in creating a healthy work environment. In G. Bauer & G. Jenny (Eds.), *Salutogenic Organizations and Change* (pp. 327–350). Springer. doi:10.1007/978-94-007-6470-5_18

Nies, M. A., Vollman, M., & Cook, T. (1996). African American women's experiences with physical activity in their daily lives. *Public Health Nursing (Boston, Mass.), 16*(1), 23–31. doi:10.1046/j.1525-1446.1999.00023.x PMID:10074819

Nixon, A. E., Mazzola, J. J., Bauer, J., Krueger, J. R., & Spector, P. E. (2011). Can work make you sick? A meta-analysis of the relationship between job stressors and physical symptoms. *Work and Stress, 25*(1), 1–22. doi:10.1080/02678373.2011.569175

Noe, M. (2021, May 11). *Calling all frontline workers and comic artists!* Graphic Medicine International Collective. https://www.graphicmedicine.org/calling-all-frontline-workers-and-comics-artists/

Noe, M., & Levin, L. (2020). *Mapping the use of comics in health education: A scoping review of the graphic medicine literature*. Graphic Medicine.

Nolan, J. M., Fee, C., Cooper, B. A., Rankin, S. H., & Blegen, M. A. (2015). Psychiatric boarding incidence, duration, and associated factors in United States emergency departments. *Journal of Emergency Nursing: JEN, 41*(1), 57–64. doi:10.1016/j.jen.2014.05.004 PMID:25034663

Nolte, A. G., Downing, C., Temane, A., & Hastings-Tolsma, M. (2017). Compassion fatigue in nurses: A metasynthesis. *Journal of Clinical Nursing, 26*(23-24), 4364–4378. doi:10.1111/jocn.13766 PMID:28231623

Nomaguchi, K. M., & Bianchi, S. M. (2004). Exercise time: Gender differences in the effects of marriage, parenthood, and employment. *Journal of Marriage and Family, 66*(2), 413–430. https://doi-org.proxy108.nclive.org/10.1111/j.1741-3737.2004.00029.x

Northouse, P. (2022). *Leadership: Theory & Practice* (9th ed.). Sage.

Nowrasteh, A., & Landgrave, M. (2020). *Immigrant Health Care Workers by Occupation and State*. Academic Press.

Nowson, C. (2020). Opportunities for innovation in nutrition education for health professionals. *BMJ Nutrition. Prevention & Health, 3*(2), 126. PMID:33521520

Nübling, M., Vomstein, M., Schmidt, S. G., Gregersen, S., Dulon, M., & Nienhaus, A. (2010). Psychosocial work load and stress in the geriatric care. *BMC Public Health, 10*(1), 428. doi:10.1186/1471-2458-10-428 PMID:20663137

Nunez-Smith, M., Curry, L. A., Bigby, J., Berg, D., Krumholz, H. M., & Bradley, E. H. (2007). Impact of race on the professional lives of physicians of African descent. *Annals of Internal Medicine, 146*(1), 45–51. doi:10.7326/0003-4819-146-1-200701020-00008 PMID:17200221

Nunnally, J. C. (1978). *Psychometric theory* (2nd ed.). McGraw-Hill.

Nuzzo, J. B., Meyer, D., Snyder, M., Ravi, S. J., Lapascu, A., Souleles, J., Andrada, C. I., & Bishai, D. (2019). What makes health systems resilient against infectious disease outbreaks and natural hazards? Results from a scoping review. *BMC Public Health, 19*(1), 1–9. doi:10.118612889-019-7707-z PMID:31623594

Nyberg, A., Bernin, P., & Theorell, T. (2005). *The impact of leadership on the health of subordinates.* Report No 1, National Institute for Working Life.

Nyblade, L., Stockton, M. A., Giger, K., Bond, V., Ekstrand, M. L., Lean, R. M., Mitchell, E. M. H., Nelson, L. R. E., Sapag, J. C., Siraprapasiri, T., Turan, J., & Wouters, E. (2019). Stigma in health facilities: Why it matters and how we can change it. *BMC Medicine, 17*(1), 25. doi:10.118612916-019-1256-2 PMID:30764806

O'Brien, W. H., & Carhart, V. (2011). Functional analysis in behavioral medicine settings. *European Journal of Psychological Assessment, 27*(1), 4-16. doi/. doi:10.1027/1015-5759/a000052

O'Brien, W. H., Horan, K. A., Singh, S., Moeller, M. A., Wasson, R. S., Jex, S. M., Matthews, R. A., & Barratt, C. L. (2019a). Relationships among training, mindfulness, and workplace injuries among nurse aides working in long-term care settings. *Occupational Health Science, 3*(1), 45–58. doi:10.100741542-018-0031-7

O'Brien, W. H., Singh, S., Horan, K. A., Moeller, M. A., Wasson, R. S., & Jex, S. M. (2019b). Group-Based Acceptance and Commitment Therapy for Nurses and Nurse Aides Working in Long-Term Care Residential Settings. *Journal of Alternative and Complementary Medicine (New York, N.Y.), 25*(7), 753–761. doi:10.1089/acm.2019.0087 PMID:31314564

O'Hara, M. A., McCann, T. A., Fan, W., Lane, M. M., Kernie, S. G., & Rosenthal, S. L. (2020). Child abuse taking its toll on the emotional well-being of pediatricians. *Clinical Pediatrics, 59*(4–5), 450–457. doi:10.1177/0009922820905865 PMID:32070135

O'Neill, J. W., Harrison, M. M., Cleveland, J., Almeida, D., Stawski, R., & Crouter, A. C. (2009). Work–family climate, organizational commitment, and turnover: Multilevel contagion effects of leaders. *Journal of Vocational Behavior*, *74*(1), 18–29. doi:10.1016/j.jvb.2008.10.004 PMID:19412351

Obrien, N., Flott, K., & Durkin, M. (2021). COVID-19: Leadership on the frontline is what matters when we support healthcare workers. *International Journal for Quality in Health Care*, *33*(1), 1–2. doi:10.1093/intqhc/mzaa153 PMID:33227137

Obuobi, S., Vela, M. B., & Callender, B. (2021). Comics as anti-racist education and advocacy. *Lancet*, *397*(10285), 1615–1617. doi:10.1016/S0140-6736(21)00940-5 PMID:33933198

Occupational Safety and Health Administration. (n.d.). *Computer workstations eTool*. United States Department of Labor. https://www.osha.gov/SLTC/etools/computerworkstations/positions.html

Oenema, A., Brug, J., & Lechner, L. (2001). Web-based tailored nutrition education: Results of a randomized controlled trial. *Health Education Research*, *16*(6), 647–660. doi:10.1093/her/16.6.647 PMID:11780705

Ohue, T., Moriyama, M., & Nakaya, T. (2011). Examination of a cognitive model of stress, burnout, and intention to resign for Japanese nurses: Cognitive model of burnout for nurses. *Japan Journal of Nursing Science*, *8*(1), 76–86. doi:10.1111/j.1742-7924.2010.00161.x

Okechukwu, C. A., Bacic, J., Velasquez, E., & Hammer, L. B. (2016). Marginal structural modelling of associations of occupational injuries with voluntary and involuntary job loss among nursing home workers. *Occupational and Environmental Medicine*, *73*(3), 175–182. doi:10.1136/oemed-2015-103067 PMID:26786757

Oliver, D. (2018). David Oliver: Moral distress in hospital doctors. *BMJ (Clinical Research Ed.)*, *k1333*. doi:10.1136/bmj.k1333

Orton, P., & Gray, D. P. (2015). Burnout in NHS staff. *Lancet*, *385*(9980), 1831. doi:10.1016/S0140-6736(15)60921-7

Orton, P., Orton, C., & Pereira Gray, D. (2012). Depersonalised doctors: A cross-sectional study of 564 doctors, 760 consultations and 1876 patient reports in UK general practice. *BMJ Open*, *2*(1), e000274. doi:10.1136/bmjopen-2011-000274

Owens, I. T. (2020). Supporting nurses' mental health during the pandemic. *Nursing*, *50*(10). https://journals.lww.com/nursing/Fulltext/2020/10000/Supporting_nurses__mental_health_during_the.13aspx

Owens, J. A. (2007). Sleep loss and fatigue in healthcare professionals. *The Journal of Perinatal & Neonatal Nursing*, *21*(2), 92–100. doi:10.1097/01.JPN.0000270624.64584.9d PMID:17505227

Ozyurek, P., Cevik, C., Kılıc, I., & Aslan, A. (2021). Effects of Day and Night Shifts on Stress, Anxiety, Quality of Life, and Oxidative Stress Parameters in Nurses. *Florence Nightingale Journal of Nursing*, *29*(1), 81–92. doi:10.5152/FNJN.2021.19141 PMID:34263226

Painter, K. (2020). Work visas: Foreign doctors in the US have more than covid-19 to fear. *BMJ (Clinical Research Ed.)*, 370. doi:10.1136/bmj.m3172 PMID:32816818

Palmer, E. (2020, May 11). Voices from the pandemic's front lines. *New York Times*. https://www.nytimes.com/2020/05/11/reader-center/coronavirus-healthcare-workers.html

Pal, R., & Yadav, U. (2020). COVID-19 pandemic in india: Present scenario and a steep climb ahead. *Journal of Primary Care & Community Health*, *11*, 1–4. doi:10.1177/2150132720939402 PMID:32644871

Pappa, S., Ntella, V., Giannakas, T., Giannakoulis, V. G., Papoutsi, E., & Katsaounou, P. (2020). Prevalence of depression, anxiety, and insomnia among healthcare workers during the COVID-19 pandemic: A systematic review and meta-analysis. *Brain, Behavior, and Immunity*, *88*, 901–907. doi:10.1016/j.bbi.2020.05.026 PMID:32437915

Park, E., Meyer, R. M., & Gold, J. I. (2020). The role of medical specialization on posttraumatic symptoms in pediatric nurses. *Journal of Pediatric Nursing*, *53*, 22–28. doi:10.1016/j.pedn.2020.03.019 PMID:32339973

Parker, A. L., Forsythe, L. L., & Kohlmorgen, I. K. (2019). TeamSTEPPS®: An evidence-based approach to reduce clinical errors threatening safety in outpatient settings: An integrative review. *Journal of Healthcare Risk Management*, *38*(4), 19–31.

Parker, R. W. (2021). Why America's Response to the COVID-19 Pandemic Failed: Lessons from New Zealand's Success. *ADMIN L. REV.*, *73*, 77–77.

Parry, D. A., Oeppen, R. S., Amin, M. S. A., & Brennan, P. A. (2018). Sleep: Its importance and the effects of deprivation on surgeons and other healthcare professionals. *British Journal of Oral & Maxillofacial Surgery*, *56*(8), 663–666. doi:10.1016/j.bjoms.2018.08.001 PMID:30173962

Parthasarathy, R., Jaisoorya, T. S., Thennarasu, K., & Murthy, P. (2021). Mental health issues among health care workers during the COVID-19 pandemic–a study from India. *Asian Journal of Psychiatry*, *58*, 102626. doi:10.1016/j.ajp.2021.102626

Partlow, P., Medeiros, K., & Mumford, M. (2015). Leader cognition in vision formation: Simplicity and negativity. *The Leadership Quarterly*, *26*(3), 448–469. Advance online publication. doi:10.1016/j.leaqua.2015.02.009

Parush, A., Wacht, O., Gomes, R., & Frenkel, A. (2020). Human factor considerations in using personal protective equipment in the COVID-19 pandemic context: Binational survey study. *Journal of Medical Internet Research*, *22*(6), e19947. https://preprints.jmir.org/preprint/19947

Passmore, S., Hemming, E., McIntosh, H. C., & Hellman, C. M. (2020). The relationship between hope, meaning in work, secondary traumatic stress, and burnout among child abuse pediatric clinicians. *The Permanente Journal*, *24*. Advance online publication. doi:10.7812/TPP/19.087 PMID:31852051

Patel, R. S., Sekhri, S., Bhimanadham, N. N., Imran, S., & Hossain, S. (2019). A review on strategies to manage physician burnout. *Cureus*, *11*(6). Advance online publication. doi:10.7759/cureus.4805 PMID:31404361

Patel, Y. M., Ly, D. P., Hicks, T., & Jena, A. B. (2018). Proportion of non-US-born and noncitizen health care professionals in the United States in 2016. *Journal of the American Medical Association*, *320*(21), 2265–2267. doi:10.1001/jama.2018.14270 PMID:30512091

Patterson, M. M., Carron, A. V., & Loughead, T. M. (2005). The influence of team norms on the cohesion–self-reported performance relationship: A multi-level analysis. *Psychology of Sport and Exercise*, *6*(4), 479–493.

Patton, M. Q. (2002). *Qualitative research and evaluation methods*. Sage Publications.

Paturel, A. (2019). *When physicians are traumatized.* American Association of Medical Colleges News. Available from: https://www.aamc.org/news-insights/when-physicians-are-traumatized

Paulauskaite, L., Farris, O., Spencer, H. M., & Hassiotis, A.EPICC-ID Group. (2021). My son can't socially distance or wear a mask: How families of preschool children with severe developmental delays and challenging behavior experienced the COVID-19 pandemic. *Journal of Mental Health Research in Intellectual Disabilities*, *14*(2), 225–236. doi:10.1080/19315864.2021.1874578

Pavez, I., Gómez, H., Laulié, L., & González, V. A. (2021). Project team resilience: The effect of group potency and interpersonal trust. *International Journal of Project Management, 39*(6), 697–708.

Payne, N. (2001). Occupational stressors and coping as determinants of burnout in female hospice nurses. *Journal of Advanced Nursing, 33*(3), 396–405. doi:10.1046/j.1365-2648.2001.01677.x PMID:11251727

Payne, N., Jones, F., & Harris, P. R. (2010). A daily diary investigation of the impact of work stress on exercise intention realisation: Can planning overcome the disruptive influence of work? *Psychology & Health, 25*(1), 111–129. doi:10.1080/08870440903337622 PMID:20391210

Pearman, A., Hughes, M. L., Smith, E. L., & Neupert, S. D. (2020). Mental health challenges of United States healthcare professionals during COVID-19. *Frontiers in Psychology, 11*, 2065. doi:10.3389/fpsyg.2020.02065 PMID:32903586

Pedrazza, M., Berlanda, S., Trifiletti, E., & Bressan, F. (2016). Exploring Physicians' Dissatisfaction and Work-Related Stress: Development of the PhyDis Scale. *Frontiers in Psychology, 7*, 187. doi:10.3389/fpsyg.2016.01238 PMID:27588013

Peiró, J. M., González-Romá, V., Tordera, N., & Mañas, M. A. (2001). Does role stress predict burnout over time among health care professionals? *Psychology & Health, 16*(5), 511–525. doi:10.1080/08870440108405524

Pelletier, K. R. (2001). A review and analysis of the clinical- and cost-effective studies of comprehensive health promotion and disease management programs at the worksite: 1998-2000 update. *American Journal of Health Promotion, 16*(2), 107–116. doi:10.4278/0890-1171-16.2.107 PMID:11727590

Peng, J., Clarkin, C., & Doja, A. (2018). Uncovering cynicism in medical training: A qualitative analysis of medical online discussion forums. *BMJ Open, 8*(10), e022883. doi:10.1136/bmjopen-2018-022883

Perle, J. G. (2015). Avoiding the clash of the titans: A literature- and experience-based discussion of considerations for preventing and managing challenging caregiver behaviors throughout child-focused family therapy. *Professional Psychology, Research and Practice, 46*(5), 366–374. doi:10.1037/pro0000028

Perle, J. G. (2021a). *A mental health provider's guide to telehealth: Providing outpatient videoconferencing services.* Routledge. doi:10.4324/9781003150473

Perle, J. G. (2021b). Training psychology students for telehealth: A model for doctoral-level education. *Journal of Technology in Behavioral Science, 6*(3), 456–459. doi:10.100741347-021-00212-8

Perry, L., Gallagher, R., & Duffield, C. (2015). The health and health behaviours of Australian metropolitan nurses: An exploratory study. *BMC Nursing, 14*(1), 1–11. doi:10.118612912-015-0091-9 PMID:26339200

Perry, L., Lamont, S., Brunero, S., Gallagher, R., & Duffield, C. (2015). The mental health of nurses in acute teaching hospital settings: A cross-sectional survey. *BMC Nursing, 14*(1), 1–8. doi:10.118612912-015-0068-8 PMID:25904820

Persson, M., & Mårtensson, J. (2006). Situations influencing habits in diet and exercise among nurses working night shift. *Journal of Nursing Management, 14*(5), 414–423. doi:10.1111/j.1365-2934.2006.00601.x PMID:16787477

Persson, R., Hansen, Å. M., Garde, A. H., Kristiansen, J., Nordander, C., Balogh, I., Ohlsson, K., Östergren, P.-O., & Ørbæk, P. (2012). Can the job content questionnaire be used to assess structural and organizational properties of the work environment? *International Archives of Occupational and Environmental Health, 85*(1), 45–55. doi:10.100700420-011-0647-2 PMID:21573960

Pessin, H., Fenn, N., Hendriksen, E., DeRosa, A. P., & Applebaum, A. (2015). Existential distress among caregivers or professionals taking care of dying patients. *Current Opinion in Supportive and Palliative Care, 9*(1), 77–86. doi:10.1097/SPC.0000000000000116

Peters, L. H., O'Connor, E. J., & Rudolf, C. J. (1980). The behavioral and affective consequences of performance-relevant situational variables. *Organizational Behavior and Human Performance*, *25*(1), 79–96. doi:10.1016/0030-5073(80)90026-4

Peterson, U., Demerouti, E., Bergström, G., Samuelsson, M., Åsberg, M., & Nygren, Å. (2008). Burnout and physical and mental health among Swedish healthcare workers. *Journal of Advanced Nursing*, *62*(1), 84–95. doi:10.1111/j.1365-2648.2007.04580.x PMID:18352967

Peters, S. E., Nielsen, K. M., Nagler, E. M., Revette, A. C., Madden, J., & Sorensen, G. (2020). Ensuring organization-intervention fit for a participatory organizational intervention to improve food service workers' health and wellbeing: Workplace organizational health study. *Journal of Occupational and Environmental Medicine*, *62*(2), e33–e45. doi:10.1097/JOM.0000000000001792 PMID:31815814

Petrocchi, N., & Cheli, S. (2019). The social brain and heart rate variability: Implications for psychotherapy. *Psychology and Psychotherapy: Theory, Research and Practice*, *92*(2), 208–223. doi:10.1111/papt.12224 PMID:30891894

Pfeffer, J., Vilendrer, S., Joseph, G., Kim, J., & Singer, S. J. (2020). Employers' Role in Employee Health: Why They Do What They Do. *Journal of Occupational and Environmental Medicine*, *62*(11), e601–e610. doi:10.1097/JOM.0000000000001967 PMID:32769791

Phillips, J. P. (2016). Workplace violence against health care workers in the United States. *The New England Journal of Medicine*, *374*(17), 1661–1669. doi:10.1056/NEJMra1501998 PMID:27119238

Phiri, L. P., Draper, C. E., Lambert, E. V., & Kolbe-Alexander, T. L. (2014). Nurses' lifestyle behaviours, health priorities and barriers to living a healthy lifestyle: A qualitative descriptive study. *BMC Nursing*, *13*(1), 1–11. doi:10.118612912-014-0038-6 PMID:25506262

Piers, R. D., Van den Eynde, M., Steeman, E., Vlerick, P., Benoit, D. D., & Van Den Noortgate, N. J. (2012). End-of-Life Care of the Geriatric Patient and Nurses' Moral Distress. *Journal of the American Medical Directors Association*, *13*(1), 80.e87–80.e13. doi:10.1016/j.jamda.2010.12.014

Piko, B. F. (2006). Burnout, role conflict, job satisfaction and psychosocial health among Hungarian health care staff: A questionnaire survey. *International Journal of Nursing Studies*, *43*(3), 311–318. doi:10.1016/j.ijnurstu.2005.05.003 PMID:15964005

Pinikahana, J., & Happell, B. (2004). Stress, burnout and job satisfaction in rural psychiatric nurses: A Victorian study. *The Australian Journal of Rural Health*, *12*(3), 120–125. doi:10.1111/j.1440-1854.2004.00572.x

Piotrkowski, C. S. (1998). Gender harassment, job satisfaction, and distress among employed white and minority women. *Journal of Occupational Health Psychology*, *3*(1), 33–43. doi:10.1037/1076-8998.3.1.33 PMID:9552270

Pipe, T. B., Bortz, J. J., Dueck, A., Pendergast, D., Buchda, V., & Summers, J. (2009). Nurse Leader Mindfulness Meditation Program for Stress Management a Randomized Controlled Trial. *The Journal of Nursing Administration*, *39*(3), 130–137. doi:10.1097/NNA.0b013e31819894a0 PMID:19590469

Pollock, A., Campbell, P., Cheyne, J., Cowie, J., Davis, B., McCallum, J., McGill, K., Elders, A., Hagen, S., McClurg, D., Torrens, C., & Maxwell, M. (2020). Interventions to support the resilience and mental health of frontline health and social care professionals during and after a disease outbreak, epidemic or pandemic: A mixed methods systematic review. *Cochrane Database of Systematic Reviews*, *2020*(11). Advance online publication. doi:10.1002/14651858.CD013779 PMID:33150970

Poulin, P. A., Mackenzie, C. S., Soloway, G., & Karayolas, E. (2008). Mindfulness training as an evidenced-based approach to reducing stress and promoting well-being among Human Services Professionals. *International Journal of Health Promotion and Education*, *46*(2), 72–80. doi:10.1080/14635240.2008.10708132

Powell, N. B., Schechtman, K. B., Riley, R. W., Li, K., Troell, R., & Guilleminault, C. (2001). The road to danger: The comparative risks of driving while sleepy. *The Laryngoscope*, *111*(5), 887–893. doi:10.1097/00005537-200105000-00024 PMID:11359171

Pratt, M., Norris, J., Lobelo, F., Roux, L., & Wang, G. (2014). The cost of physical inactivity: Moving into the 21st century. *British Journal of Sports Medicine*, *48*(3), 171–173. doi:10.1136/bjsports-2012-091810 PMID:23134760

Pridgeon, A., & Whitehead, K. (2013). A qualitative study to investigate the drivers and barriers to healthy eating in two public sector workplaces. *Journal of Human Nutrition and Dietetics*, *26*(1), 85–95. doi:10.1111/j.1365-277X.2012.01281.x PMID:22906402

Proper, K. I., & van Oostrom, S. H. (2019). The effectiveness of workplace health promotion interventions on physical and mental health outcomes—A systematic review of reviews. *Scandinavian Journal of Work, Environment & Health*, *45*(6), 546–559. doi:10.5271jweh.3833 PMID:31134284

ProQOL. (n.d.). *Helper pocket card.* https://proqol.org/helper-pocket-card

Providence Health Care. (2021, May 12). Nurses express hope, anxiety around COVID-19 in new study. *The Daily Scan.* https://thedailyscan.providencehealthcare.org/2021/05/nurses-express-hope-anxiety-around-covid-19-in-new-study/

Qiu, J., Shen, B., Zhao, M., Wang, Z., & Xie, B. (2020). *A nationwide survey of psychological distress among Chinese people in the COVID-19 epidemic: implications and policy recommendations.* Academic Press.

Qiu, X., Lan, Y., Miao, J., Wang, H., Wang, H., Wu, J., Li, G., Zhao, X., Cao, Z., Mei, J., Sun, W., Zhu, Z., Zhu, S., & Wang, W. (2021). A Comparative study on the psychological health of frontline health workers in Wuhan under and after the lockdown. *Frontiers in Psychiatry*, •••, 12.

Quick, J. C. (1999). Occupational health psychology: The convergence of health and clinical psychology with public health and preventive medicine in an organizational context. *Professional Psychology, Research and Practice*, *30*(2), 123–128. doi:10.1037/0735-7028.30.2.123

Raab, K., Sogge, K., Parker, N., & Flament, M. F. (2015). Mindfulness-based stress reduction and self-compassion among mental healthcare professionals: A pilot study. *Mental Health, Religion & Culture*, *18*(6), 503–512. doi:10.1080/13674676.2015.1081588

Rabatin, J., Williams, E., Baier Manwell, L., Schwartz, M. D., Brown, R. L., & Linzer, M. (2016). Predictors and outcomes of burnout in primary care physicians. *Journal of Primary Care & Community Health*, *7*(1), 41–43. doi:10.1177/2150131915607799 PMID:26416697

Rabelo, I., Lee, V., Fallah, M. P., Massaquoi, M., Evlampidou, I., Crestani, R., ... Severy, N. (2016). Psychological distress among Ebola survivors discharged from an Ebola treatment unit in Monrovia, Liberia–a qualitative study. *Frontiers in Public Health*, •••, 142.

Rabow, M. W., Huang, C. S., White-Hammond, G. E., & Tucker, R. O. (2021). Witnesses and victims both: Healthcare workers and grief in the time of COVID-19. *Journal of Pain and Symptom Management*, *62*(3), 647–656. doi:10.1016/j.jpainsymman.2021.01.139 PMID:33556494

Rafferty, A. E., Jimmieson, N. L., & Restubog, S. L. D. (2013). When leadership meets organizational change: The influence of the top management team and supervisory leaders on change appraisals, change attitudes, and adjustment to change. The psychology of organizational change: Viewing change from the employee's perspective, 145-172.

Raiber, K., & Verbakel, E. (2021). Are the gender gaps in informal caregiving intensity and burden closing due to COVID-19 pandemic? Evidence from the Netherlands. *Gender, Work and Organization*, *28*(5), 1926–1936. doi:10.1111/gwao.12725 PMID:34548767

Rajai, P., & Jackson, M. (2020). *How to support women of color during COVID-19 - Culture Amp Blog*. Culture Amp - Blog. https://www.cultureamp.com/blog/how-to-support-women-of-color-during-covid-19/

Raja, M., Azeem, M. U., Haq, I. U., & Naseer, S. (2020). Perceived threat of terrorism and employee outcomes: The moderating role of negative affectivity and psychological capital. *Journal of Business Research*, *110*, 316–326. doi:10.1016/j.jbusres.2020.01.026

Ramos-Morcillo, A. J., Fernández-Salazar, S., Ruzafa-Martínez, M., & Del-Pino-Casado, R. (2015). Effectiveness of a Brief, Basic Evidence-Based Practice Course for Clinical Nurses. *Worldviews on Evidence-Based Nursing*, *12*(4), 199–207. doi:10.1111/wvn.12103 PMID:26220505

Ramos, S., Costa, P., Passos, A. M., Silva, S. A., & Sacadura-Leite, E. (2020). Intervening on burnout in complex organizations – The incomplete process of an action research in the hospital. *Frontiers in Psychology*, *11*, 2203. doi:10.3389/fpsyg.2020.02203 PMID:33071844

Rana, B. U. I., & Munir, K. (2011). *Impact of stressors on the performance of employees*. Munich Personal RePEc Archive.

Rattner, N., & Towey, R. (2021, September 22). Average daily U.S. Covid deaths climb above 2,000 for the first time since March. *CNBC*. https://www.cnbc.com/2021/09/22/average-daily-us-covid-deaths-cross-2000.html

Recio-Saucedo, A., Dall'Ora, C., Maruotti, A., Ball, J., Briggs, J., Meredith, P., Redfern, O. C., Kovacs, C., Prytherch, D., Smith, G. B., & Griffiths, P. (2017). What impact does nursing care left undone have on patient outcomes? Review of the literature. *Journal of Clinical Nursing*, *27*(11-12), 2248–2259. doi:10.1111/jocn.14058 PMID:28859254

Reid, K., Flowers, P., & Larkin, M. (2005). Exploring lived experience.. *The Psychologist*, *18*(1), 20–23.

Reilly, E., Dhingra, K., & Boduszek, D. (2014). Teachers' self-efficacy beliefs, self-esteem, and job stress as determinants of job satisfaction. *International Journal of Educational Management*, *28*(4), 365–378. doi:10.1108/IJEM-04-2013-0053

Repper, J., & Carter, T. (2011). A review of the literature on peer support in mental health services. *Journal of Mental Health (Abingdon, England)*, *20*(4), 392–411. doi:10.3109/09638237.2011.583947 PMID:21770786

Rhodes, A., Ferdinande, P., Flaatten, H., Guidet, B., Metnitz, P. G., & Moreno, R. P. (2012). The variability of critical care bed numbers in Europe. *Intensive Care Medicine*, *38*(10), 1647–1653. doi:10.100700134-012-2627-8

Richardson, A., Gurung, G., Derrett, S., & Harcombe, H. (2019). Perspectives on preventing musculoskeletal injuries in nurses: A qualitative study. *Nursing Open*, *6*(3), 915–929. doi:10.1002/nop2.272 PMID:31367415

Richardson, D. M., Steeves-Reece, A., Martin, A., Hurtado, D. A., Dumet, L. M., & Goodman, J. M. (2019). Employee experiences with a newly adopted paid parental leave policy: Equity considerations for policy implementation. *Health Equity*, *3*(1), 117–123. doi:10.1089/heq.2019.0007 PMID:30989153

Richardson, N. M., Lamson, A. L., Smith, M., Eagan, S. M., Zvonkovic, A. M., & Jensen, J. (2020). Defining Moral Injury Among Military Populations: A Systematic Review. *Journal of Traumatic Stress*, *33*(4), 575–586. doi:10.1002/jts.22553

Rippe, J. M. (2020). Lifestyle Medicine Is Truly the Strong Foundation for Modern Health Care. *American Journal of Lifestyle Medicine*, *14*(5), 468–470. doi:10.1177/1559827620912165 PMID:32922230

Riskin, A., Erez, A., Foulk, T. A., Kugelman, A., Gover, A., Shoris, I., Riskin, K. S., & Bamberger, P. A. (2015). The impact of rudeness on medical team performance: A randomized trial. *Pediatrics*, *136*(3), 487–495. doi:10.1542/peds.2015-1385 PMID:26260718

Ritchie, T. D. (2014). Denial. In T. R. Levine (Ed.), *Encyclopedia of Lying and Deception*. Sage Publications. doi:10.4135/9781483306902.n107

Roberts, L. (2021). How COVID hurt the fight against other dangerous diseases. *Nature*, *592*(7855), 502–504. doi:10.1038/d41586-021-01022-x PMID:33883727

Robeznieks, A. (2021). *What physicians need to do to optimize Telehealth after pandemic*. American Medical Association. https://www.ama-assn.org/practice-management/digital/what-physicians-need-do-optimize-telehealth-after-pandemic?gclid=EAIaIQobChMIvdiajaeZ9AIVw513Ch2BZArpEAAYAiAAEgJzE_D_BwE

Robins, P. M., Meltzer, L., & Zelikovsky, N. (2009). The experience of secondary traumatic stress upon care providers working within a children's hospital. *Journal of Pediatric Nursing*, *24*(4), 270–279. doi:10.1016/j.pedn.2008.03.007 PMID:19632504

Rogers, D. (2016). Which educational interventions improve healthcare professionals' resilience? *Medical Teacher*, *38*(12), 1236–1241. doi:10.1080/0142159X.2016.1210111 PMID:27573430

Rolling, J., Mengin, A. C., Palacio, C., Mastelli, D., Fath, M., Gras, A., Von Hunolstein, J.-J., Schröder, C. M., & Vidailhet, P. (2021). COVID-19: Mental health prevention and care for healthcare professionals. *Frontiers in Psychiatry*, *12*, 566740. doi:10.3389/fpsyt.2021.566740 PMID:33833696

Roman, N. V., Mthembu, T. G., & Hoosen, M. (2020). Spiritual care–'A deeper immunity'–A response to Covid-19 pandemic. *African Journal of Primary Health Care & Family Medicine*, *12*(1). Advance online publication. doi:10.4102/phcfm.v12i1.2456 PMID:32634003

Rosen, M. A., Diazgranados, D., Dietz, A. S., Benishek, L. E., Thompson, D., Pronovost, P. J., & Weaver, S. J. (2018). Teamwork in healthcare: Key discoveries enabling safer, high-quality care. *American Psychologist, 73*(4), 433-450. 8 doi:10.1037/amp000029

Rosenbaum, L. (2020). The untold toll—The pandemic's effects on patients without Covid-19. *The New England Journal of Medicine*, *382*(24), 2368–2371. doi:10.1056/NEJMms2009984 PMID:32302076

Rosmond, R. (2005). Role of stress in the pathogenesis of the metabolic syndrome. *Psychoneuroendocrinology*, *30*(1), 1–10. doi:10.1016/j.psyneuen.2004.05.007 PMID:15358437

Rossi, R., Socci, V., Talevi, D., Mensi, S., Niolu, C., Pacitti, F., Di Marco, A., Rossi, A., Siracusano, A., & Di Lorenzo, G. (2020). COVID-19 pandemic and lockdown measures impact on mental ealth among the general population in Italy. *Frontiers in Psychiatry*, *11*, 790. doi:10.3389/fpsyt.2020.00790 PMID:32848952

Rossman, J. (2019). Cognitive-behavioral therapy for insomnia: An effective and underutilized treatment for insomnia. *American Journal of Lifestyle Medicine*, *13*(6), 544–547. doi:10.1177/1559827619867677 PMID:31662718

Rubin, R. S., Dierdorff, E. C., Bommer, W. H., & Baldwin, T. T. (2009). Do leaders reap what they sow? Leader and employee outcomes of leader organizational cynicism about change. *The Leadership Quarterly*, *20*(5), 680–688. doi:10.1016/j.leaqua.2009.06.002

Rudolph, C. W., Murphy, L. D., & Zacher, H. (2020). A systematic review and critique of research on "healthy leadership". *The Leadership Quarterly*, *31*(1), 101335. doi:10.1016/j.leaqua.2019.101335

Ruiz-Fernández, M. D., Ramos-Pichardo, J. D., Ibáñez-Masero, O., Cabrera-Troya, J., Carmona-Rega, M. I., & Ortega-Galán, Á. M. (2020). Compassion fatigue, burnout, compassion satisfaction and perceived stress in healthcare professionals during the COVID-19 health crisis in Spain. *Journal of Clinical Nursing*, *29*(21-22), 4321–4330. doi:10.1111/jocn.15469

Rushton, C. H., Batcheller, J., Schroeder, K., & Donohue, P. (2015). Burnout and Resilience Among Nurses Practicing in High-Intensity Settings. *American Journal of Critical Care*, *24*(5), 412–420. doi:10.4037/ajcc2015291

Ruyter, K., Wetzels, M., & Feinberg, R. (2001). Role stress in call centers: Its effects on employee performance and satisfaction. *Journal of Interactive Marketing*, *15*(2), 23-35. doi:10.1002/dir.1008

Ruzek, J. I., Brymer, M. J., Jacobs, A. K., Layne, C. M., Vernberg, E. M., Patricia, J., & Watson, P. J. (2007). Psychological First Aid. *Journal of Mental Health Counseling*, *29*(1), 17–49. doi:10.17744/mehc.29.1.5racqxjueafabgwp

Ryan, A.M. & Kossek, E.E. (2008), Work-life policy implementation: Breaking down or creating barriers to inclusiveness? *Human Resource Management*, *47*(2), 295-310. doi:10.1002/hrm.20213

Ryan, S. (2020). *The vitals: True nurse stories*. Marvel Comics. https://www.marvel.com/comics/issue/93069/the_vitals_true_nurse_stories_2020

Sabbath, E. L., Shaw, J., Stidsen, A., & Hashimoto, D. (2018). Protecting Mental Health of Hospital Workers after Mass Casualty Events: A Social Work Imperative. *Social Work*, *63*(3), 272–275. doi:10.1093wwy029 PMID:29701847

Sacks, E., Talajic, D., & Kim, B. (2020). *Covid chronicles*. NBC News and Upshot Studios. https://www.nbcnews.com/think/opinion/covid-chronicles-series

Sahin, T., Aslaner, H., Eker, O. O., Gokcek, M. B., & Dogan, M. (2020). Effect of COVID-19 pandemic on anxiety and burnout levels in emergency healthcare workers: a questionnaire study. doi:10.21203/rs.3.rs-32073/v1

Sahoo, S., Mehra, A., Suri, V., Malhotra, P., Yaddanapudi, L. N., Puri, G. D., & Grover, S. (2020). Lived experiences of the corona survivors (patients admitted in COVID wards): A narrative real-life documented summaries of internalized guilt, shame, stigma, anger. *Asian Journal of Psychiatry*, *53*, 102187. doi:10.1016/j.ajp.2020.102187 PMID:32512532

Saji, S., Venkatesan, S., & Callender, B. (2021). Comics in the time of a pan(dem)ic: COVID- 19, graphic medicine, and metaphors. *Perspectives in Biology and Medicine*, *64*(1), 136–154. doi:10.1353/pbm.2021.0010 PMID:33746135

Sallis, R. (2011). Developing healthcare systems to support exercise: Exercise as the fifth vital sign. *British Journal of Sports Medicine*, *45*(6), 473–474. doi:10.1136/bjsm.2010.083469 PMID:21292925

Salmon, J., Owen, N., Crawford, D., Bauman, A., & Sallis, J. F. (2003). Physical activity and dedentary behavior : A population-based study of barriers, enjoyment, and preference. *Health Psychology*, *22*(2), 178–188. doi:10.1037/0278-6133.22.2.178 PMID:12683738

Salyers, M. P., Bonfils, K. A., Luther, L., Firmin, R. L., White, D. A., Adams, E. L., & Rollins, A. L. (2017). The Relationship Between Professional Burnout and Quality and Safety in Healthcare: A Meta-Analysis. *Journal of General Internal Medicine*, *32*(4), 475–482. doi:10.100711606-016-3886-9

Sameer, A. S., Khan, M. A., Nissar, S., & Banday, M. Z. (2020). Assessment of mental health and various coping strategies among general population living under imposed COVID-lockdown across world: A cross-sectional study. *Ethics, Medicine, and Public Health*, *15*, 100571. doi:10.1016/j.jemep.2020.100571 PMID:32838000

Santa Maria, A., Wolter, C., Gusy, B., Kleiber, D., & Renneberg, B. (2019). The Impact of Health-Oriented Leadership on Police Officers' Physical Health, Burnout, Depression and Well-Being. *Policing. Journal of Policy Practice*, *13*(2), 186–200. doi:10.1093/police/pay067

Sarkar, M., & Page, A. E. (2020). Developing individual and team resilience in elite sport: Research to practice. *Journal of Sport Psychology in Action*. Advance online publication. doi:10.1080/21520704.2020.1861144

Schaufeli, W. B. (2017). Applying the Job Demands-Resources model: A "how to" guide to measuring and tackling work engagement and burnout. *Organizational Dynamics*, *46*(2), 120–132. doi:10.1016/j.orgdyn.2017.04.008

Schaufeli, W. B., Bakker, A. B., Hoogduin, K., Schaap, C., & Kladler, A. (2001). on the clinical validity of the maslach burnout inventory and the burnout measure. *Psychology & Health*, *16*(5), 565–582. doi:10.1080/08870440108405527

Schaufeli, W. B., Bakker, A. B., & Van Rhenen, W. (2009). How changes in job demands and resources predict burnout, work engagement, and sickness absenteeism. *Journal of Organizational Behavior*, *30*(7), 893–917. doi:10.1002/job.595

Schaufeli, W., & Enzmann, D. (1998). *The burnout companion to study and practice: A critical analysis*. CRC Press.

Schilgen, B., Nienhaus, A., & Mösko, M. (2020). The extent of psychosocial distress among immigrant and non-immigrant homecare nurses—A Comparative cross sectional survey. *International Journal of Environmental Research and Public Health*, *17*(5), 1635. doi:10.3390/ijerph17051635 PMID:32138277

Schmerling, R. H. (2020). *First, do no harm*. Harvard Health Publishing. https://www.health.harvard.edu/blog/first-do-no-harm-201510138421

Schoenfisch, A. L., & Lipscomb, H. J. (2009). Job characteristics and work organization factors associated with patient-handling injury among nursing personnel. *Work (Reading, Mass.)*, *33*(1), 117–128. doi:10.3233/WOR-2009-0847 PMID:19597289

Schonfeld, I. S., & Bianchi, R. (2016). Burnout and Depression: Two Entities or One?: Burnout and Depression. *Journal of Clinical Psychology*, *72*(1), 22–37. doi:10.1002/jclp.22229

Schreffler, J., Petrey, J., & Huecker, M. (2020). The impact of COVID-19 on healthcare worker wellness: A scoping review. *The Western Journal of Emergency Medicine*, *21*(5), 1059–1066. doi:10.5811/westjem.2020.7.48684

Schubert, M., Ludwig, J., Freiberg, A., Hahne, T. M., Romero Starke, K., Girbig, M., Faller, G., Apfelbacher, C., von dem Knesebeck, O., & Seidler, A. (2021). Stigmatization from work-related COVID-19 exposure: A systematic review with meta-analysis. *International Journal of Environmental Research and Public Health*, *18*(12), 6183. doi:10.3390/ijerph18126183 PMID:34201024

Schulte, E. E., Bernstein, C. A., & Cabana, M. D. (2020). Addressing faculty emotional responses during the coronavirus 2019 pandemic. *The Journal of Pediatrics*, *222*, 13–14. doi:10.1016/j.jpeds.2020.04.057 PMID:32387715

Schuster, M., & Dwyer, P. A. (2020). Post-traumatic stress disorder in nurses: An integrative review. *Journal of Clinical Nursing*, *29*(15–16), 2769–2787. doi:10.1111/jocn.15288 PMID:32372541

Schwarzer, R. (2001). Social-cognitive factors in changing health-related behaviors. *Current Directions in Psychological Science*, *10*(2), 47–51. doi:10.1111/1467-8721.00112

Schyns, B., & Schilling, J. (2013). How bad are the effects of bad leaders? A meta-analysis of destructive leadership and its outcomes. *The Leadership Quarterly*, *24*(1), 138–158. doi:10.1016/j.leaqua.2012.09.001

Seale, H., Leask, J., Po, K., & MacIntyre, C. R. (2009). "Will they just pack up and leave?"–attitudes and intended behaviour of hospital health care workers during an influenza pandemic. *BMC Health Services Research*, *9*(1), 1–8. doi:10.1186/1472-6963-9-30 PMID:19216792

Seligman, M. E., & Csikszentmihalyi, M. (2014). Positive psychology: An introduction. In *Flow and the foundations of positive psychology* (pp. 279–298). Springer.

Selman, L. E., Chao, D., Sowden, R., Marshall, S., Chamberlain, C., & Koffman, J. (2020). Bereavement Support on the Frontline of COVID-19: Recommendations for Hospital Clinicians. *Journal of Pain and Symptom Management*, *60*(2), e81–e86. doi:10.1016/j.jpainsymman.2020.04.024

Sendler, D., Rutkowska, A., & Makara-Studzinska, M. (2016). How the exposure to trauma has hindered physician's capacity to heal: Prevalence of PTSD among healthcare workers. *European Journal of Psychiatry*, *30*(4), 321–334. doi:10.7490/f1000research.1111861.1

Sevimli, S. (2020). Healthcare professionals acting ethically under the risk of stigmatization and violence during COVID-19 from media reports in Turkey. [doi:https://philpapers.org/rec/SEVHPA]. *Eubios Journal of Asian and International Bioethics; EJAIB*, *30*(5), 207–211.

Shaban, I. A., Khater, W. A., & Akhu-Zaheya, L. M. (2012). Undergraduate nursing students' stress sources and coping behaviors during their initial period of clinical training: A Jordanian perspective. *Nurse Education in Practice*, *12*(4), 204–209. doi:10.1016/j.nepr.2012.01.005 PMID:22281123

Shamia, N. A., Thabet, A. A. M., & Vostanis, P. (2015). Exposure to war traumatic experiences, post-traumatic stress disorder and post-traumatic growth among nurses in Gaza: War impact on nurses in Gaza. *Journal of Psychiatric and Mental Health Nursing*, *22*(10), 749–755. doi:10.1111/jpm.12264 PMID:26283005

Shanafelt, T. D., Balch, C. M., Bechamps, G., Russell, T., Dyrbye, L., Satele, D., Collicott, P., Novotny, P. J., Sloan, J., & Freischlag, J. (2010). Burnout and medical errors among American surgeons. *Annals of Surgery*, *251*(6), 995–1000. doi:10.1097/SLA.0b013e3181bfdab3 PMID:19934755

Shanafelt, T. D., Hasan, O., Dyrbye, L. N., Sinsky, C., Satele, D., Sloan, J., & West, C. P. (2015). Changes in burnout and satisfaction with work–life balance in physicians and the general US working population between 2011 and 2014. *Mayo Clinic Proceedings*, *90*(12), 1600–1613. doi:10.1016/j.mayocp.2015.08.023 PMID:26653297

Shanafelt, T. D., & Noseworthy, J. H. (2017). Executive leadership and physician well-being: Nine organizational strategies to promote engagement and reduce burnout. *Mayo Clinic Proceedings*, *92*(1), 129–146. doi:10.1016/j.mayocp.2016.10.004 PMID:27871627

Shang, J., Needleman, J., Liu, J., Larson, E., & Stone, P. W. (2019). Nurse staffing and healthcare associated infection, unit-level analysis. *The Journal of Nursing Administration*, *49*(5), 260–265. doi:10.1097/NNA.0000000000000748 PMID:31008835

Shapiro, G. K., Schulz-Quach, C., Matthew, A., Mosher, P., Rodin, G., de Vries, F., Hales, S., Korenblum, C., Black, S., Beck, L., Miller, K., Morita, J., Li, M., & Elliot, M. (2021, March 12). An institutional model for health care workers' mental health during COVID- 19. *NEJM Catalyst*. https://catalyst.nejm.org/doi/full/10.1056/CAT.20.0684

Shapiro, S. L., Astin, J. A., Bishop, S. R., & Cordova, M. (2005). Mindfulness-based stress reduction for health care professionals: Results from a randomized trial. *International Journal of Stress Management*, *12*(2), 164–176. doi:10.1037/1072-5245.12.2.164

Shapiro, S., Schwartz, G., & Bonner, G. (1998). Effects of mindfulness-based stress reduction on medical and premedical students. *Journal of Behavioral Medicine*, *21*(6), 581–599. doi:10.1023/A:1018700829825 PMID:9891256

Shaukat, N., Ali, D. M., & Razzak, J. (2020). Physical and mental health impacts of COVID-19 on healthcare workers: A scoping review. *International Journal of Emergency Medicine*, *13*(1), 40. doi:10.118612245-020-00299-5

Shay, J. (2014). Moral injury. *Psychoanalytic Psychology*, *31*(2), 182.

Sheahan, T. P., Sims, A. C., Leist, S. R., Schäfer, A., Won, J., Brown, A. J., Montgomery, S. A., Hogg, A., Babusis, D., Clarke, M. O., Spahn, J. E., Bauer, L., Sellers, S., Porter, D., Feng, J. Y., Cihlar, T., Jordan, R., Denison, M. R., & Baric, R. S. (2020). Comparative therapeutic efficacy of remdesivir and combination lopinavir, ritonavir, and interferon beta against MERS-CoV. *Nature Communications*, *11*(1), 1–14. doi:10.103841467-019-13940-6 PMID:31924756

Shechter, A., Diaz, F., Moise, N., Anstey, D. E., Ye, S., Agarwal, S., Birk, J. L., Brodie, D., Cannone, D. E., Chang, B., Claassen, J., Cornelius, T., Derby, L., Dong, M., Givens, R. C., Hochman, B., Homma, S., Kronish, I. M., Lee, S. A. J., ... Abdalla, M. (2020). Psychological distress, coping behaviors, and preferences for support among New York healthcare workers during the COVID-19 pandemic. *General Hospital Psychiatry*, *66*, 1–8. doi:10.1016/j.genhosppsych.2020.06.007 PMID:32590254

Shikdar, A. A., & Al-Kindi, M. A. (2007). Office ergonomics: Deficiencies in computer workstation design. *International Journal of Occupational Safety and Ergonomics*, *13*(2), 215–223. doi:10.1080/10803548.2007.11076722 PMID:17599795

Shrestha, A., Pyakurel, P., Shrestha, A., Gautam, R., Manandhar, N., Rhodes, E., Tamrakar, D., Karmacharya, B., Malik, V., Mattie, J., & Spiegelman, D. (2017). Facilitators and barriers to healthy eating in a worksite cafeteria: A qualitative study from Nepal. *Heart Asia*, *9*(2), 1–7. doi:10.1136/heartasia-2017-010956 PMID:29225703

Sianoja, M., Crain, T. L., Hammer, L. B., Bodner, T., Brockwood, K. J., LoPresti, M., & Shea, S. A. (2020). The relationship between leadership support and employee sleep. *Journal of Occupational Health Psychology*, *25*(3), 187–202. doi:10.1037/ocp0000173 PMID:31789546

Sibeoni, J., Bellon-Champel, L., Mousty, A., Manolios, E., Verneuil, L., & Revah-Levy, A. (2019). Physicians' perspectives about burnout: A systematic review and Metasynthesis. *Journal of General Internal Medicine*, *34*(8), 1578–1590. doi:10.100711606-019-05062-y PMID:31147982

Sikka, R., Morath, J. M., & Leape, L. (2015). The quadruple aim: Care, health, cost and meaning in work. *BMJ Quality & Safety*, *24*(10), 608–610. doi:10.1136/bmjqs-2015-004160 PMID:26038586

Silverman, H. J., Kheirbek, R. E., Moscou-Jackson, G., & Day, J. (2021). Moral distress in nurses caring for patients with COVID-19. *Nursing Ethics*, (7-8), 1137–1164. Advance online publication. doi:10.1177/09697330211003217 PMID:33910406

Sim, J., & Waterfield, J. (2019). Focus group methodology: Some ethical challenges. *Quality & Quantity*, *53*(6), 3003–3022. doi:10.100711135-019-00914-5

Singhania, N., Kathiravan, S., & Pannu, A. K. (2021). Acceptance of Covid-19 vaccine among healthcare personnel in India: A cross-sectional survey during the initial phase of vaccination. *Clinical Microbiology and Infection*. doi:10.1016/j.cmi.2021.03.008

Sisk, R. J. (2000). Caregiver burden and health promotion. *International Journal of Nursing Studies*, *37*(1), 37–43. doi:10.1016/S0020-7489(99)00053-X PMID:10687808

Sizmur, S., & Raleigh, V. (2018). *The risks to care quality and staff wellbeing of an NHS system under pressure*. Retrieved from https://www.picker.org/wp-content/uploads/2014/12/Risks-to-care-quality-and-staff-wellbeing-VR-SS-v8-Final.pdf

Skaal, L., & Pengpid, S. (2011). Obesity and health problems among South African healthcare workers: Do healthcare workers take care of themselves? *South African Family Practice*, *53*(6), 562. doi:10.1080/20786204.2011.10874153

Skakon, J., Nielsen, K., Vilhelm Borg, V., & Guzman, J. (2010). Are leaders' well-being, behaviours and style associated with the affective well-being of their employees? A systematic review of three decades of research. *Work and Stress*, *24*(2), 107–139. doi:10.1080/02678373.2010.495262

Sliter, K. A. (2013). Development and validation of a measure of workplace climate for healthy weight maintenance. *Journal of Occupational Health Psychology, 18*(3), 350–362. doi:10.1037/a0033132 PMID:23834449

Smirmaul, B. P., Chamon, R. F., de Moraes, F. M., Rozin, G., Moreira, A. S. B., de Almeida, R., & Guimarães, S. T. (2021). Lifestyle medicine during (and after) the COVID-19 pandemic. *American Journal of Lifestyle Medicine, 15*(1), 60–67. doi:10.1177/1559827620950276 PMID:33456421

Smith, B.W., Dalen, J., & Wiggins, K. (n.d.). The brief resilience scale: Assessing the ability to bounce back. *International Journal of Behavioral Medicine, 15,* 194–200. doi:10.1080/10705500802222972

Smith, C. S., Folkard, S., Tucker, P., & Evans, M. S. (2003). Work schedules, health, and safey. In J. C. Quick & L. E. Tetrick (Eds.), *Occupational Health Psychology Handbook* (2nd ed.). American Psychological Association.

Smith, J. A., & Osborn, M. (2003). Interpretative phenomenological analysis. In J. A. Smith (Ed.), *Qualitative psychology: A practical guide to research methods* (pp. 51–80). Sage Publications, Inc.

Smith, J. A., & Osborn, M. (2008). Interpretative phenomenological analysis. In V. Eatough & J. A. Smith (Eds.), *The Sage Handbook of Qualitative Research in Psychology* (pp. 179–194). Sage Publications.

Smith, J. A., & Osborn, M. (2015). Interpretative phenomenological analysis as a useful methodology for research on the lived experience of pain. *British Journal of Pain, 9*(1), 41–42. doi:10.1177/2049463714541642 PMID:26516556

Smith, J. L., De Nadai, A. S., Petrila, J., & Storch, E. A. (2019). Factors associated with length of stay in emergency departments for pediatric patients with psychiatric problems. *Pediatric Emergency Care, 35*(10), 716–721. doi:10.1097/PEC.0000000000001651 PMID:31593981

Smith, J., Cho, R., Martin, C., Cory, E., Smith, T., & Shouldice, M. (2021). Building skills and resilience in child abuse pediatricians: A novel program to address secondary traumatic stress. *Child Abuse & Neglect, 117*, 105082. doi:10.1016/j.chiabu.2021.105082 PMID:33930661

Sockalingam, S., Clarkin, C., Serhal, E., Pereira, C., & Crawford, A. (2020). Responding to health care professionals' mental health needs during COVID-19 through the rapid implementation of Project ECHO. *The Journal of Continuing Education in the Health Professions, 40*(3), 211–214. doi:10.1097/CEH.0000000000000311 PMID:32658015

Sofer, D. (2018). Responding to Mass Shootings: Are Hospitals and Nurses Fully Prepared? *The American Journal of Nursing, 118*(9), 18–19. doi:10.1097/01.NAJ.0000544970.28486.90 PMID:30138194

Song, Y., & Lindquist, R. (2015). Effects of mindfulness-based stress reduction on depression, anxiety, stress and mindfulness in Korean nursing students. *Nurse Education Today, 35*(1), 86–90. doi:10.1016/j.nedt.2014.06.010 PMID:25066651

Sonnentag, S., & Jelden, S. (2009). Job stressors and the pursuit of sport activities: A day-level perspective. *Journal of Occupational Health Psychology, 14*(2), 165–181. doi:10.1037/a0014953 PMID:19331478

Sorensen, G., Sparer, E., Williams, J. A. R., Gundersen, D., Boden, L. I., Dennerlein, J. T., Hashimoto, D., Katz, J. N., McLellan, D. L., Okechukwu, C. A., Pronk, N. P., Revette, A., & Wagner, G. R. (2018). Measuring best practices for workplace safety, health and wellbeing: The Workplace Integrated Safety and Health Assessment. *Journal of Occupational and Environmental Medicine, 60*(5), 430–439. doi:10.1097/JOM.0000000000001286 PMID:29389812

South, E. C., Butler, P. D., & Merchant, R. M. (2020). Toward an equitable society: Building a culture of antiracism in health care. *The Journal of Clinical Investigation, 130*(10), 5039–5041. Advance online publication. doi:10.1172/JCI141675 PMID:32692730

Spector, P. E., Fox, S., Penney, L. M., Bruursema, K., Goh, A., & Kessler, S. (2006). The dimensionality of counterproductivity: Are all counterproductive behaviors created equal? *Journal of Vocational Behavior*, *68*(3), 446–460. doi:10.1016/j.jvb.2005.10.005

Spector, P. E., & Jex, S. M. (1998). Development of four self-report measures of job stressors and strain: Interpersonal Conflict at Work Scale, Organizational Constraints Scale, Quantitative Workload Inventory, and Physical Symptoms Inventory. *Journal of Occupational Health Psychology*, *3*(4), 356–367. doi:10.1037/1076-8998.3.4.356 PMID:9805281

Spector, P. E., Yang, L. Q., & Zhou, Z. E. (2015). A longitudinal investigation of the role of violence prevention climate in exposure to workplace physical violence and verbal abuse. *Work and Stress*, *29*(4), 325–340. doi:10.1080/02678373.2015.1076537

Spilsbury, J. C., & Cooney, M. C. (1998). Immigrant Health Care Providers in the United States. Handbook of Immigrant Health, 607–627. doi:10.1007/978-1-4899-1936-6_29

Spitzmuller, M., Park, G., Van Dyne, L., Wagner, D. T., & Maerz, A. (2020). When do you benefit? Differential boundary conditions facilitate positive affect and buffer negative affect after helping others. *European Journal of Work and Organizational Psychology*, *30*(4), 482–494. doi:10.1080/1359432X.2020.1843436

Spoorthy, M. S., Pratapa, S. K., & Mahant, S. (2020). Mental health problems faced by healthcare workers due to the COVID-19 pandemic–A review. *Asian Journal of Psychiatry*, *51*, 102119. doi:10.1016/j.ajp.2020.102119 PMID:32339895

Squiers, J. J., Lobdell, K. W., Fann, J. I., & DiMaio, J. M. (2017). Physician Burnout: Are We Treating the Symptoms Instead of the Disease? *The Annals of Thoracic Surgery*, *104*(4), 1117–1122. doi:10.1016/j.athoracsur.2017.08.009

Squillace, M. R., Remsburg, R. E., Bercovitz, A., Rosenoff, E., & Branden, L. (2007). An introduction to the National Nursing Assistant Survey. *Vital and health statistics. Ser. 1, Programs and collection procedures*, (44), 1-54.

Srivastava, A., Arya, Y. K., Joshi, S., Singh, T., Kaur, H., Chauhan, H., & Das, A. (2021). Major stressors and coping strategies of internal migrant workers during the COVID-19 pandemic: A qualitative exploration. *Frontiers in Psychology*, *12*, 12. doi:10.3389/fpsyg.2021.648334 PMID:34093333

Stamm, B. H. (2010). The Concise ProQOL Manual (2nd ed.). Pocatello, ID: ProQOL.org.

Stanev, S., Bailer, J., Straker, J. K., Mehdizadeh, S., Park, R. M., & Li, H. (2012). Worker injuries and safety equipment in Ohio nursing homes. *Journal of Gerontological Nursing*, *38*(6), 47–56. doi:10.3928/00989134-20120508-01 PMID:22774234

Stangl, A. L., Earnshaw, V. A., Logie, C. H., van Brakel, W. C., Simbayi, L., Barré, I., & Dovidio, J. F. (2019). The Health Stigma and Discrimination Framework: A global, crosscutting framework to inform research, intervention development, and policy on health-related stigmas. *BMC Medicine*, *17*(1), 31. doi:10.118612916-019-1271-3 PMID:30764826

Stankevitz, K., Dement, J., Schoenfisch, A., Joyner, J., Clancy, S. M., Stroo, M., & Østbye, T. (2017). Perceived barriers to healthy eating and physical activity among participants in a workplace obesity intervention. *Journal of Occupational and Environmental Medicine*, *59*(8), 746–751. doi:10.1097/JOM.0000000000001092 PMID:28692017

Stanley, B., & Brown, G. K. (2012). Safety planning intervention: A brief intervention to mitigate suicide risk. *Cognitive and Behavioral Practice*, *19*(2), 256–264. doi:10.1016/j.cbpra.2011.01.001

Starck, A., Gutermann, J., Schouler-Ocak, M., Jesuthasan, J., Bongard, S., & Stangier, U. (2020). The relationship of acculturation, traumatic events and depression in female refugees. *Frontiers in Psychology*, *11*, 906. doi:10.3389/fpsyg.2020.00906 PMID:32528358

Starmer, A. J., Frintner, M. P., & Freed, G. L. (2016). Work–life balance, burnout, and satisfaction of early career pediatricians. *Pediatrics*, *137*(4), e20153183. Advance online publication. doi:10.1542/peds.2015-3183 PMID:27020792

Stockton, A., & King, L. (2021, February 24). Death, through a nurse's eyes. *New York Times*. https://www.nytimes.com/video/opinion/100000007578176/covid-icu-nurses-arizona.html

Stokes-Parish, J., Elliott, R., Rolls, K., & Massey, D. (2020). Angels and heroes: The unintended consequence of the hero narrative. *Journal of Nursing Scholarship*, *52*(5), 462–466. doi:10.1111/jnu.12591 PMID:32856396

Stone, A. A., Turkkan, J. S., Bachrach, C. A., Jobe, J. B., Kurtzman, H. S., & Cain, V. S. (2002). *The Science of Self-Report: Implications for Research and Practice*. Lawrence Erlbaum Associates.

Stovernik, A. C., Kirkman, B. L., Mistry, S., & Rosen, B. (2020). Bouncing back together: Toward a theoretical model of work team resilience. *Academy of Management Review*, *45*, 395–422. https://doi.org/10.5465/amr.2017.0005

Stower, H., & Guennot, M. (2021, March 15). Art in a pandemic: A digital gallery. *Nature Medicine*. https://www.nature.com/articles/d41591-021-00009-5

Stuijfzand, S., Deforges, C., Sandoz, V., Sajin, C. T., Jaques, C., Elmers, J., & Horsch, A. (2020). Psychological impact of an epidemic/pandemic on the mental health of healthcare professionals: A rapid review. *BMC Public Health*, *20*(1), 1–18. doi:10.118612889-020-09322-z PMID:32787815

Sun, L., Gao, Y., Yang, J., Zang, X.-Y., & Wang, Y.-G. (2016). The impact of professional identity on role stress in nursing students: A cross-sectional study. *International Journal of Nursing Studies*, *63*, 1–8. doi:10.1016/j.ijnurstu.2016.08.010 PMID:27565423

Sun, N., Wei, L., Shi, S., Jiao, D., Song, R., Ma, L., Wang, H., Wang, C., Wang, Z., You, Y., Liu, S., & Wang, H. (2020). A qualitative study on the psychological experience of caregivers of COVID-19 patients. *American Journal of Infection Control*, *48*(6), 592–598. doi:10.1016/j.ajic.2020.03.018 PMID:32334904

Suryadevara, V., Adusumalli, C., Adusumilli, P. K., Chalasani, S. H., & Radhakrishnan, R. (2020). Mental health status among the south Indian pharmacy students during Covid-19 pandemic quarantine period: A cross-sectional study. medRxiv.

Suryavanshi, N., Kadam, A., Dhumal, G., Nimkar, S., Mave, V., Gupta, A., Cox, S. R., & Gupte, N. (2020). Mental health and quality of life among healthcare professionals during the COVID-19 pandemic in India. *Brain and Behavior*, *10*(11), e01837. doi:10.1002/brb3.1837 PMID:32918403

Sutherland, T., Choi, D., & Yu, C. (2021). "Brought to life through imagery" – animated graphic novels to promote empathic, patient-centred care in postgraduate medical learners. *BMC Medical Education*, *21*(1), 66. doi:10.118612909-021-02491-4 PMID:33478483

Swinkels, J., van Tilburg, T., Verbakel, E., & van Groenou, M. B. (2019). Explaining the gender gap in the caregiving burden of partner caregivers. *The Journals of Gerontology. Series B, Psychological Sciences and Social Sciences*, *74*(2), 309–317. PMID:28379560

Tafvelin, S., von Thiele Schwarz, U., Nielsen, K., & Hasson, H. (2018). Employees' and line managers' active involvement in participatory organizational interventions: Examining direct, reversed, and reciprocal effects on well-being. *Stress and Health*, *35*(1), 69–80. doi:10.1002mi.2841 PMID:30303299

Taggar, S., & Ellis, R. (2007). The role of leaders in shaping formal team norms. *The Leadership Quarterly*, *18*(2), 105–120.

Tawfik, D. S., Profit, J., Webber, S., & Shanafelt, T. D. (2019). Organizational factors affecting physician well-being. *Current Treatment Options in Pediatrics*, *5*(1), 11–25. doi:10.100740746-019-00147-6 PMID:31632895

Teleghani, F., Ashouri, E., & Saburi, M. (2017). Empathy, burnout, demographic variables and their relationships in oncology nurses. *Iranian Journal of Nursing and Midwifery Research, 22*(1), 41–45. doi:10.4103/ijnmr.IJNMR_66_16 PMID:28382057

Telford, B., Fletcher, K., & Bedwell, W. (2017). Informal Learning in the Healthcare Industry. In J. E. Ellingson & R. A. Noe (Eds.), *Autonomous learning in the workplace* (pp. 219–236). Routledge. doi:10.4324/9781315674131-12

ten Hoeve, Y., Jansen, G., & Roodbol, P. (2014). The nursing profession: Public image, self- concept and professional identity. A discussion paper. *Journal of Advanced Nursing, 70*(2), 295–309. doi:10.1111/jan.12177 PMID:23711235

Teoh, K. R., Hassard, J., & Cox, T. (2020). Individual and organizational psychosocial predictors of hospital doctors' work-related well-being: A multilevel and moderation perspective. *Health Care Management Review, 45*(2), 162–172. doi:10.1097/HMR.0000000000000207 PMID:29957704

Teo, S. T. T., Nguyen, D., Trevelyan, F., Lamm, F., & Boocock, M. (2021). Workplace bullying, psychological hardiness, and accidents and injuries in nursing: A moderated mediation model. *PLoS One, 16*(1), e0244426. doi:10.1371/journal.pone.0244426 PMID:33417612

Terre, L. (2014). Clinical implications of impaired sleep. *American Journal of Lifestyle Medicine, 8*(6), 352–370. doi:10.1177/1559827614521955

Tessaro, I., Campbell, M., Benedict, S., Kelsey, K., Heisler-MacKinnon, J., Belton, L., & DeVellis, B. (1998). Developing a worksite health promotion intervention: Health Works for Women. *American Journal of Health Behavior, 22*(6), 434.

Teti, M., Epping, S., Myroniuk, T. W., & Evans-Agnew, R. (2021). HIV stigma and its metaphors: Photos, symbols, and solutions. *Journal of HIV/AIDS & Social Services, 20*(1), 97–114. doi:10.1080/15381501.2021.1911903

The Moral Injury Project. (2021). *What is moral injury*? Syracuse University. https://moralinjuryproject.syr.edu/about-moral-injury/

Thomas, M. R., Dyrbye, L. N., Huntington, J. L., Lawson, K. L., Novotny, P. J., Sloan, J. A., & Shanafelt, T. D. (2007). How Do Distress and Well-being Relate to Medical Student Empathy? A Multicenter Study. *Journal of General Internal Medicine, 22*(2), 177–183. doi:10.100711606-006-0039-6

Thum, J. S., Parsons, G., Whittle, T., & Astorino, T. A. (2017). High-Intensity Interval Training Elicits Higher Enjoyment than Moderate Intensity Continuous Exercise. *PLoS One, 12*(1), 1–11. doi:10.1371/journal.pone.0166299 PMID:28076352

Tierney, J., & Baumeister, R. F. (2019). *The power of bad: How the negativity effect rules us and how we can rule it.* Penguin.

Tiwari, V., Bhardwaj, A., Sonani, B., & Mehta, A. C. (2020). Urgent issues facing immigrant physicians in the United States in the COVID-19 era. In Annals of internal medicine (Vol. 173, Issue 10, pp. 838–839). NLM (Medline). doi:10.7326/M20-4103

Traynor, M. (2017). Critical Resilience for Nurses: An Evidence-based Guide to Survival and Change in the Modern NHS. Routledge.

Traynor, M. (2018). Guest editorial: What's wrong with resilience. *Journal of Research in Nursing, 23*(1), 5–8. doi:10.1177/1744987117751458

Tregoning, C., Remington, S., & Agius, S. (2014). Facing change: Developing resilience for staff, associate specialist, and specialty doctors. *BMJ (Clinical Research Ed.), g251*. doi:10.1136/bmj.g251

Trotochaud, K., Coleman, J. R., Krawiecki, N., & McCracken, C. (2015). Moral distress in pediatric healthcare workers. *Journal of Pediatric Nursing, 30*(6), 908–914. doi:10.1016/j.pedn.2015.03.001 PMID:25869472

Tryon, K. (2014). Healthy staff increase productivity. *Occupational Health, 66*(4), 11.

Tsao, P., & Yu, C. H. (2016). "There's no billing code for empathy" - Animated comics remind medical students of empathy: A qualitative study. *BMC Medical Education, 16*(1), 204. doi:10.118612909-016-0724-z PMID:27520824

Tsutsumi, A. (2011). Development of an evidence-based guideline for supervisor training in promoting mental health: Literature review. *Journal of Occupational Health, 53*(1), 1–9. doi:10.1539/joh.R10002 PMID:21079372

Turan, B., Hatcher, A. M., Weiser, S. D., Johnson, M. O., Rice, W. S., & Turan, J. M. (2017). Framing Mechanisms Linking HIV-Related Stigma, Adherence to Treatment, and Health Outcomes. *American Journal of Public Health, 107*(6), 863–869. doi:10.2105/AJPH.2017.303744 PMID:28426316

Turgut, B. (2018). Ocular ergonomics for the computer vision syndrome. *Journal of Eye and Vision, 1*(2), 1–2. https://www.imedpub.com/articles/ocular-ergonomics-for-the-computer-vision-syndrome.php?aid=22200

Tyagi, N. (2021). Aligning organizational culture to enhance managerial effectiveness of academic leaders: An interface for employee engagement and retention. *International Journal of Educational Management, 35*(7), 1387–1404. Advance online publication. doi:10.1108/IJEM-10-2020-0447

Tyagi, N., & Moses, D. B. (2020). Developing and validating the antecedents of managerial effectiveness: Factorial constitution in institutions of higher learning. *International Journal of Leadership in Education, 0*(0), 1–21. doi:10.1080/13603124.2020.1762003

Tyagi, N., Moses, D. B., & Rana, S. (2017). Influence of Organizational Justice on Managerial Effectiveness in Institutions of Higher Learning. *Productivity, 58*(3), 286–299.

U.S. Census Bureau. (2016). *US census bureau QuickFacts: Ohio*. Retrieved from www.census.gov/search-results.html?q=ohio&page=1&stateGeo=none&searchtype=web&cssp=SERP&_charset_=UTF-8

U.S. Census Bureau. (2019). *2019 American Consumer Survey*. Retrieved from https://www.census.gov/programs-surveys/acs/

U.S. Department of Agriculture and U.S. Department of Health and Human Services. (2020). *Dietary Guidelines for Americans, 2020-2025* (9th ed.). DietaryGuidelines.gov.

U.S. Department of State. (n.d.). *Employment-Based Immigrant Visas*. Retrieved July 5, 2021, from https://travel.state.gov/content/travel/en/us-visas/immigrate/employment-based-immigrant-visas.html

U.S. Department of Veterans Affairs. (2018, September 24). *How Common is PTSD in Veterans*. National Center for PTSD. https://www.ptsd.va.gov/understand/common/common_veterans.asp

Udaya, B. B., Pokharel, S., Munikar, S., Wagle, C. N., Adhikary, P., Shahi, B. B., Thapa, C., Bhandari, R. P., Adhikari, B., & Thapa, K. (2021). Anxiety and depression among people living in quarantine centers during COVID-19 pandemic: A mixed-method study from western Nepal. *PLoS One, 16*(7), e0254126. doi:10.1371/journal.pone.0254126 PMID:34242319

Uhl Bien, M., & Russ, M. (2009). Complexity leadership in bureaucratic forms of organizing: A meso model. *The Leadership Quarterly, 20*(4), 631–650. doi:10.1016/j.leaqua.2009.04.007

Ungar, N., Sieverding, M., Weidner, G., Ulrich, C. M., & Wiskemann, J. (2016). A self-regulation-based intervention to increase physical activity in cancer patients. *Psychology Health and Medicine, 21*(2), 163–175. doi:10.1080/13548506.2015.1081255 PMID:26367803

United States Government Accountability Office. (2020). *Distance learning: Challenges providing services to K-12 English learners and students with disabilities during COVID-19.* https://www.gao.gov/assets/gao-21-43.pdf

University of Colorado Anschutz Medical Campus. (2020, May 18). *Tell your story with COVID-19 narratives.* https://medschool.cuanschutz.edu/physical-medicine-and-rehabilitation/newsdetail/news-and-media-2020/tell-your-story-with-covid-19-narratives

Uthayaratana, T., Taephant, N., & Pisitsungkagarn, K. (2019). Four Noble Truths based problem solving: A therapeutic view. *Mental Health, Religion & Culture, 22*(2), 119–129. doi:10.1080/13674676.2018.1512565

Vagni, M., Maiorano, T., Giostra, V., & Pajardi, D. (2020). Hardiness, stress and secondary trauma in italian healthcare and emergency workers during the COVID-19 pandemic. *Sustainability, 12*(14), 5592. doi:10.3390u12145592

Valizadeh, L., Zamanzadeh, V., Gargari, R. B., Ghahramanian, A., Tabrizi, F. J., & Keogh, B. (2016). Pressure and protective factors influencing nursing students' self-esteem: A content analysis study. *Nurse Education Today, 36,* 468-472. .nedt.2015.10.019 doi:10.1016/j

Van Cappellen, P., Rice, E. L., Catalino, L. I., & Fredrickson, B. L. (2018). Positive affective processes underlie positive health behaviour change. *Psychology & Health, 33*(1), 77–97.

Van den Broeck, A., De Cuyper, N., De Witte, H., & Vansteenkiste, M. (2010). Not all job demands are equal: Differentiating job hindrances and job challenges in the Job Demands-Resources model. *European Journal of Work and Organizational Psychology, 19*(6), 735–759. doi:10.1080/13594320903223839

van Dorssen-Boog, P., de Jong, J., Veld, M., & Van Vuuren, T. (2020). Self-leadership among healthcare workers: A mediator for the effects of job autonomy on work engagement and health. *Frontiers in Psychology, 11,* 1420. doi:10.3389/fpsyg.2020.01420 PMID:32765341

Van Moi, M. M. C., Kompanje, E. J. O., Benoit, D. D., Bakker, J., & Nijkamp, M. D. (2015). The prevalence of compassion fatigue and burnout among healthcare professionals in intensive care units: A systematic review. *PLoS One, 10*(8), e0136955. doi:10.1371/journal.pone.0136955 PMID:26322644

van Rossem, C., Spigt, M. G., Kleijsen, J. R., Hendricx, M., van Schayck, C. P., & Kotz, D. (2015). Smoking cessation in primary care: Exploration of barriers and solutions in current daily practice from the perspective of smokers and healthcare professionals. *The European Journal of General Practice, 21*(2), 1–7. doi:10.3109/13814788.2014.990881 PMID:25649048

Vanyo, L., Sorge, R., Chen, A., & Lakoff, D. (2017). Posttraumatic stress disorder in emergency medicine residents. *Annals of Emergency Medicine, 70*(6), 898–903. doi:10.1016/j.annemergmed.2017.07.010 PMID:28826753

Varajao, J., Fernandes, G., Amaral, A., & Gonçalves, A. M. (2021). Team Resilience Model: An Empirical Examination of Information Systems Projects. *Reliability Engineering & System Safety, 206,* 107303.

Varvogli, L., & Darviri, C. (2011). Stress management techniques: Evidence-based procedures that reduce stress and promote health. *Health Science Journal, 5*(2), 74.

Vera, M., Rodríguez-Sánchez, A. M., & Salanova, M. (2017). May the force be with you: Looking for resources that build team resilience. *Journal of Workplace Behavioral Health, 32,* 119–138. doi:10.1080/15555240.2017.1329629

Vidyarthi, P. R., Singh, S., Erdogan, B., Chaudhry, A., Posthuma, R., & Anand, S. (2016). Individual deals within teams: Investigating the role of relative i-deals for employee performance. *The Journal of Applied Psychology, 101*(11), 1536–1552. doi:10.1037/apl0000145 PMID:27513681

Vignoli, M., Nielsen, K., Guglielmi, D., Tabanelli, M. C., & Violante, F. S. (2017). The importance of context in screening in occupational health interventions in organizations: A mixed methods study. *Frontiers in Psychology*, *8*, 1347. doi:10.3389/fpsyg.2017.01347 PMID:28848468

Vindrola-Padros, C., Andrews, L., Dowrick, A., Djellouli, N., Fillmore, H., Bautista Gonzalez, E., ... Johnson, G. (2020). Perceptions and experiences of healthcare workers during the COVID-19 pandemic in the UK. *BMJ Open*, *10*(11), e040503. doi:10.1136/bmjopen-2020-040503

Vizheh, M., Qorbani, M., Arzaghi, S. M., Muhidin, S., Javanmard, Z., & Esmaeili, M. (2020). The mental health of healthcare workers in the COVID-19 pandemic: A systematic review. *Journal of Diabetes and Metabolic Disorders*, *19*(2), 1967–1978. doi:10.100740200-020-00643-9 PMID:33134211

Vogel, M., Braungardt, T., Meyer, W., & Schneider, W. (2012). The effects of shift work on physical and mental health. *Journal of Neural Transmission (Vienna, Austria)*, *119*(10), 1121–1132. doi:10.100700702-012-0800-4 PMID:22488445

Wald, H. S. (2020). Optimizing resilience and wellbeing for healthcare professions trainees and healthcare professionals during public health crises–Practical tips for an 'integrative resilience' approach. *Medical Teacher*, *42*(7), 744–755. do i:10.1080/0142159X.2020.1768230 PMID:32449867

Waldman, J. D., Kelly, F., Aurora, S., & Smith, H. L. (2004). The shocking cost of turnover in health care. *Health Care Management Review*, *29*(1), 2–7. doi:10.1097/00004010-200401000-00002 PMID:14992479

Walsh, R. (2011). Lifestyle and mental health. *The American Psychologist*, *66*(7), 579–592. doi:10.1037/a0021769 PMID:21244124

Wang, C., Grassau, P., Lawlor, P. G., Webber, C., Bush, S. H., Gagnon, B., Kabir, M., & Spilg, E. G. (2020). Burnout and resilience among Canadian palliative care physicians. *BMC Palliative Care*, *19*(1), 169. doi:10.118612904-020-00677-z PMID:33158428

Wang, C., Pan, R., Wan, X., Tan, Y., Xu, L., Ho, C. S., & Ho, R. C. (2020). Immediate psychological responses and associated factors during the initial stage of the 2019 coronavirus disease (COVID-19) epidemic among the general population in China. *International Journal of Environmental Research and Public Health*, *17*(5), 1729. doi:10.3390/ijerph17051729 PMID:32155789

Wang, Y., Beydoun, M. A., Min, J., Xue, H., Kaminsky, L. A., & Cheskin, L. J. (2020). Has the prevalence of overweight, obesity and central obesity levelled off in the United States? Trends, patterns, disparities, and future projections for the obesity epidemic. *International Journal of Epidemiology*, *49*(3), 810–823. doi:10.1093/ije/dyz273 PMID:32016289

Ward, K. P., Shaw, S. A., Chang, M., & El-Bassel, N. (2018). Social support moderates the association between traumatic life events and depression among migrant and nonmigrant men in Almaty, Kazakhstan. *Journal of Traumatic Stress*, *31*(5), 698–707. doi:10.1002/jts.22324 PMID:30338586

Wardle, J., Steptoe, A., Oliver, G., & Lipsey, Z. (2000). Stress, dietary restraint and food intake. *Journal of Psychosomatic Research*, *48*(2), 195–202. doi:10.1016/S0022-3999(00)00076-3 PMID:10719137

Watanabe, N., Horikoshi, M., Shinmei, I., Oe, Y., Narisawa, T., Kumachi, M., Matsuoka, Y., Hamazaki, K., & Furukawa, T. A. (2019). Brief mindfulness-based stress management program for a better mental state in working populations - happy nurse project: A randomized controlled trial¶¶. *Journal of Affective Disorders*, *251*, 186–194. doi:10.1016/j.jad.2019.03.067 PMID:30927579

Waterman, S., Hunter, E. C. M., Cole, C. L., Evans, L. J., Greenberg, N., Rubin, G. J., & Beck, A. (2018). Training peers to treat Ebola centre workers with anxiety and depression in Sierra Leone. *The International Journal of Social Psychiatry*, *64*(2), 156–165. doi:10.1177/0020764017752021 PMID:29432085

Weaver-Hightower, M. (2013). Sequential art for qualitative research: Making comics to make meaning of the social world. In C. Syma & R. Weiner (Eds.), *Graphic novels, comics, and education* (pp. 260–273). McFarland.

Wegge, J., Shemla, M., & Haslam, S. A. (2014). Leader behavior as a determinant of health at aork: Specification and evidence of five key pathways. *German Journal of Human Resource Management, 28*(1–2), 6–23. doi:10.1177/239700221402800102

Weick, K. E. (1995). *Sensemaking in Organizations*. Sage Publications, Inc.

Weierter, S. J. (1997). Who wants to play "follow the leader?" A theory of charismatic relationships based on routinized charisma and follower characteristics. *The Leadership Quarterly, 8*(2), 171-193.

Weiss, A. K., & Ludwig, S. (2019). Physician well-being: Special considerations in pediatrics. *Current Problems in Pediatric and Adolescent Health Care, 49*(11), 100657. Advance online publication. doi:10.1016/j.cppeds.2019.100657 PMID:31542326

Wenzel, J., Shaha, M., Klimmek, R., & Krumm, S. (2011). Working through grief and loss: Oncology nurses' perspectives on professional bereavement. *Oncology Nursing Forum, 38*(4), E272–E282. doi:10.1188/11.ONF.E272-E282 PMID:21708522

West, C. P., Dyrbye, L. N., & Shanafelt, T. D. (2018). Physician burnout: Contributors, consequences and solutions. *Journal of Internal Medicine, 283*(6), 516–529. doi:10.1111/joim.12752 PMID:29505159

Whitehead, P. B., Herbertson, R. K., Hamric, A. B., Epstein, E. G., & Fisher, J. M. (2015). Moral Distress Among Healthcare Professionals: Report of an Institution-Wide Survey: Moral Distress. *Journal of Nursing Scholarship, 47*(2), 117–125. doi:10.1111/jnu.12115

Whysall, Z., Haslam, C., & Haslam, R. (2006). Implementing health and safety interventions in the workplace: An exploratory study. *International Journal of Industrial Ergonomics, 36*(9), 809–818. doi:10.1016/j.ergon.2006.06.007

Wiener, L., Rosenberg, A. R., Pennarola, B., Fry, A., & Weaver, M. (2021). Navigating the terrain of moral distress: Experiences of pediatric end-of-life care and bereavement during COVID-19. *Palliative & Supportive Care, 19*(2), 129–134. doi:10.1017/S1478951521000225 PMID:33648612

Wilkinson, E. (2015). UK NHS staff: Stressed, exhausted, burnt out. *Lancet, 385*(9971), 841–842. doi:10.1016/S0140-6736(15)60470-6

Willan, J., King, A. J., Jeffery, K., & Bienz, N. (2020). Challenges for NHS hospitals during covid-19 epidemic. *BMJ (Clinical Research Ed.), m1117*. doi:10.1136/bmj.m1117

Willard-Grace, R., Hessler, D., Rogers, E., Dube, K., Bodenheimer, T., & Grumbach, K. (2014). Team Structure and Culture Are Associated With Lower Burnout in Primary Care. *Journal of the American Board of Family Medicine, 27*(2), 229–238. doi:10.3122/jabfm.2014.02.130215

Williams, I. (2007). *What is "graphic medicine"?* Graphic Medicine International Collective. https://www.graphicmedicine.org/why-graphic-medicine/

Williams, C. L., & Berry, J. W. (1991). Primary prevention of acculturative stress among refugees: Application of psychological theory and practice. *The American Psychologist, 46*(6), 632–641. doi:10.1037/0003-066X.46.6.632 PMID:1952422

Williams, I. (2011). Autography as auto-therapy: Psychic pain and the graphic memoir. *The Journal of Medical Humanities, 32*(4), 353–366. doi:10.100710912-011-9158-0 PMID:21898054

Williams, I. C. (2012). Graphic medicine: Comics as medical narrative. *Medical Humanities, 38*(1), 21–27. doi:10.1136/medhum-2011-010093 PMID:22282425

Williams, I. M., & Lewis, W. G. (2020). Stress in the workplace for healthcare professionals. *Physiological Reports*, *8*(13). Advance online publication. doi:10.14814/phy2.14496 PMID:32744802

Williamson, V., Murphy, D., & Greenberg, N. (2020). COVID-19 and experiences of moral injury in front-line key workers. *Occupational Medicine*, *70*(5), 317–319. doi:10.1093/occmed/kqaa052

Williamson, V., Murphy, D., Phelps, A., Forbes, D., & Greenberg, N. (2021). Moral injury: The effect on mental health and implications for treatment. *The Lancet. Psychiatry*, *8*(6), 453–455. doi:10.1016/S2215-0366(21)00113-9 PMID:33743196

Williamson, V., Stevelink, S. A. M., & Greenberg, N. (2018). Occupational moral injury and mental health: Systematic review and meta-analysis. *The British Journal of Psychiatry*, *212*(6), 339–346. doi:10.1192/bjp.2018.55 PMID:29786495

Williams, R. D., Brundage, J. A., & Williams, E. B. (2020). Moral injury in times of COVID-19. *Journal of Health Service Psychology*, *46*(2), 65–69. doi:10.100742843-020-00011-4 PMID:32363349

Wilson, W., Raj, J. P., Rao, S., Ghiya, M., Nedungalaparambil, N. M., Mundra, H., & Mathew, R. (2020). Prevalence and predictors of stress, anxiety, and depression among healthcare workers managing COVID-19 pandemic in India: A nation-wide observational study. *Indian Journal of Psychological Medicine*, *42*(4), 353–358. doi:10.1177/0253717620933992 PMID:33398224

Winston, J., Johnson, C., & Wilson, S. (2008). Barriers to healthy eating by National Health Service (NHS) hospital doctors in the hospital setting: Results of a cross-sectional survey. *BMC Research Notes*, *1*(1), 1–7. doi:10.1186/1756-0500-1-69 PMID:18755022

Wong, H., Wong, M. C., Wong, S. Y., & Lee, A. (2010). The association between shift duty and abnormal eating behavior among nurses working in a major hospital: A cross-sectional study. *International Journal of Nursing Studies*, *47*(8), 1021–1027. doi:10.1016/j.ijnurstu.2010.01.001 PMID:20116059

Wong, T. W., Yau, J. K., Chan, C. L., Kwong, R. S., Ho, S. M., Lau, C. C., Lau, F. L., & Lit, C. H. (2005). The psychological impact of severe acute respiratory syndrome outbreak on healthcare workers in emergency departments and how they cope. *European Journal of Emergency Medicine*, *12*(1), 13–18. doi:10.1097/00063110-200502000-00005 PMID:15674079

Wood, M. (2020). *How Pink-Collar Jobs Have Changed Since 1940.* Retrieved February 19, 2022. https://internationalwim.org/how-pink-collar-jobs-have-changed-since-1940/

Woodhead, E.L., Northrop, L., & Edelstein, B. (2016). Stress, social support, and burnout among long-term care nursing staff. *Journal of Applied Gerontology, 35*(1), 84-105. DOI: 10.1177/0733464814542465

Woo, T., Ho, R., Tang, A., & Tam, W. (2020). Global prevalence of burnout symptoms among nurses: A systematic review and meta-analysis. *Journal of Psychiatric Research, 123*, 9–20. doi:10.1016/j.jpsychires.2019.12.015 PMID:32007680

World Health Organization. (2003). *Consensus document on the epidemiology of severe acute respiratory syndrome (SARS) WHO/CDS/CSR/GAR/2003*. Retrieved from https://www.who.int/csr/sars/en/WHOconsensus.pdf

World Health Organization. (2020a). *Attacks on health care in the context of COVID-19.* Retrieved from https://www.who.int/news-room/feature-stories/detail/attacks-on-health-care-in-the-context-of-covid-19

World Health Organization. (2020b). *Keep health workers safe to keep patients safe.* Retrieved from https://www.who.int/news/item/17-09-2020-keep-health-workers-safe-to-keep-patients-safe-who

World Health Organization. (2022). *Weekly epidemiological update on COVID-19 - 8 March 2022.* Retrieved on March 11, 2022 from https://www.who.int/publications/m/item/weekly-epidemiological-update-on-covid-19---8-march-2022

Wright, J. D., Donley, A. M., Gualtieri, M. C., Strickhouser, S. M., & Wright, J. D. (2016). Food deserts: What is the problem? What is the solution? *Social Science and Public Policy*, *53*(2), 171–181. doi:10.100712115-016-9993-8

Wright, T. A., & Cropanzano, R. (1998). Emotional exhaustion as a predictor of job performance and voluntary turnover. *The Journal of Applied Psychology*, *83*(3), 486–493. doi:10.1037/0021-9010.83.3.486

Wu, Y., Wang, J., Luo, C., Hu, S., Lin, X., Anderson, A. E., Bruera, E., Yang, X., Wei, S., & Qian, Y. (2020). A comparison of burnout frequency among oncology physicians and nurses working on the frontline and usual wards during the COVID-19 epidemic in Wuhan, China. *Journal of Pain and Symptom Management*, *60*(1), e60-e65. .1016/j,painsymman.2020.04.008 doi:https://doi.org/10

Wylde, C. M., Mahrer, N. E., Meyer, R. M. L., & Gold, J. I. (2017). Mindfulness for novice pediatric nurses: Smartphone application versus traditional intervention. *Journal of Pediatric Nursing*, *36*, 205–212. doi:10.1016/j.pedn.2017.06.008 PMID:28888505

Wynd, C. A., & Ryan-Wenger, N. A. (2004). Factors predicting health behaviors among army reserve, active duty army, and civilian hospital employees. *Military Medicine*, *169*(12), 942–947. doi:10.7205/MILMED.169.12.942 PMID:15646182

Xiang, Y. T., Yang, Y., Li, W., Zhang, L., Zhang, Q., Cheung, T., & Ng, C. H. (2020). Timely mental health care for the 2019 novel corona virus outbreak is urgently needed. *The Lancet. Psychiatry*, *7*(3), 228–229. doi:10.1016/S2215-0366(20)30046-8 PMID:32032543

Xiao, H., Zhang, Y., Kong, D., Li, S., & Yang, N. (2020). Social capital and sleep quality in individuals who self-isolated for 14 days during the coronavirus disease 2019 (COVID-19) outbreak in January 2020 in China. *Medical Science Monitor*, *26*, e923921–e1. doi:10.12659/MSM.923921 PMID:32194290

Xiao, W., Lin, X., Li, X., Xu, X., Guo, H., Sun, B., & Jiang, H. (2021). The influence of emotion and empathy on decisions to help others. *SAGE Open*, *11*(2). doi:10.1177/21582440211014513

Xujun, Z., Yue, G., Mengjing, C., Lorann, S., & Huiyun, X. (2015). Needlestick and sharps injuries among nurses at a teaching hospital in China. *Workplace Health & Safety*, *63*(5), 219–225. doi:10.1177/2165079915580035 PMID:26031696

Yancy, C. W. (2020). COVID-19 and African Americans. *Journal of the American Medical Association*. doi:10.1001/jama.2020.6548

Yang, T., Guo, Y., Ma, M., Li, Y., Tian, H., & Deng, J. (2017). Job stress and presenteeism among Chinese healthcare workers: The mediating effects of affective commitment. *International Journal of Environmental Research and Public Health*, *14*(9), 978. doi:10.3390/ijerph14090978 PMID:28850081

Yang, T., Shen, Y.-M., Zhu, M., Liu, Y., Deng, J., Chen, Q., & See, L.-C. (2015). Effects of Co-Worker and Supervisor Support on Job Stress and Presenteeism in an Aging Workforce: A Structural Equation Modelling Approach. *International Journal of Environmental Research and Public Health*, *13*(1), 72. doi:10.3390/ijerph13010072 PMID:26703705

Yang, X., Yu, Y., Xu, J., Shu, H., Liu, H., Wu, Y., ... Shang, Y. (2020). Clinical course and outcomes of critically ill patients with SARS-CoV-2 pneumonia in Wuhan, China: A single-centered, retrospective, observational study. *The Lancet. Respiratory Medicine*, *8*(5), 475–481. doi:10.1016/S2213-2600(20)30079-5 PMID:32105632

Yang, Y., & Hayes, J. A. (2020). Causes and consequences of burnout among mental health professionals: A practice-oriented review of recent empirical literature. *Psychotherapy (Chicago, Ill.)*, *57*(3), 426–436. doi:10.1037/pst0000317 PMID:32463274

Yard, E., Radhakrishnan, L., Ballesteros, M. F., Sheppard, M., Gates, A., Stein, Z., Hartnett, K., Kite-Powell, A., Rodgers, L., Adjemian, J., Ehlman, D. C., Holland, K., Idaikkadar, N., Ivey-Stephenson, A., Martinez, P., Law, R., & Stone, D. M. (2021). Emergency department visits for suspected suicide attempts among persons aged 12–25 years before and during the COVID-19 pandemic: United States, January 2019–May 2021. *Morbidity and mortality weekly report*, *70*(24), 888–894. doi:10.15585/mmwr.mm7024e1 PMID:34138833

Yates, M., & Samuel, V. (2019). Burnout in oncologists and associated factors: A systematic literature review and meta-analysis. *European Journal of Cancer Care*, *28*(3), 1–19. doi:10.1111/ecc.13094 PMID:31090179

Yellow Horse, A. J. (2021). Anti-Asian racism, xenophobia, and Asian American health during COVID-19. *The COVID-19 Crisis: Social Perspectives*, 195–206. doi:10.4324/9781003111344-21

Yong, E. (2020, November 13). No one is listening to us. *The Atlantic*. https://www.theatlantic.com/health/archive/2020/11/third-surge-breaking-healthcare-workers/617091/

Young, A., Froggatt, K., & Brearley, S. G. (2017). 'Powerlessness' or 'doing the right thing' – Moral distress among nursing home staff caring for residents at the end of life: An interpretive descriptive study. *Palliative Medicine*, *31*(9), 853–860. doi:10.1177/0269216316682894

Young, K. P., Kolcz, D. L., O'Sullivan, D. M., Ferrand, J., Fried, J., & Robinson, K. (2020). Health Care Workers' Mental Health and Quality of Life During COVID-19: Results From a Mid-Pandemic, National Survey. *Psychiatric Services (Washington, D.C.)*, *72*(2), 122–128. doi:10.1176/appi.ps.202000424 PMID:33267652

Yu, M. (2018). Roles of graphic pathographies in clinical training. *AMA Journal of Ethics*, *20*(2), 115–121. doi:10.1001/journalofethics.2018.20.2.peer1-1802 PMID:29460763

Zablotsky, B., Black, L. I., Maenner, M. J., Schieve, L. A., Danielson, M. L., Bitsko, R. H., Blumberg, S. J., Kogan, M. D., & Boyle, C. A. (2019). Prevalence and trends of developmental disabilities among children in the United States: 2009–2017. *Pediatrics*, *144*(4), 1–21. doi:10.1542/peds.2019-0811 PMID:31558576

Zaçe, D., Hoxhaj, I., Orfino, A., Viteritti, A. M., Janiri, L., & Di Pietro, M. L. (2021). Interventions to address mental health issues in healthcare workers during infectious disease outbreaks: A systematic review. *Journal of Psychiatric Research*, *136*, 319–333. doi:10.1016/j.jpsychires.2021.02.019 PMID:33636688

Zadeh, S., Gamba, N., Hudson, C., & Wiener, L. (2012). Taking care of care providers: A wellness program for pediatric nurses. *Journal of Pediatric Oncology Nursing*, *29*(5), 294–299. doi:10.1177/1043454212451793 PMID:22907685

Zapka, J. M., Lemon, S. C., Magner, R. P., & Hale, J. (2009). Lifestyle behaviours and weight among hospital-based nurses. *Journal of Nursing Management*, *17*(7), 853–860. doi:10.1111/j.1365-2834.2008.00923.x PMID:19793242

Zea, M. C., Asner-Self, K. K., Birman, D., & Buki, L. P. (2003). The abbreviated multidimensional acculturation scale: Empirical validation with two Latino/Latina samples. *Cultural Diversity & Ethnic Minority Psychology*, *9*(2), 107–126. doi:10.1037/1099-9809.9.2.107 PMID:12760324

Zettle, R. D., Hayes, S. C., Barnes-Holmes, D., & Biglan, A. (2016). *The Wiley handbook of contextual behavioral science*. John Wiley & Sons.

Zhang, J., Wu, W., Zhao, X., & Zhang, W. (2020). Recommended psychological crisis intervention response to the 2019 novel corona virus pneumonia outbreak in China: A model of West China Hospital. *Precision Clinical Medicine*, *3*(1), 3–8. doi:10.1093/pcmedi/pbaa006

Zhang, Q., Mu, M.-c., He, Y., Cai, Z.-l., & Li, Z.-c. (2020). Burnout in emergency medicine physicians: A meta-analysis and systematic review. *Medicine*, *99*(32), e21462. doi:10.1097/MD.0000000000021462

Zhang, W., & Lane, B. S. (2013). Promoting neonatal staff nurses' comfort and involvement in end of life and bereavement care. *Nursing Research and Practice*, *365329*, 1–5. Advance online publication. doi:10.1155/2013/365329 PMID:23606955

Zhang, Y., Wang, C., Pan, W., Zheng, J., Gao, J., Huang, X., Cai, S., Zhai, Y., Latour, J. M., & Zhu, C. (2020). Stress, Burnout, and Coping Strategies of Frontline Nurses During the COVID-19 Epidemic in Wuhan and Shanghai, China. *Frontiers in Psychiatry*, *11*(October), 1–9. doi:10.3389/fpsyt.2020.565520 PMID:33192686

Zipf, A. L., Polifroni, E. C., & Beck, C. T. (2021). The experience of the nurse during the COVID-19 pandemic: A global meta-synthesis in the year of the nurse. *Journal of Nursing Scholarship*. Advance online publication. doi:10.1111/jnu.12706 PMID:34738314

Zohar, D. (1997). Predicting burnout with a hassle-based measure of role demands. *Journal of Organizational Behavior: The International Journal of Industrial, Occupational and Organizational Psychology and Behavior*, *18*(2), 101–115.

Zubatsky, M., Runyan, C., Gulotta, S., Knight, J. R., & Pettinelli, J. D. (2020). Burnout among behavioral health providers in integrated care settings. *Families, Systems & Health*, *38*(1), 74–82. doi:10.1037/fsh0000456 PMID:31789532

Zuckerman, N. (2014). Shift work, stress, and violence: Shift work. In T. Gorman (Ed.), *Controlling health hazards to hospital workers: A reference guide* (pp. 126–129). Baywood Publishing Co., Inc. doi:10.2190/NS.23.Suppl

Zunker, C., Cox, T. L., Wingo, B. C., Knight, B., Jefferson, W. K., & Ard, J. D. (2008). Using formative research to develop a worksite health promotion program for African American women. *Women & Health*, *48*(2), 189–207. doi:10.1080/03630240802313514 PMID:19042216

About the Contributors

Clint A. Bowers, PhD, is a Pegasus Professor of Psychology and at the University of Central Florida. His recent research is in the area of technology-based teaching. Current research projects include technology-based prevention and treatment interventions for mental illness. He has published numerous refereed journal articles and book chapters in the area of training and has edited three books related to training and technology.

Deborah C. Beidel, Ph.D., ABPP is Trustee Chair and Pegasus Professor of Psychology and Medical Education and the Executive Director of UCF RESTORES, a clinical research center dedicated o changing the way that we understand, diagnose, and treat posttraumatic stress disorder and other trauma disorders. She has provided psychological support interventions at a number of mass casualty events across the United States.

Madeline R. Marks is an assistant professor at the University of Maryland, School of Medicine, Department of Psychiatry. Prior to graduate training, she worked as a volunteer and professional EMT for 6 years. While currently not "on the road," she maintains her certifications. Dr. Marks' interests are in the development, research, and dissemination of prevention, intervention, and training protocols with a focus on stress injuries in first responders and healthcare workers. Additionally, she is interested in the use of technology as a delivery mechanism for prevention, intervention, and training protocols. Currently, Dr. Marks is tasked with developing a proactive consultation model between the psychiatry team and the Adams R. Cowley Shock Trauma Center. The focus is on trauma-informed care and equitable access to mental health care.

Kristin Horan is an Assistant Professor in Industrial Organizational Psychology at the University of Central Florida. Her research interests relate to Occupational Health Psychology (OHP), specifically OHP interventions, OHP in vulnerable occupations and populations, and the relationship between work and health behaviors.

* * *

Melyssa Allen, MA, DipACLM, attended the University of Central Florida where she received her Bachelor's degrees in Biology and Psychology and her Master's degree in Clinical Psychology. She is also a board-certified lifestyle medicine professional and currently pursuing her board-certification in health and wellness coaching. Melyssa is an esteemed member of the Lake Nona Performance Club Medical

Advisory Council and serves in a leadership role with the American College of Lifestyle Medicine as the Secretary for the Fitness and Medicine member interest group.

Tracey C. Arnold is an Assistant Professor in the School of Nursing at Southern Connecticut State University. She earned her associate degree from Three Rivers Community Technical College, her bachelors degree from the University of Louisiana at Lafayette, and her master's degree (nursing education) from Western Governors University. She is currently pursuing her PhD from the University of Connecticut. She has 20+ years of clinical nursing experience working in critical care and the emergency department. She has seen the negative affect in both herself and her colleagues. As such, her doctoral studies have focused on the negative affect of healthcare providers through the publication of manuscripts, presentations at nursing conferences, and pending dissertation work.

Claire Baniak, PsyD, is a pediatric psychologist with WVU Medicine Children's Neurodevelopmental Center and assistant professor of Behavioral Medicine and Psychiatry and Pediatrics in the WVU School of Medicine. She received her doctorate in clinical psychology with an emphasis on children, adolescents, and families at Spalding University in Louisville, KY. She completed her predoctoral internship through the Lewisville Independent School District in Lewisville, TX, and her postdoctoral fellowship in neurodevelopment through the WVU Medicine Children's Neurodevelopmental Center. Dr. Baniak has an extensive background diagnosing, evaluating, and treating children with Autism Spectrum Disorder and other neurodevelopmental disabilities. She has worked in community, medical, and school-based settings. Dr. Baniak enjoys collaborating with multidisciplinary partners to help raise awareness and understanding of Autism Spectrum Disorder, neurodevelopmental disabilities, and general child development. In her free time, she enjoys hiking with her husband, baking, and reading.

Claire Burnett is a third-year Ph.D. student in the Industrial-Organizational Psychology program at Georgia Tech. She received her B.S. in Psychology from the University of Georgia. Her research interests are in leadership behaviors and follower health outcomes, with a particular emphasis on follower sleep outcomes.

Jennifer Chavanovanich received her Ph.D. in Cross-Cultural and Industrial/Organizational Psychology from Brunel University, London, UK, where she completed her dissertation on acculturation of employees in Thailand and England. In 2019, she joined the faculty of psychology at Chulalongkorn University, Thailand, as a lecturer. Her research interests focus on cross-cultural I/O psychology including acculturation, diversity, and work attitudes and behaviors in organizations. Dr. Chavanovanich's current research projects also examine topics on homelessness, sexual harassment in the workplace, and online trolling.

Marit Christensen is an associate professor of work and organizational psychology at the Department of Psychology of the Norwegian University of Science and Technology. Her professional interests include positive occupational health psychology, health promotion, organizational interventions, and development of measuring tools for the psychosocial working environment.

Christa Cook's program of research focuses on examining barriers and facilitators to engagement in HIV care, from prevention to viral suppression, and how public health nurses can facilitate transitions to improve individual and population healthcare. Her work has been funded by the National Institutes of Health, the National Institute on Alcohol Abuse and Alcoholism, and the Florida Department of Health, and she has published and presented widely. She is a 2019 recipient of a Pabst Steinmetz Foundation Arts & Wellness Innovation Award for a collaboration with faculty in the UCF College of Arts and Humanities to develop data-driven comics to educate providers about HIV discrimination and stigma. Her methodological expertise is in qualitative methods, and she leads a qualitative research colloquium at UCF that provides peer evaluation and expert support for faculty and graduate students engaging in qualitative research from multiple disciplines (public health, medicine, engineering, education, anthropology) and universities.

Marco De Angelis is Junior Assistant Professor at the Department of Psychology, Alma Mater Studiorum – University of Bologna. Member of the Human Factors, Risk and Safety - Research Unit. His scientific interests focus on the promotion of mental health and psychosocial well-being at work, the implementation of multilevel interventions, digital solutions and the acceptance of new technologies. Additional research interests are related to human factors, safety and risk management in high-risk occupational environments. He is active part of the EU-H2020 H-WORK project coordinating team.

Cooper Drose received his B.S. in Psychology from the University of Georgia. He is a second year PhD student in Industrial-Organizational Psychology at Georgia Tech. His research interests include leadership behaviors, team dynamics, and personality at work.

Ilaria Rita Faiulo is a work, organizational, and personnel psychologist and practitioner in occupational health at the Health & Safety O.U. of the Azienda Unità Sanitaria Locale di Bologna.

Keaton Fletcher is an Assistant Professor of Industrial-Organizational Psychology at the Georgia Institute of Technology. His research focuses on occupational health psychology, leadership, teams, and training.

Lorna French received her BA in Psychology and Physiology from the University of Oxford in 2013. She worked in mental health within the UK National Health Service (NHS) from 2013, and received her Doctorate in Clinical Psychology from the University of Surrey in 2021. Her thesis research focused on burnout and moral injury in NHS staff, and was developed through work in a COVID Staff Support Service.

Davide Giusino is a PhD Candidate at the Human Factors, Risk and Safety - Research Unit, Department of Psychology of the Alma Mater Studiorum – University of Bologna, with the scholarship "Digital-based interventions for teams in the workplace", funded under the EU-H2020 research and innovation project "H-WORK: Multilevel Interventions to Promote Mental Health in SMEs and Public Workplaces". His research domain covers work and organizational psychology, occupational health psychology, and human factors and ergonomics. His scientific interests relate to mental health and psychosocial well-being in working environments, particularly in healthcare and academia.

Paul Hanna is the Research Director in Clinical Psychology at the University of Surrey. His research expertise is in community psychology, theoretical and critical psychology, mental health/wellbeing, distress, and qualitative methods. Paul has published in a wide range of academic journals and has authored two books.

Nathan Holic is the author of *Bright Lights, Medium-Sized City*, a hybrid novel (comics, watercolors, choose your own adventure!) from Burrow Press that attempts to cram as much of Orlando between two covers as possible. He is also the author of *The Things I Don't See* (a novella published by Main Street Rag), *American Fraternity Ma*n (a novel published by Beating Windward Press), and the University of Central Florida campus history (Arcadia Publishing), and is the editor of the anthology series *15 Views of Orlando* (Burrow Press), At UCF, he serves as the Graphic Narrative Editor at *The Florida Review.* His fiction, nonfiction, and comics have been widely published in print and online. Visit his personal web site at nathanholic.com for a list of publications and appearances.

Catherine Huckle is a Chartered Clinical Psychologist with 15 years of experience of working within the NHS. She works as a Senior Teaching Fellow on the PsychD Clinical Psychology training programme at the University of Surrey and is admissions lead and chair of the Equality, Diversity and Inclusion Committee.

Siw Tone Innstrand is a professor in occupational health psychology at the Department of Psychology of the Norwegian University of Science and Technology. Director of the Center for Health Promotion Research. Her scientific interests relate to interaction between work and family, occupational health, work environment, health promotion, intervention research, and quantitative methods.

Somboon Jarukasemthawee, Ph.D., is a lecturer in Clinical/Counseling Psychology at the Faculty of Psychology, Chulalongkorn University. Dr. Jarukasemthawee has a research interest in how Eastern philosophies can be integrated into mindfulness psychotherapies, cognitive behavioral therapy for Thais, psychological distress (depression, anxiety, and stress), and positive psychological functions (well-being, acceptance, compassion, and grit). They currently teach courses on Cognitive-Behavioral Therapy and Evidence-Based Psychology Therapies to postgraduate psychology students and Theories of Personality Psychology for undergraduate psychology students. Dr. Jarukasemthawee is a Clinical Psychologist licensed in Thailand.

Maria Kalantzis is a second-year doctoral student in the Clinical Psychology Doctoral Program at Bowling Green State University. Maria grew up in Bolingbrook, Illinois, a suburb of Chicago, and in 2020 completed her Bachelor of Science (honors) in Psychology at North Central College. Maria completed an institutionally grant-funded project as a part of her honors thesis to study the cultural differences within eating behaviors in Scottish and American college students. Maria is currently a doctoral student in the clinical psychology program at Bowling Green State University. Maria's master's thesis examined how perceived discrimination impacts disordered and emotional eating in women of color, and how personal and social resources impact such relationships.

Stephany Lora is an assistant professor at WVU. She specializes in pediatric psychology.

Jennifer Ludrosky, PhD, is an assistant professor and clinical psychologist at the West Virginia University School of Medicine.

Anu Malik is working as an Assistant Professor at The LNM Institute of Information Technology, Jaipur. She did a Ph.D. from the Indian Institute of Technology, Kanpur. Her research interests focus on health psychology, organizational behavior, and other allied areas. As a researcher, she has published articles in reputed journals and presented papers in prestigious national and international conferences.

Greta Mazzetti is an Assistant Professor in Work and Organizational Psychology at the Department of Education Studies of the Alma Mater Studiorum – University of Bologna. Her research interests include employability, job insecurity, workaholism, work engagement, job burnout, soft skills, emotional contagion, and job and individual resources.

Joseph Mazzola is currently an Associate Professor of Psychology and Director of Industrial-Organizational Psychology Master's Program at Meredith College. He received is M.A. at Bowling Green State University. His research and teaching focus is on stress measurement and management, promoting healthy behaviors in the workplace, and qualitative/mixed methodology. He has been published in several scholarly journals and books, including Work & Stress, Journal of Occupational Health Psychology, and Stress & Health.

Janelle Mentrikoski, PhD, is a pediatric psychologist and associate professor in the Department of Behavioral Medicine and Psychiatry at the West Virginia University School of Medicine. She received her doctorate in clinical psychology from West Virginia University. Dr. Mentrikoski completed her internship training in pediatric psychology at University of Louisville School of Medicine in Louisville, KY and her fellowship training in pediatric psychology at Akron Children's Hospital in Akron, OH. Dr. Mentrikoski has clinical and research experiences with a variety of pediatric populations, including burn injuries, cystic fibrosis, and pain disorders.

Karina Nielsen is Chair in Work Psychology at the Institute of Work Psychology, Sheffield University Management School, University of Sheffield. Her research interests fall in the category of changing organisations, including participatory organizational interventions, evaluation design, employee well-being, leadership, and qualitative, quantitative, and mixed methods research designs.

William H. O'Brien, Ph.D., ABPP, is a Professor of Psychology in the Clinical Psychology Training Program at Bowling Green State University and the Fulbright Distinguished Chair of Social Sciences to China/Thailand 2020-2021. Dr. O'Brien is board certified in cognitive behavioral psychology by the American Board of Professional Psychology. Dr. O'Brien's research is focused on basic and applied research in contextual behavioral science; functional analysis and clinical decision making; Acceptance and Commitment Therapy; occupational health psychology; clinical psychophysiology; and the integration of Eastern and Western perspectives in clinical psychology.

Vidhi Patel, PhD, is a Researcher-Instructor at the Center for Health Innovations and Outcomes Research, Institute of Health System Science, Northwell Health, the largest health system serving the New York metropolitan area and Assistant Professor, Zucker School of Medicine, Hofstra/Northwell. She has received her doctorate from Hofstra University in Applied Organizational Psychology. She also holds a master's degree in Industrial/Organizational Psychology and MBA in Management and Marketing. Her expertise includes grant writing, quantitative and qualitative analysis, experimental and quasi-experimental research methods, and designing and implementing community based-participatory research studies aimed at improving quality of life in the minority/vulnerable communities. In 2020, she was the recipient of Researcher-in-Training award from AWSM (Advancing Women in Science and Medicine), New York. She is part of numerous research studies and activities aimed at improving patient-centered health outcomes, specifically those in the older adults and suffering from chronic illnesses such as type 2 diabetes.

Jonathan Perle, PhD, ABPP, is a board-certified clinical child and adolescent psychologist, Associate Professor, and Director of Telepsychology with the Department of Behavioral Medicine and Psychiatry at the West Virginia University School of Medicine. He has significant experience providing youth-focused clinical assessment and intervention within diverse clinical settings (e.g., medical centers, primary care, schools, university clinics) and roles (e.g., interdisciplinary, multidisciplinary, outpatient, inpatient). In addition to his current responsibilities that include teaching, supervising, and conducting research, Dr. Perle provides both face-to-face and virtual psychological care. His clinical and research interests focus on childhood attention-deficit/hyperactivity disorder, childhood disruptive behavior disorders, integrated healthcare, and telehealth.

Kullaya Pisitsungkagarn, Ph.D., is an Assistant Professor in the Psychology Department at Chulalongkorn University, Thailand. She received her Ph.D. in Educational Psychology from University of Texas at Austin 2004, and her DPsych. in Clinical/Counseling Psychology at University of Queensland in 2011. She obtained clinical licensure in Australia and Thailand. Her research interests include depression, anxiety, body image and eating behavior, Cognitive Behavioral Therapy (CBT), Acceptance and Commitment Therapy (ACT), and clinical assessment. Dr. Pisitsungkagarn is active in disseminating her research works at the international level.

E. Carol Polifroni is a Professor in the School of Nursing at the University of Connecticut. She earned her bachelor's degree from Saint Anselm College, her master's degree from New York University, and her doctorate in education from Rutgers: The State University of New Jersey. She teaches classes in leadership and management, administration, contemporary topics, policy, and philosophy of science to undergraduate, graduate, and doctoral students. She has 40+ years of nursing experience specializing in critical care, administration, and education. She views concepts through a lens of possibility and change, and has focused her recent research experiences on the positive affect of meaning and joy.

Sajedeh Rabipour is one of the youngest researchers in mental health quality and environmental conditions. Her main research interest is therapeutical psychiatric.

Blake Scott came to UCF in 2002, having previously taught at the University of Florida, Penn State University, and the University of Oklahoma. When UCF created the Department of Writing & Rhetoric in 2011, he became its founding Associate Chair and Director of Degree Programs, leading the creation of three new undergraduate programs (including a B.A. in Writing & Rhetoric). At UCF, he has served as Vice Chair of the Faculty Senate (2020-present), United Faculty of Florida Grievance Chair, Provost Fellow (2012-2013), and Faculty Excellence Fellow (2017-2018). In this latter role, helped Faculty Excellence advance a number of faculty development and advancement initiatives--including a new Associate Professor Mentoring Communities program and Faculty Development Conference track--

identified through the COACHE survey. He has also worked on and, in some cases, helped lead of parts of other university initiatives, including those associated with the Foundations of Excellence Transfer Initiative, Quality Enhancement Program, and revision of University Promotion & Tenure Guidelines.

Rajbala Singh is working as an Associate Professor, Department of Humanities and Social Sciences, The LNM Institute of Information Technology, Jaipur, India. She has earned a Ph.D. from the Indian Institute of Technology, Kanpur, India, and has teaching and research experience of more than ten years. She has published her research in refereed journals and presented research papers in national and international conferences of repute. Her teaching and research interest include health psychology, social psychology, psychology of technology, and other allied areas.

Maeher Sukhija is a UCF Honors freshman and a Burnetts Medical Scholar. She is majoring in Biomedical Sciences and minoring in Art. She hopes to become an ER doctor, and was inspired to do so by her time volunteering at Advent Health Hospital and Moffitt Cancer Center.

Kathryn Sunderman is a doctoral student in clinical psychology at the University of Central Florida. Her research interests are in the area of trauma and PTSD in veterans and first responders.

Jonah Swinson graduated with a Bachelor of Science degree from Liberty University. From there, he went onto receive a Master of Science in Sport and Performance Psychology from Florida State University. Jonah is currently pursuing a doctorate in Clinical Psychology from the University of Central Florida. Jonah is a member of the UCF RESTORES lab and is mentored by Dr. Clint Bowers. His research interests include methods of training psychologists and fostering psychological resilience.

Navneesh Tyagi is an assistant professor at the Noida Institute of Engineering and Technology, Greater Noida, India. She is a PhD in Management and has qualified UGC NET (IR) 2013, UGC NET (Management) 2012. She has published two books and 13 research papers in various ABDC, SCOPUS, and UGC-approved journals.

Preeti Tyagi is an assistant professor in ICRI, Dehradun, and Ph.D. supervisor in Zee Himgiri University, Dehradun, India. She is a Ph.D. in Management and also possesses M.Com and MBA degrees. She has published various research papers in SCOPUS and UGC-approved journals.

Myia S. Williams, Ph.D., is a Research Industrial/Organizational Psychologist in the Institute of Health Systems Science at Northwell Health, an Assistant Professor at the Donald and Barbara Zucker School of Medicine at Hofstra University and Research Instructor at the Feinstein Institute of Medical Research. She holds a PhD in Applied Organizational Psychology from Hofstra University. She is actively involved in research on the impact of COVID-19 on the mental health of healthcare professionals; addressing health disparities through culturally tailored interventions for historically underserved racial/ethnic minority and immigrant populations; and organizational and interpersonal factors that impact the diversification of the physician workforce. In 2019 and 2020, she received a Researcher-In Training Award and Educational Advancement Award, respectively from Advancing Women in Science and Medicine. She is originally from the beautiful Caribbean island of St. Lucia.

Ashley T. Winch is a doctoral student in clinical psychology at the University of Central Florida. Her research interests are in the area of trauma in children.

Aislinn Woody served 7 years in the US Coast Guard. She earned her BS in Exercise Science from the University of Massachusetts Boston in 2015 and a BS in Nursing from Northeastern University in 2016. She has since worked in a variety of acute and post-acute settings. Aislinn is currently a graduate fellow and PhD student at the University of Central Florida with a research focus on substance use and harm reduction.

Index

I

J

L

M

N

O

P

Q

R

S

T

W

www.ingramcontent.com/pod-product-compliance
Lightning Source LLC
LaVergne TN
LVHW060300011026
849161LV00011B/2746